Principles of Nuclear Medicine

Majid Assadi • Hojjat Ahmadzadehfar
Hans-Jürgen Biersack

Principles of Nuclear Medicine

Self-Assessment and Board Review

Springer

Majid Assadi
Department of Nuclear Medicine
Bushehr University of Medical Sciences
Bushehr
Iran

Hojjat Ahmadzadehfar
Department of Nuclear Medicine
University Hospital Bonn
Bonn
Germany

Hans-Jürgen Biersack
Department of Nuclear Medicine
Univerity Hospital Bonn
Bonn, Nordrhein-Westfalen
Germany

ISBN 978-3-319-91700-9 ISBN 978-3-319-91701-6 (eBook)
https://doi.org/10.1007/978-3-319-91701-6

Library of Congress Control Number: 2018955704

This Springer imprint is published by the registered company Springer Nature Switzerland AG
The registered company address is: Gewerbestrasse 11, 6330 Cham, Switzerland

Preface

Principles of Nuclear Medicine: Self-Assessment and Board Review features more than 4000 review questions along with answers through the 9 chapters and 133 subsections.

This guidebook has almost everything required for preparation for the national and international nuclear medicine exams. It serves as both a study guide and an in-depth review. This study tool is intended to be used in a simple method to help readers by providing questions to evaluate their understanding of the material. It can stand alone if the reader has already been exposed to the more comprehensive material at some time in the past and is simply looking for a quick review.

Readers find in the book three main purposes. One is to allow the reader to evaluate their current level of nuclear medicine understanding and assessing possible weak points for further study. Second, it includes subsections to the textbooks, should the reader wish to pursue a more in-depth study of specific topics. Finally, practice exams help to familiarize the reader with the process of taking multiple-choice examinations.

Moreover, it has made every effort to include questions from the entire spectrum of nuclear medicine fields from basic to clinical fields. Some questions require profound knowledge in basic and clinical nuclear medicine, which are both critical for the accomplishment of the diagnostic and therapeutic missions.

This book will be useful to scientists and physicians associated with nuclear medicine fields, e.g., radiologists, oncologists, medical physics, radiopharmacists, and radiobiologists, and also they may find this to be a valuable resource. Nuclear medicine is core knowledge in several fields; therefore they may benefit from basic education in many aspects of nuclear medicine.

Bushehr, Iran — Majid Assadi
Bonn, Germany — Hojjat Ahmadzadehfar
Bonn, Germany — Hans J. Biersack

Contents

1 Nuclear Medicine in Tumor Diagnosis

1.1 Radiopharmaceuticals for Cancer Imaging: Nature, Mechanisms of Localization, and Molecular Targets

1. A species of an atomic nucleus characterized by its mass number, atomic number, and nuclear energy state provided that the mean life in that state is long enough to be observable:
   (a) Nuclide
   (b) Radionuclide
   (c) Radioisotope
   (d) Radiopharmaceutical

2. Radionuclides used in nuclear medicine are synthesized by the following methods *except*:
   (a) Thermal neutron reactor
   (b) Cyclotron
   (c) Fission reactor
   (d) Vapor condensation

3. All of the following radioisotopes can be used in SPECT *except*:
   (a) ^{53}Se
   (b) ^{76}Br
   (c) ^{67}Ga
   (d) ^{123}I

4. The decay mode of all of the following radionuclides is electron capture (EC) *except*:
   (a) ^{67}Ga
   (b) ^{201}Tl
   (c) ^{111}In
   (d) ^{99m}Tc

M. Assadi et al., *Principles of Nuclear Medicine*,
https://doi.org/10.1007/978-3-319-91701-6_1

5. Which radiopharmaceutical requires heating for preparation?
   (a) ^{99m}Tc-tetrofosmin
   (b) ^{99m}Tc-sulfur colloid
   (c) ^{123}I-MIBG
   (d) ^{99m}Tc-RBC

6. Which isotope is a beta emitter?
   (a) ^{15}O
   (b) ^{3}H
   (c) ^{13}C
   (d) ^{64}Cu

7. Choose the isotope with the shortest half-life.
   (a) ^{13} N
   (b) ^{15} O
   (c) ^{82} Rb
   (d) ^{11} C

8. The mean effective life of an ideal gamma-emitting radiopharmaceutical should be approximately ... times of the duration of the diagnostic procedure.
   (a) 2
   (b) 3
   (c) 1.5
   (d) 1

9. What is the minimum target-to-nontarget ratio of an ideal gamma-emitting radiopharmaceutical for planar and SPECT imaging, respectively?
   (a) 5:1, 2:1
   (b) 4:1, 3:1
   (c) 2:1, 1:1
   (d) 3:1, 2:1

10. What is the spatial resolution of the most clinical PET scanners?
   (a) 3–4 mm
   (b) 4–5 mm
   (c) 5–7 mm
   (d) 6–8 mm

11. What is the sensitivity of PET?
   (a) 10^{-11}–10^{-12} moles/I
   (b) 10^{-7}–10^{-8} moles/I
   (c) 10^{-15}–10^{-16} moles/I
   (d) 10^{-5}–10^{-6} moles/I

12. An imaging type that does not depend on precise biological or cellular markers but is more of a reflection of functional status is called:
    (a) Surrogate imaging
    (b) Tissue microenvironment imaging
    (c) Targeted imaging
    (d) a and b

13. Compared with normal tissue, tumors show increased values of the following parameters *except*:
    (a) Hexokinase level
    (b) Glut-1
    (c) Glut mRNA/protein
    (d) Glucose-6-phosphatase activity

14. All of the following radiopharmaceuticals are used in the imaging of tumor hypoxia *except*:
    (a) ^{123}I-AZA
    (b) ^{99m}Tc-HL91
    (c) ^{62}CU-ATSM
    (d) ^{18}F-α-methyltyrosine (FMT)

15. An imaging radiopharmaceutical for tumor apoptosis:
    (a) ^{18}F-MISO
    (b) $^{11}C\text{-}CO_2$
    (c) ^{99m}Tc-annexin V
    (d) ^{62}Cu-ATSM

16. Murine monoclonal antibody Fab′ fragment is used in:
    (a) ^{111}In-satumomab pendetide (OncoScint)
    (b) ^{99m}Tc-CEA (arcitumomab)
    (c) ^{111}In capromab pendetide (ProstaScint)
    (d) ^{111}In-ibritumomab tiuxetan (Zevalin)

17. Which protein is associated with multidrug resistance (MDR) to chemotherapeutic agents?
    (a) P-glycoprotein (P-gp)
    (b) Lung resistance protein (LRP)
    (c) Breast cancer resistance protein (BCRP)
    (d) All of the above

18. Which one does NOT affect the tumor uptake of FDG?
    (a) Physical activity
    (b) Blood insulin level
    (c) Surrounding temperature
    (d) Body mass index

19. In which tumor is FDG-PET the least applicable?
    (a) Lymphoma
    (b) Head and neck cancer
    (c) Prostate cancer
    (d) Colorectal cancer

20. The uptake mechanism of $^{15}O-H_2O$ and ^{67}Cu-PTSM is associated with... and ^{18}F-fluoromisonidazole with..., respectively.
    (a) Tumor flow, tumor flow
    (b) Hypoxia, tumor flow
    (c) Tumor flow, hypoxia
    (d) Hypoxia, hypoxia

21. All of the following mechanisms mediate the tumoral uptake of FDG *except*:
    (a) Increase in the expression of glucose transporters on the cell surface
    (b) Increase in hexokinase activity
    (c) Increase in glucose-6-phosphatase activity
    (d) a and b

22. One hour after injection, FDG is normally distributed in all of the following organs *except*:
    (a) Large intestine
    (b) Brain
    (c) Heart
    (d) Kidney and urinary tract

23. About myocardial uptake in FDG-PET scan:
    (a) Myocardial uptake depends on the nutrition of the patient
    (b) Insulin increases myocardial and muscular uptake
    (c) Glucose transporter 4 (GluT-4) is expressed in the myocardium
    (d) All of the above

24. All of the following statements regarding the effects of blood sugar on the FDG-PET scan are correct *except*:
    (a) Invasive insulin treatment increases the muscular uptake and decreases the tumoral uptake of FDG.
    (b) High blood sugar competitively inhibits the tumoral uptake of FDG.
    (c) The appropriate approach to diabetic patients is NOT yet defined.
    (d) Fasting and administration of insulin for cases with high blood sugar are recommended in most centers.

25. Which of the following variables is strongly associated with the tumoral uptake of FDG?
    (a) Cell proliferation
    (b) Number of viable cells
    (c) Ratio of cytoplasm to nucleus
    (d) a and b

26. Which of the following mechanisms justifies the increased uptake of ^{11}C-methionine in cancer cells?
    (a) Phosphorylation
    (b) Decarboxylation
    (c) Hexokinase activity
    (d) Transmethylation

27. The observation of ^{11}C-methionine uptake in all organs in the PET scan is considered normal *except*:
    (a) Kidneys
    (b) Lungs
    (c) Liver
    (d) Pancreas

28. What is the meaning of stereospecificity of the radiotracer uptake in brain tumors?
    (a) If BBB is normal, the D isoform of the radiotracer will be more localized in brain tumors than the L isoform.
    (b) If BBB is normal, the L isoform of the radiotracer will be more localized in brain tumors than the D isoform.
    (c) If BBB is abnormal, the L isoform of the radiotracer will be more localized in brain tumors than the D isoform.
    (d) If BBB is abnormal, the D isoform of the radiotracer will be more localized in brain tumors than the L isoform.

29. What is the choice reagent for the study on the amino acid entrance into tumoral cells?
    (a) Aminocyclohexanecarboxylate (ACHC)
    (b) Aminocyclopentane carboxylic acid (ACPC)
    (c) Methionine
    (d) a and b

30. Which of the following PET radiotracers is NOT used as a DNA precursor?
    (a) Fluoroethyl uracil ([18F] FEU)
    (b) ^{67}Cu-PTSM
    (c) Carbon-11-thymidine
    (d) Adenosine ^{18}F-

31. Which of the following PET radiotracers better predicts the therapeutic efficacy of cancer treatment?
    (a) FDG
    (b) ^{67}Cu-PTSM
    (c) $^{15}O-H_2O$
    (d) ^{18}F-fluorodeoxyuridine (FLT)

32. All of the following radiotracers can be used for the evaluation of tumor flow *except*:
    (a) $^{15}O\text{-}CO$
    (b) $^{15}O\text{-}CO_2$
    (c) $^{15}O\text{-}H_2O$
    (d) ^{66}Cu-PTSM

33. What are the recommended radiotracers to determine the tumor volume and the tumor distribution volume, respectively?
    (a) ^{66}Cu-PTSM, $^{15}O\text{-}CO_2$
    (b) $^{15}O\text{-}CO$, $^{15}O\text{-}H_2O$
    (c) $^{15}O\text{-}CO_2$, $^{15}O\text{-}CO$
    (d) ^{66}Cu-PTSM, $^{15}O\text{-}CO$

34. Labeled ligands are designed against specific receptors. 16α-[^{18}F]-fluoro-17β-estradiol (FES) is one of these ligands and is indicated for the diagnosis of:
    (a) Kidney cancer
    (b) Breast cancer
    (c) Testis cancer
    (d) Kidney cancer

35. The greater the FDG uptake is, the worse the prognosis *except* in:
    (a) RCC
    (b) HCC
    (c) Juvenile pilocytic astrocytomas
    (d) Choriocarcinoma

36. The ability to study polyamine metabolism in tumor cells is demonstrated by using:
    (a) ^{11}C-putrescine
    (b) ^{11}C-thymidine
    (c) ^{18}F-fluorocholine
    (d) ^{18}F-fluorothymidine

37. It appears to be a promising agent for the imaging of membrane synthesis:
    (a) ^{18}F-fluorocholine
    (b) ^{11}C-thymidine
    (c) ^{11}C-putrescine
    (d) ^{18}F-fluorothymidine

38. Which of the following radioisotopes is recommended for the labeling of monoclonal antibodies for PET imaging?
    (a) ^{68}Ga
    (b) ^{124}I
    (c) ^{18}F
    (d) ^{11}C

1.1.1 Answer

	A	B	C	D
1	*			
2				*
3		*		
4				*
5		*		
6		*		
7			*	
8			*	
9	*			
10				*
11	*			
12				*
13				*
14				*
15			*	
16		*		
17				*
18				*
19			*	
20			*	
21			*	
22	*			
23				*
24				*
25				*
26				*
27		*		
28		*		
29				*
30		*		
31				*
32	*			
33		*		
34		*		
35			*	
36	*			
37	*			
38		*		

1.2 Radionuclide Imaging of Hepatic Tumors

1. FDG-PET appears to be a valuable method for the following studies *except*:
   (a) Histologic grading of HCC
   (b) Tumor viability
   (c) Monitoring the effect of therapy
   (d) Tumor vascularity

2. ^{99m}Tc-RBC scintigraphy for the diagnosis of hepatic cavernous hemangioma (HH):
   (a) Is the most sensitive noninvasive method
   (b) Is the most specific noninvasive method
   (c) Its sensitivity does not depend on lesion size
   (d) It cannot differentiate HHs from vascular tumors

3. Which of the following situations is NOT a false-positive finding of hepatic cavernous hemangioma (HH)?
   (a) HCC
   (b) Angiosarcoma
   (c) Metastasis
   (d) FNH

4. All of the following statements regarding FNH are correct *except*:
   (a) Diameter is smaller than 5 cm.
   (b) No need for treatment.
   (c) OCPs cause its development.
   (d) It may leave a central scar.

5. All of the following statements regarding the diagnostic methods in FNH are correct *except*:
   (a) 30–70% of all FNHs have either normal or increased ^{99m}Tc-colloid uptake.
   (b) Its detectability by ^{99m}Tc-IDA scintigraphy is greater than that by CT or MRI.
   (c) On ^{18}F FDG-PET, FNH may show a normal or an increased uptake.
   (d) ^{99m}Tc-NGA SPECT is useful for the differential diagnosis of FNH and malignant hepatic tumors.

6. About liver tumors:
   (a) Tc colloid is rarely uptaken in FNH.
   (b) Tc colloid is always uptaken in hepatocellular adenoma.
   (c) The possibility of detection of FNH by ^{99m}Tc-IDA is higher than that by CT and MRI.
   (d) The gallium scan is NOT used for the evaluation of liver tumors because of the natural hepatic uptake.

7. ^{99m}Tc-RBC scan is performed for a 49-year-old patient with ambiguous pains in the RUQ. A reduced uptake in the perfusion phase and an increased uptake in the blood-pool phase are observed. What are the most probable diagnosis and the strength point of the method?
   (a) Metastasis, high specificity
   (b) Metastasis, high sensitivity
   (c) Cavernous hemangioma, high specificity
   (d) Cavernous hemangioma, high sensitivity

8. Hepatosplenic scintigraphy is performed for a 54-year-old woman with a positive HBS antigen and high alpha-fetoprotein. Decreased focal activity in the left lobe is observed in the perfusion and static phases. In addition, an increased uptake is found in the bone marrow. What is the most probable diagnosis?
   (a) Hepatocellular carcinoma
   (b) Pseudotumor
   (c) Metastasis with the origin of the colon
   (d) Metastasis with the origin of the testis

9. Multiple hypodense lesions are found in the CT scan, which shows tracer uptake in the perfusion and static phases of the sulfur colloid scan, of a 45-year-old woman. What is the most probable diagnosis?
   (a) Focal nodular hyperplasia
   (b) Hepatic adenoma
   (c) Hepatic hemangioma
   (d) Hepatoma

10. All of the following statements regarding cavernous hemangioma are true *except*:
   (a) Its density on the CT scan is the same as that of the aorta.
   (b) Its prevalence in women is greater than that in men.
   (c) Rarely ruptures.
   (d) Fluid–fluid level formation is common.

11. A hypoecho region is found in the hepatosplenic scan with sulfur colloid of a 65-year-old man with pain in the RUQ. Hb of 9.6 and WBC of 14,000 are reported in the laboratory tests. The gallium scan shows reduced activity in the same region. What is the most probable diagnosis?
   (a) Liver metastasis due to melanoma
   (b) Adenoma
   (c) Amoebiasis abscess
   (d) Pyogenic abscess

12. An increased activity of caudate lobe is reported in the hepatosplenic scan with sulfur colloid of a 65-year-old woman. What is the most probable diagnosis?
    (a) Focal nodular hyperplasia
    (b) Thrombosis of the inferior vena cava
    (c) Thrombosis of the superior vena cava
    (d) Thrombosis of hepatic veins

13. Which method is NOT indicated for the detection of recurrent hepatocellular carcinoma?
    (a) Measurement of alpha-fetoprotein
    (b) Gallium scan
    (c) Octreoscan
    (d) Measurement of the carcinoembryonic antigen

14. A large focal lesion with no uptake is observed in the right hepatic lobe in the hepatosplenic scan of an old woman with weight loss. What is the most probable diagnosis?
    (a) Adenoma
    (b) Metastasis of breast cancer
    (c) Metastasis of colon cancer
    (d) Amoebiasis abscess of the liver

15. Hepatosplenic scintigraphy of a 45-year-old patient shows a focal increase in activity in the right hepatic lobe in the angiography phase, which is cold in the static images. A shift of the colloid to the spleen and the bone marrow is also observed. What is the most probable diagnosis for hepatic cold lesion?
    (a) Cholangiocarcinoma
    (b) Hemangioma
    (c) Hamartoma
    (d) Pseudotumor

16. Which line describes the liver size with Riedel's lobe in the anterior scintigraphy view?
    (a) A vertical line dividing the distance between the right dorsal edge and the xiphoid into half
    (b) An oblique line from the lateral edge of the right lobe until the end of the inferior Riedel's lobe
    (c) A line from the left medial lobe until the end of the right inferior lobe
    (d) A line from the dome region until the end of the inferior Riedel's lobe

17. Hepatic scintigraphy of a 38-year-old woman shows vascular lesions in the angiography phase that uptakes the radiotracer in the static phase. What is the most probable diagnosis?
    (a) Focal nodular hyperplasia
    (b) Hepatic abscess
    (c) Hemangioma
    (d) Hepatocellular carcinoma

18. A photopenic focus, which occupies most of the right hepatic lobe, is observed in the anterior view of the sulfur colloid liver scintigraphy of a 9-year-old child. Moreover, the labeled RBC scintigraphy shows increased perfusion in the margins of the mentioned defect, with central photopenia and mixed components in the delayed images. Its activity is greater than that of a normal liver tissue but less than that of the cardiac pool. What is the most probable diagnosis?
    (a) Cavernous hemangioendothelioma
    (b) Mesenchymal hamartoma
    (c) Capillary hemangioma
    (d) Hepatoma

19. The spleen is NOT observed in the hepatobiliary scan with ^{99m}Tc-sulfur colloid. The patient reports no further surgery except for kidney transplantation. Furthermore, Howell–Jolly bodies are NOT present in the hematological evaluation. What is the most probable diagnosis?
    (a) Splenic hypofunction
    (b) Sudden occlusion of the splenic artery
    (c) Transplanted kidney rejection
    (d) Heart failure

20. A 3 cm × 3 cm photopenic lesion is observed in the ^{99m}Tc-SC scan of a patient's liver. In addition, the gallium scan shows a homogenous liver uptake. What is the most probable diagnosis?
    (a) Adenoma
    (b) Abscess
    (c) Hemangioma
    (d) Pseudotumor

21. A mass with a size of 3.2 cm in the liver is observed in the sonography of a 78-year-old man with a history of hepatic cirrhosis. This mass had NO uptake in the ^{99m}Tc-SC but showed an uptake I and then ^{68}Ga scan performed 3 days prior. What is the most probable diagnosis?
    (a) HCC
    (b) Regenerative nodule
    (c) FNH
    (d) Adenoma

22. Which of the following lesions is able to mimic the pattern of a cyst in the hepatic arterial perfusion scintigraphy (HAPS) using ^{99m}Tc-MAA?
    (a) Hepatic arteriovenous fistula
    (b) Cavernous hemangioma
    (c) Hepatoma
    (d) Liver metastasis

23. Pseudotumors:
    (a) Are observed as very small lesions in the hepatic scan
    (b) Can be simply misdiagnosed as hepatoma
    (c) Finally metastasize to other organs
    (d) Display significant hyperemia and increased activity

24. Select the most appropriate imaging method for liver diseases:
    (a) Liver dome can be better evaluated by sonography.
    (b) Obesity decreases the echogenicity on sonography and the activity in hepatic isotopic scintigraphy but increases the contrast of a CT scan.
    (c) Multiple surgical clips or sutures have NO effect on CT scan images.
    (d) Motion of the patient has NO effect on CT scan images.

25. What is the most common tumor causing diffuse infiltration of the liver?
    (a) Melanoma
    (b) Colon carcinoma
    (c) Breast carcinoma
    (d) Lung cancer

26. A 36-year-old woman with a history of administration of oral contraceptives (OCP) comes to your department. Her sonography shows a hypoechoic mass with a size of 4 cm in the right border of the right liver lobe. Furthermore, a mild increased activity in comparison with the surrounding liver parenchymal tissue is observed in the ^{99m}Tc-sulfur colloid scintigraphy. What is most likely the diagnosis?
    (a) Hepatic adenoma
    (b) Focal nodular hyperplasia
    (c) Single hepatic metastasis
    (d) Unusual hemangioma

27. Which phrase is NOT correct about the application of the ^{99m}Tc-RBC scan for liver hemangioma?
    (a) The scan can be false negative if the hemangioma is large with thrombosis and fibrosis.
    (b) Blood vessels are the most important differential diagnosis in SPECT.
    (c) The regional uptake being equal or greater than the adjacent blood vessels indicates a positive scan.
    (d) The angiography phase is the most important phase of the study for diagnosis.

28. Howell–Jolly bodies in the peripheral blood smear with a normal hepatobiliary scan are reported for a patient. What is the most probable diagnosis?
    (a) Treated iron deficiency anemia
    (b) Extensive splenic infiltration due to lymphoma
    (c) Polycythemia vera
    (d) Acute thrombosis of the portal vein

29. What is the pattern of hepatic focal fatty infiltration in different imaging modalities?
    (a) Hyperechoic lesion on sonography
    (b) Increase in activity in the sulfur colloid scan
    (c) No uptake in the ^{133}Xe scan
    (d) High attenuation in CT

30. RBC scintigraphy is performed for a child with a suspected tumor of vascular origin. The angiography phase shows a large liver and an apparent increase in perfusion. In addition, multiple regions of increased activity are observed in the delayed images. What is the most probable diagnosis?
    (a) Cavernous hemangioendothelioma
    (b) Capillary hemangioma
    (c) Mesenchymal hamartoma
    (d) Hepatoblastoma

31. In primary hepatocellular carcinoma in cirrhotic patients:
    (a) The sulfur colloid scan with an angiography phase is helpful.
    (b) The specificity of the CT scan is very high.
    (c) Less than 40% of patients with this cancer are cirrhotic.
    (d) The gallium scan alone is sensitive and specific for the diagnosis.

32. Focal hepatic lesions with low attenuation are reported in the CT scan of an alcoholic patient, but the sulfur colloid scan shows an increased uptake in these regions. What is the most probable diagnosis?
    (a) Regenerated nodule
    (b) Fatty infiltration
    (c) Metastasis
    (d) Granulomatosis

33. A patient is referred with hepatic lesions, but the primary workup is NOT helpful. Which of the following methods is recommended for further evaluation?
    (a) MRI
    (b) CT scan
    (c) Sonography
    (d) FDG-PET scan

34. This disease can cause false-positive findings in the FDG-PET imaging of the liver:
    (a) Hemangioma
    (b) Adenoma
    (c) Low-grade HCC
    (d) Nodular lymphoid hyperplasia (pseudolymphoma)

35. All of the following statements regarding the role of PET in cholangiocarcinoma are true *except*:
    (a) PET is highly sensitive to the detection of gallbladder carcinoma.
    (b) PET sensitivity to carcinomatosis is limited.
    (c) Sensitivity to infiltrative cholangiocarcinoma is much higher than that to nodular cholangiocarcinoma.
    (d) In patients with cholangiocarcinoma and gallbladder carcinoma, PET/CT findings change the management protocol in 17% patients.

36. Which segments are separated by the ligamentum teres fissure in the anatomical partitioning of the liver segments?
    (a) VIII and IVa segments; IVa and II segments
    (b) IV and IVb segments
    (c) VIII and IVa segments
    (d) IVa and IVb segments

37. All of the following statements are true *except*:
    (a) Density of a normal liver on the CT scan is equal to or greater than that of the spleen.
    (b) Enhancement of a normal liver during the portal phase is equal to or greater than that of the spleen.
    (c) The signal of a normal liver on T2W is greater than that of the spleen.
    (d) The signal of a normal liver on T1W is greater than that of the spleen.

38. All of the following statements regarding liver masses are correct *except*:
    (a) The halo sign of a liver mass on ultrasonography is more likely suggestive of a benign process.
    (b) Metastatic liver masses usually have low vascularity.
    (c) A hyperechoic metastatic mass in the liver is more likely suggestive of adenocarcinoma of the colon.
    (d) Cystic liver metastases are rare.

39. Which of the following statements regarding liver cavernous hemangioma is false?
    (a) It is more common in women than in men.
    (b) It is the most common benign liver mass.
    (c) It does not have a remarkable annual growth.
    (d) It is usually multiple.

40. All of the following statements regarding hepatoma are correct *except*:
    (a) It is more common in men than in women.
    (b) It is more common in cirrhosis following hepatitis rather than in alcoholic cirrhosis.
    (c) It rarely infiltrates into the hepatic and portal veins.
    (d) Calcification rarely occurs in this tumor.

41. Which of the following tumors is less likely to metastasize to the liver?
    (a) Colon tumors
    (b) Thyroid tumors
    (c) Lung tumors
    (d) Breast tumors

42. Which of the following items is located between the left and the right liver lobes?
    (a) Coronary ligament
    (b) Ligamentum teres
    (c) Middle hepatic vein
    (d) Triangular ligament

1.2.1 Answer

	A	B	C	D
1				*
2		*		
3				*
4			*	
5			*	
6			*	
7			*	
8	*			
9	*			
10				*
11			*	
12				*
13			*	
14			*	
15				*
16	*			
17	*			
18		*		
19		*		
20		*		
21	*			
22		*		
23		*		
24	*			
25			*	
26		*		
27				*
28	*			
29	*			
30	*			

31	*			
32	*			
33	*			
34				*
35			*	
36	*			
37			*	
38	*			
39				*
40			*	
41		*		
42			*	

1.3 PET in Lymphoma and Malignant Melanoma

1. What is the most important benefit of the PET scan in lymphoma?
   (a) Staging
   (b) Restaging
   (c) Extranodal involvement
   (d) a and c

2. Lymphadenopathy:
   (a) Multiple lymph nodes (8–10 mm) in the retroperitoneum are abnormal.
   (b) The maximum diameter of lymph nodes in the pelvis is 12 mm.
   (c) The maximum diameter of lymph nodes in the gastrohepatic ligament is 10 mm.
   (d) The maximum diameter of lymph nodes in the porta hepatis is 10 mm.

3. Which organ is an unusual site for the metastasis of melanoma?
   (a) Spleen
   (b) Lung
   (c) Liver
   (d) Brain

4. In which stage of melanoma does the PET scan have the most effect?
   (a) II
   (b) III
   (c) IV
   (d) I

5. Which item is required for the preparation for FDG-PET of a patient with malignancy?
   (a) Imaging for at least 30 min after radiotracer injection
   (b) Fasting
   (c) Administration of at least 20 mCi FDG
   (d) Administration of glucose in diabetic patients

6. Which of the following patients benefits most from FDG-PET?
   (a) A 53-year-old woman with lingual SCC for primary staging
   (b) A 44-year-old man with malignant melanoma with a thickness of 1 mm in the metatarsus for the evaluation of metastasis
   (c) A 20-year-old boy with lymphoma for the evaluation of the possible involvement of the bone marrow
   (d) A 63-year-old man for the confirmation of a recurrent mucinous tumor of the rectum

7. Which of the following findings is observed in the radionuclide scintigraphy of the spleen in the splenic metastasis of melanoma?
   (a) Splenomegaly and a reduced uptake
   (b) Normal size and a reduced uptake
   (c) Splenomegaly or normal size with a reduced uptake
   (d) Splenomegaly with multiple photopenic lesions

8. Which of the following items results in the lower tumor uptake of ^{18}F-FDG?
   (a) Tumors with high growth fractions
   (b) Hyperglycemia
   (c) Inflammation
   (d) Recent chemotherapy

9. Diffuse uptake of FDG in the thyroid is NOT observed in:
   (a) Subacute thyroiditis
   (b) Chronic inflammation
   (c) Autoimmune disease
   (d) Lymphoma

10. A patient with malignant melanoma thicker than 1 mm and without a palpable lymph node is evaluated. In which of the following conditions is FDG-PET NOT applied?
    (a) Treatment setup after tumor relapse
    (b) Evaluation of a distant metastasis
    (c) Restaging after a primary CT scan
    (d) Evaluation of a regional lymph node metastasis

11. A standardized uptake value (SUV) is used to determine the malignancy of tumors. Choose the correct item about SUV.
    (a) Different values are obtained according to the image processing algorithm.
    (b) Evaluation of the tumor size and location is NOT necessary.
    (c) The unit of SUV is gram per minute.
    (d) b and c.

12. A 66-year-old man diagnosed with melanoma is referred. What is the recommended scan for evaluating the local–regional involvement of a lymph node for biopsy?
    (a) Radioimmunoscintigraphy
    (b) Lymphoscintigraphy
    (c) Lymphangiography with methylene blue
    (d) PET/CT

13. A patient with lymphoma is referred for staging. What is the preferred method for evaluating the involvement of the spleen?
    (a) FDG-PET
    (b) Contrast CT
    (c) Sonography
    (d) MRI

14. ^{18}F-FDG scan is performed 4 days after cytokine therapy for leukemia. A diffuse increase in uptake is observed in the bone marrow. What is the most common cause of this finding?
    (a) Diffuse relapse of the tumor
    (b) Increased metabolic activity
    (c) Hyperglycemia
    (d) Artifact due to the interaction of cytokines with FDG

15. About the diagnosis of lymphatic lesions in a patient with Hodgkin's disease:
    (a) The CT scan outcome is NOT influenced by lesion size.
    (b) CT scan and lymphangiography better show the margin of lesion than gallium scan.
    (c) The gallium scan is more efficient in detecting the involved lymph nodes smaller than 10 mm.
    (d) Abdominal lymph nodes are better observed in the gallium scan than chest lymphatic lesions.

16. In which type of low-grade lymphoma is FDG-PET indicated?
    (a) Small lymphocytic lymphoma
    (b) Low-grade follicular NHL
    (c) Mantle cell lymphoma
    (d) MALT lymphoma

17. A 65-year-old woman with a skin lesion on her neck (2.3 mm in thickness) is referred. Biopsy and pathology reports are indicative of melanoma. Which of the following items is the most probable?
    (a) The patient is considered low risk, and the possible involvement of the lymph node is 2–3%.
    (b) The patient is considered low risk, and the possible involvement of the lymph node is 10%.
    (c) The patient is considered high risk, and the possible involvement of the lymph node is 50–70%.
    (d) The patient is considered an intermediate risk, and the possible involvement of the lymph node is 20–50%.

18. Which of the following activities does NOT interfere with the interpretation of the scan during an FDG-PET scan?
    (a) Closing the eyes
    (b) Reading
    (c) Speaking
    (d) Chewing gum

19. A 38-year-old man weighing 70 kg with a history of Hodgkin's lymphoma is referred for an ^{18}F-FDG scan. What are the recommended radiotracer dose and time of scan?
    (a) 15 mCi, 60 min after injection
    (b) 10 mCi, 30 min after injection
    (c) 25 mCi, 4 h after injection
    (d) 15 mCi, 24 h after injection

20. ^{18}F-FDG:
    (a) Although it is a glucose analog, it is excreted from the kidneys unlike glucose.
    (b) There is NO relationship between the perfusion and the tumoral uptake of FDG.
    (c) Fasting is NOT required for FDG-PET.
    (d) It enters the cellular metabolic cycle like glucose.

21. What is the mechanism of FDG-6-phosphate accumulation in tumoral cells?
    (a) Decrease in the density of glucose transporters on the cell surface
    (b) Decrease in mitochondrial glucose metabolism
    (c) Increase in the glucose-6-phosphate level compared with normal tissue
    (d) Increase in the expression or activity of hexokinase

22. To which tumor is the PET scan the most sensitive for diagnosis?
    (a) Liver metastasis of colorectal carcinoma
    (b) Brain metastasis of colorectal tumors
    (c) Lymphatic involvement in intermediate-risk melanoma
    (d) Colorectal mucinous adenocarcinoma

23. What is the main reason for the low accumulation of ^{18}F-FDG in the liver and renal cells?
    (a) Presence of phosphatase
    (b) Lack of phosphorylation of ^{18}F-FDG
    (c) Inappropriate intracellular pH
    (d) Hydrophilicity of the cell membrane

24. For optimal PET image quality, the glucose level should be:
    (a) $\leq$200 mg/dl
    (b) $\leq$150 mg/dl
    (c) $\leq$126 mg/dl
    (d) $\leq$100 mg/dl

25. Which diet given before PET examination can optimize the uptake and decrease the myocardial uptake?
    (a) Low carbohydrate/high protein/high fat
    (b) High carbohydrate/low protein/high fat
    (c) Low carbohydrate/low protein/low fat
    (d) High carbohydrate/high protein/high fat

26. All of the following PET scan times are true *except*:
    (a) Post-biopsy—1 week
    (b) Post-surgery—6 weeks
    (c) Post-granulocyte colony-stimulating factor (G-CSF)—1 week to 1 month
    (d) Post-radiofrequency ablation—2–6 months

27. In the standardized uptake value (SUV) calculation:
    (a) Earlier imaging provides high SUV results.
    (b) Earlier scans are usually associated with smaller measurement errors.
    (c) The SUV plateaus early following therapeutic interventions.
    (d) The SUV is underestimated in obese patients.

28. Which factor can affect the result of the standardized uptake value (SUV)?
    (a) Partial volume effects
    (b) Background activity
    (c) Reconstruction parameter
    (d) All of the above

29. Extensive diffused bone marrow uptake in FDG-PET imaging is NOT seen in:
    (a) Chemotherapy
    (b) Erythropoietin therapy
    (c) Myelodysplastic syndrome
    (d) Chronic myeloid leukemia

30. All of the following statements regarding PET in the staging of lymphoma are true *except*:
    (a) In HD, PET is the most useful in stage IV of the disease.
    (b) In NHL, PET can be of value in any stage.
    (c) PET may be of potential value in mantle cell lymphoma.
    (d) Overall, PET changes the management of 14% of HD patients on average.

31. Which subtype of Hodgkin's disease demonstrates the highest FDG uptake?
    (a) Mixed cellularity subtype
    (b) Nodular sclerosis
    (c) Nodular lymphocytic predominance
    (d) Mucosa-associated lymphoid type (MALT)

32. Which subtype of non-Hodgkin's lymphoma has poor FDG uptake?
    (a) Follicular lymphoma
    (b) Marginal zone lymphoma
    (c) Small-cell lymphocytic lymphoma
    (d) Peripheral T-cell lymphoma

33. All of the following statements regarding PET in the therapy response of lymphoma are true *except*:
    (a) A positive FDG-PET study is highly predictive of residual/recurrent disease.
    (b) Follow-up scans are necessary for patients with negative PET and NHL.
    (c) The NPV of midtreatment in HD is high (at least 94%).
    (d) Follow-up scans are necessary in patients with stage I and II HD and negative PET.

34. All of the following statements regarding PET in melanoma are true *except*:
    (a) Lung metastases in melanoma are usually very small and undetectable by PET.
    (b) Liver MRI is significantly more sensitive than PET for liver metastases from melanoma.
    (c) Melanin content influences lesion detectability by PET.
    (d) PET is a standard modality in evaluating recurrent melanoma.

35. What is the most common location of extranodal lymphoma?
    (a) CNS
    (b) Lung
    (c) GI
    (d) GU

36. Which statement regarding stomach lymphoma is NOT true?
    (a) It makes up 20% stomach cancers.
    (b) It is the most common region of primary lymphoma in the GI.
    (c) Its prognosis is worse than that of stomach carcinoma.
    (d) It may have a polypoid pattern.

37. Regarding the application of PET in lymphoma:
    (a) An increase in protein synthesis is found in lymphoma; therefore, ^{11}C-tryptophan is indicated for imaging.
    (b) The higher uptake of FDG indicates poor prognosis.
    (c) PET is NOT capable of detecting splenic lymphoma.
    (d) The high uptake of FDG in the thymus is a specific finding for thymic lymphoma.

38. All of the following statements regarding the application of PET scan in lymphoma are correct *except*:
    (a) PET is NOT indicated for evaluating the involvement of the bone marrow in lymphomas.
    (b) The conventional modalities for the staging of lymphoma include physical examination; CT of the chest, abdomen, and pelvis; bone scintigraphy; and bone marrow biopsy.
    (c) Both Hodgkin's disease and non-Hodgkin's lymphoma exhibit a marked FDG uptake, and FDG imaging is useful in both staging and therapeutic monitoring.
    (d) The degree of FDG uptake in untreated patients seems to be a better prognostic factor than the degree of ^{67}Ga uptake.

39. PET scan is indicated for melanoma for all of the following purposes *except*:
    (a) Initial evaluation of intermediate-risk patients
    (b) Initial evaluation of high-risk patients
    (c) Evaluation of suspected recurrence
    (d) Evaluation of a metastatic disease

40. If the goal is to evaluate the response to chemotherapy with FDG and ^{11}C-methionine, a metabolic response is defined as a decrease in the tumor SUV to a level below … of the baseline.
    (a) 20%
    (b) 30%
    (c) 70%
    (d) 55%

41. A 48-year-old woman underwent total excision of a tumor in the left tibia, and the pathology report indicates malignant melanoma. Lymphadenopathy of the left inguinal is observed in the physical examination, and biopsy confirms malignant melanoma. What is the best method for staging?
    (a) CT scan of the abdomen and pelvis + chest X-ray + brain MRI
    (b) CT scan of the abdomen and pelvis + chest X-ray + bone scan
    (c) Whole-body PET/CT scan
    (d) CT scan of the abdomen, pelvis, and thorax

42. In which stages of melanoma is the sentinel lymph node biopsy (SLNB) or the selective resection of lymph nodes indicated?
    (a) T1a and higher
    (b) T2b and higher
    (c) T3a and higher
    (d) T1b and higher

43. Which of the following statements regarding nodal and extranodal lymphomas is NOT correct?
    (a) Approximately two-thirds of lymphoma cases are nodal, and one-third of the cases are extranodal.
    (b) Nodal lymphomas are initially localized, whereas extranodal forms are usually diffused.
    (c) Nodal lymphomas are usually follicular, whereas extranodal forms are diffuse large B cells.
    (d) In similar conditions, the treatment and prognosis of nodal and extranodal lymph nodes are completely identical.

44. Which of the following statements is NOT correct regarding a patient diagnosed with lymphoma and having a positive PET scan during and after completion of chemotherapy?
    (a) The PET scan must be performed with short intervals because of the high incidence of false-positive findings for tumor recurrence.
    (b) Other diagnostic modalities are recommended because of the high incidence of recurrence.
    (c) PET is valuable for diffuse large B-cell lymphoma, but limited information is available about the benefits of PET scan in other forms of the disease.
    (d) The patient undergoes salvage chemotherapy because of the high probability of the diagnosis of tumor recurrence as a NO response to the treatment in the PET scan.

45. Regarding the involvement of lymph nodes in Hodgkin's disease:
    (a) Splenic involvement, even minor, indicates a high risk for extranodal lymphoma.
    (b) The probability of involvement of a mesenteric lymph node is greater than that of a para-aortic lymph node in subdiaphragmatic Hodgkin's disease.
    (c) The bilateral involvement of cervical lymph nodes without the involvement of mediastinal lymph nodes is a common presentation of the disease.
    (d) The spleen is usually NOT involved when the disease has progressed to the liver.

46. All of the following lymph nodes are hypodense on the CT scan *except*:
    (a) Tuberculosis
    (b) Lymphoma
    (c) Seminoma
    (d) Nonseminomatous carcinoma

1.3.1 Answer

	A	B	C	D
1				*
2	*			
3	*			
4		*		
5		*		
6			*	
7			*	
8	*			
9	*			
10				*
11	*			
12		*		
13	*			
14		*		
15		*		
16		*		
17				*
18	*			
19	*			
20	*			
21				*
22	*			
23	*			
24		*		
25	*			
26				*
27			*	
28				*
29	*			
30	*			
31	*			
32			*	
33				*
34			*	
35			*	
36			*	
37		*		
38	*			
39	*			
40				*
41	*			
42				*
43		*		
44				*
45	*			
46			*	

1.4 Parathyroid Imaging

1. All of the following conditions can predispose to secondary hyperparathyroidism *except*:
   (a) Osteomalacia
   (b) Malabsorption syndrome
   (c) Renal tubular disorders
   (d) Conn's syndrome

2. What is the extremely rare location of parathyroid adenoma?
   (a) Close to the aortic arch
   (b) Thymus
   (c) Neck
   (d) Carotid sheath 13

3. False-positive ^{99m}Tc-MIBI parathyroid images have NOT been seen in:
   (a) Sarcoidosis
   (b) Lymphoma
   (c) Thyroglossal duct cyst
   (d) Thyroid carcinoma

4. Which of the following conditions is the result of a usually positive parathyroid scan?
   (a) Parathyroid carcinoma
   (b) Sarcoidosis
   (c) Tertiary hyperparathyroidism
   (d) All of the above

5. A parathyroid scan is requested for evaluating recurrence in a patient who underwent parathyroidectomy. The patient is taking levothyroxine and labetalol. Which method is NOT recommended?
   (a) Administration of the study at two phases
   (b) SPECT
   (c) Imaging in the oblique and lateral views
   (d) Administration of two radioisotopes

6. A parathyroid scan is requested for a patient who underwent parathyroidectomy, and a suspicious finding is observed in the mediastinum. Which method can help to obtain a better diagnosis?
   (a) Octreoscan
   (b) MRI
   (c) CT scan without contrast
   (d) SPECT/CT

7. Which of the following findings is observed in ^{99m}Tc-MIBI if oxyphil cells dominate in parathyroid adenoma?
   (a) Decreased uptake, decreased retention
   (b) Increased uptake, increased retention
   (c) Increased uptake, decreased retention
   (d) Decreased uptake, increased retention

8. About the ^{99m}Tc-MIBI scan for a patient suspected of having parathyroid adenoma:
   (a) SPECT has the best outcome for the localization of the parathyroid.
   (b) The separate localization of the thyroid with the ^{123}I scan is necessary.
   (c) The best time for imaging is 10 min after administration.
   (d) Levothyroxine must be discontinued 2 weeks before the test.

9. If the goal is to treat primary hyperparathyroidism, which of the following imaging techniques will be applied before the "minimally invasive parathyroidectomy"?
   (a) Sonography
   (b) Thyroid scan with ^{99m}Tc-MIBI
   (c) MRI
   (d) CT scan

10. Surgical therapy has been unsuccessful for a patient with primary hyperparathyroidism. What is the imaging method of choice for the localization of the lesion before the second surgery?
    (a) Sonography with CT scan
    (b) ^{99m}Tc-MIBI scan with MRI
    (c) ^{99m}Tc-MIBI scan with CT scan
    (d) Sonography with ^{99m}Tc-MIBI scan

11. In hyperparathyroidism:
    (a) The intensity of hypercalcemia is NOT related to the size of the adenoma.
    (b) A low number of oxyphil cells in the adenoma can produce false-negative scan results.
    (c) A high iodine regime can cause false-negative or false-positive scan results.
    (d) False-negative scan results are NOT observed in large adenomas.

12. In parathyroid scintigraphy:
    (a) ^{201}Tl uptake in the parathyroid is higher than that in the surrounding thyroid tissue.
    (b) Large adenomas with a rapid clearance can cause false-negative findings.
    (c) ^{11}C-methionin is NOT helpful in the detection of problematic cases.
    (d) Scan accuracy of the diagnosis of an adenoma is similar to that of hyperplasia.

13. ^{99m}Tc-MIBI scan is performed for a 49-year-old woman suspected of having parathyroid adenoma with serum calcium of 10.8 mg/dl and serum phosphor of 3.3 mg/dl. What is the most common source of the false-positive results in the scan?
    (a) Differentiated thyroid carcinoma
    (b) Solid nodule of the thyroid
    (c) Thyroid lymphoma
    (d) Sarcoidosis

14. What is the reason for the accumulation of ^{201}Tl in parathyroid adenoma?
    (a) High density of the mitochondria in this tumor
    (b) Increase in cellularity and vascularity of this tumor
    (c) High level of glucose hexokinase in this tumor
    (d) High density of potassium receptors that absorb thallium

15. In a parathyroid scan:
    (a) The washout of ^{99m}Tc-MIBI in the parathyroid is slower than that of thallium.
    (b) The washout of ^{99m}Tc-MIBI in the parathyroid is faster than that in the thyroid.
    (c) The activity of ^{99m}Tc-MIBI in a normal thyroid is greater than that of thallium.
    (d) ^{99m}Tc-MIBI alone has low sensitivity in the diagnosis of parathyroid adenoma.

16. What is the relationship between radiopharmaceutical uptake and adenoma properties in the scan of a patient with suspected adenoma?
    (a) An inverse relationship is found between the ^{99m}Tc-MIBI localization in the adenoma and lesion size.
    (b) An inverse relationship is found between the ^{99m}Tc-MIBI uptake and the intensity of the mitochondria.
    (c) An inverse relationship is found between the ^{99m}Tc-MIBI localization in the adenoma and its function.
    (d) A direct relationship is found between the ^{99m}Tc-MIBI retention and the intensity of oxyphil cells.

17. A parathyroid scan is requested for a patient with a history of bone pain and a high level of serum PTH. Which item is correct?
    (a) Application of two isotopes (technetium and thallium) is recommended.
    (b) The sensitivity of the ^{99m}Tc-MIBI scan in parathyroid hyperplasia is greater than 95%.
    (c) The specificity of the ^{99m}Tc-MIBI scan in parathyroid adenoma is less than 60%.
    (d) The application of one isotope in the second phase is recommended.

18. Choose the correct phrase about parathyroid scan.
    (a) The accumulation of ^{99m}Tc-MIBI is NOT related to the size and activity of an adenoma.
    (b) The histology of an adenoma is NOT related to the level of the ^{99m}Tc-MIBI uptake.
    (c) The dual-tracer ^{99m}Tc-MIBI and SPECT in the primary phase of the dual-phase scan increase the sensitivity of this method.
    (d) If the size of the parathyroid glands is identical, the sensitivity of the dual-phase ^{99m}Tc-MIBI scan in primary and secondary hyperparathyroidism is similar.

19. BMD is −2.7 for a 56-year-old patient, with serum calcium of 12 mg/dl, PTH level twice that of the normal value, and serum creatinine of 0.9 mg/dl. What is the recommended therapeutic approach?
    (a) Parathyroid surgery
    (b) Diuretic
    (c) Limitation of calcium intake
    (d) Follow-up without treatment

20. What is the most common cause of primary hyperparathyroidism?
    (a) Parathyroid adenoma
    (b) Chief cell hyperplasia
    (c) Follicular cell hyperplasia
    (d) Parathyroid carcinoma

21. About the evaluation of a parathyroid adenoma in a parathyroid scan:
    (a) The scan sensitivity for adenomas below 100 mg is low.
    (b) Levothyroxine is recommended before the scan to reduce the thyroid uptake of ^{99m}Tc-MIBI.
    (c) ^{201}Tl uptake in parathyroid adenoma is three times greater than that in the thyroid.
    (d) A semiquantitative analysis is required for interpreting the scan.

22. In a parathyroid scan with technetium–sestamibi:
    (a) The technetium–thallium subtraction scan is more sensitive than the ^{123}I-Tc-MIBI subtraction for the diagnosis of parathyroid hyperplasia.
    (b) The technetium–sestamibi scan immediately after injection is sufficient for the diagnosis of parathyroid adenoma.
    (c) A high intensity of the mitochondria in the parathyroid adenoma cells increases the sestamibi uptake and prolongs its washout.
    (d) Sestamibi can efficiently distinguish parathyroid adenoma and cancer.

23. What is the radiopharmaceutical of choice for the diagnosis of parathyroid adenoma in PET scan?
    (a) ^{11}C-methionine
    (b) FLT
    (c) ^{11}C-L-DOPA
    (d) ^{11}C-5MTP

24. What is the mechanism of the ^{99m}Tc-MIBI accumulation in parathyroid adenoma in comparison with that in thyroid tissue?
    (a) Increase in the permeability of the cell membrane
    (b) High density of the mitochondria
    (c) Decrease in cell degradation
    (d) Decrease in the cAMP activity

25. Which of the following items is NOT included in the false-positive results of parathyroid scintigraphy with ^{99m}Tc-MIBI?
    (a) Thyroid cystic nodule
    (b) Sarcoidosis
    (c) Thyroid carcinoma
    (d) Lymphoma

26. Identify the correct statement regarding abnormal parathyroid tissue.
    (a) MRI can be applied for the differential diagnosis of a parathyroid adenoma of soft tissue from lesions with thyroid origin.
    (b) An abnormal parathyroid tissue in primary hyperthyroidism is better detected than that in secondary hyperparathyroidism of the same size with nuclear medicine techniques.
    (c) An abnormal parathyroid tissue is presented as a hyperechoic lesion in high-resolution ultrasound.
    (d) CT is NOT appropriate for evaluating an abnormal parathyroid tissue in the retrosternal and retrotracheal regions.

27. Which of the following parameters does NOT affect the parathyroid pattern in the dual-phase ^{99m}Tc-MIBI scan?
    (a) Administration of the thyroid hormone
    (b) The number of oxyphilic cells in parathyroid adenoma
    (c) Utilization of SPECT
    (d) Delayed imaging of more than 2 h after injection

28. Parathyroid surgery has been revolutionized because of novel diagnostic methods. Which of the following methods has NOT had an important role in this transformation?
    (a) Rapid measurement of free serum calcium during surgery
    (b) ^{99m}Tc-MIBI parathyroid imaging
    (c) Rapid measurement of PTH during surgery
    (d) Localization of the parathyroid pathology by gamma probe

29. About primary hyperparathyroidism:
    (a) It is more common in men than in women, and its prevalence does NOT change with age.
    (b) Currently, most patients are asymptomatic or present non-specific symptoms at the time of diagnosis.
    (c) Most patients demonstrate adenoma in more than one gland.
    (d) The polyclonal proliferation of mutated cells is the main reason for parathyroid adenoma.

30. If the goal is to diagnose parathyroid hyperplasia, which of the following methods is less sensitive?
    (a) CT scan
    (b) Sonography
    (c) ^{99m}TcO4-^{201}Tl subtraction
    (d) MRI

31. Which of the following statements is NOT correct about parathyroid glands?
    (a) The prevalence of ectopic glands is higher in the lower parathyroid glands than in the upper ones.
    (b) The parathyroid glands originate from the third and fourth pharyngeal arches.
    (c) The superior parathyroid glands are usually larger.
    (d) Extra parathyroid glands may be observed in 2–6.5% of adults.

32. Which of the following statements is NOT correct?
    (a) The parathyroid hormone increases calcium absorption from the GI, osteoclastic activity, and reabsorption of phosphate and calcium from renal tubules.
    (b) The chief cells responsible for PTH production have two active and inactive forms with a ratio of 1:3 under a normal condition.
    (c) Hyperparathyroidism is observed after thyroidectomy.
    (d) Primary hyperparathyroidism may be due to singular or multiple adenomas or hyperplasia.

33. Novel techniques have been developed for measuring calcium. What is the main purpose of imaging in hyperparathyroidism?
    (a) Detection of bone presentation of the disease
    (b) Detection of renal presentation of the disease
    (c) Identification of the source of production of the extra PTH
    (d) All of the above

34. Which of the following imaging techniques is NOT used any more in parathyroid scan because of its low sensitivity and quality of images?
    (a) 75Se scan
    (b) ^{99m}Tc-^{201}Tl subtraction scan
    (c) ^{131}I-toluidine blue-^{99m}Tc scan
    (d) BB5-G1 monoclonal antibody scan

35. Regarding ectopic parathyroid adenoma in the mediastinum:
    (a) ^{99m}Tc-MIBI scan does NOT have a high diagnostic value.
    (b) It has a very high signal on the MRI with STIR sequence.
    (c) It is NOT differentiated from a lymph node on the IV contrast CT scan of the mediastinum.
    (d) Planar and SPECT images on the ^{99m}Tc-MIBI scan have similar accuracy.

36. Which of the following statements regarding parathyroid adenoma is correct?
    (a) Hyperechoic and homogenous on sonography
    (b) Hypervascular on Doppler sonography
    (c) Same or less signal rather than fast on the T2W MRI
    (d) Cystic degeneration or calcification is common

1.4.1 Answer

	A	B	C	D
1				*
2	*			
3			*	
4				*
5				*
6		*		
7		*		
8	*			
9		*		
10		*		
11		*		
12		*		
13		*		
14		*		
15	*			
16				*
17				*
18			*	
19	*			
20	*			
21	*			
22			*	
23	*			
24		*		
25	*			
26		*		
27	*			
28	*			
29		*		
30			*	
31	*			
32	*			
33			*	
34	*			
35		*		
36		*		

1.5 Adrenocortical Scintigraphy

1. What is the gold standard technique for adrenal imaging?
   (a) Adrenal CT
   (b) Adrenal scintigraphy
   (c) PET
   (d) Venography with venous sampling

2. All are radiopharmaceuticals for adrenocortical imaging *except*:
   (a) ^{75}Selenomethylnorcholestrol (Scintadren)
   (b) ^{11}C-metomidate
   (c) ^{131}I-metyrapone
   (d) ^{11}C-methionine

3. Which organ does NOT appear in the normal FDG-PET scan for the evaluation of the adrenal medulla?
   (a) Adrenal medulla
   (b) Salivary glands
   (c) Heart
   (d) Liver

4. What changes in the adrenal cortex scan are induced by glucocorticoid-producing carcinoma of the adrenal cortex?
   (a) Adrenals are NOT observed on both sides.
   (b) No uptake is observed in the adrenal with tumor.
   (c) A remarkable increase in adrenal uptake especially on the right side.
   (d) A remarkable bilateral increase in adrenal uptake.

5. Which of the following situations or drugs results in a decreased adrenal uptake in adrenal cortex scintigraphy?
   (a) Hypercholesterolemia
   (b) Oral contraceptives
   (c) Diuretics
   (d) Exogenous ACTH

6. Only one adrenal gland is observed in the NP-59 scan of a patient. Which diagnosis is the least possible?
   (a) Remnant adrenal
   (b) Adrenal adenoma
   (c) Severe hypercholesterolemia
   (d) Ectopic adrenocortical tissue

7. What is the radiopharmaceutical of choice for observing the normal adrenal medulla in the sympathomedullary scan?
   (a) ^{123}I-MIBG
   (b) ^{11}C-epinephrine
   (c) ^{18}F-FDG
   (d) ^{11}C-HED

8. What is the best time for adrenal cortex imaging with ^{131}I-NP59?
   (a) 3–5 h after injection
   (b) Immediately after injection
   (c) 6 h after injection
   (d) 24 h after injection

9. The dexamethasone suppression test is NOT indicated for the diagnosis of:
   (a) Gonadal hyperfunction
   (b) Adrenal hyperandrogenism
   (c) Hyperaldosteronism
   (d) Cushing's syndrome

10. Adrenal cortex scintigraphy with 59NP is requested for a 48-year-old woman with symptoms of Cushing's syndrome. Both adrenal glands are observed in the scan, but the radiopharmaceutical uptake is dissymmetric. What is the most common source of Cushing's syndrome according to the scan results?
    (a) ACTH-independent nodular hyperplasia
    (b) Adrenal carcinoma
    (c) Adrenal adenoma
    (d) Ectopic ACTH production by pulmonary cancer

11. Which of the following radiopharmaceuticals is used for the better observation of the adrenal medulla?
    (a) ^{123}I-MIBG
    (b) ^{11}C-epinephrin
    (c) ^{18}F-FDG
    (d) ^{131}I-MIBG

12. A 59NP scan is requested for a 49-year-old man with suspected Cushing's syndrome. Only 1 day after injection, a faint bilateral activity with right adrenal dominancy is observed. What is the most probable diagnosis?
    (a) Adenoma of the right adrenal
    (b) Normal adrenal
    (c) Bilateral hyperplasia
    (d) Carcinoma of the right adrenal

13. About neuroendocrine imaging:
    (a) The adrenal is mostly observed in the ^{123}I-MIBG scan.
    (b) Observation of the hypophysis activity in the octreotide scan is always considered abnormal.
    (c) The medullar uptake of ^{18}F-FDG is NOT observed in a normal adrenal gland.
    (d) ^{123}I-MIBG and ^{131}I-MIBG have similar sensitivity in the diagnosis of pheochromocytoma and paraganglioma.

14. A patient with low renin, high aldosterone, and hypokalemia is referred. What it is the scan of choice for the localization of an adrenal lesion?
    (a) 59NP scan with dexamethasone suppression
    (b) 59NP scan
    (c) 59NP scan with ACTH stimulation
    (d) ^{123}I-MIBG scan

15. About incidentaloma of the adrenal gland:
    (a) Radio-cholesterol uptake indicates a benign lesion.
    (b) It has an obvious clinical presentation.
    (c) An increasing secretion of cortisol is usually observed.
    (d) It is accidentally detected in the 59NP scan for the first time.

16. The dexamethasone suppression test in 59NP imaging is NOT indicated for the diagnosis of which disease?
    (a) Adrenal hyperandrogenism
    (b) Cushing's syndrome
    (c) Hyperaldosteronism
    (d) Gonadal hyperfunction

17. Which item is NOT correct about the application of PET in neuroendocrine tumors?
    (a) ^{18}F-FDG-PET is specifically useful in tumors with low proliferation.
    (b) ^{11}C-5HTP is used for the screening of the abdomen and the thorax when the octreotide scan is negative.
    (c) The octreotide scan is the method of choice when deciding on somatostatin therapy and is preferred over PET.
    (d) ^{67}Ga-DOTATATE is used in somatostatin scintigraphy with PET.

18. Which drug is required to be discontinued before adrenal scan with MIBG?
    (a) Amitriptyline
    (b) Atenolol
    (c) Phenoxybenzamine
    (d) Diuretics

19. None of the adrenals is observed in the ^{131}I-59NP scan of a patient with Cushing's syndrome. What is the most probable diagnosis?
    (a) Adrenal carcinoma
    (b) ACTH-dependent adrenal hyperplasia
    (c) ACTH-independent adrenal hyperplasia
    (d) Adrenal adenoma

20. Which of the following methods for the imaging of the adrenal medulla can better observe normal adrenal glands in a scan?
    (a) ^{123}I-MIBG
    (b) ^{131}I-MIBG
    (c) ^{11}C-HED PET
    (d) ^{11}C-epinephrine PET

21. Laboratory tests confirm Cushing's syndrome in a patient, and a 7 cm mass is observed in the left adrenal in the abdominal CT scan. If this mass is due to carcinoma, how is the pattern of the adrenal cortex scintigraphy described?
    (a) Appearance of the left adrenal gland with absence of the right adrenal
    (b) Appearance of the right adrenal with absence of the left adrenal
    (c) Bilateral absence of the adrenal glands
    (d) Appearance of both adrenals with higher intensity on the left side

22. Which of the following findings indicates adenoma of the right adrenal cortex in a patient with hyperaldosteronism (Conn's syndrome)?
    (a) Increased uptake in the right adrenal with dexamethasone administration.
    (b) Increased uptake in the right adrenal without dexamethasone administration.
    (c) Bilateral increase in adrenal uptake.
    (d) Both adrenals are not observed.

23. Which item is NOT correct about the 59NP adrenal cortex scintigraphy?
    (a) Scan must be performed on the first to the third day in patients with suspected Cushing's syndrome.
    (b) The scan is performed on the third to the fifth day in patients under suppression.
    (c) 59NP is the radiotracer of choice.
    (d) After dexamethasone is discontinued on the fifth day, the scan is repeated on the seventh day.

24. In which condition is the 59NP adrenal scan the least valuable?
    (a) Evaluation of a patient with suspected Cushing's syndrome with increased ACTH
    (b) Differentiation of neoplasm and hyperplasia in patients with primary hyperaldosteronism
    (c) Determination of the probability of malignancy in an asymptomatic adrenal mass (incidentaloma)
    (d) Diagnosis of hypofunctional adrenal tissue in patients with Addison's disease

25. A mass in the left adrenal is detected by abdominal CT scan. The 59NP scan shows an increased uptake in the left adrenal despite the normal results of the adrenal function tests. What is the most probable diagnosis?
    (a) Adrenal cancer
    (b) Benign adenoma
    (c) Metastasis
    (d) Adrenal cyst

26. Which organ appears abnormal in 59NP scintigraphy?
    (a) Kidneys
    (b) Adrenal
    (c) Liver
    (d) Gallbladder

27. All of the following statements regarding FDG-PET imaging in adrenals are true *except*:
    (a) FDG-PET has high accuracy in detecting adrenal metastases from lung cancer.
    (b) An SUV cutoff of 3.1 can be used to differentiate metastases from adenomas.
    (c) FDG uptake differs between lipid-rich and lipid-poor adenomas.
    (d) PET sensitivity in the characterization of adrenal lesions with known malignancy is equal to that of MRI and is superior to that of CT.

28. Which of the following adrenal cortex diseases is ACTH dependent?
    (a) Bilateral hyperplasia
    (b) Bilateral nodular hyperplasia
    (c) Carcinoma
    (d) Unilateral adenoma

29. In adrenal cortex carcinoma:
    (a) None of the adrenals are observed in the scan.
    (b) It is ACTH dependent.
    (c) One of the adrenals has a normal pattern, and the one with carcinoma does NOT appear in the scan.
    (d) It is observed as multiple nodules in both adrenals.

30. What is the most appropriate modality for the diagnosis of adrenal enlargement?
    (a) CT scan
    (b) FDG-PET
    (c) MRI
    (d) ^{131}I MIBG scintigraphy

31. All of the following statements regarding adrenal adenoma are correct *except*:
    (a) Benign and asymptomatic adrenal masses are incidentally seen in 3–5% of the population.
    (b) Non-hyperfunctioning adenomas are usually smaller than 4 cm.
    (c) It is a well-marginated and low-density (10 HU) mass on the CT scan without contrast.
    (d) MRI and CT scan are capable of differentiating benign from malignant masses.

32. A patient with lung cancer is found to have an adrenal mass. The MRI using an in-phase/out-of-phase (IP/OP) signal shows no changes. What is the next appropriate modality?
    (a) Contrast CT scan
    (b) Scintigraphy
    (c) Biopsy
    (d) IV contrast MRI

33. A patient with bronchogenic cancer is found to have a 3 cm mass in the right adrenal. Which of the following has the most diagnostic sensitivity for differentiating adrenal adenoma from adrenal metastatic defects?
    (a) Contrast CT scan
    (b) Contrast MR
    (c) Chemical shift MRI
    (d) FDG-PET scan

34. Which type of Cushing's syndrome exhibits a high bilateral adrenal uptake in NP-59 scintigraphy?
    (a) Ectopic ACTH
    (b) Cushing disease
    (c) Cushing's syndrome
    (d) Adrenal carcinoma

35. A 49-year-old patient with symptoms of Cushing's syndrome is referred. The plasma level of ACTH is high and insuppressible with high-dose dexamethasone. What is the first diagnostic study?
    (a) Chest CT scan, CXR
    (b) Brain MRI, skull X-ray
    (c) Abdominal and pelvic CT scan, IVP
    (d) Octreotide receptor scintigraphy

1.5.1 Answer

	A	B	C	D
1				*
2				*
3	*			
4	*			
5	*			
6			*	
7	*			
8	*			
9	*			
10	*			
11	*			
12		*		
13			*	
14	*			
15	*			
16		*		
17	*			
18	*			
19	*			
20	*			

21			*	
22	*			
23	*			
24	*			
25		*		
26	*			
27			*	
28	*			
29	*			
30	*			
31				*
32				*
33				*
34	*			
35	*			

1.6 Gallium Scintigraphy in Tumor Diagnosis and Management

1. In non-Hodgkin's lymphoma, the following factors have been shown to affect ^{67}Ga uptake *except*:
   (a) Histology
   (b) Lactoferrin receptor status
   (c) Transferrin receptor status
   (d) Presence of a large cell component

2. If a cycle of chemotherapy is initiated every 4 weeks, when is the best time for ^{67}Ga scintigraphy?
   (a) 2 weeks prior to the next chemotherapy cycle
   (b) 1 week prior to the next chemotherapy cycle
   (c) 3–4 days prior to the next chemotherapy cycle
   (d) 1–2 days prior to the next chemotherapy cycle

3. What are the main prognostic factors in Hodgkin's lymphoma (HL) and non-Hodgkin's lymphoma (NHL), respectively?
   (a) Clinical stage, clinical stage
   (b) Clinical stage, histology subtype
   (c) Histology subtype, clinical stage
   (d) Histology subtype, histology subtype

4. What is the overall specificity of ^{67}Ga scintigraphy in Hodgkin's lymphoma (HL) and non-Hodgkin's lymphoma (NHL), respectively?
   (a) 93%, 89%
   (b) 89%, 93%
   (c) 100%, 100%
   (d) 93%, 93%

5. This condition reduces the soft tissue uptake of ^{67}Ga:
   (a) Iron overload
   (b) AIDS
   (c) Hormones
   (d) Chemotherapy

6. ^{67}Ga scintigraphy for the staging of lymphoma is:
   (a) Superior to CT and MRI
   (b) Superior to CT and equivalent to MRI
   (c) Superior to MRI and equivalent to CT
   (d) Equivalent to CT and MRI

7. The panda pattern on ^{67}Ga scintigraphy indicates:
   (a) Salivary and lacrimal gland uptake in sarcoidosis disease
   (b) Pulmonary hilar uptake in sarcoidosis disease
   (c) Salivary and pulmonary hilar uptake in Sjögren's syndrome
   (d) Pulmonary hilar uptake in Sjögren's syndrome

8. Evaluation of the response to chemotherapy with gallium scan is requested for a lymphoma case. What is the minimum interval between the last chemotherapy and gallium scan?
   (a) 24 h
   (b) 3 days
   (c) 10 days
   (d) 1 month

9. What is the most important mechanism of gallium uptake in chronic joint inflammation?
   (a) Binding to transferrin receptors
   (b) Increased vascular permeability
   (c) Leukocyte accumulation
   (d) Increased vascular pool

10. ^{67}Ga is commonly uptaken in all of the following items *except*:
    (a) Kaposi's sarcoma
    (b) Sarcoidosis
    (c) Non-small-cell lung cancer
    (d) Wegner's granulomatosis

11. An abnormal uptake of ^{67}Ga is observed in a pulmonary lesion in a patient with AIDS. This finding is NOT indicative of:
    (a) Kaposi's sarcoma
    (b) Tuberculosis
    (c) Lymphoma
    (d) *Pneumocystis carinii* pneumonia

12. Abnormal absorption is NOT observed in the ^{67}Ga scan of a patient with Hodgkin's lymphoma. However, a decreased uptake in the liver and an increased uptake in the kidneys are observed. What is the most probable diagnosis?
    (a) Administration of oral Fe
    (b) Acute renal failure
    (c) Chronic renal failure
    (d) Increased serum albumin

13. In which of the following diseases does ^{G}Ga have the least diagnostic sensitivity?
    (a) Tumor of the head and neck
    (b) Melanoma
    (c) Sarcoma of soft tissue
    (d) Hepatocellular carcinoma

14. Which type of lymphoma histologies has the least chance of ^{67}Ga uptake?
    (a) Low-grade NHL
    (b) High-grade NHL
    (c) Burkitt's lymphoma
    (d) High-grade HD

15. Gallium scan:
    (a) After the first 6 h, changes in the serum gallium will NOT alter the activity of lesions in the scan.
    (b) Desferrioxamine does NOT significantly change the diagnosis of infections in the scan.
    (c) Desferrioxamine is used for the stimulation of intestinal excretion of Ga.
    (d) Maximum uptake in normal tissue is observed in the scan after 6 h.

16. Ga scan in pulmonary tumors:
    (a) Tumors with a dimension of at least 2 cm have the lowest limit of detection.
    (b) This scan is usually important for the detection of tumors in the basal parts of the lung.
    (c) Ga scan has low sensitivity but high specificity in the diagnosis of pulmonary tumors.
    (d) Ga scan has higher sensitivity and specificity than the simple radiography of the chest.

17. A 7-year-old child with major thalassemia, history of several transfusions, and confirmed iron overload is subjected to ^{67}Ga scan for suspected soft tissue infection. What is the most expected outcome of the gallium scan?
    (a) Increased uptake in bones
    (b) Significant uptake in the salivary glands
    (c) Decreased uptake in the kidneys
    (d) Significant uptake in the lacrimal glands

18. Gallium scan is performed for a patient with metastatic melanoma. A low uptake is shown in the metastasis to which organ:
    (a) Brain
    (b) Liver
    (c) Bone
    (d) Spleen

19. Gallium scan is performed for tumor detection in a patient with esophageal cancer. Which view has the highest diagnostic sensitivity?
    (a) Left lateral view
    (b) Left bending posterior view
    (c) Right bending anterior view
    (d) Posterior view

20. A 58-year-old man diagnosed with squamous cell lung carcinoma measuring 4.5 cm in the right upper lobe with bilateral hydrothorax is referred. The patient has NO history of chemotherapy or radiotherapy. Gallium scan is performed for further evaluation, but a notable uptake in the tumor region is NOT observed in sequential images. Which item is correlated with the absence or reduced uptake of gallium?
    (a) Hydrothorax
    (b) Tumor size (4.5 cm)
    (c) Tumor region (upper lobe)
    (d) Poor prognosis and shorter life

21. A patient with bronchogenic carcinoma and a history of recent extensive chest and neck radiotherapy is evaluated. Which finding in the gallium scan represents the posttreatment changes?
    (a) Increased diffuse uptake in the pulmonary tissue
    (b) Increased tumor uptake
    (c) Decreased radiopharmaceutical accumulation in the salivary glands
    (d) Decreased diffuse uptake in bone

22. The goal is to conduct an oncologic evaluation by gallium scan. What are the appropriate dose of radiopharmaceutical and the time of the first image acquisition?
    (a) 7–10 mCi, 72 h
    (b) 3–5 mCi, 24 h
    (c) 4–5 mCi, 48 h
    (d) 10–12 mCi, 48 h

23. An 8-year-old child with a history of leukemia and chemotherapy and with pain in the RUQ is referred. A mass is observed in the right lobe of the liver in the CT scan. Gallium scan and sulfur colloid scan are requested. Which scan pattern and diagnosis are the most common?
    (a) Decreased sulfur colloid uptake and increased gallium scan due to abscess
    (b) Decreased uptake in both scans due to regional leukemic infiltration
    (c) Decreased sulfur colloid uptake and increased gallium scan due to regional leukemic infiltration
    (d) Decreased uptake in both scans due to abscess

24. In which tumor is gallium uptake unusual?
    (a) Parathyroid adenoma
    (b) Gastric adenocarcinoma
    (c) Ewing sarcoma
    (d) Multiple myeloma

25. An increased uptake in the skeleton and kidneys is observed in a child 48 h after the injection of a radiopharmaceutical in the gallium scan. What is the most probable blood disorder?
    (a) Hemolytic
    (b) Aplastic
    (c) Iron deficiency
    (d) Hypoblastic

26. Bilateral pulmonary uptake is observed in the 72 h gallium scan of a 68-year-old man. What is the most probable diagnosis?
    (a) Normal finding
    (b) Diffuse bilateral metastasis
    (c) Diffuse bilateral infection and inflammation
    (d) Kaposi's sarcoma

27. A decreased physiologic uptake in soft tissue and bones and a significant increase in renal uptake are observed in a 72 h gallium scan. Which item justifies such a finding?
    (a) Iodine-containing contrast CT
    (b) Tumoral involvement of the kidney
    (c) Gadolinium
    (d) Desferal

28. Which statement is correct about the application of CT, MRI, and gallium scan in evaluating response to treatment?
    (a) Gallium scan at the end of treatment is the best predictive method for prolonged remission.
    (b) Gallium scan after a chemotherapy cycle is the best predictive method for prolonged remission.
    (c) CT scan at the end of treatment is the best predictive method for prolonged remission.
    (d) MRI after a chemotherapy cycle is the best predictive method for prolonged remission.

29. Gallium mostly binds to … after intravenous injection.
    (a) Hemoglobin
    (b) Transferrin
    (c) Albumin
    (d) Lipoproteins

30. In which disease is splenic uptake greater than liver uptake in the gallium scan?
    (a) Sepsis
    (b) Hematological neoplasms
    (c) Splenic sarcoidosis
    (d) All of the above

31. What is the scan of choice for the evaluation of response to treatment in chronic bone infection?
    (a) Gallium scan
    (b) CT scan
    (c) Bone scan
    (d) FDG-PET

32. A patient with Hodgkin's lymphoma underwent radiotherapy 3 months ago, and gallium scan is requested to evaluate recurrence. Which of the following is correct?
    (a) The scan must be performed after another 2 months.
    (b) A positive scan is more valuable than a negative scan for this patient.
    (c) If the scan is positive, it must be repeated after 2 months.
    (d) The diagnostic accuracy of gallium scan is 50% in this patient.

33. A patient with lung cancer with mediastinal involvement underwent radiotherapy and chemotherapy. Gallium scan is requested to evaluate the response to treatment. Which item is considered abnormal when observed in this patient?
    (a) High uptake in inguinal glands
    (b) Diffuse pulmonary uptake
    (c) Mediastinal uptake
    (d) Renal uptake

34. A 59-year-old man diagnosed with lymphoma is referred for ^{68}Ga scan. Which item is correct?
    (a) 48 h images are preferred over 72 h images.
    (b) The incidence of false-negative findings decreases with the increase in gallium dose.
    (c) High-energy collimators canNOT be used for imaging when the medium energy collimator is NOT available.
    (d) The application of two peaks of energy enhances the image quality in comparison with that of three peaks.

35. Which item is NOT correct about the role of ^{67}Ga in the diagnosis of lymphoma?
    (a) Gallium scan has the highest sensitivity in the diagnosis of lymphocytic lymphoma.
    (b) ^{67}Ga scan can help in the diagnosis, staging, and evaluation of response to treatment in patients with lymphoma.
    (c) Gallium scan has the highest sensitivity in the diagnosis of Burkitt's lymphoma.
    (d) Gallium scan is especially valuable in the detection of recurrences.

36. ^{67}Ga is NOT indicated for the imaging of which tumors:
    (a) Hepatoma and melanoma
    (b) Gastric and large intestinal adenocarcinoma
    (c) Lymphoma and Hodgkin's disease
    (d) Pulmonary adenocarcinoma and head and neck tumors

37. A patient who is hospitalized for analgesic abuse experiences fever and abdominal pain. Gallium scan is performed to rule out abdominal abscess. Only severe diffused bilateral renal uptake is observed in the 48 h and 72 h images. What is the most probable diagnosis?
    (a) Interstitial nephritis
    (b) Nephritic syndrome
    (c) Lobar nephronia
    (d) Renal abscess

38. Gallium scan is performed 48 h after injection for a patient with a transplanted kidney. Diffuse pulmonary uptake and uptake in the adrenals and eyes are reported in the scan. What is the most probable diagnosis?
    (a) Hodgkin's lymphoma
    (b) Cytomegalovirus infection
    (c) Grade II sarcoidosis
    (d) Mycobacterium tuberculosis infection

39. Gallium scan is performed for a patient with lymphoma. The radiotracer uptake in bones is higher than normal, and the liver and intestines do NOT appear clearly. Which of the following factors is the least possible?
    (a) Previous chemotherapy
    (b) Desferrioxamine treatment
    (c) Previous transfusion
    (d) Iron therapy

40. In which of the following organs is gallium uptake NOT considered normal in children?
    (a) Epiphysis
    (b) Heart
    (c) Cranial base in infants
    (d) Thymus

41. Gallium scan for the evaluation of sarcoidosis:
    (a) Liver and spleen involvement can be easily evaluated by gallium scan.
    (b) A negative gallium scan and a normal serum ACE level are suggestive of an inactive disease.
    (c) An increase in the lacrimal gland uptake is specific for the diagnosis of sarcoidosis.
    (d) NO relationship exists between the intensity of pulmonary uptake of gallium and the prognosis of sarcoidosis.

42. In which of the following conditions is gallium scintigraphy of lymphoma NOT indicated?
    (a) Staging of Hodgkin's and non-Hodgkin's lymphoma
    (b) Differentiation between Hodgkin's and non-Hodgkin's lymphoma
    (c) Evaluation and detection of metastatic lesions
    (d) Evaluation of therapeutic effects

43. Regarding the rebound phenomenon in gallium scan:
    (a) Discontinuation of antibiotics in infection
    (b) Discontinuation of chemotherapy in lymphoma
    (c) Discontinuation of chemotherapy in Hodgkin's disease
    (d) Discontinuation of corticosteroids in sarcoidosis

44. Regarding the ^{67}Ga scan in pulmonary diseases:
    (a) The focal bibasilar uptake of gallium is observed in idiopathic pulmonary fibrosis.
    (b) Gallium is NOT uptaken in amiodarone toxicity with normal CXR.
    (c) Gallium scan effectively shows the activity of sarcoidosis.
    (d) Gallium uptake is related to CXR abnormality in AIDS-associated Kaposi's sarcoma.

45. Gallium scintigraphy is indicated for the differential diagnosis of all items *except*:
    (a) Differentiation between Hodgkin's and non-Hodgkin's lymphoma
    (b) Differentiation between a malignant tumor of the maxillary sinus and chronic sinusitis
    (c) Differentiation between recurrent head and neck tumor after radiation and necrotic tissue
    (d) Differentiation between the mesothelium and increased pleural thickness

46. If the goal is to evaluate the ^{67}Ga citrate uptake in the para-aortic lymph nodes of a patient with cancer, which of the following gallium energies is better detected in the scan?
    (a) 288 keV
    (b) 91 and 92 keV
    (c) 184 and 296 keV
    (d) 294 keV

47. Which of the following statements is NOT correct about the application of gallium in lymphoma and leukemia?
    (a) Gallium uptake is high in ALL and CLL with B-cell origin.
    (b) Gallium scan is effective in determining Hodgkin's lymphoma, histiocytic lymphoma, and Burkitt's lymphoma.
    (c) Gallium uptake is high in low-grade follicular lymphoma.
    (d) Gallium uptake is low in high-grade diffuse immunoblastic lymphoma.

48. Sonography and CT scan of a patient with abdominal pain are normal. However, gallium scan shows abnormal accumulation of the radiotracer with ambiguous margins in the RUQ. What is the most probable diagnosis?
    (a) Abscess
    (b) Phlegmon
    (c) Tumor
    (d) Infectious cyst

49. Diffuse pulmonary uptake and increased bone and renal uptake are reported in the gallium scan. What is the most probable diagnosis?
    (a) Chronic anemia
    (b) Iron overload
    (c) Recent chemotherapy
    (d) Sarcoidosis

50. What is the most important factor for the increase in diagnostic efficacy of gallium?
   (a) Delayed imaging
   (b) SPECT
   (c) Higher doses of gallium
   (d) Multiple pulse height analyzers

51. What is the correct order (highest to lowest sensitivity) of the sensitivity of the gallium scan for different lymphomas?
   (a) Hodgkin's, histiocytic, lymphocytic, Burkitt's
   (b) Histiocytic, Burkitt's, lymphocytic, Hodgkin's
   (c) Lymphocytic, Hodgkin's, Burkitt's, histiocytic
   (d) Burkitt's, Hodgkin's, histiocytic, lymphocytic

52. Which of the following diseases show the greatest uptake of thallium?
   (a) Intermediate-grade lymphoma
   (b) High-grade lymphoma
   (c) Low-grade lymphoma
   (d) Hodgkin's lymphoma

53. Which of the following items does NOT describe the advantages of gallium SPECT imaging over planar scan?
   (a) Better specificity
   (b) Better resolution
   (c) Better sensitivity
   (d) Better accuracy

54. What is the method of choice for evaluating the involvement of mediastinal lymph nodes?
   (a) CT scan
   (b) PET/CT
   (c) Mediastinoscopy
   (d) Gallium scan

55. Which of the following diseases shows the highest uptake of gallium?
   (a) Primary extranodal seminoma
   (b) Metastatic seminoma
   (c) Teratoma
   (d) Embryonal cell carcinoma

56. Gallium scan is requested for tumor localization in an 18-year-old boy with a history of Hodgkin's lymphoma. What is the recommended scan protocol?
   (a) High-energy collimator; whole-body images at 24, 48, and 72 h; SPECT
   (b) High-energy collimator; whole-body images at 96 and 120 h; SPECT
   (c) Medium-energy collimator; whole-body images at 96 and 120 h; SPECT
   (d) Medium-energy collimator; whole-body images at 24, 48, and 72 h; SPECT

57. What changes are induced in a gallium biological distribution when an antineoplastic drug is administered before gallium injection?
    (a) Decreased uptake in soft tissue and bone, increased uptake in the kidney
    (b) Decreased uptake in tumor and bone, increased uptake in the kidney
    (c) Decreased uptake in soft tissue and tumor, increased uptake in bone
    (d) Decreased uptake in soft tissue and kidney, increased uptake in bone

1.6.1 Answer

	A	B	C	D
1		*		
2			*	
3		*		
4			*	
5				*
6		*		
7	*			
8				*
9	*			
10	*			
11	*			
12	*			
13	*			
14	*			
15		*		
16				*
17	*			
18	*			
19	*			
20	*			
21	*			
22	*			
23	*			
24	*			
25	*			
26			*	
27				*
28		*		
29		*		
30				*
31	*			
32		*		
33			*	
34		*		
35	*			
36		*		

37	*			
38		*		
39		*		
40		*		
41		*		
42		*		
43				*
44			*	
45	*			
46			*	
47			*	
48		*		
49			*	
50		*		
51				*
52			*	
53	*			
54			*	
55	*			
56			*	
57			*	

1.7 Thallium-201 Chloride: A Tumor-Imaging Agent

1. What is the cutoff of the 201Tl tumor index for predicting malignant brain tumors and histopathological results?
   (a) 2.5
   (b) 2
   (c) 1.5
   (d) 3

2. ^{201}Tl tumor imaging is the most valuable in the:
   (a) Pelvis
   (b) Abdomen
   (c) Mediastinum
   (d) Peripheral bone

3. Which lung carcinoma uptakes less ^{201}Tl than ^{67}Ga?
   (a) Oat cell carcinoma
   (b) Adenocarcinoma
   (c) Non-small-cell lung cancer (NSCLC)
   (d) a and b

4. Compare ^{201}Tl, ^{67}Ga, and ^{99m}Tc-MDP bone scans if the goal is to evaluate the response to preoperative chemotherapy in bone and soft tissue sarcomas.
   (a) ^{67}Ga is the most reliable of the three and more accurate than CT/MRI.
   (b) ^{201}Tl is the most reliable of the three and more accurate than CT/MRI.
   (c) ^{67}Ga is the most reliable of the three but less accurate than CT/MRI.
   (d) ^{201}Tl is the most reliable of the three but less accurate than CT/MRI.

5. Which condition in AIDS patients almost always takes up either ^{201} Tl or ^{67}Ga?
   (a) Kaposi's sarcoma
   (b) Acute opportunistic infection
   (c) *Pneumocystis carinii*
   (d) Tuberculosis

6. Which one is considered a limitation for thallium in detecting the recurrences of differentiated thyroid cancers?
   (a) Inconsistency with Tg
   (b) SPECT cannot be performed for the accurate localization of the lesion
   (c) Detection of abdominal and pulmonary metastases
   (d) All of the above

7. In which of the following tumors is thallium scan NOT recommended?
   (a) Tumor of the head and neck
   (b) Melanoma
   (c) Tumor of soft tissue
   (d) Pulmonary tumors

8. Which method is very accurate for the follow-up of patients with osteosarcoma after chemotherapy?
   (a) Ga scan
   (b) MIBI scan
   (c) Three-phase bone scan
   (d) Octreoscan

9. The goal is to evaluate viability and tumor grading in a 48-year-old man with a history of surgery and chemotherapy for brain tumor. What is the recommended radiopharmaceutical?
   (a) ^{67}Ga
   (b) ^{99m}Tc-HMPAO
   (c) ^{201}Tl
   (d) ^{99m}Tc-labeled glucoheptonate

10. About the uptake of ^{201}Tl and ^{99m}Tc-MIBI:
   (a) The uptakes of ^{201}Tl and potassium are similar.
   (b) Digitalis inhibits the uptake of ^{201}Tl.
   (c) ^{99m}Tc-MIBI is uptaken by the Na/K ATPase system.
   (d) Furosemide inhibits the uptake of ^{99m}Tc-MIBI.

11. In which tumor does the severe uptake of gallium predict a poor prognosis?
   (a) Renal cell carcinoma
   (b) Bronchogenic carcinoma
   (c) Anaplastic adenocarcinoma (lung)
   (d) Lymphoma

12. ^{201}Tl function in the body is similar to which ion?
   (a) Na+
   (b) K
   (c) Ca++
   (d) Mg++

13. A patient with a brain tumor in the medial region near the lateral ventricle is referred. What is the scan of choice to distinguish infection from malignancy?
   (a) ^{18}FDG
   (b) ^{99m}Tc-MIBI
   (c) ^{201}Tl
   (d) ^{99m}Tc-ECD

14. A patient with suspected hilar adenopathy is subjected to thorax scintigraphy with gallium and thallium. If the adenopathy is due to benign inflammatory lesions, how will the patterns of the gallium and thallium scans appear, respectively?
   (a) Increased uptake, increased uptake
   (b) No uptake, increased uptake
   (c) No uptake, no uptake
   (d) Increased uptake, no uptake

15. Regarding the evaluation of brain tumors by thallium and ^{99m}Tc-MIBI scans:
    (a) ^{99m}Tc-MIBI scintigraphy is NOT valuable in the therapeutic monitoring of glioma tumors in adults.
    (b) Although the photon flux of ^{99m}Tc-MIBI is greater than that of thallium, the differentiation of the choroid plexus from a tumor is sometimes problematic.
    (c) The differentiation between high-grade and low-grade glioma is NOT possible with a brain thallium scan.
    (d) The relative thallium uptake in a brain tumor to a healthy cortex in children is greater than that of ^{99m}Tc-MIBI.

16. Which part of a tumor shows the highest thallium uptake in a diagnostic scan regardless of the time of injection?
    (a) Mitochondria
    (b) Tumoral fluid
    (c) Nucleus
    (d) Microsome

17. Which of the following statements is NOT correct about sarcoma of bone and soft tissue?
    (a) ^{99m}Tc-MIBI shows more regions of uptake than thallium.
    (b) Gallium uptake is weakly associated with successful chemotherapy.
    (c) Thallium and MIBI are greatly associated with successful chemotherapy (approximately 100%).
    (d) A bone scan 2 weeks after chemotherapy is relatively associated with response to treatment.

18. Which brain lesion does NOT uptake thallium?
    (a) Lymphoma
    (b) Toxoplasmosis
    (c) Glioma
    (d) Meningioma

19. In which of the following tumors is thallium scan the least indicated?
    (a) Brain tumors
    (b) Tumors of the urinary tract
    (c) Soft tissue sarcoma
    (d) Bone sarcoma

1.7.1 Answer

	A	B	C	D
1			*	
2				*
3			*	
4		*		
5				*
6			*	
7		*		
8		*		
9			*	
10		*		
11	*			
12		*		
13			*	
14				*
15		*		
16		*		
17				*
18		*		
19		*		

1.8 MIBG in the Diagnosis of Neuroendocrine Tumors

1. Which antihypertensive drug may be administered to control hypertension prior to MIBG scintigraphy?
   (a) Phenoxybenzamine
   (b) Labetalol
   (c) Metoprolol
   (d) Diltiazem

2. In which organ is the ^{131}I-MIBG uptake NOT considered a normal finding in a 3-month-old child?
   (a) Heart
   (b) Spleen
   (c) Liver
   (d) Bone

3. Compared with radioiodinated MIBG, somatostatin receptor scintigraphy provides better sensitivity in the detection of carcinoid metastatic lesions of all regions *except*:
   (a) Ocular
   (b) Thoracic
   (c) Spleen
   (d) Liver

4. MIBG scan is recommended for a patient with hypertension and asthma. The patient is taking nifedipine, salbutamol, beclomethasone, and amitriptyline. Which of the mentioned drugs is NOT necessary to be discontinued?
   (a) Nifedipine
   (b) Salbutamol
   (c) Beclomethasone
   (d) Amitriptyline

5. Which of the following findings is considered abnormal in an MIBG scan?
   (a) Cerebellar uptake
   (b) Bilateral symmetric uptake in the upper thorax in children
   (c) No uptake in the heart
   (d) Slight uptake in the vertebrae

6. In an MIBG scan, in which part of the brain is the focal accumulation of the radiotracer considered abnormal?
   (a) Pituitary
   (b) Cerebellum
   (c) Basal ganglia
   (d) Thalamus

7. In which of the following conditions does ^{131}I-MIBG have the highest diagnostic sensitivity?
   (a) Medullary thyroid cancer
   (b) Carcinoid tumor
   (c) Neuroblastoma
   (d) Pituitary adenoma

8. Which type of carcinoid tumors is the most probable to demonstrate a positive MIBG scan?
   (a) Hindgut.
   (b) Foregut.
   (c) Midgut.
   (d) The probability of positive scan is equal for all of the above.

9. Adrenal pheochromocytoma complies with the rule of 10s. In which of the following items is this role NOT correct?
   (a) 10% sporadic
   (b) 10% of children
   (c) 10% malignancy
   (d) 10% bilateral

10. The observation of which of the following organs is considered abnormal in the MIBG scan?
    (a) Brain
    (b) Thymus
    (c) Lung
    (d) Ovary

11. Which method is the most specific for diagnosing a patient with high VMA in 24 h urine?
    (a) Octreotide scan
    (b) Abdominal sonography
    (c) Abdominal CT scan
    (d) MIBG scan

12. In adrenal scintigraphy:
    (a) The adrenal medulla is always observed in a PET scan with ^{11}C-epinephrin and ^{18}F-FDG.
    (b) The uptake of ^{131}I-MIBG in the adrenal medulla is common.
    (c) In a ^{123}I-MIBG scan, an uptake in the adrenal medulla is observed in 20% of normal subjects.
    (d) The primary regions of a ^{131}I-MIBG uptake are the liver, spleen, and brain.

13. Pheochromocytoma:
    (a) It is malignant in 40% of cases.
    (b) 10% of cases are children.
    (c) It is bilateral in 70% of cases.
    (d) It is a form of MEN syndrome in 60% of cases.

14. About the application of PET in neuroblastoma and pheochromocytoma:
    (a) No specific radiopharmaceutical is identified.
    (b) ^{131}I-MIBG imaging is preferred over PET.
    (c) Similar to MIBG, PET requires imaging in several days.
    (d) FDG-PET is used for the localization of the tumor.

15. Compare ^{131}I-MIBG with MRI and CT if the goal is to diagnose paraganglioma.
    (a) Higher specificity, higher sensitivity
    (b) Lower specificity, higher sensitivity
    (c) Higher specificity, lower sensitivity
    (d) Lower specificity, lower sensitivity

16. A child with a history of surgery for neuroblastoma and localized bone pain is referred. Which method is recommended to evaluate bone metastasis?
    (a) MIBG scan
    (b) Bone scan
    (c) Bone scan and MIBG scan
    (d) X-ray and measurement of VMA

17. All of the following drugs interfere with the MIBG uptake by competing for granular uptake *except*:
    (a) Norepinephrine
    (b) Serotonin
    (c) Guanethidine
    (d) Phenylpropanolamine

18. Neuroblastoma with abdominal mass is diagnosed in a 2-year-old child. Which of the following studies is recommended to determine the prognosis and response to treatment?
    (a) ^{123}I-MIBG SPECT/CT
    (b) Planar ^{123}I-MIBG
    (c) ^{123}I-MIBG SPECT
    (d) CT scan

19. A 49-year-old man with refractory hypertension is suspected to have pheochromocytoma. Abdominal CT scan is normal, and the levels of serum catecholamines and metanephrines are normal. The physician asks about the diagnostic value of the ^{131}I-MIBG scan for this patient. What is your answer?
    (a) Somatostatin receptor scintigraphy is recommended.
    (b) Abdominal MRI is recommended.
    (c) ^{131}I-MIBG scan is the choice imaging method.
    (d) It is NOT indicated.

20. About the MIBG scan for evaluating neuroblastoma:
    (a) This scan is less sensitive than CT in detecting liver metastasis.
    (b) If this scan is normal, bone scan will NOT be required.
    (c) This scan is less valuable than CT and MRI for staging.
    (d) This scan is less sensitive than bone scan in the diagnosis of bone involvement.

21. Which of the following drugs has the least effect on the adrenal uptake of MIBG?
    (a) Clonidine
    (b) Amitriptyline
    (c) Reserpine
    (d) Cocaine

22. Which of the following organs shows the highest intensity in an MIBG scan (with regular method and low dose) in a healthy subject?
    (a) Heart
    (b) Liver
    (c) Lung
    (d) Spleen

23. In an MIBG scan:
    (a) Reserpine and tricyclic antidepressants increase the adrenal uptake.
    (b) The radiation of ^{131}I-MIBG is 25 times greater than that of ^{123}I-MIBG.
    (c) Octreotide is an alternative to MIBG.
    (d) SSRI administration before and after the scan is NOT recommended.

24. Which of the following items is NOT correct about pheochromocytoma?
    (a) It is bilateral in 10% of cases.
    (b) It is familial in 90% of cases.
    (c) Pediatric cases comprise 10% of the patients.
    (d) Recurrence in 5–10 years is reported in 10% of cases.

25. A 39-year-old woman with a history of palpitation, headache, and paroxysmal hypertension comes to your office. In the laboratory findings, VMA level in the urine is high, but her CT scan is unremarkable. What is the best next step for this patient?
    (a) MRI
    (b) FNA of adrenals
    (c) Assessment of other secondary causes
    (d) ^{131}I MIBG scintigraphy

26. Pheochromocytoma:
    (a) Angiography is a diagnostic in this tumor.
    (b) Ectopic pheochromocytoma may cause renal artery stenosis.
    (c) Calcification is rather common in this tumor.
    (d) If it located in the mediastinum, the usual location is the paratracheal region.

27. In which type of neuroblastoma metastases does the MIBG scan NOT provide valuable information?
    (a) MIBG scan can help in all of the abovementioned situations.
    (b) Soft tissue.
    (c) Bone.
    (d) Bone marrow.

28. What percentage of patients with carcinoid tumor gives a positive MIBG scan?
    (a) 50%
    (b) 30%
    (c) 90%
    (d) 70%

1.8.1 Answer

	A	B	C	D
1	*			
2				*
3				*
4			*	
5				*
6	*			
7			*	
8			*	
9	*			
10		*		
11				*
12			*	
13		*		
14				*
15			*	
16			*	
17				*
18	*			
19				*
20	*			
21	*			
22		*		
23			*	
24		*		
25				*
26		*		
27	*			
28				*

1.9 Peptide-Receptor Scintigraphy in Oncology

1. What is the dominant somatostatin receptor subtype in tumors?
   (a) Sst2
   (b) Sst3
   (c) Sst1
   (d) Sst5

2. A 47-year-old woman with a history of abdominal pain from 6 months ago is recently experiencing intermittent diarrhea. Flushing of the face, dyspnea, and wheezing occur after physical activity. The measurement of which of the following markers is critical for the diagnosis?
   (a) Serum vasoactive intestinal peptide (VIP)
   (b) Serum C-peptide
   (c) 24 h urine 5-HIAA (5-hydroxyindolacetic acid)
   (d) Serum calcitonin

3. Octreoscan is recommended for:
   (a) Acromegaly
   (b) Nonfunctioning pituitary tumor
   (c) Zollinger–Ellison syndrome
   (d) Insulinoma

4. The receptors for cholecystokinin (CCK) have been demonstrated in the following tumors *except*:
   (a) Medullary thyroid carcinoma
   (b) Small-cell lung cancer
   (c) Gastrointestinal tumors
   (d) Differentiated thyroid cancer

5. Gastrin-releasing peptide (GRP) receptor scintigraphy with ^{99m}Tc-bombesin is indicated for:
   (a) Differentiated thyroid cancer
   (b) Insulinoma
   (c) Prostate cancer
   (d) Non-small-cell lung cancer

6. In which tumor does ^{111}In-pentetreotide have higher sensitivity than ^{131}I-MIBG?
   (a) Pheochromocytoma
   (b) Neuroblastoma
   (c) Carcinoid tumor
   (d) b and c

7. Which statement is false about ^{99m}-Tc-Neotect?
   (a) Imaging is performed 24 h after administration.
   (b) It is a somatostatin analog.
   (c) It is indicated for the discrimination of a benign lesion from a malignant lesion.
   (d) It has a simple protocol for preparation.

8. Which organ does NOT uptake ^{111}In-octreotide?
   (a) Heart
   (b) Spleen
   (c) Pituitary
   (d) Intestine

9. ^{111}In-octreotide:
   (a) It is a 5-amino acid peptide.
   (b) Compared with MIBG, it provides higher sensitivity for the localization of pheochromocytoma and neuroblastoma.
   (c) It can be used for the treatment of neuroendocrine tumors because of the bremsstrahlung X-ray.
   (d) It has the highest affinity to the somatostatin receptor subtype 2.

10. Which of the following tumor markers is used for the diagnosis and follow-up of carcinoid tumors?
    (a) 5HT (5-hydroxytryptamine)
    (b) 5HTP (5-hydroxytryptophan)
    (c) 51-L-DOPA (51-dihydroxyphenylalanine)
    (d) 5HTIAA (5-hydroxyindoleacetic acid)

11. Which of the following radiopharmaceuticals is more specific for the somatostatin receptors?
    (a) [^{177}Lu-DOTA] octreotate
    (b) [^{111}In-DTPA] octreotide
    (c) ^{90}Y-DOTATOC
    (d) ^{111}In-DOTATOC

12. Which of the following lesions does NOT express the somatostatin receptors?
    (a) Sarcoidosis
    (b) Thyroid in Grave's disease
    (c) Undifferentiated glioblastoma
    (d) Hodgkin's disease

13. Which item is NOT correct about PET application in neuroendocrine tumors?
    (a) ^{11}C-5HTP is used for chest and abdominal screening when the octreotide scan is negative.
    (b) Octreotide scan is used for making treatment decisions on somatostatin PET.
    (c) ^{68}Ga-octreotide is used for somatostatin PET scintigraphy.
    (d) ^{18}F-FDG-PET is especially helpful in tumors with low proliferation.

14. Which type of carcinoid tumor produces peptide hormones such as ACTH and HCG instead of serotonin?
    (a) Midgut originated carcinoid
    (b) Hindgut originated carcinoid
    (c) Foregut originated carcinoid
    (d) Pancreas originated carcinoid

15. Which radiopharmaceutical is the least suitable for delayed images of a pancreas transplantation?
    (a) ^{99m}Tc-MAG3
    (b) ^{99m}Tc-DTPA
    (c) ^{99m}Tc-MIBI
    (d) ^{99m}Tc-HMPAO

16. About ^{111}In-octreotide and ^{177}Lu-octreotate in the treatment of neuroendocrine tumors:
    (a) ^{177}Lu is a pure beta emitter.
    (b) Liver radiation with ^{177}Lu-octreotate is greater than that with ^{111}In-octreotide.
    (c) The affinity of octreotate to type 2 somatostatin receptors is greater than that of octreotide.
    (d) Kidney radiation with ^{177}Lu-octreotate is greater than that with ^{111}In-octreotide.

17. Which of the SPECT specifications increases by the fusion of octreotide SPECT and CT scan in a patient with neuroendocrine tumors?
    (a) Sensitivity
    (b) Specificity
    (c) Negative predictive value
    (d) All of the above

18. Which item is NOT correct about the effects of somatostatin?
    (a) Stimulation of hormone secretion
    (b) Immunomodulation
    (c) Neurotransmitter effect
    (d) Antiproliferation effect in tumors

19. An increased hilar, mediastinal, and parotid uptake is reported in the somatostatin receptor scintigraphy of a 39-year-old woman with uveitis. However, chest X-ray and thorax CT scan are normal. What is the most probable diagnosis?
    (a) Tuberculosis
    (b) Sarcoidosis
    (c) Aspergillosis
    (d) Wegener's granulomatosis

20. The accumulation of [^{111}IN-DTPA-D-Phe] octreotide in tumors is directly related to the level of somatostatin receptor expression. In which of the following tumors is the octreotide scan positive despite the absence of these receptors?
    (a) Gastrinoma
    (b) Insulinoma
    (c) Non-small-cell lung carcinoma
    (d) Non-Hodgkin's lymphoma

21. In which of the following lesions is the sensitivity of [^{111}In—DTPA-D-Phe] octreotide imaging NOT favorable?
    (a) Gastrinoma
    (b) Hodgkin's disease
    (c) Ophthalmic Grave's disease
    (d) Insulinoma

22. Octreotide mainly inhibits somatostatin binding to … somatostatin receptors.
    (a) Type II
    (b) Type I
    (c) Type III
    (d) Type IV

23. The normal features of somatostatin receptor scintigraphy (SRS) include the visualization of the following organs *except*:
    (a) Spleen
    (b) Liver
    (c) Hypophysis
    (d) Lung

24. What is the main reason for the appearance of the kidneys in somatostatin receptor scintigraphy (SRS)?
    (a) Expression of the somatostatin receptors on the renal tubules
    (b) Expression of the somatostatin receptors on the vasa racta
    (c) Binding of the labeled peptide to tubular cells after glomerular filtration
    (d) a and b

25. Which of the following statements is NOT correct about the diagnostic and therapeutic roles of somatostatin receptor scintigraphy (SRS) for pituitary tumors?
    (a) The diagnostic value of SRS in pituitary tumors is limited.
    (b) SRS is capable of predicting an appropriate response to octreotide in patients with acromegaly.
    (c) The radiation exposure rate in SRS is at least two times greater than that in angiography.
    (d) Octreotide treatment is NOT effective in nonfunctioning pituitary tumors.

26. What is the first diagnostic method for a patient with suspected Zollinger–Ellison syndrome?
    (a) CT scan
    (b) MRI
    (c) Endoscopic sonography
    (d) Somatostatin receptor scintigraphy (SRS)

27. The imaging of which pancreatic tumor with somatostatin receptor scintigraphy (SRS) has NOT been successful?
    (a) Gastrinoma
    (b) Glucagonoma
    (c) VIPoma
    (d) Insulinoma

28. All of the following statements regarding the diagnostic role of somatostatin receptor scintigraphy (SRS) in tumors are correct *except*:
    (a) The probability of a positive SRS in pheochromocytoma is greater than that in neuroblastoma.
    (b) The greater the differentiation of medullary thyroid cancer is, the higher the probability of a positive SRS.
    (c) SRS is positive in most cases of differentiated and anaplastic thyroid cancer.
    (d) SRS is more valuable than CT and sonography in patients with supradiaphragmatic Hodgkin's disease.

29. Which of the following tumors expresses somatostatin receptors with the highest probability?
    (a) Glioblastoma multiform (GBM)
    (b) Poorly differentiated astrocytoma
    (c) Astrocytoma with a negative epidermal growth factor receptor (EGFR)
    (d) Astrocytoma with a positive epidermal growth factor receptor (EGFR)

30. In Grave's hyperthyroidism, the accumulation of radiolabeled octreotide in the thyroid gland is markedly increased and correlated with the serum levels of:
    (a) Free thyroxin
    (b) Thyrotropin-binding inhibitory immunoglobulin
    (c) Thyroid-binding globulin (TBG)
    (d) a and b

1.9.1 Answer

	A	B	C	D
1	*			
2			*	
3			*	
4				*
5			*	
6			*	
7	*			
8	*			
9				*
10				*
11	*			
12			*	
13				*
14			*	
15	*			
16			*	
17		*		
18	*			

19		*		
20			*	
21				*
22	*			
23				*
24			*	
25			*	
26				*
27				*
28	*			
29			*	
30				*

1.10 Diagnostic Role of Radiolabeled Antibodies in Cancer

1. All of the following monoclonal antibodies for radioimmunoscintigraphy are used for colorectal cancer *except*:
   (a) PR1A3
   (b) C46
   (c) B72.3
   (d) Anti-c erb2

2. The anti-epidermal growth factor receptor (anti-EGFR) for radioimmunoscintigraphy is used in:
   (a) Breast cancer
   (b) Brain tumor
   (c) Leukemia
   (d) Ovarian cancer

3. The ability of certain cells to change their surface antigenic composition is called:
   (a) Avidity
   (b) Affinity
   (c) Antigen modulation
   (d) Hybridoma technique

4. The replacement of the constant domains of a murine mAb with the human equivalent is used in:
   (a) CDR-grafted trastuzumab
   (b) Chimeric trastuzumab
   (c) CDR-grafted rituximab
   (d) Chimeric rituximab

5. How long are the half-life and the gamma-ray energy of ^{123}I?
   (a) 23 h, 159 keV
   (b) 13 h, 159 keV
   (c) 67 h, 89 keV
   (d) 23 h, 171 keV

6. For radioimmunoscintigraphy:
   (a) No informed signed consent is required.
   (b) No skin test is recommended.
   (c) There is no need to exclude patients with a history of allergy to exogenous protein.
   (d) There is no need to exclude patients with severe atypical predisposition.

7. Radioimmunoscintigraphy (RIS) in colorectal cancer:
   (a) It is more specific but less sensitive than FDG-PET for liver metastases.
   (b) It is more specific and sensitive than FDG-PET for liver metastases.
   (c) It has the same sensitivity and specificity as FDG-PET in abdominal metastases.
   (d) It is less specific and sensitive than FDG-PET for distant metastases.

8. The sensitivity of ^{99m}Tc-Mab, such as SM3, in ovarian cancer is:
   (a) 92%
   (b) 100%
   (c) 76%
   (d) 75%

9. In breast cancer:
   (a) ^{99m}Tc-MIBI combined with mammography is becoming the method of choice for improving the positive predictive value (PPV).
   (b) MRI has good specificity.
   (c) If radioimmunoscintigraphy (RIS) with ^{99m}Tc-hHMFG1 is negative and the axillary nodes are impalpable, then sentinel node imaging will NOT be required to rule out axillary involvement.
   (d) FDG-PET has no definite clinical role in the diagnosis of axillary lymph node involvement.

10. Radioimmunoscintigraphy (RIS) provides low clinical benefit in:
    (a) Breast cancer
    (b) Prostate cancer
    (c) Bladder cancer
    (d) Lung cancer

11. What is the method of choice for medullary thyroid carcinoma?
    (a) RIS with anti-calcitonin mAb
    (b) ^{111}In-DMSA(V)
    (c) ^{99m}Tc-DMSA(V)
    (d) ^{111}In-octreotide imaging

12. Radioimmunoscintigraphy (RIS) in all of the following situations remains the nuclear medicine method of choice *except*:
    (a) Prostate cancer
    (b) Impalpable axillary nodes in breast cancer
    (c) Impalpable axillary nodes in ovarian cancer
    (d) Colorectal cancer

13. In a scan with labeled antibodies:
    (a) The maximum intestinal absorption occurs after 48 h.
    (b) Non-specific uptakes do NOT change in the first 24 h.
    (c) Splenic uptake is higher than hepatic uptake.
    (d) Tumor uptake always increases with time.

14. Which statement about ^{111}In chloride is NOT correct?
    (a) It is distributed along with erythrocytes in the bone marrow.
    (b) It has a high affinity for transferrin.
    (c) In comparison with Fe, a negligible ratio of the administered dose remains in erythrocytes after 1 week.
    (d) Its hepatic and splenic uptakes indicate erythropoiesis in these regions.

15. Regarding ^{111}In-OncoScint:
    (a) Patients must be tested with HAMA before the second injection.
    (b) It is developed against TAG-72, and all prostate cancers respond to this drug.
    (c) The liver, spleen, and lungs are the main parts for radiodrug absorption.
    (d) It has a short half-life in blood.

16. ^{99m}Tc-anti-CEA is indicated for:
    (a) Ovarian cancer
    (b) Prostate cancer
    (c) Colorectal cancer
    (d) Pulmonary cancer

17. What is the reason for the HAMA reaction?
    (a) Mouse-derived antibody
    (b) Pyrogen in the kit
    (c) Immune reaction to human cell antibody
    (d) Allergy to 111Indium

18. ^{111}In-satumomab pendetide is suitable for the imaging of:
    (a) Breast cancers
    (b) Neuroendocrine tumors
    (c) Lymphoscintigraphy
    (d) Extrahepatic metastasis of colon and ovarian cancers

19. ^{99m}Tc-labeled fragment A radioimmunoscintigraphy (RIS) is different from 111In-labeled complete antibody RIS in:
    (a) Higher blood and hepatic activity
    (b) Lower renal activity
    (c) More rapid blood clearance
    (d) Greater internal radiation

20. Which of the following tumors undergoes radioscintigraphy conducted by ^{111}In-anti-CEA?
    (a) Brain tumors
    (b) Osteosarcoma
    (c) Tumor of squamous cells of the head and neck
    (d) Colorectal cancer

21. Which of the following items is required for ProstaScint immunoscintigraphy?
    (a) Injection of the radiopharmaceutical immediately after preparation and mixing with ^{111}In
    (b) Acquisition of 24 h images after injection
    (c) Additional injection of other radiopharmaceuticals
    (d) Slow intravenous injection of the radiopharmaceutical in 5 min

22. Which of the following radiopharmaceuticals is indicated for the evaluation of soft tissue metastasis in a 68-year-old man with prostate cancer?
    (a) Satumomab pendetide
    (b) Capromab pendetide
    (c) Arcitumomab
    (d) OncoScint

23. … is produced in response to an antigen and specifically reacts with the antigen.
    (a) Hapten
    (b) Immunogene
    (c) Adjuvant
    (d) Antibody

24. Which of the following findings in a patient with a history of colorectal cancer is NOT an indication for OncoScint scan?
    (a) Routine follow-up of a patient with CEA and normal CT scan
    (b) Presence of resectable recurrence without evidence of other diseases
    (c) Presence of suspicious findings in the abdominal CT scan
    (d) Increase in CEA with normal abdominal and pelvic CT scan

25. A patient with colorectal cancer is subjected to OncoScint CR/OV imaging. An increase in uptake in the liver, spleen, and bone marrow and an intensive uptake in the kidneys and bladder are reported. What is the most probable diagnosis?
    (a) Micrometastasis of these organs
    (b) Higher dose of the radiotracer
    (c) Higher amount of HAMA
    (d) Deiodination of the radiotracer

26. Regarding Tc-monoclonal antibody imaging:
    (a) The diagnosis of renal lesions is difficult because of the higher uptake in this organ.
    (b) Continuous photopenic lesions in the liver are indicative of hepatic metastasis.
    (c) The appearance of the thyroid is due to the catabolism of the radiotracer in this organ.
    (d) Abnormality in the 10th min images is a typical finding of malignant lesions.

27. Which of the following variables is represented by the affinity of antigen to antibody?
    (a) Specificity
    (b) Sensitivity
    (c) Avidity
    (d) Accuracy

28. Antibody against which antigen results in a better response in the immunoscintigraphy of prostate cancer?
    (a) Acid phosphatase
    (b) Nucleus of prostate cells
    (c) Cytoplasmic membrane of prostate cells
    (d) Prostate-specific antigen

29. Which of the following statements is NOT correct about HAMA?
    (a) Its serum concentrations remain constant for a long time.
    (b) It is usually produced in 12 weeks after injection of the antibody.
    (c) Its production is dose dependent.
    (d) It may interfere with the subsequent immunotherapy.

30. Which of the following statements is NOT correct about anti-CD20?
    (a) CD20 antigen is NOT found in bone marrow stem cells.
    (b) It is a chimeric antibody with a low probability of producing HAMA.
    (c) ^{131}I-anti-CD20 is used before ^{90}Y-anti CD20 for the treatment of large heterogeneous tumors.
    (d) ^{111}In-anti-CD20 imaging is mandatory before ^{90}Y-anti-CD20 therapy.

31. A 69-year-old man underwent surgery for rectal cancer. After 1 year, the CT scan shows perisacral density, which is interpreted as a surgical scar. What is the recommended radiotracer for scintigraphy if the goal is to rule out tumor recurrence with high confidence?
    (a) Nofetumomab merpentan (Verluma)
    (b) Imciromab (Myoscint)
    (c) Satumomab pendetide (OncoScint)
    (d) Capromab pendetide (ProstaScint)

32. What is the main indication for ^{111}In-satumomab pendetide?
    (a) Imaging of breast tumors
    (b) Imaging of extrahepatic ovarian metastasis of colon cancers
    (c) Imaging of neuroendocrine tumors
    (d) Imaging of lymph ducts

33. All of the following items describe the advantages of monoclonal antibody compared with polyclonal antibody in imaging *except*:
    (a) Increased specificity
    (b) Maximum sensitivity
    (c) Feasible preparation
    (d) Capability to connect with the nontarget antigens

34. In monoclonal antibody imaging:
    - It refers to the interaction between a single binding site and antigen.
    - Its in crease in binding afforded by multivalency is crucial in the course of a normal immune response.
    (a) Affinity, affinity
    (b) Avidity, avidity
    (c) Affinity, avidity
    (d) Avidity, affinity

35. All of the following immunoglobulins have three constant heavy fragments (CH1, CH2, and CH3) *except*:
    (a) IgA
    (b) IgD
    (c) IgG
    (d) IgE

36. If intact ^{111}In-labeled antibodies are used, how long after injection should imaging be performed?
    (a) 12–24 h
    (b) 24–48 h
    (c) 48–72 h
    (d) 72–96 h

37. Which of the following organs shows the higher activity with Tc-antibody fragment than with In-antibody fragment?
    (a) Kidneys
    (b) Bone marrow
    (c) Liver
    (d) Blood pool

38. If the goal is to inject a second dose of OncoScint, what are the permitted and contraindicated levels of HAMA, respectively? (The component antibody of 87.3 targets the glycoprotein TAG-72.)
    (a) Less than 20, more than 200
    (b) Less than 100, more than 300
    (c) Less than 40, more than 200
    (d) Less than 50, more than 400

39. A 72-year-old man with a history of surgery for prostate cancer is referred for ProstaScint scan because of suspected recurrence. What is the recommended scan protocol?
    (a) Planar and SPECT scans in 12 h and 72 h
    (b) Planar and SPECT scans in 30 min, 24 h, 72 h, and 96 h
    (c) Planar and SPECT scans in 30 min, 72 h, and 120 h
    (d) Planar and SPECT scans in 30 min and 96 h

1.10.1 Answer

	A	B	C	D
1				*
2		*		
3			*	
4				*
5		*		
6		*		
7	*			
8		*		
9				*
10			*	
11				*
12				*
13				*
14				*
15	*			
16			*	
17	*			
18				*
19			*	
20			*	
21				*
22		*		
23				*
24	*			
25			*	
26	*			
27		*		
28				*
29	*			
30			*	
31			*	
32		*		
33		*		
34			*	
35				*
36				*
37	*			
38				*
39			*	

1.11 Cancer Cell Biology: The Basics of Nuclear Oncology Imaging

1. Which radiopharmaceutical is NOT used for assessing multidrug resistance (MDR)?
   (a) ^{11}C-colchicine
   (b) ^{11}C-verapamil
   (c) ^{11}C-daunorubicin
   (d) ^{124}I-IAZG

2. All of the following compounds are used in apoptotic imaging *except*:
   (a) Annexin V
   (b) Antisense enzyme inhibitors
   (c) Caspase enzyme inhibitors
   (d) Thrombospondin

3. In most experimental tumors studies, the percentage of hypoxic cells is:
   (a) 50–60%
   (b) 40–50%
   (c) 20–30%
   (d) 10–20%

1.11.1 Answer

	A	B	C	D
1				*
2				*
3				*

1.12 Differential Thyroid Carcinoma

1. What is the least possible region of localization of distant metastases in differentiated thyroid cancer?
   (a) Lung
   (b) Bone
   (c) Brain
   (d) Liver

2. In former iodine-deficient countries that now belong to iodine-sufficient areas:
   (a) The incidence of DTC has increased, and histopathology has changed from follicular to papillary.
   (b) The incidence of DTC has decreased, and histopathology has changed from follicular to papillary.
   (c) The incidence of DTC has increased, and histopathology has changed from papillary to follicular.
   (d) The incidence of DTC has decreased, and histopathology has changed from papillary to follicular.

3. Which statement regarding the epidemiology of DTC is NOT correct?
   (a) Clinical incidence increases with age.
   (b) The highest incidence rates are being reported in low-iodine supply areas.
   (c) The female-to-male ratio in papillary DTC is higher than that in follicular DTC.
   (d) DTC mortality is higher in iodine-deficient regions than in areas with adequate iodine supply.

4. Lymph node metastasis in DTC is:
   (a) More frequent in females than males; more frequent in younger patients that older (>50 years) patients
   (b) More frequent in males than females; more frequent in older (>50 years) patients than younger patients
   (c) More frequent in males than females; more frequent in younger patients than older (>50 years) patients
   (d) More frequent in females than males; more frequent in older (>50 years) patients than younger patients

5. All of the following statements regarding the sonographic findings of DTC are true *except*:
   (a) Most DTCs are hypoechogenic on ultrasonography.
   (b) Hyperechogenic nodules exclude DTC.
   (c) No characteristic echo pattern is defined for DTC.
   (d) Echo-free nodules exclude DTC in most cases.

6. The highest statistical parameter in the detection of DTC using US-FNAB is:
   (a) Negative predictive value (NPV)
   (b) Positive predictive value (PPV)
   (c) Specificity
   (d) Sensitivity

7. What is the method of choice in cases with a cytological diagnosis of follicular proliferation?
   (a) CT
   (b) ^{18}F-PET
   (c) MRI
   (d) Thyroid scintigraphy

8. Thyroid hormone medication in DTC patients leads to:
   (a) Tumor regression
   (b) Reduction of recurrence following surgery and radioiodine therapy
   (c) a and b
   (d) None of the above

9. At what stage and dose is adjuvant external radiotherapy in DTC patients recommended?
   (a) T3/N1 stage, total dose: 20–30 Gy
   (b) T4/N1 stage, total dose: 50–60 Gy
   (c) T4/N0 stage, total dose: 50–60 Gy
   (d) T3/N0 stage, total dose: 20–30 Gy

10. Which item regarding the administration of recombinant TSH for the follow-up of patients with differentiated thyroid cancer is NOT correct?
    (a) It is intravenously (IV) injected.
    (b) The recommended dose is 0.9 mg.
    (c) It is prescribed on days 1 and 2.
    (d) ^{131}I is administered on day 3.

11. In patients with well-differentiated thyroid cancer, which of the following variables is associated with longer survival life?
    (a) Male
    (b) Papillary cancer with tall cell variant
    (c) Younger patients
    (d) Aneuploidy of cells

12. In which of the following conditions is the administration of rhTSH better than the discontinuation of T4 on a whole-body scan with ^{131}I?
    (a) Brain metastasis
    (b) Notable remnant in the thyroid
    (c) Chronic use of steroids
    (d) All of the above

13. A patient is suffering from differentiated thyroid cancer. Which finding does NOT indicate a poor prognosis after surgery?
    (a) High TG
    (b) Increase in FDG volumetric accumulation in the tumor zone
    (c) Change in tumor type
    (d) Uptake of ^{131}I in metastases

14. Which of the following methods is recommended for assessing the differentiation of a lesion in a patient with well-differentiated thyroid carcinoma?
    (a) ^{124}I PET
    (b) ^{123}I SPECT-CT
    (c) MRI
    (d) ^{18}F-FDG-PET

15. A follow-up evaluation is performed for a patient with differentiated thyroid cancer. The hTg level with the administration of rhTSH is 10 ng/μl, and the whole-body scan with ^{131}I is negative. What is the next step?
    (a) Measurement of anti-TG
    (b) Follow-up after 6 months
    (c) Control of serum TSH
    (d) Scan after treatment with ^{131}I

16. What is the main limitation of a whole-body scan with Tl-201 or ^{99m}-Tc-MIBI in patients with differentiated thyroid carcinoma?
    (a) Scan has low sensitivity.
    (b) Thyroid residual tissues after surgery are NOT observed.
    (c) Bone lesions are NOT observed.
    (d) Scan causes serum Tg changes.

17. In ^{18}FDG-PET for thyroid carcinomas:
    (a) Thyroid lymphoma causes the absence of a diffused uptake in the thyroid.
    (b) The focal uptake of FDG in a thyroid nodule canNOT confidently distinguish between benign and malignant tissues.
    (c) Hürthle cell carcinoma is determined by the remarkable increase in FDG uptake.
    (d) Thyroid cancers with minimum cellular differentiation have a minimum chance for FDG uptake.

18. About the follow-up of patients with differentiated thyroid cancers:
    (a) Stunning is a phenomenon in which the initial diagnostic dose (3–5 mCi) decreases the therapeutic ^{131}I dose.
    (b) The rate of recurrence is negligible 5 years after treatment.
    (c) ^{201}Tl and ^{123}I have similar sensitivity for the detection of thyroid residual tissue.
    (d) ^{123}I scan after surgery has high sensitivity for the detection of distant metastases.

19. Anaplastic thyroid carcinoma is considered a stage IV disease in the presence of:
    (a) Cervical lymphadenopathy.
    (b) Lung or bone metastasis.
    (c) Anaplastic thyroid carcinoma is considered stage IV at the time of presentation.
    (d) None.

20. What is the radiotracer of choice for the detection of residual tissue of differentiated thyroid cancer after surgery?
    (a) ^{201}Tl
    (b) ^{99m}Tc-pertechnetate
    (c) ^{123}I
    (d) ^{18}F-FDG

21. A patient with a single thyroid nodule and a palpable lymph node is subjected to thyroid scintigraphy. An extra-thyroid uptake is observed in this lymph node. What is the most probable diagnosis?
    (a) Pyramidal lobe
    (b) Activity in the esophagus
    (c) Radiopharmaceutical impurity
    (d) Thyroid cancer metastasis

22. Choose the correct item about thyroglobulin.
    (a) Thyroglobulin secretion from a malignant tissue is NOT TSH dependent.
    (b) Aside from the thyroid, low amounts of thyroglobulin are also synthesized in the liver.
    (c) Thyroglobulin antibodies have NO effect on the measurement of thyroglobulin mRNA.
    (d) Thyroglobulin is specific but insensitive in the diagnosis of residual thyroid carcinoma.

23. Which organ does NOT show the physiological uptake of ^{131}I?
    (a) Gallbladder
    (b) Nose
    (c) Bladder
    (d) Intestines

24. In which of the following conditions does ^{18}F-FDG have the highest application in evaluating thyroid cancer?
    (a) Low TG, positive WBS
    (b) High TG, positive WBS
    (c) Low TG, negative WBS
    (d) High TG, negative WBS

25. Which method is the most reliable for the diagnosis of tumor recurrence in the follow-up of patients with differentiated thyroid cancer?
    (a) Measurement of thyroglobulin without the discontinuation of levothyroxine
    (b) Whole-body scan with ^{131}I after the discontinuation of levothyroxine
    (c) Measurement of thyroglobulin after the discontinuation of levothyroxine
    (d) Whole-body scan with ^{201}Tl without the discontinuation of levothyroxine

26. PET scan is performed for a 16-year-old patient with thyroid cancer. A region with FDG uptake is observed in the mediastinum, and the whole-body scan with 131I is negative. What is the most probable diagnosis?
    (a) Undifferentiated tissue of thyroid cancer
    (b) Thyroiditis in the residual thyroid
    (c) Relapse of differentiated thyroid cancer
    (d) Uptake in the thymus with hyperplasia

27. About the whole-body scan with 131I:
    (a) Thymus uptake is an unusual finding and indicates metastasis.
    (b) The incidence of artifacts decreases with the increase of radioiodine dose.
    (c) Artifacts because of iodine secretion from salivary glands are usually observed in the elderly.
    (d) The radioiodine uptake in the parotid glands is longer than that in the submandibular glands.

28. FDG-PET is performed for a patient with colon cancer, and a diffuse uptake of FDG is observed in the thyroid. Which item is NOT correct?
    (a) Normal variant for this finding.
    (b) Subclinical chronic inflammation of the thyroid.
    (c) If a palpable nodule of the thyroid is present, then it is benign according to the scan finding.
    (d) Lymphoma or autoimmune disease in the thyroid.

29. A patient with a history of thyroidectomy is referred 6 months after the surgery. The whole-body scan with radioiodine is negative, but the serum Tg is greater than 50 ng/ml in two repeats. What is the recommended intervention?
    (a) Administration of 30 mCi of 131I
    (b) Whole-body scan with thallium
    (c) Controlling the disease for another 6 months
    (d) Repeat of chest X-ray

30. Which of the following scans has the most diagnostic value for the detection of differentiated thyroid cancer?
    (a) 131I whole-body scan
    (b) ^{18}F-FDG-PET scan
    (c) ^{124}I-PET scan
    (d) ^{124}I PET/CT scan

31. About the ^{18}F-FDG uptake in the thyroid:
    (a) Glucose is the primary source of energy in the thyroid; therefore, an FDG uptake is usually observed.
    (b) In thyroid lymphoma, nonuniformity and reduction of thyroid uptake are indicative of inflammatory lesions.
    (c) The intensity of the FDG uptake is directly related with the level of differentiation of thyroid cancer.
    (d) A notable uptake is randomly observed in the thyroid.

32. A whole-body scan is performed 1 week after the administration of 150 mCi of radioiodine in a patient with a progressively increasing Tg. Which of the following organs is the most probable to demonstrate activity?
    (a) Parotids
    (b) Lingual and sublingual salivary glands
    (c) Submandibular salivary glands
    (d) Nasal mucosa

33. What is the main disadvantage of ^{123}I administration over 131I on the whole-body scan of a patient with differentiated thyroid cancer?
    (a) The possibility of the stunning phenomenon
    (b) Prolongation of levothyroxine discontinuation
    (c) Higher dose of the radiopharmaceutical
    (d) Lower sensitivity for the detection of distant metastasis

34. Which of the following methods is the most reliable in detecting tumor recurrence in the follow-up of patients with differentiated thyroid cancer?
    (a) Thyroglobulin measurement without discontinuing levothyroxine
    (b) Whole-body scan with 131I after discontinuing levothyroxine
    (c) Thyroglobulin measurement after discontinuing levothyroxine
    (d) Whole-body scan with ^{201}Tl without discontinuing levothyroxine

35. A patient is referred for follow-up evaluation after subtotal thyroidectomy. A significant uptake of ^{131}I in the neck is observed, but the thallium scan is normal. What is the most probable diagnosis?
    (a) Residual papillary carcinoma
    (b) Scar and fibrous tissue
    (c) Residual normal tissue
    (d) Residual medullary carcinoma

36. About the evaluation of thyroid tumors with 131I and PET scan:
    (a) Tumors with a lower FDG uptake and a higher 131I uptake are more malignant.
    (b) Tumors with a higher FDG uptake and a higher 131I uptake are more benign.
    (c) Tumors with a lower FDG uptake and a lower 131I uptake are more malignant.
    (d) Tumors with a higher FDG uptake and a lower 131I uptake are more malignant.

37. A patient with a history of differentiated thyroid cancer and total thyroidectomy for tumor progression from a capsule is referred. Residual cancer is indicated by ^{131}I uptake in which region?
    (a) Superior to the lobe with tumor
    (b) Lateral to the involved lobe
    (c) In the involved lobe
    (d) Upper thyroid midline

38. Which of the following cancers is associated with Hashimoto's thyroiditis?
    (a) Lymphoma
    (b) Anaplastic carcinoma
    (c) Medullary carcinoma
    (d) Follicular cancer

39. What is the most sensitive factor for detecting the recurrence of differentiated thyroid cancer?
    (a) ^{131}I-whole body scan
    (b) ^{99m}Tc-MIBI whole-body scan
    (c) Serum thyroglobulin
    (d) Precise clinical examination

40. A patient with follicular thyroid cancer underwent surgery and iodine therapy. One year later, the ^{131}I whole-body scan is negative, but the Tg concentration is high. Which of the following items is correct about the FDG-PET scan for this patient?
    (a) Tg concentration has NO effect on the FDG uptake.
    (b) The size of the FDG-avid lesion is an independent prognostic factor.
    (c) An increase in TSH decreases the sensitivity of scan.
    (d) A negative scan excludes metastasis.

41. PET imaging of the thyroid gland:
    (a) A diffuse thyroid uptake is usually associated with Grave's disease.
    (b) The normal SUV has a mean of 1.5 ± 0.2.
    (c) The focal uptake is usually due to a malignant nodule.
    (d) A mild diffuse uptake is commonly due to Hashimoto's thyroiditis.

42. In patients with elevated thyroglobulin and a negative whole-body radioiodine scan, the following issue should be considered in determining whether PET would be useful:
    (a) Surgical candidate
    (b) Anatomical imaging
    (c) Previous radioiodine exposure
    (d) All of the above

43. PET is useful in:
    (a) Hürthle cell subtype of follicular cancer
    (b) Insular cell subtype of follicular cancer
    (c) Papillary and follicular carcinoma
    (d) All of the above

44. In which of the following regions is the probability of metastasis of the early stages of papillary thyroid cancer high?
    (a) Mediastinal lymph node
    (b) Lungs
    (c) Pretracheal lymph node
    (d) Bones

45. If a patient does NOT take thyroxin, what level of thyroglobulin does NOT require further evaluation for potential metastases?
    (a) Less than 15 ng/ml
    (b) Less than 25 ng/ml
    (c) Less than 30 ng/ml
    (d) Less than 10 ng/ml

46. What is the maximum dose of ^{131}I for the treatment of differentiated thyroid cancer in one session?
    (a) 300 mCi
    (b) 100 mCi
    (c) 175 mCi
    (d) 200 mCi

47. What is the best therapeutic approach for differentiated thyroid cancer?
    (a) Lobectomy followed by thyroxin treatment
    (b) Total thyroidectomy and thyroxin treatment
    (c) Lobectomy, isthmectomy, and thyroxin treatment
    (d) Near-total thyroidectomy, radioactive iodine therapy, and thyroxin treatment

48. The worst prognosis of DTC is seen in patients with … metastasis.
    (a) Lung
    (b) Bone
    (c) Liver
    (d) Mediastinal lymph nodes

49. All of the following findings indicate an increased risk of malignancy in thyroid nodules *except*:
    (a) Solid in nature
    (b) Presence of a hypoecho on sonography
    (c) Punctate calcification
    (d) Peripheral hypervascularity

50. Which of the following statements is NOT correct about the application of different scans in thyroid carcinomas?
    (a) The sensitivity of the ^{131}I whole-body scan is greater than its specificity in the diagnosis of thyroid carcinomas and metastasis.
    (b) Hürthle cell carcinoma presents the 201Tl and ^{99m}Tc-MIBI uptakes but NOT the ^{131}I uptake.
    (c) The ^{99m}Tc-DMSA (V) scan can be used for the identification of metastases of a differentiated thyroid carcinoma (DTC).
    (d) If the calcitonin level is greater than 1000 pg/ml, 201Tl and ^{99m}Tc-MIBI scans are sensitive and specific for the medullary thyroid cancer.

51. Which of the following scans is especially valuable for the evaluation of a thyroid lymphoma?
    (a) ^{99m}Tc-MIBI scan
    (b) Gallium scan
    (c) ^{131}I scan
    (d) ^{99m}Tc-pertechnetate scan

52. Which of the following statements is NOT correct about papillary thyroid carcinoma?
    (a) It can be multicentric in 20–80% of the cases.
    (b) Punctate shadowing calcification is reported.
    (c) Nodules are usually hyperechoic.
    (d) The disease metastasizes through the lymphatic system.

53. About well-differentiated thyroid cancer:
    (a) It is 2.5 times more prevalent in men than in women.
    (b) At the time of diagnosis, the median age of the patients in follicular cancer is lower than that in the papillary cancer.
    (c) At the time of diagnosis, the median age of women is lower than that of men.
    (d) It is two times more prevalent in dark skins than in bright skins.

54. Regarding thyroid tumors:
    (a) All anaplastic carcinomas are considered stage IV.
    (b) TNM staging does NOT have an applied value in differentiated cancers.
    (c) N2 represents the bilateral lymphatic involvement.
    (d) N3 represents the involvement of the lymph nodes on the opposite side.

1.12.1 Answer

	A	B	C	D
1				*
2	*			
3		*		
4			*	
5		*		
6	*			
7		*		
8			*	
9		*		
10	*			
11			*	
12				*
13				*
14	*			
15			*	

	A	B	C	D
16		*		
17		*		
18	*			
19			*	
20			*	
21				*
22			*	
23	*			
24				*
25			*	
26	*			
27			*	
28			*	
29		*		
30				*
31				*
32		*		
33				*
34			*	
35			*	
36				*
37			*	
38	*			
39			*	
40		*		
41		*		
42				*
43				*
44			*	
45				*
46	*			
47				*
48		*		
49			*	
50				*
51	*			
52			*	
53		*		
54	*			

1.13 Medullary Thyroid Cancer

1. Medullary thyroid carcinoma:
   (a) About 10% of it is hereditary.
   (b) Familial MTC is inherited as an autosomal recessive trait.
   (c) The hereditary MTC gene is in chromosome 10.
   (d) Families with familial MTC develop the other tumors associated with the MEN syndrome.

2. Find the correct statement about MTC.
   (a) Every case of MTC should be offered a genetic testing.
   (b) All first-degree family members of every case of MTC should be offered a genetic testing.
   (c) Screening of family members with pentagastrin screening tests is required.
   (d) The timing of surgery in children with the MTC gene is an obvious issue.

3. All substances in MTC may increase *except*:
   (a) Somatostatin
   (b) Substance P
   (c) CEA
   (d) AFP

4. Distant metastasis in MTC is rarely found in:
   (a) Liver
   (b) Skeleton
   (c) Lung
   (d) Brain

5. Which MRI sequence is effective for the demonstration of a recurrent disease in MTC patients?
   (a) T2 MRI
   (b) T1 MRI
   (c) STIR
   (d) FLAIR

6. The normal distribution of ^{99m}Tc-DMSA(V) in 2 h is NOT observed in:
   (a) Skeleton
   (b) Heart
   (c) Pituitary
   (d) Adrenal

7. ^{99m}Tc-DMSA(V) in MTC:
   (a) Has more activity in bone than in soft tissue.
   (b) Its main role is in early diagnosis.
   (c) It is not taken up by DTCs.
   (d) Its sensitivity is about 90%.

8. Regarding the application of various radiopharmaceuticals in MTC:
   (a) CT scan is more sensitive than ^{99m}Tc-MIBI in the detection of recurrence in the chest.
   (b) ^{99m}Tc-MIBI is more sensitive than ^{99m}Tc bone scan in the detection of bone metastases.
   (c) ^{99m}Tc-MIBI has the least sensitivity compared with ^{201}Tl and ^{99m}Tc-DMSA(V).
   (d) ^{99m}Tc-DMSA(V) is the most sensitive radionuclide imaging agent available.

9. Which test is the most promising in MTC cases?
   (a) ^{111}In-anticalcitonin antibody
   (b) ^{131}I-anti-CEA antibody
   (c) ^{131}I-MIBG
   (d) ^{201}Tl

10. Nephrotoxicity is a major concern of:
    (a) ^{111}In-anticalcitonin antibody
    (b) ^{131}I-anti-CEA antibody
    (c) CCK-B/gastrin receptor imaging
    (d) ^{131}I-MIBG

11. Which test is the most sensitive in the follow-up of medullary thyroid cancer?
    (a) ^{201}Tl
    (b) ^{99m}Tc-MIBI
    (c) ^{99m}Tc-DMSA (V)
    (d) ^{131}I-MIBG

12. What is the most sensitive method to detect the recurrence of medullary thyroid cancer?
    (a) ^{111}In-octreotide
    (b) I-^{131} MIBG
    (c) Pentagastrin-stimulated calcitonin
    (d) FDG-PET

13. Which of the following radiotracers is NOT indicated for the evaluation of metastatic medullary thyroid cancer?
    (a) ^{123}I-MIBG
    (b) ^{18}F-FDG
    (c) ^{131}I-anti-AFP antibody
    (d) ^{111}In-octreotide

14. Which of the following situations causes a false-negative outcome in the Tc-99m-(V)-DMSA scan of medullary thyroid carcinoma?
    (a) Low anti-CEA
    (b) Severe increase in serum phosphorus
    (c) Minor increase in serum calcitonin
    (d) Amyloid precipitation in the tumor

15. Calcitonin:
    (a) Is used as a tumor marker to determine differentiated thyroid cancer
    (b) Is undetectable in patients with thyroidectomy
    (c) Is secreted from thyroid follicular cells along with the thyroid hormone
    (d) Two stimulatory tests with normal results after total thyroidectomy indicate a cure in patients with MENII

16. What is the screening method of choice for a subject with a familial history of medullary thyroid cancer?
    (a) Sonography
    (b) Thyroid scan with technetium
    (c) Thyroid scan with ^{131}I
    (d) MRI

17. Which radiotracer is the least valuable in evaluating the metastatic lesions of medullary thyroid cancer?
    (a) ^{111}In-octreotide
    (b) ^{131}I-MIBG
    (c) ^{131}I
    (d) ^{99m}Tc-DMSA (V)

18. Choose the correct statement about medullary thyroid carcinoma.
    (a) Metastatic liver lesions can be efficiently detected by ^{111}In-octreotide scintigraphy.
    (b) This disease can be treated by total thyroidectomy and cervical lymphadenectomy.
    (c) There is NO difference between the level of calcitonin and that of carcino-embryonic antigen in its well-differentiated and non-differentiated forms.
    (d) Serum calcitonin decreases immediately after thyroidectomy.

19. Regarding the treatment of medullary thyroid carcinoma:
    (a) Subtotal thyroidectomy is sufficient.
    (b) Radical neck dissection increases life expectancy.
    (c) Serum calcitonin may remain high for a few months after successful treatment.
    (d) MIBG treatment never produces a complete response.

20. What is the most appropriate management for patients with medullary thyroid carcinoma (MTC)?
    (a) Aggressive chemotherapy
    (b) Aggressive surgery
    (c) Therapeutic dose of radioactive iodine (^{131}I)
    (d) Definitive external radiotherapy

21. MEN-2b syndrome is composed of all of the following components *except*:
    (a) Medullary thyroid carcinoma
    (b) Primary hyperparathyroidism
    (c) Pheochromocytoma
    (d) Neurofibromatosis

22. ^{99m}Tc-DMSA (V):
    (a) It shows the bone metastasis only in medullary thyroid cancer.
    (b) ^{99m}Tc-DMSA (V) scan before surgery is required for patients with medullary thyroid cancer.
    (c) ^{99m}Tc-DMSA (V) uptake in bone metastases is more intense than that in soft tissue.
    (d) The biodistribution of 186Re-DMSA (V) is similar to that of ^{99m}Tc-DMSA (V) with less renal retention.

23. In which region is the sensitivity of the ^{201}Tl scan the highest for the detection of recurrent medullary thyroid cancer?
    (a) Lung
    (b) Liver
    (c) Heart
    (d) Neck

24. In which region is the sensitivity of ^{99m}Tc-MIBI less than that of CT scan if the goal is to detect medullary thyroid cancer metastasis in this area?
    (a) Liver
    (b) Neck
    (c) Head
    (d) Chest

25. Identify the correct statement regarding medullary thyroid cancer (MTC).
    (a) Patients with familial history of the disease have the highest probability for MTC.
    (b) Total thyroidectomy is NOT necessarily required for the hereditary form of the disease, and lobectomy of the involved organ is the maximum extent of thyroidectomy.
    (c) TSH suppression by administering thyroid hormones is necessary after thyroidectomy.
    (d) The protocol of surgical management and follow-up is similar for the spontaneous and familial forms of the disease.

1.13.1 Answer

	A	B	C	D
1			*	
2	*			
3				*
4				*
5			*	
6				*
7			*	
8				*
9		*		

10			*	
11			*	
12			*	
13			*	
14			*	
15				*
16	*			
17			*	
18		*		
19			*	
20		*		
21		*		
22		*		
23				*
24	*			
25				*

1.14 Breast Scintigraphy

1. What is the most specific diagnostic tool for breast cancer?
   (a) Mammography
   (b) Digitization of mammograms with artificial neural network analysis
   (c) MRI
   (d) Monoclonal antibodies

2. ^{201}Tl scintigraphy in breast cancer:
   (a) It can be a valuable tool for the differentiation between benign and malignant lesions.
   (b) The diagnostic accuracy of SPECT is better than that of planar.
   (c) The concentration of ^{201}Tl mainly depends on tumor grading, receptor status, and lymphatic/vascular invasion.
   (d) It may have a significant role in evaluating the involvement of the metastatic axillary lymph node.

3. Which benign breast lesion exhibits a remarkable focal ^{99m}Tc-MIBI uptake (false positive)?
   (a) Papilloma
   (b) Fibrous hyperplasia
   (c) Abscess
   (d) Fibroadenoma

4. All of the following radiopharmaceuticals have been used in breast cancer *except*:
   (a) ^{99m}Tc-DTPA
   (b) ^{99m}Tc-sulfur colloid
   (c) ^{99m}Tc-DMSA
   (d) Gallium-67 citrate

5. Which of the following situations is NOT an indication for breast scintigraphy?
   (a) Those with non-diagnostic mammography
   (b) Those who present an axillary mass that is found to be squamous cell carcinoma
   (c) Those with mass abnormalities in the breast
   (d) Those who require the assessment of therapeutic response

6. Which of the following approaches can be applied to increase the sensitivity of scintimammography?
   (a) Scintimammography in the prone position instead of in the supine position
   (b) Delayed scintimammography instead of early radiography
   (c) SPECT scintimammography instead of planar scintimammography
   (d) All of the above

7. Which item on the sensitivity of scintimammography with ^{99m}Tc-MIBI is correct?
   (a) It cannot detect lesions smaller than 10 mm.
   (b) Sensitivity slightly decreases in fatty breasts.
   (c) Similar sensitivity is observed in both palpable and non-palpable lesions.
   (d) It has lower sensitivity but higher specificity than MRI.

8. If the goal is to detect malignancy, which patient is NOT an appropriate candidate for breast scan with ^{99m}Tc-MIBI?
   (a) A patient with a history of breast radiotherapy
   (b) A patient with a history of breast lumpectomy
   (c) Previous administration of chemotherapy for malignancy before lumpectomy
   (d) Concurrent dense mass in the breast and axillary adenopathy

9. A 3 cm mass is found in the left breast of a 32-year-old woman. A dense breast is reported in the mammography because of fibrocystic tissue. Which one is the most suitable for the evaluation of malignancy of the tumor?
   (a) 18 F-FDG
   (b) MRI
   (c) CT
   (d) ^{99m}Tc-MIBI

10. In which of the following conditions is scintimammography with ^{99m}Tc-MIBI NOT indicated?
    (a) Dense breast
    (b) A lesion smaller than 10 mm
    (c) Palpable mass with normal mammography
    (d) Breast implant

11. In ^{99m}Tc-MIBI scintimammography:
    (a) Rapid clearance indicates good response to chemotherapy.
    (b) An increase in the uptake in deep lesions is considered one of the disadvantages of the lateral view.
    (c) The sensitivity of thallium scan is higher than that of ^{99m}Tc-MIBI when the goal is to detect malignant breast lesions.
    (d) SPECT increases the precision of tumor detection but results in high false-positive outcomes.

12. In ^{99m}Tc-MIBI scintimammography:
    (a) Thallium scan is preferred over ^{99m}Tc-MIBI because of its higher sensitivity.
    (b) Delayed clearance of the tumor indicates a weak response to chemotherapy.
    (c) The lateral view can overlook miss small lesions in the medial parts of the breast.
    (d) SPECT decreases the number of false-positive cases.

13. Which item is the least important in the tissue uptake of ^{99m}Tc-MIBI?
    (a) Trafficking of lysosomes
    (b) P-glycoprotein multidrug resistance system
    (c) Positive charge of the molecule
    (d) Lipophilicity of the molecule

14. What is the most important prognostic factor in breast cancer?
    (a) Tumor size
    (b) Involvement of the axillary lymph nodes
    (c) Positive or negative estrogen receptor
    (d) Histology of the tumor

15. In which item is PET scan the least helpful in the evaluation of a patient with breast cancer?
    (a) Detection of recurrence
    (b) Evaluation of response to treatment
    (c) Detection of metastasis
    (d) Primary diagnosis

16. A patient with a mass in the breast and a history of radiotherapy for breast cancer of the opposite side is referred. What is the next diagnostic step?
    (a) Whole-body scan with thallium
    (b) Whole-body scan with ^{99m}Tc-MIBI
    (c) Biopsy
    (d) Mammography

17. Diagnosis of breast cancer:
    (a) Diagnostic sensitivity of ^{18}FDG-PET is similar to that of ^{99m}Tc-MIBI.
    (b) All palpable masses of the breast are detectable by mammography.
    (c) The diagnostic sensitivity of ^{99m}Tc-MIBI is less than that of ^{201}Tl.
    (d) Benign fibrocystic breast cancer is efficiently detectable by thallium scan.

18. What is the recommended method of diagnosis for a 28-year-old woman with suspected breast lymphoma?
    (a) Gallium SPECT scan
    (b) Mammography
    (c) Sonography
    (d) Sampling with aspiration

19. In which of the following malignancies is FDG-PET indicated for the evaluation of response to chemotherapy during treatment (without the need for completing chemotherapy)?
    (a) Breast cancer
    (b) Pulmonary adenocarcinoma
    (c) Non-Hodgkin's lymphoma
    (d) Hodgkin's lymphoma

20. FDG-PET is performed for a 55-year-old woman with breast cancer on the right side. The only abnormality is the primary tumor in the right breast, but no lesion is observed in the right axillary. What is the next step?
    (a) Lymphoscintigraphy and biopsy of the right sentinel lymph node
    (b) Sonography of the right axillary to confirm the absence of lymphadenopathy
    (c) Referral for surgical mastectomy without surgery of the right axillary
    (d) MRI evaluation of the right axillary

21. In ^{99m}Tc-MIBI scintimammography:
    (a) 10 mCi of radiopharmaceutical is sufficient.
    (b) Injection is performed on the veins of the hand on the same side.
    (c) The prone position is preferred.
    (d) Imaging begins 4–6 h after injection.

22. FDG-PET scan is performed to evaluate metastasis in a woman with breast cancer. An axillary nodule is found with SUV > 3. What is the best recommendation for this patient?
    (a) This finding has a low-positive predictive value; therefore, the patient should NOT be treated.
    (b) The diagnostic sensitivity of FDG-PET in axillary metastasis is high; therefore, the patient must be treated.
    (c) This finding has a high-positive predictive value; therefore, the patient must be treated.
    (d) The diagnostic accuracy of FDG-PET in axillary metastasis is greater than 95%; therefore, the patient must be treated.

23. What is the recommended method for the evaluation of a palpable dense breast mass of a young woman?
    (a) Mammography
    (b) Needle aspiration biopsy
    (c) ^{201}Tl scan
    (d) ^{99m}Tc-MIBI

24. Which item is correct about ^{99m}Tc-MIBI and drug resistance of malignancies?
    (a) The slow clearance of ^{99m}Tc-MIBI from breast cancer is predictive of an inappropriate response to chemotherapy.
    (b) P-glycoprotein acts as an accumulating agent for the chemotherapy agent in the cell.
    (c) Inhibition of P-glycoprotein increases the wash-out rate of ^{99m}Tc-MIBI from malignant tumors.
    (d) Chemotherapy-resistant tumors highly express P-glycoprotein on the cell surface.

25. About ^{99m}Tc-MIBI imaging of breast cancer:
    (a) It is recommended as a screening method.
    (b) The specificity of this method for malignancy is higher than that of mammography.
    (c) The sensitivity of this method is suitable for lesions smaller than 1 cm.
    (d) ^{99m}Tc-MIBI is NOT uptaken in hypo-proliferative breast diseases.

26. A 58-year-old woman with a breast tumor underwent biopsy, and the report indicates adenocarcinoma. Therefore, she is referred for a ^{99m}Tc-MIBI breast scan. A high uptake in the corresponding tumor is observed in the 10 min scan, and the scan 100 min after the radiotracer injection shows a severe decrease in uptake. This scan pattern is indicative of:
    (a) An appropriate response to chemotherapy
    (b) An extensive cell proliferation
    (c) Highly differentiated tumoral cells
    (d) An inappropriate response to chemotherapy

27. A myocardial perfusion scan with ^{99m}Tc-MIBI is conducted for a 59-year-old woman. A focal increase in uptake is observed in the upper region exterior to the heart's location. What is the most probable diagnosis?
    (a) Carcinoma of the left breast
    (b) Pulmonary carcinoma
    (c) Thyroid metastatic foci
    (d) All of the above

28. Which of the following interventions is recommended to improve the scan results in ^{99m}Tc-MIBI mammography?
    (a) Acquisition of delayed images 60–90 min after injection
    (b) Injection I then lower limb veins in patients with a history of radiotherapy
    (c) Imaging in the supine position for the better localization of the medial quarter lesions
    (d) Lower dose of radiotracer to reduce the interference of cardiac activity

29. Z-^{131}I-MIVE (MIVE: methoxy-iodo-vinyl-estradiol) uptake in breast cancer is directly related to the expression of which hormone receptor?
    (a) Progesterone
    (b) Androgen
    (c) Estrogen
    (d) Glucocorticoid

30. What is the screening method of choice for the evaluation of non-symptomatic patients with suspected breast cancer?
    (a) Mammography
    (b) Sonography
    (c) MRI
    (d) ^{99m}Tc-MIBI breast scintigraphy

31. What is the main reason for the tumoral uptake of ^{99m}Tc-MIBI?
    (a) Vascular leakage
    (b) Lipophilicity of the radiotracer
    (c) High density of the mitochondria
    (d) Negative charge of the radiotracer

32. Receptor imaging has been given attention recently in the study of breast cancers. Which of the following item is NOT correct about this method?
    (a) 50–70% of breast cancer cases express somatostatin receptors.
    (b) ^{18}F-labeling of steroid molecules induces little changes in their structure and is practical for the evaluation of breast cancer.
    (c) 16-α-^{123}I-estradiol imaging has produced satisfactory results for the evaluation of primary tumors and recurrence of breast cancer.
    (d) The sensitivity of breast scintigraphy with somatostatin receptor is greater than that of ^{99m}Tc-MIBI.

33. Which of the following statements is NOT correct about the evaluation of resistance to chemotherapy?
    (a) Mitochondrial accumulation of ^{99m}Tc-MIBI does NOT induce cytotoxicity.
    (b) The MDR gene on chromosome 7 encodes P-glycoprotein, which expels the drugs from cells.
    (c) P-glycoprotein expression and drug resistance can be evaluated by the wash-out rate of MIBI from the tumor.
    (d) Verapamil and quinidine inhibit the P-glycoprotein pump.

34. The false-negative findings of breast cancer on PET imaging include:
    (a) Fibroadenoma
    (b) Ductal adenoma
    (c) Fibrous dysplasia
    (d) Invasive lobular carcinoma

35. PET is the most valuable for the staging of breast cancer in the following conditions *except*:
    (a) Primary tumor T3 or T4.
    (b) Stage II disease.
    (c) The primary lesion is medial or superior.
    (d) Neoadjuvant therapy is planned without axillary dissection or sentinel node sampling.

36. Which of the following patients is the most likely to develop breast cancer?
    (a) Woman who delivered her first child at 25 years old
    (b) Woman who delivered her first child at 29 years old
    (c) Woman who has NOT experienced pregnancy up to now
    (d) Woman who delivered her first child at 38 years old

37. Which of the following items is NOT considered an indication for ^{99m}Tc-MIBI scan in breast cancer?
    (a) Prediction of response to treatment
    (b) Evaluation of the patient after lumpectomy
    (c) Evaluation of high-risk patients (with genetic susceptibility or a history of malignant breast lesions)
    (d) Suspicious mammography in a patient who is psychologically worried about breast cancer

38. In ^{99m}Tc-MIBI scintimammography:
    (a) The MDR can cause false-negative findings.
    (b) It is NOT sensitive enough to detect lesions smaller than 2 cm.
    (c) The sensitivity of this test for the involvement of an axillary lymph node is high.
    (d) The total sensitivity of the scan in the detection of palpable malignant lesions is less than 80%.

39. Which of the following situations is NOT considered an indication for ^{99m}Tc-MIBI scan?
    (a) Medullar thyroid cancer
    (b) Prediction of response to chemotherapy in breast cancer
    (c) Detection of the recurrence of brain tumors
    (d) High-grade lymphoma

40. A 36-year-old woman is presented with a suspected malignant mass. What is the best modality for the evaluation?
    (a) Sonography
    (b) Mammography
    (c) PET
    (d) MRI

41. Which of the following statements regarding the application of FDG-PET in breast cancer is NOT correct?
    (a) Low uptake of FDG is commonly observed in fibrocystic diseases.
    (b) PET is a valuable modality for the staging of axillary lymph nodes.
    (c) Glucose transporter 1 (GluT-1) is commonly expressed in breast cancers.
    (d) PET is valuable even in patients who underwent mastectomy and silicon implantation.

42. What is the role of axillary dissection and drainage in patients with invasive ductal breast cancer?
    (a) It has a therapeutic role in all patients with positive lymphatic involvement and increases the survival rate.
    (b) It is therapeutic in all patients regardless of the involvement of lymph nodes and increases the survival rate.
    (c) It only provides information on the regional axillary involvement and prognosis but does NOT change the survival rate.
    (d) It has a therapeutic role in some patients with a positive lymphatic involvement and increases the survival rate.

43. Which of the following prognostic factors is the most important in breast cancer?
    (a) Involvement of the axillary lymph nodes
    (b) Size of the primary tumor
    (c) Location of the tumor
    (d) HER2 positivity

44. A 69-year-old woman with a mass in the left axillary region is referred. The biopsy report indicates well-differentiated adenocarcinoma, but there is NO pathologic finding in the CXR, mammography, breast sonography, and CT scan of the abdomen, pelvis, and thorax. Which of the following diagnostic studies is the most helpful?
    (a) Random biopsy of the breast
    (b) PET scan
    (c) Breast MRI
    (d) Measurement of CEA and CA 15-3

45. Which agent is the most appropriate for the scintigraphy of a patient with poorly differentiated neuroendocrine cancer and negative octreotide results?
    (a) HTP
    (b) ^{11}C-L-DOPA
    (c) ^{18}F-Fluoro-DOPA
    (d) FDG

1.14.1 Answer

	A	B	C	D
1				*
2	*			
3				*
4			*	
5		*		
6	*			
7				*
8				*
9				*
10		*		
11				*
12			*	
13	*			
14		*		
15				*
16			*	
17	*			
18				*
19	*			

20	*			
21			*	
22			*	
23		*		
24				*
25		*		
26				*
27				*
28			*	
29			*	
30	*			
31			*	
32				*
33				*
34				*
35		*		
36			*	
37			*	
38	*			
39				*
40		*		
41		*		
42				*
43	*			
44			*	
45				*

1.15 Pediatric Tumors

1. Neuroblastoma rarely metastasizes to the:
   (a) Bone
   (b) Liver
   (c) Soft tissue
   (d) Lung

2. Neuroblastoma:
   (a) Its extra-adrenal occurrence is reported in only 10% of children.
   (b) 17% of the primary tumor site is in the pelvic sympathetic side chain.
   (c) The disease is rare after age 4.
   (d) The deletion of chromosome 1p36 is a prognostic factor in the treatment.

3. A pathologic lesion taking up ^{131}I-MIBG in a child is most likely to be a:
   (a) Ganglioneuroma
   (b) Pheochromocytoma
   (c) Retinoblastoma
   (d) Neuroblastoma

4. ^{99m}Tc-N-pyridoxyl-5-methyltryptophan (PMT) is used in:
   (a) Neuroblastoma
   (b) Hepatoblastoma
   (c) Rhabdomyosarcoma
   (d) Osteosarcoma

5. Lymphoma in children:
   (a) NHL is usually low grade and has good prognosis.
   (b) Gallium scan is preferred to be conducted with 10 mCi of radiotracer and 7-day delayed images.
   (c) NHL in the mediastinum is indistinguishable from AML.
   (d) ^{99m}Tc-MIBI is NOT recommended to control the thymic rebound.

6. Role of scintigraphy in neuroblastoma:
   (a) Abnormal findings in the MDP bone scan are higher than those in the MIBG scan.
   (b) Ovoid epiphysis in the bone scan of a child younger than 18 months indicates a suspected metastasis.
   (c) The possibility of an MDP uptake in the primary tumors of neuroblastoma with thoracic origin is greater than that of those with abdominal origin.
   (d) Metastasis is NOT included in the differential diagnosis if epiphysis is wedge shaped in the bone scan.

7. What is the recommended method for the evaluation of tumor viability in a patient with sarcoma of soft tissue?
   (a) Color Doppler sonography
   (b) ^{99m}Tc-MIBI scan
   (c) CT scan
   (d) MRI

8. Gallium scan is performed for a young boy with a mass in the distal femoral metaphysis. A region with an increased uptake and a central decrease in activity (doughnut sign) is observed in the scan. What is the most probable diagnosis?
   (a) Low-grade osteosarcoma
   (b) High-grade osteosarcoma
   (c) Osteomyelitis
   (d) Bone metastasis

9. Identify the most common malignancy in children in the corresponding anatomical regions.
   (a) Large intestine: carcinoid
   (b) Biliary system: leiomyosarcoma
   (c) Urinary tract: rhabdomyosarcoma
   (d) Small intestine: lymphoma

10. A 3-year-old child with strabismus is referred. Which of the following methods is recommended for the evaluation of the intra-orbital progression of retinoblastoma?
    (a) CT
    (b) MRI
    (c) Bone scan
    (d) Gallium scan

11. Hepatic scan shows a metastasis for a 9-month-old infant. What is the most common cause of this disease?
    (a) Retinoblastoma
    (b) Osteosarcoma
    (c) Pheochromocytoma
    (d) Neuroblastoma

12. Bone scan is NOT indicated for the diagnosis of which tumor in children?
    (a) Rhabdomyosarcoma
    (b) Neuroblastoma
    (c) Lymphoma
    (d) Ewing sarcoma

13. An abnormal abdominal uptake is observed in the MIBG scan of a child with an unknown tumor. What is the most probable tumor?
    (a) Neuroblastoma
    (b) Ephroblastoma
    (c) Lymphoma
    (d) Hepatoblastoma

14. All of the following scan patterns are observed in children with leukemia *except*:
    (a) Increase in mastoid uptake in the gallium scan
    (b) Absence of the gallbladder in the biliary scan
    (c) Decrease in clearance of MAG3 in the renal scan
    (d) Increase in the metaphyseal uptake in long bones in the bone scan

15. Which of the following statements is NOT correct about pheochromocytoma?
    (a) Malignancy is determined only with the identification of metastasis and invasion.
    (b) ^{131}I-MIBG is the treatment of choice.
    (c) The higher the level of the tumoral dopamine secretion is, the higher the tumor grade.
    (d) The incidence of malignancy in children and in extra-adrenal pheochromocytoma is high.

16. Which of the following statements is NOT correct about pediatric thyroid malignancy?
    (a) Papillary carcinoma is the most common malignancy.
    (b) Thyroid malignancy in children is more invasive than that in adults.
    (c) The probability of malignancy of a cold nodule in children is similar to that in adults.
    (d) Somatostatin receptor imaging is reported to be successful in medullary cancer.

17. Which of the following radiotracers has the least diagnostic value in pediatric neuroblastoma if the goal is to detect metastasis in the cranium and upper abdomen, respectively?
    (a) ^{11}C-epinephrine, FDG-PET
    (b) In-octreotide, ^{11}C-epinephrine
    (c) ^{99m}Tc-MDP, FDG-PET
    (d) FDG-PET, In-pentetreotide

18. What is the most common primary biliary tumor in children?
    (a) Lymphoma
    (b) Hepatoblastoma
    (c) Rhabdomyosarcoma
    (d) Hepatocellular carcinoma

19. Which of the following items is NOT an indication for PET scan in the evaluation of pediatric neoplasms?
    (a) Determination of the histologic grade of astrocytoma before initial surgery or surgery from recurrence
    (b) Differentiation of focal infection from focal lymphoma in acquired immune deficiency patients
    (c) Differentiation of recurrent or persistent tumor from radiation necrosis
    (d) Differentiation of a viable tumor from the surrounding edema of the tumor

20. In which location of astrocytomas can tumor-imaging tracers be used in the same way in children as in adults?
    (a) Cerebral hemispheres
    (b) Brain stem
    (c) Optic pathway
    (d) Basal ganglions

21. Which item describes the applied characteristics of ^{11}C-methionine in children?
    (a) Accumulation in high-grade astrocytoma
    (b) Accumulation in grade II astrocytoma
    (c) Differentiation of tumor recurrence from radiotherapy-induced effects
    (d) All of the above

22. Which of the following items is NOT correct about pilocytic astrocytoma?
    (a) It is more common in the middle fossa.
    (b) It shows a minor uptake of FDG and thallium.
    (c) It is similar to a low-grade brain tumor.
    (d) Cerebellar hemispheres are the most common site of involvement.

23. Which of the following statements is NOT correct about ependymoma?
    (a) Neurofibromatosis 1 (NF-1) is observed in 5–15% of patients.
    (b) It is commonly observed in the posterior fossa.
    (c) Infratentorial and supratentorial forms comprise 60% and 40% of the cases, respectively.
    (d) An intense uptake of FDG and ^{201}Tl does NOT always occur.

24. Which of the following statements is NOT correct about medulloblastoma?
    (a) It is considered as primitive neuroectodermal tumors (PNET).
    (b) Recurrence is common but NOT metastasis.
    (c) It is usually infratentorial, and drop metastasis is observed in this type of PNET.
    (d) FDG-PET studies and thallium SPECT studies demonstrate the consistent localization of radiopharmaceuticals in new or recurrent PNET.

25. What is the method of choice for the diagnosis of heterotopia?
    (a) rCBF PET
    (b) rCMRglc
    (c) MRI
    (d) CT

26. All of the following statements regarding tuberous sclerosis are correct *except*:
    (a) An increased FDG uptake is observed in cortical tuberous lesions.
    (b) Seizure is common and difficult to control.
    (c) FDG is NOT capable of distinguishing between epileptogenic and non-epileptogenic forms.
    (d) α-[C11] methyl-L-tryptophan (AMT) is capable of distinguishing between epileptogenic and non-epileptogenic forms.

27. In which of the following pediatric renal cancers should an appropriate management include bone X-ray, bone scan, and bone marrow biopsy?
    (a) Wilms' tumor (favorable histology)
    (b) Wilms' tumor with focal anaplasia
    (c) Wilms' tumor with diffuse anaplasia
    (d) Clear cell sarcoma of kidney

28. In which of the following signs related to pediatric neuroblastoma is MRI the least helpful?
    (a) Intratumoral calcification
    (b) Perivascular involvement
    (c) Tumoral infiltration into the spinal canal
    (d) Bone marrow involvement

29. Infants with neuroblastoma in stage IV-S have a good prognosis. Which of the following organ metastases is not included in this stage?
    (a) Liver
    (b) Bone marrow
    (c) Skin
    (d) Bone

30. In patients with poorly differentiated carcinoma of unknown origin, which of the following diagnostic tests has the least specificity for the localization of the original tumor?
    (a) CT scan of the thorax and abdomen
    (b) Measurement of the beta HCG and AFP serum levels
    (c) Measurement of the CA 15-3, CA 19-9, CA 125, and CEA serum levels
    (d) PET scan

31. All of the following statements about neuroblastoma are correct *except*:
    (a) Neuroblastoma is the most common solid neurologic tumor in childhood, and it usually metastasizes to the bone.
    (b) Primary thorax tumors exhibit more MDP uptake than abdominal tumors.
    (c) MIBG scintigraphy alone is recommended for the staging and monitoring of children with neuroblastoma.
    (d) A radionuclide skeletal survey should be the primary investigation.

32. All of the following items are characteristics of Ewing sarcoma *except*:
    (a) It is commonly observed in the diaphysis of wide bones.
    (b) A nonhomogenous uptake of ^{99m}Tc-MDP is observed in the bone scan.
    (c) Arteriovenous malformation is NOT reported.
    (d) The angiography phase of the bone scan shows higher flow than that of blood pool.

33. All of the following statements about Langerhans cell histiocytosis are correct *except*:
    (a) Langerhans cell histiocytosis (formerly called histiocytosis X) is the term used to describe three diseases with histiocytic hyperproliferation.
    (b) Both bone scan and X-ray are required for the evaluation of patients.
    (c) Only 90% of pediatric cases show bone lesions.
    (d) Bone scan shows an increased uptake in the corresponding lytic lesion in the X-ray.

34. What is the most sensitive method for the detection of bone marrow metastasis?
    (a) Whole-body FDG-PET scan
    (b) Whole-body bone scan
    (c) Whole-body MRI
    (d) CT scan

35. All of the following statements about retinoblastoma are correct *except*:
    (a) It is dominantly bilateral.
    (b) It is common in men and in specific races.
    (c) Whole-body radionuclide skeletal scintigraphy is NOT indicated for the determination of the extent of orbital involvement.
    (d) MRI is the imaging method of choice for intraocular retinoblastoma.

36. Imaging of spinal cord tumors, primary or metastatic, includes:
    (a) Gallium scan
    (b) MRI
    (c) Bone scan
    (d) FDG-PET

37. Which of the following statements about pediatric tumors is NOT correct?
    (a) Lymphoma is the most common head and neck tumor.
    (b) Rhabdomyosarcoma is the most common non-ocular tumor of the orbit.
    (c) The most common primary biliary malignancy is cholangiosarcoma.
    (d) Lymphoma is the most common neoplasm involving the thoracic region.

38. What is the method of choice for investigating the tumoral involvement of pulmonary parenchyma, vessels, or mediastinum?
    (a) MRI
    (b) FDG-PET
    (c) HRCT with contrast
    (d) MRI with contrast

39. What are the patterns of hepatoblastoma and hepatocellular carcinoma in the ^{99m}Tc-sulfur colloid, Tc-IDA, and gallium scans, respectively?
    (a) Decreased uptake, decreased uptake, usually decreased uptake
    (b) Decreased uptake, decreased uptake, usually increased uptake
    (c) Decreased uptake, increased uptake, usually decreased uptake
    (d) Increased uptake, decreased uptake, usually increased uptake

40. If splenic photopenic regions are reported in the ^{99m}Tc-sulfur colloid scan, what are the most probable diagnoses for two children with lymphoma and leukemia, respectively?
    (a) Usually hematoma, disease involvement
    (b) Disease involvement, usually infection or hematoma
    (c) Usually infection, disease involvement
    (d) Disease involvement, disease involvement

41. All of the following statements about Wilms' tumor are correct *except*:
    (a) It is the fifth common tumor, the most common neoplasm of the genitourinary tract, and the most common solid abdominal tumor in children.
    (b) Six years is the most common age of involvement.
    (c) It is bilateral in 5–10% of cases.
    (d) The ^{99m}Tc-sulfur colloid scan shows an increased uptake in an enlarged spleen.

42. All of the following statements about testis tumors are correct *except*:
    (a) More than 50% of testicular tumors, including seminoma and endodermal sinus tumors, demonstrate increased gallium activity.
    (b) Seminoma is the most common tumor associated with cryptorchidism.
    (c) Endodermal sinus tumor is the most common childhood testicular tumor.
    (d) Most of the testis tumors appear before 25 years old.

43. All of the following statements about neuroblastoma are correct *except*:
    (a) The survival rate is optimal in younger ages (less than 14–24 months).
    (b) Abdomen is the most common region of involvement.
    (c) Metastatic involvement of the skeletal system is common in neuroblastoma.
    (d) Thorax neuroblastomas have the poorest prognosis.

44. Which of the following diseases rarely shows significant calcification?
    (a) Neuroblastoma of the thorax
    (b) Ganglioneuroblastoma of the thorax
    (c) Ganglioneuroma of the thorax
    (d) b and c

45. What is the most common region of rhabdomyosarcoma in children?
    (a) Hepatobiliary system
    (b) Genitourinary system
    (c) Head and neck
    (d) Extremities

46. This scan may be the best modality for the detection of a recurrent and metastatic disease in cases with malignant fibrous histiocytoma:
    (a) Bone scan
    (b) ^{99m}Tc-MIBI scan
    (c) Gallium scan
    (d) ^{201} Tl scan

47. What is the most common site of presentation of Ewing tumor?
    (a) Scapula
    (b) Spine
    (c) Femur
    (d) Tibia

48. What is the most common pediatric malignancy?
    (a) Leukemia
    (b) Lymphoma
    (c) Neuroblastoma
    (d) Rhabdomyosarcoma

49. What is the most common form of leukemia in children?
    (a) AML
    (b) CML
    (c) CLL
    (d) ALL

50. Which pattern of ^{99m}Tc-sulfur colloid scan in a child with leukemia represents the post-chemotherapy state?
    (a) Reduction of Tc-sulfur colloid extraction by the liver
    (b) Normal uptake and hepatosplenomegaly
    (c) Reduced hepatosplenic uptake of the tracer
    (d) Focal intrahepatic or intrasplenic lesion

51. Non-Hodgkin's lymphoma (NHL) in children is similar to:
    (a) ALL
    (b) AML
    (c) NHL in adults
    (d) Hodgkin's disease in adults

52. All of the following statements about non-Hodgkin's lymphoma (NHL) in children are correct *except*:
    (a) It comprises 6% of all pediatric cancers and 60% of pediatric lymphomas.
    (b) It is malignant and shows metastasis at the time of clinical presentation.
    (c) Mediastinal NHL is more dangerous than its abdominal form.
    (d) The mediastinum and abdomen are the most and second most common sites of localization, respectively.

53. Which of the following factors in a child with neuroblastoma is NOT indicative of a favorable prognosis?
    (a) Stage IV
    (b) DNA index more than 1.1
    (c) Age below 2 years
    (d) Amplified N-myc

54. Which of the following studies is NOT necessary for the staging of rhabdomyosarcoma in children?
    (a) MIBG scan
    (b) CT scan or MRI of the primary region of tumor
    (c) Bone scan and bone marrow biopsy
    (d) Thoracic CT scan

55. A young adult is evaluated for a mass in the tibial soft tissue. The cytology report indicates a lymphoma with relative skeletal differentiation, and the pathology report indicates rhabdomyosarcoma. Which form of rhabdomyosarcoma is the most probable?
    (a) Embryonal rhabdomyosarcoma
    (b) Pleomorphic rhabdomyosarcoma
    (c) Alveolar rhabdomyosarcoma
    (d) Small-cell rhabdomyosarcoma

56. Which of the following imaging methods is the most specific for the detection of bone metastases of neuroblastoma?
    (a) Conventional X-ray
    (b) MRI
    (c) Bone scan with technetium
    (d) ^{123}I MIBG

57. Which of the following items is NOT considered as a prognostic factor for neuroblastoma?
    (a) Age
    (b) P53 mutation
    (c) Differentiation of tumor
    (d) High level of serum ferritin (>142)

58. In Ewing sarcoma:
    (a) PET/CT detects the tumor regression and progression even before the identification of morphological changes.
    (b) Disease progression is characterized by a 30% increase in SUV.
    (c) Patients with extraosseous Ewing sarcoma should receive the same treatment indicated for the classical Ewing tumor with similar therapeutic response rates.
    (d) All of the above.

59. Which region of Ewing sarcoma is the most common in children?
    (a) Tibia
    (b) Sacroiliac
    (c) Femur
    (d) Humerus

60. What is the required dose of FDG for PET imaging in infants?
    (a) 100 mCi/kg
    (b) 300 μCi/kg
    (c) 1 mCi/kg
    (d) 500 μCi/kg

61. Indolent lymphomas are rare in children. All of the following items belong to indolent lymphomas *except*:
    (a) Extranodal marginal zone lymphoma
    (b) Large cell lymphoma
    (c) Small lymphocytic lymphoma
    (d) Peripheral T-cell lymphoma

62. Metastasis to which organ is the least probable in retinoblastoma?
    (a) Lungs
    (b) Bone
    (c) Central nervous system (CNS)
    (d) Bone marrow

1.15.1 Answer

	A	B	C	D
1				*
2				*
3				*
4		*		
5		*		
6			*	
7		*		
8		*		
9				*
10		*		
11	*			
12			*	
13	*			
14				*
15		*		
16			*	
17				*
18			*	
19	*			
20	*			
21				*
22		*		
23	*			
24		*		
25			*	
26	*			
27				*
28	*			
29				*
30			*	

31			*	
32				*
33			*	
34	*			
35		*		
36		*		
37			*	
38			*	
39		*		
40		*		
41				*
42	*			
43				*
44	*			
45			*	
46			*	
47			*	
48	*			
49				*
50	*			
51	*			
52				*
53				*
54	*			
55			*	
56				*
57		*		
58				*
59			*	
60		*		
61		*		
62				*

1.16 Functional Analysis of Cancer Therapy Effects on Other Organs

1. The onset of doxorubicin-induced cardiomyopathy is induced by:
   (a) Apoptosis
   (b) Aponecrosis
   (c) Necrosis
   (d) Hypoxia
2. The diagnosis of anthracycline-associated cardiotoxicity may be confirmed by the detection of wall motion abnormalities especially in the:
   (a) Inferolateral ventricular wall
   (b) Anterior ventricular wall
   (c) Anteroseptal ventricular wall
   (d) Inferoseptal ventricular wall
3. Anthracycline-associated cardiotoxicity:
   (a) Usually develop a reversible left ventricular dysfunction.
   (b) LVEF using cardiac-gated SPECT remains the most used parameter to evaluate cardiotoxicity.
   (c) Stopping the anthracycline therapy is recommended after an absolute 15% decrease in LVEF.
   (d) Adverse anthracycline effects on the cardiac function may be reduced by the iron-chelating bispiperazinedione ICRF-187.
4. In radiation-induced cardiac damage:
   (a) A reversible perfusion lesion on the ^{201}Tl SPECT is anatomically correlated with epicardial coronary vessels.
   (b) Abnormal cardiac ^{123}I-MIBG parameters are found in the early period after thoracic irradiation.
   (c) LVEF tends to decrease shortly after irradiation.
   (d) LVEF recovery is observed only 4 months later.
5. Vanishing kidney on the DMSA scan is seen in:
   (a) Radiation nephropathy
   (b) Chemotherapy-induced tubular injury
   (c) ^{90}Y-radioimmunotherapy
   (d) Surgical manipulation
6. Chemotherapy-associated pulmonary toxicity causes the following problems *except*:
   (a) Alveolar epithelial disruption
   (b) Focal necrosis of type II pneumocytes
   (c) Intra-alveolar fluid
   (d) Protein leakage

7. Regarding the adverse lung effects induced by thoracic irradiation:
   (a) Radiation pneumonitis appears 6 months after irradiation.
   (b) Loss of lung ventilation is more pronounced than perfusion.
   (c) ^{111}In-pentetreotide is a sensitive tracer for the detection of radiation pneumonitis.
   (d) ^{67}Ga is NOT abnormal in asymptomatic irradiated patients.

8. In bone and bone marrow radiation:
   (a) Bone scintigraphy shows a diffuse decrease in uptake.
   (b) Bone marrow scintigraphy shows a diffuse decrease in uptake.
   (c) Bone uptake in nonirradiated areas tends to decrease.
   (d) Bone marrow regeneration is significantly greater in patients over 8 years old.

9. Regarding adverse brain effects:
   (a) Most radiation injuries occur in functioning mature nerve cells.
   (b) Chemotherapy may act on the vasculoconnective tissue stroma.
   (c) Chemotherapy acts directly on the glial cells.
   (d) The administration of interleukin 2 may be associated with the development of cerebral infarction.

10. In the evaluation of cancer therapy:
    (a) Irradiated thyroid dysfunction may be seen in patients receiving >26 Gy to the thorax.
    (b) The most common chemotherapy-associated liver injury is seen with methotrexate and 6-mercaptopurine.
    (c) ^{99m}Tc-colloid can help in cases with chemotherapy-associated hepatic veno-occlusive disease.
    (d) All of the above.

11. Which of the following complications is due to the radiotherapy and chemotherapy of children?
    (a) Stroke and cognitive dysfunction (in brain radiotherapy)
    (b) Heart tumors (in chest radiotherapy)
    (c) Cholecystitis (in abdominal radiotherapy)
    (d) Acute myasthenia (in radiotherapy of extremities)

12. About pneumonitis due to radiation:
    (a) ^{67}Ga scan in 50% of clinical cases is abnormal.
    (b) A simple chest X-ray is always normal.
    (c) Perfusion scan shows more defects than ventilation scan after the fifth month.
    (d) ^{111}In-pentreotide is NOT sensitive for diagnosis.

13. A 15-year-old child is subjected to chemotherapy with a nephrotoxic agent. What is the recommended scan for the evaluation of renal function?
    (a) MAG3 with ERPF determination
    (b) DMSA with the evaluation of the difference in function between the kidneys
    (c) DTPA with GFR determination
    (d) GHA with furosemide administration and determination of split function

14. About the study of pediatric rhabdomyosarcoma with ^{111}In-AMA scan:
    (a) A positive scan requires confirmation; a negative scan excludes the disease.
    (b) A positive scan does NOT require confirmation; a negative scan does NOT exclude the disease.
    (c) A positive scan does NOT require confirmation; a negative scan excludes the disease.
    (d) A positive scan requires confirmation; a negative scan does NOT exclude the disease.

15. If a child is subjected to chemotherapy or radiotherapy of the thorax, an ejection fraction below … is indicative of the discontinuation of treatment, and an ejection fraction below … is predictive of irreversible cardiac damages, respectively.
    (a) 60%, 50%
    (b) 50%, 40%
    (c) 55%, 45%
    (d) 45%, 35%

16. What are the most common benign and malignant tumors in the region of radiotherapy, respectively?
    (a) Osteochondroma, osteosarcoma
    (b) Osteochondroma, chondrosarcoma
    (c) Osteoblastoma, chondroblastoma
    (d) Osteoblastoma, osteosarcoma

17. What is the main mechanism of the deleterious effects of radiation on the myocardium?
    (a) Direct damage to myocytes
    (b) Coronary artery fibrosis
    (c) Diffuse interstitial fibrosis
    (d) Coronary artery thrombosis

18. Which of the following drugs is the most probable to induce cardiotoxicity?
    (a) MTX
    (b) BCNU
    (c) 5FU
    (d) Melphalan

19. Considering the cardiotoxicity of doxorubicin, echocardiography for the evaluation of left ventricular function in patients without an underlying heart disease must be started when the cumulative dose is …
    (a) 400 mg/m^2
    (b) 550 mg/m^2
    (c) 200 mg/m^2
    (d) From the beginning of the drug treatment

1.16.1 Answer

	A	B	C	D
1	*			
2			*	
3				*
4			*	
5	*			
6		*		
7			*	
8			*	
9			*	
10				*
11	*			
12			*	
13			*	
14				*
15		*		
16	*			
17			*	
18			*	
19	*			

1.17 Use of Intraoperative Probes in Surgical Oncology

1. Radioimmuno-guided surgery (RIGS) is extensively studied in:
   (a) Colorectal cancer
   (b) Ovarian cancer
   (c) Breast cancer
   (d) Melanoma

2. What is the most suitable radioisotope for radioimmuno-guided surgery (RIGS)?
   (a) 125I
   (b) ^{123}I
   (c) ^{111}In
   (d) ^{99m}Tc

3. In this cancer, lymph node dissection is generally considered the standard care:
   (a) Melanoma
   (b) Head and neck cancer
   (c) Invasive breast cancer
   (d) Vulvar cancer

4. What is the most common crystal used in intraoperative probes?
   (a) Cadmium telluride (CdTe)
   (b) Thallium-activated sodium iodide [Na(Tl)]
   (c) Csl(Na)
   (d) Bgo

5. Sentinel node (SN) mapping in melanoma has a false-negative rate of:
   (a) <5.5%
   (b) <4.6%
   (c) <2.7%
   (d) <7.8%

6. Radioguided occult lesion localization (ROLL) is used in:
   (a) Penile cancer
   (b) Breast cancer
   (c) Head and neck cancer
   (d) Melanoma

7. In the surgery of minimally invasive parathyroid adenoma, which variable is the least important for gamma-probe selection?
   (a) Energy resolution
   (b) Sensitivity
   (c) Spatial resolution
   (d) Shielding

8. Gamma probe:
   (a) Sensitivity of the scintillation detector is better than that of the ionizing chamber.
   (b) Energy resolution of the ionizing chamber is better than that of the scintillation detector.
   (c) Energy resolution is more important than sensitivity of the system.
   (d) All of the above.

9. Which item about the application of surgical probes is NOT correct?
   (a) NaI crystals are typically used in scintillation probes.
   (b) Energy resolution is highly dependent on the design of the probe.
   (c) Bismuth germanate crystals are generally used in semiconducting probes.
   (d) Semiconducting detectors have a better energy resolution than scintillation detectors.

10. A gamma probe is extensively used for the identification of the sentinel node and for radio-guided surgery. Which of the following items about the selection and application of a gamma probe is NOT correct?
   (a) Probes with angular tips are the most user-friendly.
   (b) The use of collimators should be avoided as much as possible.
   (c) Weight, size, and shape of the probe are critical.
   (d) Scintillation detector is better than semiconductor probes in the evaluation of small lesions.

1.17.1 Answer

	A	B	C	D
1	*			
2	*			
3			*	
4	*			
5			*	
6		*		
7	*			
8				*
9			*	
10				*

1.18 Lymphatic Mapping and Sentinel Node Biopsy

1. The trapping of radiolabeled particles in the sentinel node by macrophages depends on all of the following variables *except*:
   (a) Route of administration
   (b) Particle size
   (c) Number of particles
   (d) Dosage of the radiopharmaceutical

2. Which radiopharmaceutical has the smallest particle size for lymphoscintigraphy?
   (a) ^{99m}Tc-DTPA mannosyl dextran
   (b) 198Au-colloid
   (c) ^{99m}Tc-nanocolloidal albumin
   (d) ^{99m}Tc-human serum albumin

3. Which anatomical region has the least predictability of drainage using lymphoscintigraphy?
   (a) Upper trunk
   (b) Lower trunk
   (c) Head and neck
   (d) Posterior trunk

4. The reason that may explain an absent or faint sentinel node uptake:
   (a) Patient age
   (b) Tumor involvement of the sentinel node
   (c) Insufficient number of particles
   (d) All of the above

5. The overall survival rate of melanoma is:
   (a) 20%
   (b) 40%
   (c) 60%
   (d) 80%

6. The sentinel nodes that are situated outside the known anatomic basins in melanoma patients (3.1–22%):
   (a) In-transit nodes
   (b) Interval nodes
   (c) Extra-anatomic nodes
   (d) All of the above

7. The most drainage to the axilla is from which part of the breast?
   (a) Upper outer quadrant
   (b) Lower inner quadrant
   (c) Center
   (d) Lower outer quadrant

8. The least sentinel node in the internal mammary chain region is seen in which part of the breast?
   (a) Upper outer quadrant
   (b) Lower outer quadrant
   (c) Lower inner quadrant
   (d) Center

9. The overall survival rate of patients with breast cancer and isolated internal mammary chain metastases is:
   (a) Higher than that of patients with isolated axillary lymph node involvement
   (b) Lower than that of patients with isolated axillary lymph node involvement
   (c) Similar to that of patients with isolated axillary lymph node involvement
   (d) None

10. Lymphatic mapping has been attempted in the followings situations *except*:
    (a) Esophageal cancer
    (b) Carcinoid
    (c) Small bowel cancer
    (d) Pheochromocytoma

11. Non-axillary drainage is the least observed in which of the following injections for the diagnosis of sentinel node?
    (a) Intradermal
    (b) Subcutaneous
    (c) Peritumoral
    (d) Intratumoral

12. Choose the correct statement regarding sentinel node.
    (a) Sentinel node is the nearest node to the primary tumor.
    (b) Sentinel node is the hottest node in the field.
    (c) Sentinel node is the first node in the field.
    (d) All of the above.

13. Regarding sentinel node:
    (a) In peritumoral injection, delayed imaging is necessary.
    (b) In intradermal injection, the sentinel node usually appears in 1 h.
    (c) Both.
    (d) None.

14. What is the most important factor determining the indication for SLNB in patients with melanoma?
    (a) Pigmentation rate
    (b) Mitotic rate
    (c) Ulceration
    (d) Breslow thickness

15. In which anatomical regions is the lymphatic drainage of melanoma the most and least predicted, respectively?
    (a) Head and neck–upper extremities
    (b) Trunk–lower extremities
    (c) Upper extremities–trunk
    (d) Lower extremities–head and neck

16. Which of the following is NOT an advantage of sentinel lymph node (SLN) biopsy over axillary lymph node dissection (ALND)?
    (a) Standard practical protocol
    (b) Lower morbidity
    (c) Possibility for immunohistochemistry
    (d) Possibility for multiple incisions

17. Which of the following areas of injection does NOT show the drainage pathway of inguinal lymph nodes, external iliac, and para-aorta?
    (a) Metatarsus
    (b) Vulva
    (c) Penis
    (d) Prostate

18. Radiocolloid accumulation is observed in a chain including three lymph nodes in a patient with breast cancer. In 5 min images, the node with the shortest distance from injection site has the highest activity, and in 20 min images, the node with the longest distance shows more activity. Which one is the sentinel node?
    (a) Both nodes with the shortest and longest distance
    (b) Node with the shortest distance
    (c) Middle node
    (d) Node with the longest distance

19. Which characteristic is required for the method of choice in the detection and evaluation of the sentinel lymph node in breast cancer?
    (a) Low negative predictive value
    (b) High positive predictive value
    (c) High negative predictive value
    (d) Low positive predictive value

20. Which method is used to increase the possibility of simultaneously detecting the sentinel lymph node in the axillary and internal mammary?
    (a) Combined intradermal and deep subdermal injections
    (b) Subareolar injection only
    (c) Intradermal injection only
    (d) Combined intradermal and deep intradermal injections

21. What is the difference between intradermal and subcutaneous injection of a radiopharmaceutical in the lymphoscintigraphy of malignant melanoma?
    (a) Intradermal injection is easier.
    (b) Observing the drainage pathway is less problematic in intradermal injection.
    (c) No significant difference can be found between intradermal and subcutaneous injection.
    (d) Rapid movement of the radiopharmaceutical in intradermal injection.

22. The goal is to observe the sentinel lymph node in lymphoscintigraphy. Which of the following radiopharmaceuticals results in the most rapid observation of this node because of its small particle size?
    (a) Tc-antimony sulfur colloid
    (b) Tc-sulfur colloid
    (c) Tc-phytate
    (d) Tc-HAS

23. The most sentinel nodes in the internal mammary chain region is seen in tumors located in the following part of the breast:
    (a) Upper outer quadrant
    (b) Inner quadrant
    (c) Lower outer quadrant
    (d) Center

24. Which of the following radiopharmaceuticals is associated with in vivo colloid formation in lymphoscintigraphy?
    (a) ^{99m}Tc-sulfur colloid
    (b) ^{99m}Tc-HAS-nanocolloid
    (c) ^{99m}Tc-stannous phytate
    (d) ^{99m}Tc-antimony sulfide colloid

25. A patient with posterior melanoma near the head of the right scapula is subjected to lymphoscintigraphy. The axillary lymph nodes of both sides are observed in the scan. What is the next step?
    (a) Bilateral biopsy of the observed lymph nodes
    (b) Bilateral dissection because of the bilateral lymphatic metastasis
    (c) Expected view, no specific intervention is required
    (d) Biopsy of the observed lymph nodes on the right side

26. Variable radiopharmaceuticals are used for lymphoscintigraphy. What are the radiopharmaceuticals of choice for the observation of lymphatic vessels (drainage pathway) and for the determination of the sentinel lymph node, respectively? (noncolloid, HAS and dextran; colloid, sulfur colloid)
    (a) Noncolloid, noncolloid
    (b) Colloid, colloid
    (c) Colloid, noncolloid
    (d) Noncolloid, colloid

27. In the process of lymphoscintigraphy of breast cancer, imaging before any operation is strongly recommended because in ... of patients, more than one sentinel node can be visualized.
    (a) 10%
    (b) 40%
    (c) 20%
    (d) 30%

28. The lymph node is NOT observed in 4–6 h images after injection in the internal mammary lymphoscintigram. Which of the following items is the most probable?
    (a) Bilateral parasternal abnormality
    (b) Technical error and inadequate bilateral injection
    (c) Abnormality of distal ipsilateral nodes
    (d) Normal anatomic submanubrial cross-drainage

29. Which nodes are identified as intercalated nodes?
    (a) Popliteal lymph nodes in the lymphoscintigraphy of lesions in the lower limbs
    (b) Secondary lymph nodes in the lymphoscintigraphy of melanoma
    (c) Lymph nodes in an abnormal anatomic pathway in lymphoscintigraphy
    (d) Axillary lymph nodes in the lymphoscintigraphy of lesions in the upper limbs

30. Isotopic lymphoscintigraphy:
    (a) Abnormal lymph nodes are observed as the regions with high uptakes.
    (b) Only superficial lymphatic nodes can be evaluated with this method.
    (c) The involved lymph nodes can be detected even if their size is normal.
    (d) This technique has a high-radiation dose and morbidity.

31. A patient suffering from breast cancer is a candidate for axillary lymphoscintigraphy. What happens to the scan result with the presence of inflammation in these nodes, and what is the recommended method of correction?
    (a) False-positive finding, regional massage, or delayed imaging.
    (b) False-negative finding, increase in the dose and volume of the radiotracer.
    (c) False-negative finding, no specific intervention is suggested.
    (d) No effect on the scan result; therefore, no specific intervention is required.

32. What is the range of the injected particle size in lymphoscintigraphy?
    (a) More than 2000 mm
    (b) Less than 100 mm
    (c) Less than 2 mm
    (d) More than 1000 mm

33. What is the reason for the absence of lymph nodes in the lymphoscintigraphy with intra-parenchymal injection in a patient with breast cancer?
    (a) Particle size of 5–100 nm
    (b) Injected dose of 100 MBq
    (c) Imaging 2 h after injection
    (d) High specific activity of the particles

34. Which of the following statements about the evaluation of sentinel lymph node (SLN) in breast cancer is NOT correct?
   (a) The count of SLN is ideally ten times that of the background count.
   (b) The optimal sensitivity of the test is achieved with the synchronization of the probe and blue dye imaging.
   (c) The learning curve phenomenon is one of the reasons for the varying reports from different centers.
   (d) SLN is always the hottest lymph node.

1.18.1 Answer

	A	B	C	D
1	*			
2				*
3			*	
4				*
5				*
6				*
7			*	
8	*			
9			*	
10				*
11		*		
12			*	
13			*	
14				*
15				*
16	*			
17				*
18	*			
19			*	
20	*			
21				*
22	*			
23		*		
24				*
25	*			
26				*
27			*	
28		*		
29	*			
30			*	
31			*	
32		*		
33			*	
34				*

1.19 PET Imaging of Head and Neck Cancer

1. The anterior cervical nodes in the head and neck lymph node classification are categorized in:
   (a) Level III
   (b) Level IV
   (c) Level V
   (d) Level VI

2. Regarding PET imaging:
   (a) Proceeding is inadvisable if the serum glucose level exceeds 200 mg/dl (11 mmol/l).
   (b) Gum chewing should be allowed.
   (c) The uptake period between FDG injection and the start of imaging should be at least 45 min.
   (d) Recent radiation may cause inflammation lasting 2 months.

3. What is the best indication for FDG-PET imaging in head and neck malignancies?
   (a) Unknown primary
   (b) Restaging/recurrence
   (c) Assessing treatment response
   (d) Surveillance and follow-up

4. Regarding head and neck cancers:
   (a) A negative PET scan can exclude metastatic neck disease.
   (b) Squamous cell cancers of the middle cervical nodes likely metastasize from below the clavicle.
   (c) The sensitivity of PET scan for detecting a recurrent disease is higher than its specificity.
   (d) It is probably prudent to wait at least 1 month following surgery before undergoing PET imaging.

5. Which is the best indication for FDG-PET in a patient with head and neck tumor?
   (a) Metastasis without diagnosis of a primary tumor
   (b) A tumor with N0
   (c) Response to treatment
   (d) Follow-up

6. A 69-year-old man with a history of SCC of the neck underwent complete treatment. A focal abnormal uptake in the neck is observed in FDG-PET 1 year after treatment, but a non-specific finding is reported in the biopsy. What is the next step?
   (a) Repeat of biopsy
   (b) CT of neck
   (c) MRI of neck
   (d) Further evaluation is NOT required

7. Head and neck tumors:
   (a) CT scan, clinical examination, and endoscopy provide anatomical data similar to those of PET for the staging of the primary tumor.
   (b) The sensitivity of the PET scan is similar to that of the CT scan, MRI, and sonography for the evaluation of a local node.
   (c) The sensitivity of the PET scan for the detection of a residual disease after treatment is similar to that of a needle biopsy.
   (d) Radiation-induced hypermetabolism interferes with the detection of tumor recurrence by PET scan.

8. A patient following IV contrast for CT scan has developed nausea, vomiting, and urticaria. What is the most appropriate management?
   (a) Intravenous corticosteroid administration
   (b) Half-an-hour observation
   (c) Reassurance and discharge
   (d) Subcutaneous epinephrine

9. Which of the following statements regarding the application of PET in head and neck cancers is NOT correct?
   (a) PET is significantly prior to MRI for presurgical staging.
   (b) The accuracy of PET for the detection of tumor recurrence is greater than (about two times) that of CT and MRI.
   (c) The accuracy of PET for the staging of a nodal disease is greater than that of CT and MRI.
   (d) b and c.

10. In which of the following situations is follow-up alone recommended for a suspected recurrent head and neck tumor although the tumor is suitable for curable treatment?
    (a) Negative findings of the head and neck PET study
    (b) Positive findings of the head and neck PET study
    (c) Positive findings of the head and neck PET study but negative findings of the whole-body PET scan
    (d) Positive findings of the head and neck PET scan with distant metastatic lesions in whole-body PET scan

11. Head and neck PET scan and whole-body PET scan are positive for a patient with suspected recurrence of head and neck cancer. Which statement regarding the necessity of a biopsy for this patient is correct?
    (a) All lesions require confirmation with biopsy.
    (b) Confirmation with biopsy is NOT required.
    (c) Only intense lesions require confirmation.
    (d) Some lesions (e.g., multiple bone or pulmonary lesions) do NOT require confirmation, but some other lesions do.

12. What is the most commonly used imaging modality for the staging of head and neck squamous cell carcinomas (HNSCCs)?
    (a) CT without iodine contrast
    (b) CT with iodine contrast
    (c) MRI with gadolinium-based contrast
    (d) PET/CT

13. Tumor metabolism can be at the baseline level of soft tissue as early as.... after chemotherapy in responding HNSCC patients.
    (a) 12–16 months
    (b) 12–24 months
    (c) 2 months
    (d) 1 week

14. What is the most common site of distant recurrence in HNSCC patients?
    (a) Colon
    (b) Lung
    (c) Liver
    (d) Kidney

15. Which of the following studies is critical for the staging of nasopharyngeal cancer?
    (a) Bone scan
    (b) Thoracic CT scan
    (c) Panendoscopy
    (d) PET scan

16. Which area is the most common region of metastasis in head and neck cancers?
    (a) Liver
    (b) Bone
    (c) Lungs
    (d) Brain

17. Which of the following items is recommended for the reduction of FDG muscular uptake artifact in evaluating head and neck malignancies?
    (a) Imipramine administration
    (b) Extension of the head and neck during FDG uptake
    (c) Chewing gum before FDG injection
    (d) Diazepam administration

1.19.1 Answer

	A	B	C	D
1				*
2	*			
3				*

4			*	
5				*
6	*			
7				*
8		*		
9	*			
10	*			
11				*
12		*		
13				*
14		*		
15			*	
16			*	
17				*

1.20 External Beam Radiotherapy Treatment Planning with PET

1. In respiratory correlation for PET imaging:
   (a) Respiratory motion causes a blurring effect in PET imaging.
   (b) Motion artifacts lead to an underestimation of lesion size.
   (c) Motion artifacts lead to an overestimation of the corresponding standardized uptake value (SUV).
   (d) Breath-hold techniques are more interventional than respiratory gating techniques for the reduction of respiratory motion.

2. Respiratoryt motion:
   (a) Decreases image contrast.
   (b) Affects the detection of lesion.
   (c) The smearing artifact results in the overestimation of the metabolic target volume (MTV).
   (d) All of the above.

3. All the following statements regarding PET for therapy response are true *except*:
   (a) The goal of late prediction using PET imaging is to predict the future outcome.
   (b) Defined responses are usually specific to particular tumors, time intervals, and treatment methods.
   (c) A negative posttreatment PET scan typically has a lower predictive value than a negative midtreatment scan.
   (d) A negative posttreatment PET scan can differentiate between a few log units and many log units of tumor cell killing.

4. The effect of PET on the radiation therapy planning (RTP) process can be seen in:
   (a) A more accurate staging
   (b) Delineating the accurate volume and the extent of the disease
   (c) Dose painting and theragnostic imaging
   (d) All of the above

5. What is the most appropriate imaging method for determining the field of radiotherapy in low-grade glioma?
   (a) CT scan with contrast
   (b) T1-weighted MRI with gadolinium injection
   (c) T2-weighted MRI with gadolinium injection
   (d) PET scan

6. Which of the following statements about intensity-modulated radiotherapy (IMRT) is correct?
   (a) Radiation exposure of healthy organs is more important than that of the tumor in inverse planning.
   (b) The absorbed dose of different regions in a planning target volume (PTV) is different in IRMT.
   (c) The optimal dose distribution in IRMT is due to its excellent beam flatness.
   (d) Optimal dose distribution is defined as an input for a dose-monitoring computer in inverse planning.

1.20.1 Answer

	A	B	C	D
1	*			
2				*
3				*
4				*
5			*	
6				*

1.21 PET in Aerodigestive Tumors

1. Regarding solitary pulmonary nodule (SPN):
   (a) Calcification in radiography favors a malignant etiology.
   (b) About 60% of SPNs are malignant.
   (c) Popcorn calcification is suggestive of a benign pathology.
   (d) The current standard approach is to perform PET/CT for initial evaluation.

2. Observing the SPNs over the next few months to confirm that they do not change in size is necessary, but this is a common problem in all of the following tumors *except*:
   (a) Carcinoid tumors
   (b) Bronchoalveolar cancers (BAC)
   (c) Mucinous tumors
   (d) Small-cell lung carcinoma

3. All of the following regions are common sites of distant metastasis with the origin of lung cancer *except*:
   (a) Adrenal glands
   (b) Brain
   (c) Bone
   (d) Spleen

4. FDG-PET in esophageal cancer has a limited role in:
   (a) Assessment of the aggressiveness of the tumor
   (b) Prognosis of the patient
   (c) Identification of the lymph node metastasis
   (d) Identification of the primary tumor

5. It is generally accepted that FDG uptake … after radiation is usually associated with colorectal tumor recurrence.
   (a) 1 month
   (b) 2 months
   (c) 4 months
   (d) 6 months

6. Regarding the effect of PET on the treatment of colorectal cancer:
   (a) It changes the treatment in >30% of patients and changes the stage in 20%.
   (b) It changes the treatment in >15% of patients and changes the stage in 12%.
   (c) It changes the treatment in >10% of patients and changes the stage in 8%.
   (d) It changes the treatment in >5% of patients and changes the stage in 3%.

7. In pancreatic cancer:
   (a) The use of PET to detect peritoneal lesions is limited.
   (b) The major advantage of PET is its sensitivity in comparison with CT.
   (c) Patients with obvious metastases on CT require PET.
   (d) Those with a fasting blood sugar >100 mg/dl can have low sensitivity levels.

8. In hepatocellular carcinoma:
   (a) Abscesses with granulomatous inflammation have an FDG uptake greater than that of a normal liver.
   (b) Regenerative nodules have an FDG uptake greater than that of a normal liver.
   (c) PET detects many of the well-differentiated HCC lesions.
   (d) A lesion that is suspected for malignancy detected by PET should be considered for urgent therapy.

9. Which item is considered a limitation of FDG-PET in patients with colorectal carcinoma?
   (a) Lower sensitivity for the detection of mucinous than for non-mucinous tumors
   (b) Application in primary staging
   (c) Detection of recurrences
   (d) All of the above

10. In which of the following tumors does FDG-PET have the least sensitivity?
    (a) Colorectal carcinoma
    (b) Stomach carcinoma
    (c) Pancreas adenocarcinoma
    (d) Hepatocellular carcinoma

11. A 3 cm nodule in the right lung is found in the chest radiography of a 65-year-old male smoker who is currently suffering from chronic cough. This nodule does NOT show an uptake in ^{18}F-FDG-PET. What is the next step?
    (a) Follow-up with CT scan
    (b) Gallium scan
    (c) Biopsy with the aid of bronchoscopy
    (d) Repeat of chest radiography after 6 months

12. In which of the following items is 18F-FDG-PET preferred over CT scan in a patient with esophageal cancer?
    (a) Diagnosis of the primary tumor
    (b) Diagnosis of the regional progression of the tumor
    (c) Diagnosis of distant metastasis
    (d) Determination of the surgical field

13. A 59-year-old man with non-small-cell lung cancer is subjected to FDG-PET for primary staging, and stage II is determined by the scan results. What is the next step?
    (a) Bone scan for a more accurate staging
    (b) Thoracoscopy and evaluation of the lymph node in the opposite site
    (c) Bone marrow aspiration
    (d) Beginning of treatment

14. In which of the following conditions is FDG-PET NOT helpful in the evaluation of a patient with colorectal cancer?
    (a) Preoperative evaluation of the tumor thickness
    (b) Increase in carcinoembryonic antigen (CEA) with a normal abdominal CT scan
    (c) Evaluation of a solitary hepatic lesion detected by sonography
    (d) Changes in the resection site of the CT scan and relapse of GI symptoms after surgery and treatment

15. About the application of PET in esophageal cancer:
    (a) In countries with a high incidence of tuberculosis, PET is useful in the staging of esophageal cancer.
    (b) The efficiency of FDG-PET for the detection of the primary tumor of the esophagus is limited.
    (c) Metastasis of the small lymph nodes near the primary tumor is always detected.
    (d) ^{11}C-cholin PET in the upper abdomen is more sensitive than ^{18}F-FDG-PET in the detection of small metastases.

16. What is the radiopharmaceutical of choice for the evaluation of multidrug resistance in pulmonary tumors?
    (a) ^{201}Tl
    (b) DMSA (V)
    (c) Somatostatin
    (d) ^{99m}Tc-MIBI

17. PET scan is performed for a patient with a pulmonary nodule. Imaging demonstrates an SUV of 1.3 for the images of the nodule zone with a negative scan. Therefore, a biopsy is performed because of the clinical suspect, and the result is positive lung cancer. Which item does NOT justify these findings?
    (a) Bronchoalveolar carcinoma
    (b) Carcinoid tumor
    (c) Partial volume lesion
    (d) Tuberculosis

18. A patient with a history of colorectal cancer with an increased CEA level is referred. What is the recommended method for the diagnosis and staging?
    (a) FDG-PET plus radioimmunoscintigraphy
    (b) FDG-PET plus CT
    (c) CT plus radioimmunoscintigraphy
    (d) ^{11}C-choline PET plus CT

19. A 53-year-old patient with NSSLC is subjected to chemotherapy. What is the best prognostic factor for the estimation of survival?
    (a) Posttreatment PET scan
    (b) Clinical status
    (c) CT response
    (d) Pretreatment performance status

20. What is the best prognostic value in the PET scan of a patient with lung cancer?
    (a) Tumor location
    (b) SUV
    (c) Tumor size
    (d) Central necrosis of tumor

21. CT scan and PET scan are used for the staging and estimation of prognosis in a patient with non-small-cell lung cancer (NSCLC). Which item is correct?
    (a) PET scan after treatment better predicts survival than CT scan.
    (b) FDG uptake in the tumor (SUV) is not related to malignancy or prognosis.
    (c) Patients with an SUV of less than five have a significantly low survival rate.
    (d) PET scan is NOT a quantitative method for the evaluation of the biological effects of anticancer treatments.

22. A patient with colorectal cancer, high possibility of relapse, and metastasis is a candidate for surgery. Which modality offers the highest diagnostic accuracy?
    (a) CT scan
    (b) Measurement of CEA
    (c) Sonography
    (d) ^{18}FDG-PET

23. Diagnosis of suspected pulmonary cancer:
    (a) PET and CT scan have similar diagnostic accuracy for the differentiation of benign and malignant cancers.
    (b) Conventional imaging methods are currently replaced by PET.
    (c) Patients with a positive PET scan of the chest do NOT need extensive surgery for staging.
    (d) PET scan is the gold standard for the evaluation of a solitary pulmonary nodule.

24. A 69-year-old woman is subjected to radiotherapy because of pharyngeal cancer. Five months later, PET scan is performed to evaluate the efficiency of the treatment. The results show an increased uptake with SUV = 4.9 in the tumor region. What is the most probable cause of this finding?
    (a) Recent radiotherapy
    (b) Superimposed infection
    (c) Failure of therapy
    (d) Presence of fibrosis and necrosis in the tumor

25. Which item about the SUV and survival of patients with NSCLC is correct?
    (a) SUV is NOT important in survival rate.
    (b) Patients with SUV > 10 show better disease-free survival.
    (c) Patients with SUV < 5 show better disease-free survival.
    (d) Patients with SUV > 15 show better disease-free survival.

26. In which of the following conditions is ^{18}F-FDG-PET economical for the evaluation of a solitary pulmonary nodule?
    (a) Low pretest probability and evidence of malignancy in CT scan
    (b) High pretest probability and evidence of malignancy in CT scan
    (c) Low pretest probability and evidence of a benign lesion in CT scan
    (d) High pretest probability and low risk of surgical complication

27. Which item about the evaluation of esophageal cancer with FDG-PET is NOT correct?
    (a) The intensity of FDG uptake in the primary tumor provides prognostic value.
    (b) It has more sensitivity than CT scan in detecting primary esophageal cancer.
    (c) It is preferred over CT plus ultrasonography for evaluating the involvement of local lymph nodes.
    (d) Severe esophagitis can cause a false-positive outcome.

28. A single pulmonary nodule with an intermediate size is observed in chest X-ray of the right lung of a patient with a low economic and social level. Transthoracic needle aspiration (TTNA) indicates negative results for malignancy. In addition, this region shows an increased uptake with SUV > 2.6 in the FDG-PET scan. Which item is recommended for this patient?
    (a) A more accurate evaluation is required according to the FDG-PET findings.
    (b) Negative TTNA completely rejects malignancy and further evaluation is not required.
    (c) SUV > 2.5 in the FDG-PET of this patient indicates malignancy.
    (d) The lifestyle of this patient decreases the possibility of a false-positive finding on FDG-PET scan.

29. Which of the following organs is NOT a common site of lung cancer spread?
    (a) Adrenal glands
    (b) Bone marrow
    (c) Brain
    (d) Pancreas

30. Which of the following modalities is the most valuable for the staging of pulmonary cancer?
    (a) CT
    (b) PET
    (c) PET/CT
    (d) Visual side-by-side review of PET and CT

31. In which of the following conditions is FDG-PET recommended for the evaluation of a single pulmonary nodule?
    (a) Low pretest probability for malignancy
    (b) Intermediate pretest probability for malignancy
    (c) High pretest probability for malignancy
    (d) Very high pretest probability for malignancy

32. In which of the following situations is FDG-PET NOT valuable for the evaluation of pulmonary cancer?
    (a) Staging
    (b) Bone metastasis
    (c) Brain metastasis
    (d) Adrenal metastasis

33. A 59-year-old man with a history of smoking for 12 years, hemoptysis, and a single pulmonary nodule in lung radiography is referred for ^{18}F-FDG scan. The nodules show an uptake with an SUV of 6. Furthermore, laboratory tests show Na, 132; K, 3.6; and Ca, 8.9. What is the most probable diagnosis?
    (a) Pulmonary SCC
    (b) Tuberculosis
    (c) Hamartoma
    (d) Small-cell lung cancer

34. A 62-year-old man with a history of colon cancer is referred with CEA threefold that of the normal value. ^{18}F-FDG scan is less sensitive than CT scan in which part if the goal is to identify metastasis?
    (a) Liver
    (b) Retroperitoneal
    (c) Lung
    (d) Abdominal lymphadenopathy

35. CXR reveals opacity with distinct margins without atelectasis and lymphadenopathy in a 32-year-old woman. This lesion appears on the CT scan with clear margins and without calcification. The patient has a 12-year history of smoking (half a pack per day). The lesion shows an uptake in ^{18}F-FDG-PET with an SUV of 1.5. Which item is correct?
    (a) This pulmonary lesion is malignant with high probability.
    (b) This pulmonary lesion is a benign lesion with high probability.
    (c) Benign and malignant lesions canNOT be distinguished because of the uptake on the scan.
    (d) ^{99m}Tc-deoretide scan is recommended.

36. A 56-year-old patient diagnosed with pulmonary cancer is subjected to ^{18}FDG-PET scan. A radiotracer uptake is observed in the pulmonary tumor, and no other abnormal activity is found. What is the next appropriate intervention for staging?
    (a) Mediastinal angiography
    (b) Mediastinoscopy
    (c) Mediastinal MRI
    (d) No further intervention is required

37. FDG-PET scan is performed for a patient with a pulmonary lesion, and the results show an SUV of two. Which of the following items is the least possible?
    (a) Pulmonary TB
    (b) Pulmonary carcinoid
    (c) Non-small-cell lung carcinoma
    (d) Bronchoalveolar carcinoma

38. An abnormal increase in the tumor uptake is observed on the FDG-PET scan of a 73-year-old man with history of colorectal cancer. Therefore, he is subjected to radiotherapy. How long after the completion of radiotherapy can an uptake in the follow-up scan indicate tumor recurrence?
    (a) 3 months
    (b) 9 months
    (c) 6 months
    (d) 12 months

39. Which of the following finding in solitary nodules indicates a benign lesion?
    (a) FDG uptake
    (b) Anti-CEA mAb uptake
    (c) Calcification in the CXR
    (d) Irregular and unclear margins in the CXR

40. What is the most reliable method for the staging of bronchogenic mediastinal carcinoma?
    (a) FDG-PET
    (b) Mediastinoscopy
    (c) MRI
    (d) CT

41. What is the most important role of FDG-PET in colorectal cancer?
    (a) Diagnosis before surgery
    (b) Initial staging
    (c) Differentiation of operable and inoperable diseases
    (d) Accurate localization of the primary lesion

42. Which of the following items describes the features of PET imaging for lung cancer?
    (a) Very high specificity for detecting a malignant nodule
    (b) High accuracy for T staging of the primary tumor
    (c) High diagnostic value for brain metastasis in asymptomatic patients
    (d) Very high negative predictive value for low-risk patients

43. A 69-year-old man with esophageal squamous cell cancer underwent surgery and chemotherapy. Four months later, you are consulted to evaluate a residual tumor. What is the recommended method?
    (a) High-resolution ultrasonography
    (b) Endoscopic ultrasound-guided FNA
    (c) High-resolution CT scan
    (d) ^{18}F-FDG-PET/CT

44. Which of the following items regarding the normal mean SUV value is true?
    (a) The normal liver has a mean SUV of 3.2 ± 0.8.
    (b) The normal spleen has a mean SUV of 2.4 ± 0.6.
    (c) The normal pancreas has a mean SUV of 2.0 ± 0.5.
    (d) All of the above.

45. Which of the following statements regarding the role of PET in solitary pulmonary nodules is NOT true?
    (a) With a pretest probability of 80%, the probability of malignancy is still 14% with a negative PET.
    (b) Considering the pretest probability of malignancy with a negative PET scan result is important.
    (c) A negative PET result is usually more accurate than a positive result.
    (d) PET/CT relative to PET alone has a significantly high sensitivity.

46. What is the most common false-negative malignant pulmonary nodule in PET imaging?
    (a) Bronchoalveolar carcinoma
    (b) Differentiated adenocarcinoma
    (c) Mucoepidermoid carcinoma
    (d) Carcinoid

47. In lung base nodules:
    (a) PET/CT should be used with caution in nodules near the hemidiaphragms.
    (b) A photopenic respiratory misregistration artifact is observed.
    (c) SUV can be artifactually decreased in these nodules.
    (d) All of the above.

48. What is the most useful indication of PET imaging in the mediastinal staging of non-small-cell lung cancer?
    (a) In patients without enlarged mediastinal nodes on CT
    (b) In patients with enlarged mediastinal nodes on CT
    (c) In clinical stage I (peripheral) tumors
    (d) b and c

49. What is the limited role of PET imaging in the distant staging of non-small-cell lung cancer?
    (a) Clinical stage IV
    (b) Clinical stage III
    (c) Clinical Stage II
    (d) In clinical stage I (peripheral) tumors

50. If the goal is the mediastinal staging of non-small-cell lung cancer, all of the following statements regarding the comparison of PET with other modalities are true *except*:
    (a) PET is superior to CT for N0, N2, and N3 diseases but not for N1 diseases.
    (b) PET has a lower frequency of false-positive findings in the upper mediastinal nodes.
    (c) PET has a lower frequency of false-negative findings in adenocarcinoma.
    (d) PET has a lower frequency of false-negative findings in squamous cell carcinoma.

51. If the goal is the mediastinal staging of non-small-cell lung cancer, all of the following statements regarding the comparison of PET/CT with other modalities are true *except*:
    (a) PET/CT is superior to PET for T (tumor) staging.
    (b) PET/CT is ideally suited for assessing chest wall and mediastinal invasion.
    (c) PET/CT has superior specificity to PET alone for left hilar, subaortic, and right paratracheal nodes.
    (d) PET/CT has superior accuracy to PET alone for subcarinal and interlobar nodes.

52. All of the following statements regarding the role PET in mesothelioma are true *except*:
    (a) PET may have limited sensitivity for the determination of the extent of a local tumor.
    (b) The primary value of PET is to identify extra-thoracic metastases and obviate thoracotomy.
    (c) A localized fibrous tumor of the pleura typically has a high uptake (SUV > 2.5).
    (d) Most benign pleural processes have an SUV < 2.2.

53. Regarding the role PET in gastric cancer, all of the following statements are true *except*:
   (a) Signet ring cell and mucinous carcinomas have a low FDG uptake.
   (b) Poorly differentiated tumors may appear to have a low uptake because of infiltration in the gastric wall.
   (c) Well-differentiated tumors may appear to have a high uptake because of mass formation.
   (d) The amount of uptake in the primary tumor correlates well with the histopathology.

54. In detecting primary esophageal cancer:
   (a) PET can accurately determine the T stage.
   (b) Adenocarcinomas and squamous cell carcinomas generally have a similar degree of FDG uptake.
   (c) PET can detect T1a tumors.
   (d) PET is useful for the evaluation of primary esophageal tumors.

55. What is the most cost-effective method for the staging of esophageal cancer?
   (a) PET
   (b) Endoscopic ultrasound (EUS)
   (c) MRI
   (d) a and b

56. What is the standard imaging modality for primary gastrointestinal stromal tumor (GIST)?
   (a) PET
   (b) CT
   (c) MRI
   (d) Endoscopic ultrasound (EUS)

57. In which of the following gastrointestinal (GI) tumors is the clinical indication of FDG-PET well established and its value supported by a large amount of clinical experience and literature?
   (a) Gastric cancer
   (b) Recurrence of esophageal cancer
   (c) Gastrointestinal stromal tumor (GIST)
   (d) Therapy response of esophageal cancer

58. Regarding the role PET in pancreatic masses and adenocarcinoma, all of the following statements are true *except*:
   (a) The sensitivity for periampullary neoplasms is less than that for neoplasm elsewhere in the pancreas.
   (b) PET is more effective than CT for lesions >4 cm.
   (c) If CT shows no discrete mass, a positive PET will be highly predictive for malignancy.
   (d) If CT is indeterminate, a positive PET will be less specific for malignancy but very sensitive.

59. Regarding the characteristics of malignant versus inflammatory masses in the pancreas:
    (a) Inflammatory lesions are usually more focal than diffuse.
    (b) The absence of clinical and laboratory findings of acute pancreatitis rules out an inflammatory etiology for a pancreatic mass.
    (c) The majority of patients with chronic pancreatitis have positive PET exams.
    (d) The possibility of malignancy should still be pursued in patients with chronic pancreatitis and positive PET.

60. Which FDG uptake pattern in colorectal cancer is usually secondary to inflammation?
    (a) Nodular colonic uptake
    (b) Segmental uptake
    (c) Diffuse uptake
    (d) a and b

61. PET/CT frequently adds staging information in:
    (a) Upper rectal cancers
    (b) Middle rectal cancers
    (c) Lower rectal cancers
    (d) Entire rectal cancers

62. All of the following statements about solitary pulmonary nodules are correct *except*:
    (a) The accuracy of the FDG-PET scan for the discrimination of benign and malignant nodules with a diameter of less than 1 cm is high.
    (b) The incidence of malignancy in subjects over 35 years old is high.
    (c) Simple radiography and CT are the most commonly used methods for diagnosis.
    (d) Calcification in radiography indicates a benign tumor.

63. In which of the following tumors does PET/CT have the most probability of failure in detection?
    (a) Salivary gland tumors
    (b) SCC of the larynx
    (c) Ductal carcinoma of the breast
    (d) Adenocarcinoma of the pancreas

64. Which of the following statements regarding PET/CT in colon cancer is true?
    (a) It is an appropriate modality to assess regional lymph nodes.
    (b) It is not useful for the differentiation of adenomatous polyps from cancers.
    (c) It cannot help in the diagnosis of tumoral recurrence in the anastomosis site because of postsurgical changes.
    (d) PET alone (without CT) is sensitive enough for the diagnosis of liver metastases.

65. Which of the following statements about lung cancer is true?
    (a) Approximately 60% of small-cell lung cancer and 30–40% of non-small-cell lung cancer are in stage IV at the time of detection.
    (b) PET scanning is NEITHER capable of detecting lesions smaller than 15 mm NOR a standard method for the assessment of lung tumors.
    (c) Sputum cytology is a test with a positive predictive value of about 80% and a sensitivity rate of 60–80% for the detection of lung tumors.
    (d) The histologic types are based on the analysis by IHC and molecular structures.

66. A patient with thymoma is operated by a thoracic surgeon. During operation, the surgeon realizes that the pericardium is also involved. Pericardial involvement is confirmed in the pathology report. What is the next best step?
    (a) 45 Gy radiation with anterior–posterior mediastinal fields
    (b) 50 Gy radiation with anterior–posterior mediastinal and supraclavicular fields
    (c) Cisplatin-based chemotherapy
    (d) Follow-up of the patient with PET scan

67. A 39-year-old man with nonseminomatous germ cell tumor of the mediastinum underwent initial therapy. CT scan shows a remarkable decrease in size (size is 3 cm post-therapy). In addition, the serum levels of the tumor markers are reduced but are not in the normal ranges. What further evaluation is indicated?
    (a) If the PET scan is unremarkable, then he will be observed.
    (b) Surgical resection of the mass
    (c) Salvage chemotherapy with a platinum-based regimen
    (d) Intraoperative radiotherapy to the mass

68. A large, well-marginated solitary pulmonary nodule (5 cm in diameter) in the periphery of the right lung is found incidentally in the chest X-ray of a 29-year-old man. What should be your next step in management?
    (a) Conduct a CT-guided biopsy immediately
    (b) Prescribe an antibiotic therapy for 2 weeks and a control chest X-ray
    (c) Perform a lung CT scan with lesion densitometry and abdominal sonography
    (d) Prescribe a control chest X-ray after 3 months

69. In all of following conditions, further correlation with thoracic HRCT is recommended *except*:
    (a) Densitometry of the solitary pulmonary nodule
    (b) Ruling out of lung metastasis
    (c) Emphysema diagnosis
    (d) Diagnosis of lung involvement in immunocompromised patients

70. What is the maximum normal size of the main pulmonary artery on the CT scan?
(a) 30 mm
(b) 15 mm
(c) 20 mm
(d) 35 mm

71. Which of the following metastatic lung cancers has the least growing rate?
(a) Choriocarcinoma
(b) Breast cancer
(c) Seminoma
(d) Osteogenic sarcoma

72. What is the most appropriate modality for the detection of metastatic involvement of the mediastinal lymph node in bronchogenic carcinoma?
(a) CT scan
(b) Chest X-ray + CT scan
(c) PET/CT
(d) MRI

73. An indeterminate nodule larger than 10 mm is found in the right lung on the HRCT of a patient. In which of the following situations is contrast CT or PET scan required before surgery and biopsy?
(a) If the lesion is solid
(b) If the lesion is ground glass accompanied with a solid component
(c) If the lesion is ground glass without a solid component
(d) It is necessary in all of the above situations

74. Which of the following statement regarding thymoma is true?
(a) The most common tumor in the anterior mediastinum.
(b) Present in 10–28% of cases accompanied with myasthenia gravis.
(c) MRI is more sensitive than CT scan for the detection of local invasion.
(d) ^{131}I-MIBG is used to asses this tumor.

75. A solitary pulmonary nodule is found on the lung CT scan of a 37-year-old patient. Which of the following findings is usually suggestive of a benign etiology rather than a malignant process?
(a) Eccentric calcification
(b) Intralesional fat
(c) Diameter smaller than 1 cm
(d) Circular shape

76. Which of the following calcification patterns in a solitary pulmonary nodule (SPN) is suggestive of malignancy?
(a) Eccentric
(b) Laminated
(c) Concentric
(d) Popcorn

77. Which of the following methods is the best modality for differentiating fibrosis from a residual tumor?
    (a) MRI with contrast
    (b) PET
    (c) Multidetector CT (MDCT)
    (d) SPECT

78. A pulmonary nodule 9 mm in size is found on the CT scan of a low-risk patient (nonsmoker or with no history of cancer). What is the next best approach?
    (a) CT-guided biopsy
    (b) Resection of the involved segment
    (c) Repeat CT scan 6 months later
    (d) Chest X-ray 3 months later

79. What is the best modality for the diagnosis of liver metastasis?
    (a) PET
    (b) CT with contrast
    (c) CT without contrast
    (d) MRI

80. What is the most sensitive modality for the diagnosis of secreting tumors of the pancreas?
    (a) CT scan
    (b) Octreotide scintigraphy
    (c) MRI
    (d) Selective angiography of the pancreas

81. All of the following statements regarding GIST are correct *except*:
    (a) Prevalence in the small bowel is lesser than that in the stomach.
    (b) With the same size, they are more aggressive in the stomach than in the bowel.
    (c) Malignant tumors are usually larger than 5 cm.
    (d) Malignant tumors are usually heterogeneous.

82. All of the following statements regarding colorectal cancers are correct *except*:
    (a) The most common GI cancer.
    (b) Endosonography is the best way for the local staging of a rectal tumor.
    (c) CT scan is the best modality to detect tumoral recurrence in the abdomen.
    (d) About 20% of colorectal cancers are seen in the rectosigmoid region.

83. Which of the following situations is the cause of a solitary pulmonary nodule?
    (a) Bronchial carcinoma
    (b) Metastasis
    (c) Lung abscess and infectious granuloma
    (d) All of the above

84. All of the following statements regarding lung calcification are true *except*:
    (a) Lung hamartoma usually has a popcorn-like appearance on chest X-ray.
    (b) Calcification is common in tuberculoma and fungal granuloma.
    (c) CXR can always diagnose a calcification.
    (d) A homogenous calcification in a solitary pulmonary nodule indicates a benign process.

85. Which of the following statements regarding a solitary pulmonary nodule in the upper right lung lobe on the CXR of a smoking man is true?
    (a) Organized patterns of calcification are more likely to be detected in a malignant nodule.
    (b) Calcification within a nodule is more likely to be detected in a malignant nodule.
    (c) The most likely diagnosis is bronchial carcinoma.
    (d) If the lesion was not present in his CXR in the previous year, the lesion would more likely be benign.

86. All of the following conditions are associated with malignant probability in a solitary pulmonary nodule *except*
    (a) Calcification
    (b) Size greater than 4 cm
    (c) Cavitation
    (d) Lobulated border

87. What is the most common cause of multiple pulmonary nodules?
    (a) Lung abscess
    (b) Inactive tuberculoma
    (c) Hamartoma
    (d) Metastasis

88. Which of the following statements regarding the role of CT scan in solitary pulmonary nodules is false?
    (a) The presence of a marked calcification within a nodule is suggestive of the ruling out of a malignant process.
    (b) CT scan cannot help in the assessment of a calcified nodule observed on the CXR.
    (c) A pulmonary nodule less than 1 cm should be resected by surgery.
    (d) CT scan is useful in the estimation of the growth rate of small pulmonary nodules.

89. Which of the following statement regarding mediastinal masses is false?
    (a) Thyroidal masses are the most common mediastinal masses.
    (b) Neurogenic masses are the most common masses of the posterior mediastinum.
    (c) MRI is the best modality to evaluate mediastinal masses.
    (d) Mediastinal calcification is observed in malignant lymphadenopathy and benign processes.

90. What is the best modality for assessing an enlarged hilar of the lungs?
    (a) Chest X-ray
    (b) PET
    (c) Gallium scintigraphy
    (d) CT scan

91. What is the most common cause of bilateral hilar lymphadenopathy?
    (a) Tuberculosis
    (b) Fungal disease
    (c) Lymphoma
    (d) Sarcoidosis

92. All of the following statements regarding neoplastic lung diseases are true *except*:
    (a) Cavitation is seen in squamous cell lung cancer.
    (b) Only a large lymphadenopathy in the carina region is seen on the CXR.
    (c) CT scan is the best modality for the diagnosis of carcinomatous lymphangitis.
    (d) CT scan is the best modality for the assessment of a Pancoast tumor.

93. Which of the following radiotracers shows a higher uptake in large cell lung carcinoma than in squamous cell lung carcinoma?
    (a) FDG
    (b) ^{11}C-methionine
    (c) ^{11}C-thymidine
    (d) $^{15}O\text{-}H_2O$

94. Which of the following statements about the application of FDG-PET in lung cancer is NOT correct?
    (a) Active tuberculosis and fungal infections are among the false-positive findings of PET in lung cancer.
    (b) PET is a reliable and economic method for the evaluation of a solitary pulmonary nodule.
    (c) A negative PET scan does NOT exclude cancer in nodules smaller than 1 cm specifically located in the lung apex.
    (d) a and b.

95. Describe the sensitivity and accuracy of FDG-PET scan in comparison with those of transthoracic needle aspiration biopsy (TTNAB), respectively.
    (a) Higher sensitivity, equal accuracy
    (b) Higher sensitivity, lower accuracy
    (c) Equal sensitivity, lower accuracy
    (d) Lower sensitivity and accuracy

96. If the goal is to determine the stage of the mediastinal lymph nodes in lung cancer, how can the sensitivity, specificity, and accuracy of FDG-PET be described in comparison with those of CT scan, respectively?
    (a) FDG-PET has higher sensitivity and specificity but equal accuracy.
    (b) FDG-PET has higher sensitivity and specificity but lower accuracy.
    (c) FDG-PET has higher sensitivity, specificity, and accuracy.
    (d) FDG-PET has lower sensitivity and specificity but equal accuracy.

97. Which of the following statements regarding the role of FDG-PET in the management of lung cancers is NOT correct?
    (a) Surgery is possible if the mediastinal PET is negative.
    (b) PET is capable of identifying lymph node involvement even when the nodes are NOT enlarged.
    (c) Tumoral involvement can be ruled out if enlarged lymph nodes in the CT scan do NOT uptake FDG.
    (d) Surgery will NOT be possible if the mediastinal PET is positive.

98. Which of the following variables is lower in tumoral cells than in normal cells in the PET evaluation of a tumoral tissue?
    (a) Regional flow
    (b) Oxygen consumption
    (c) Oxygen extraction fraction
    (d) b and c

99. Which of the following forms of bone metastasis is best detected by FDG-PET scan?
    (a) Lytic metastasis
    (b) Sclerotic metastasis
    (c) Mixed metastasis
    (d) a and c

100. Which of the following patients must be candidated for surgery?
    (a) Abdominal CT scan shows an operable colorectal cancer, but PET is negative.
    (b) Abdominal CT scan shows an operable colorectal cancer, and PET shows multiple positive lesions.
    (c) Abdominal CT scan shows multiple colorectal lesions, and PET shows multiple positive lesions.
    (d) Abdominal CT scan shows an operable colorectal cancer, and PET is positive in the corresponding regions.

101. Which of the following statements regarding the application of PET in colorectal cancer is NOT correct?
   (a) The role of PET in the management of primary disease has been established.
   (b) The accuracy of PET for the detection of liver metastases is high.
   (c) Diagnosis of tumor recurrence is the main priority of the PET scan in comparison with the CT scan in the follow-up of colorectal cancers.
   (d) PET may show a false-positive uptake in normal intestine without any explained reason.

102. Which of the following statements regarding the application of PET in pancreas cancer is NOT correct?
   (a) PET shows an increased uptake of ^{11}C-methionine and ^{11}C-tryptophan in pancreatic cancer.
   (b) Decreased uptake of ^{11}C-acetate is specific for pancreatic cancer.
   (c) $^{15}O\text{-}H_2O$ PET scan shows a higher flow of pancreatic cancer than normal tissue.
   (d) All items are false.

103. Regarding the application of PET in pancreatic cancer:
   (a) The accuracy of PET for the identification of pancreatic lesions is similar to that of CT scan.
   (b) PET is effective in the characterization of lesions and in the detection of metastasis.
   (c) FDG-PET is an ideal method for the discrimination of benign and malignant pancreatic lesions.
   (d) The incidence of false-negative findings is high.

104. Although some of the hepatomas are observed as hot spots on the PET scan, approximately 50% of the cases are NOT. What is the reason for such a controversy?
   (a) Low K3 constant coefficient
   (b) Low K4 constant coefficient
   (c) High methylation
   (d) High K4 constant coefficient

105. Which of the following statements regarding the application of PET in hepatoma is NOT correct?
   (a) FDG uptake decreases after treatment and is preferred over CT in therapeutic monitoring.
   (b) Survival of patients with a high K4/K3 ratio is high.
   (c) K3 > 0.025 is always associated with the presence of a tumor.
   (d) K3 is related to dephosphorylation of the tumor.

106. What is the correct formula for the calculation of the standardized uptake value (SUV)?
   (a) Mean ROI activity (mCi/ml) × body surface area (BSA)/injected dose (mCi)
   (b) Mean ROI activity (mCi/ml) × body weight (kg)/injected dose (mCi)
   (c) Injected dose (mCi)/mean ROI activity (mCi/ml) × body weight (kg)
   (d) Mean ROI activity (mCi/ml)/injected dose (mCi)) × body weight (kg)

107. All of the following statements regarding the role of PET scan in lung cancers are correct *except*:
   (a) The sensitivity and specificity of PET for the evaluation of lung nodules are greater than 80%.
   (b) The sensitivity of PET is high enough to consider the negative result of PET to rule out malignancy in a population with a low-to-moderate risk for malignancy.
   (c) The negative results of transbronchial or transthoracic biopsy of lung nodules are definitely indicative for the ruling out of malignancy.
   (d) PET scan is more accurate for the evaluation of lung nodules in parenchymal tissue than for the evaluation of nodules near the vital mediastinal structures.

108. What is the probability of malignancy of a pulmonary nodule with a negative PET scan?
   (a) 1%
   (b) 2%
   (c) 5%
   (d) 10%

109. The TNM system is used for the staging of lung cancers. PET is NOT effective in:
   (a) T stage
   (b) N stage
   (c) M stage
   (d) a and b

110. What are the sensitivity and specificity rates of PET scan, respectively, if the goal is to detect metastasis or recurrence of colorectal cancer?
   (a) 90%, more than 70%
   (b) 70%, more than 90%
   (c) Sensitivity and specificity of more than 90%
   (d) Sensitivity and specificity of more than 80%

111. In which of the following types of colorectal cancer is the sensitivity of PET low?
   (a) Gastrointestinal stromal tumors (GISTs)
   (b) Squamous cell carcinoma
   (c) Lymphoma
   (d) Mucinous adenocarcinoma

112. If the goal is to detect the metastasis of colorectal cancer, PET is more sensitive than CT scan in all of the following regions *except*:
    (a) Abdomen
    (b) Retroperitoneal space
    (c) Lung
    (d) Pelvis

113. Most colorectal cancers are located in which following parts of the colon and rectum?
    (a) Caecum and ascending colon
    (b) Rectosigmoid
    (c) Transverse colon
    (d) Descending colon

114. All of the following statements properly describe CT colonography in colorectal assessment *except*:
    (a) CT colonography has a high sensitivity of 96%, which is equivalent to colonoscopy for lesions ≥10 mm.
    (b) Patient preparation for CT colonography is different from that for conventional colonoscopy.
    (c) CT colonoscopy lacks accuracy in identifying lesions smaller than 5 mm.
    (d) CT colonography is less suitable for patients with a high risk for carcinoma.

115. PET scan is generally important for the evaluation of colorectal cancers for all of the following purposes *except*:
    (a) Differentiation of posttreatment changes from the recurrent tumor
    (b) Differentiation of benign and malignant lesions (indeterminate lymph node and hepatic and pulmonary lesions)
    (c) Preoperative evaluation
    (d) Evaluation of patients with increasing tumor markers in the absence of a known source

116. In the PET scan of lung cancers:
    (a) The accuracy of the differentiation of treatment-induced changes from a recurrent disease with PET is high.
    (b) The sensitivity of mediastinoscopy is greater than that of PET scan for the detection of the involvement of mediastinal lymph nodes in lung cancer.
    (c) PET has been shown to be effective in the screening of patients with lung cancer for brain metastases, especially when they are asymptomatic.
    (d) PET findings result in patient management changes in 10% of cases.

117. The diagnosis of mediastinal masses by MRI:
    (a) The injection of contrast media is required for the evaluation of vascular lesions.
    (b) MRI does NOT provide more information than CT in the detection of posterior mediastinal lesions or spinal involvement.
    (c) The injection of contrast media is NOT necessarily required for the evaluation of dissecting an aneurysm of the aorta by MRI, and coronal, sagittal, and oblique views can be prepared without reconstruction.
    (d) The accuracy of MRI for the detection of calcification of mediastinal tumors is greater than that of fat deposits.

118. All of the following statements regarding the role of PET/CT in gastric cancer are true *except*:
    (a) T staging is best evaluated with PET/CT.
    (b) In peritoneal metastases, PET/CT has poor sensitivity of 35%.
    (c) Intestinal-type tumors have higher 18F-FDG uptake than diffuse.
    (d) PET/CT has high specificity for detecting lymph node metastases.

119. Which of the following items does NOT properly describe the characteristics of ground glass density?
    (a) Pulmonary vessels are NOT observed in the lesion.
    (b) It represents an active inflammatory disease or edema.
    (c) It is identified by a granular pattern.
    (d) Air bronchogram is absent.

120. Which of the following structures is NOT included in the posterior mediastinum?
    (a) Inferior vena cava
    (b) Azygos
    (c) Thoracic duct
    (d) Esophagus

121. Lobar anatomy of the lung:
    (a) The left upper lobe consists of the lateral, medial, apicoposterior, and anterior segments.
    (b) The right upper lobe consists of the superior, inferior, and apical segments.
    (c) The right medial lobe consists of two inferior and superior segments.
    (d) The left lower lobe consists of the lateral, posterior, and anteromedial basal segments and a superior segment.

122. Which of the following items are included in false-negative findings if the goal is to detect malignant cells by PET?
    (a) Bronchoalveolar cell CA
    (b) Tissue infection or inflammation
    (c) Wegener's granuloma
    (d) Coal miner's lung

123. Pulmonary hilum consists of:
 (a) Pulmonary arteries and veins
 (b) Main bronchi and lymphatics
 (c) Upper lobe arteries and veins
 (d) Lower lobe arteries and veins

124. What is the main limitation of MRI for the evaluation of lung tumors in comparison with CT scan?
 (a) Estimation of tumor size
 (b) Precise localization of the tumor
 (c) Detection of nodules adjacent to the hilar vessels
 (d) Detection of vascular and mediastinal metastasis

125. What is the most common histological subtype of cancers with the origin of small intestine?
 (a) Lymphoma
 (b) Gastrointestinal stromal tumor (GIST)
 (c) Adenocarcinoma
 (d) Carcinoid tumor

126. Regarding the role of PET/CT in gastric cancer:
 (a) PET/CT is the modality of choice in defining the resectability of gastric cancer.
 (b) For nodal (N) staging, PET/CT has higher diagnostic performance than CECT.
 (c) PET/CT has high sensitivity and specificity in the detection of recurrent gastric cancers.
 (d) CECT has higher sensitivity than PET/CT and lower specificity than PET/CT in the detection of peritoneal metastases.

127. A 57-year-old man with a history of descending colon cancer, stage T3N1M0, is referred 7 months after surgery and chemotherapy, with CEA = 18. Repeat of the test after 1 month shows CEA = 30, but CT scan of the thorax, abdomen, and pelvis and colonoscopy are normal. What is the next recommended intervention?
 (a) Repeat of CEA after 1 month
 (b) Diagnostic laparotomy
 (c) FDG-PET scan
 (d) Repeat of CEA and CT scan of the thorax, abdomen, and pelvis after 4 months

128. A 58-year-old woman with small-cell lung cancer (SCLC) is referred after bronchoscopy. Which of the following statements is NOT correct?
 (a) PET scan can replace bone scan, if it is available.
 (b) Bone marrow biopsy is recommended for high LDH and the presence of myelophthisis in the peripheral blood smear in a limited stage.
 (c) Thoracic CT scan and brain MRI are indicated if the patient is symptomatic.
 (d) A very low level of pleural effusion on the same side of the lesion does NOT necessarily increase the stage of the disease.

129. In which of the following cancers is low physical activity considered a risk factor?
    (a) Breast and colon
    (b) Endometrium and ovary
    (c) Prostate and kidney
    (d) Pancreas and gallbladder

130. What is the gold standard imaging method for the identification of pulmonary metastasis due to primary bone cancers?
    (a) Chest X-ray
    (b) Spiral CT scan
    (c) MRI with contrast
    (d) FDG-PET scan

131. Regarding the role of PET/CT in cholangiocarcinoma:
    (a) a. PET has low sensitivity for the detection of intrahepatic cholangiocarcinoma.
    (b) PET has high sensitivity for extrahepatic cholangiocarcinoma.
    (c) PET has high sensitivity for the detection of lymph node metastases.
    (d) The workup of cholangiocarcinoma is mainly by CECT and MRI with cholangiopancreatography.

132. Which of the following studies is NOT included in the standard tests for the evaluation of patients with metastasis of unknown origin?
    (a) Pulmonary CT scan
    (b) Bone scan
    (c) Abdominal CT scan
    (d) PET scan

133. Which of the following receptors is overexpressed in more than 70% of non-small-cell lung carcinomas (NSCLC), especially adenocarcinoma?
    (a) ERBB2 (Her2/neu)
    (b) Gastrin-releasing peptide (GRP) receptor
    (c) Epithelial growth factor (EGF)
    (d) RAS family (N-RAS, H-RAS, and K-RAS)

134. Which of the following imaging modalities provides the most valuable information for the detection of mediastinal invasion of NSCLC?
    (a) MRI
    (b) Triple-phase spiral CT scan
    (c) FDG-PET scan
    (d) Comparative PET and CT scan

135. Which of the following imaging modalities provides the most accurate and valuable information for the detection of occult metastases of lung cancer (NSCLC or SCLC)?
    (a) Spiral CT scan with contrast
    (b) MRI with gadolinium
    (c) FDG-PET scan
    (d) Comparative PET scan with CT or MRI

136. Which of the following statements regarding small-cell lung carcinoma (SCLC) is NOT correct?
    (a) Liver and adrenal metastases are usually asymptomatic and may be diagnosed with a high level of LDH, alkaline phosphatase, and transaminases.
    (b) Brain metastases detected in MRI or CT scan are usually accompanied by neurologic symptoms.
    (c) Bone metastasis is usually lytic and associated with severe bone pain and increased alkaline phosphatase.
    (d) Endovascular metastasis, tumor embolus, or lymphangitic spread may be associated with dyspnea.

137. A 64-year-old man underwent surgery for colon cancer 4 years ago. Subsequently, he was subjected to FOLFOX adjuvant chemotherapy for 6 months because of stage T3N1M0, but he was NOT closely followed up until recently. Total colonoscopy is normal, CEA is 79, and CT scan only shows a low-density lesion of 4 cm in the sixth hepatic segment. Previous CT scan 19 months ago reported the corresponding lesion as hemangioma. What is the next recommended intervention?
    (a) PET scan
    (b) Repeat of CT scan after 6–8 weeks
    (c) Repeat of CEA after 6–8 weeks
    (d) Fine-needle biopsy of the lesion

138. A young patient with previously treated osteosarcoma is referred with multiple pulmonary nodules in the CXR. What is the recommended intervention?
    (a) Repeat of treatment without biopsy
    (b) Biopsy for confirmation of metastasis
    (c) Close follow-up if the general condition is favorable
    (d) Beginning of treatment after a positive PET scan

139. A patient with a 3 cm tumor in the right lung is referred, and further evaluation demonstrates the tumoral involvement of lymph nodes in the left lung. What is the stage of the disease?
    (a) IIIB
    (b) IV
    (c) IIIA
    (d) IIB

140. Lymphatic drainage in esophageal tumors:
    (a) Lymphatic drainage of the upper one-third of esophageal thoracic tumors goes to the cervical and upper mediastinal nodes.
    (b) Lymphatic drainage of the medial one-third of esophageal tumors goes to the paratracheal, hilar subcarinal pericardial, and periesophageal nodes.
    (c) Involvement of the celiac, lower mediastinal, and cervical lymph nodes is reported in distal esophageal tumors.
    (d) All of the above.

141. Involvement of pulmonary hilum of the opposite side in NSCLC indicates tumor stage of:
   (a) T4
   (b) N2
   (c) N3
   (d) M1

142. If the goal is to evaluate a patient with pulmonary cancer, in which of the following assessments is PET scan limited in comparison with CT scan?
   (a) Involvement of the mediastinal lymph nodes
   (b) Tumor progress to the mediastinum
   (c) Tumor relapse
   (d) Response to radiotherapy

143. Which variable has the least effect on the differentiation of a normal GI uptake from malignancies in FDG-PET?
   (a) Agreement with CT
   (b) SUV
   (c) Uptake pattern
   (d) Physical examination and history

144. Which statement about the calculation of SUV in ^{18}F-FDG-PET oncology is correct?
   (a) The sensitivity and specificity of SUV are comparable with the activity ratio in pulmonary lesions.
   (b) Serum glucose correction is NOT required.
   (c) Delayed imaging after 2.5 h does NOT change the results.
   (d) Lean body weight is NOT critical.

145. A 65-year-old woman underwent surgery and chemotherapy 5 years ago because of mucinous adenocarcinoma of the colon. The patient is referred with a 3 cm left para-aortic tumor on the CT scan and normal PET scan. What are the most appropriate interpretation and recommended intervention, respectively?
   (a) Possibility of recurrence, biopsy
   (b) Nonviable mass, follow-up with CT scan
   (c) Possibility of recurrence, follow-up with FDG-PET
   (d) Nonviable tumor, follow-up with FDG-PET

146. Which of the following radiotracers is indicated for the evaluation of pancreatic cancer?
   (a) 75Se-seleno-methionine
   (b) 125I-fibrinogen
   (c) ^{111}In-WBC
   (d) ^{67}Ga

1.21.1 Answer

	A	B	C	D		A	B	C	D		A	B	C	D
1			*		51			*		101	*			
2				*	52				*	102				*
3				*	53				*	103		*		
4				*	54		*			104				*
5				*	55				*	105				*
6	*				56		*			106				*
7	*				57			*		107			*	
8	*				58		*			108	*			
9	*				59				*	109	*			
10				*	60		*			110	*			
11	*				61			*		111				*
12			*		62	*				112			*	
13				*	63				*	113		*		
14	*				64			*		114		*		
15		*			65	*				115			*	
16				*	66	*				116	*			
17				*	67		*			117			*	
18		*			68			*		118	*			
19	*				69		*			119	*			
20		*			70	*				120	*			
21	*				71		*			121				*
22				*	72			*		122	*			
23			*		73	*				123			*	
24	*				74	*				124		*		
25			*		75			*		125			*	
26	*				76	*				126				*
27			*		77		*			127			*	
28	*				78			*		128			*	
29				*	79				*	129	*			
30			*		80				*	130		*		
31		*			81		*			131				*
32			*		82				*	132		*		
33				*	83				*	133			*	
34			*		84			*		134	*			
35		*			85			*		135				*
36				*	86	*				136			*	
37			*		87				*	137	*			
38			*		88			*		138	*			
39			*		89			*		139	*			
40		*			90				*	140				*
41			*		91				*	141			*	

42				*	**92**				*	**142**		*		
43				*	**93**		*			**143**		*		
44				*	**94**			*		**144**	*			
45				*	**95**	*				**145**	*			
46		*			**96**			*		**146**	*			
47				*	**97**				*	**147**				
48	*				**98**			*		**148**				
49				*	**99**				*	**149**				
50				*	**100**				*	**150**				

1.22 PET in Gynecological Tumors

1. In breast cancer:
   (a) Invasive lobular carcinomas in PET imaging are usually more false negative than invasive ducal carcinomas.
   (b) Currently, PET imaging can significantly reduce unnecessary invasive procedures.
   (c) PET imaging can contribute to an improved diagnosis of noninvasive breast cancer.
   (d) PET is superior to bone scan in the detection of osteoblastic breast cancer metastases.

2. In breast cancer:
   (a) Invasive ductal carcinoma is the most common histologic type.
   (b) It is most frequently found in the upper outer quadrant.
   (c) Sentinel node biopsy seems to be the method of choice in the early stages of the disease.
   (d) All of the above.

3. In ovarian cancer:
   (a) Most ovarian metastatic lesions originate from the lung.
   (b) Most palpable adnexal masses are malignant.
   (c) PET can definitely rule out a borderline malignancy in patients with an asymptomatic adnexal mass.
   (d) PET may be particularly useful in the detection of metastatic lesions intimately associated with the bowel wall.

4. Which of the following imaging modalities is a very sensitive method for the assessment of regional node involvement in cervical cancer?
   (a) PET scan
   (b) MRI scan
   (c) CT scan
   (d) Intravaginal ultrasonography

1.22.1 Answer

	A	B	C	D
1	*			
2				*
3				*
4		*		

1.23 PET Imaging in Pediatric Oncology

1. Regarding radiation safety issues:
   (a) The percent uptake of injected FDG in the brain of pediatrics is lower than that of adults.
   (b) Urine excretion of FDG in pediatrics is less than that in adults.
   (c) The whole-body effective dose in pediatrics is higher than that in adults.
   (d) The whole-body effective dose in pediatrics is higher than that in ^{99m}Tc-DMSA.

2. SUV in children is … compared with adults and is … in heavier patients than in those with normal body habitus.
   (a) Lower, lower
   (b) Higher, lower
   (c) Higher, higher
   (d) Lower, higher

3. In neuroblastoma:
   (a) Abdominal neuroblastomas are called dumbbell tumors.
   (b) At the time of diagnosis, it already shows visible metastatic involvement.
   (c) The inhibition of the MYCN oncogene and diploid chromosomal content is an adverse prognostic marker.
   (d) Stage 4S only applies to infants >1 year old.

4. In neuroblastoma:
   (a) MIBG scan has an accuracy of 70% for the detection of a recurrent tumor.
   (b) Octreoscan is suboptimal in the upper abdomen.
   (c) FDG-PET is worse than MIBG for soft tissue and extracranial skeletal disease.
   (d) Disease in the calvarium is always detected by FDG-PET.

5. What is the most common site of osteogenic sarcoma?
   (a) Proximal tibia
   (b) Proximal humerus
   (c) Distal femur
   (d) Proximal fibula

6. In rhabdomyosarcoma:
   (a) Most cases have detectable distant metastases.
   (b) Alveolar histopathology is an adverse prognostic factor.
   (c) FDG-PET is important for the initial staging of the disease.
   (d) CT scan has the ability to show bone marrow metastases.

7. The most common sites of distant metastasis in Wilms' tumor are:
   (a) Lung and liver
   (b) Lung and bone
   (c) Liver and bone
   (d) Liver and brain

8. The most common site of distant metastasis in hepatoblastoma is:
   (a) Lung
   (b) Liver
   (c) Brain
   (d) Bone

1.23.1 Answer

	A	B	C	D
1		*		
2				*
3		*		
4		*		
5			*	
6		*		
7	*			
8	*			

1.24 PET in Genitourinary Tumors: Prostate, Bladder, Testicular, and Renal Cancer

1. PET in genitourinary tumors:
   (a) FDG-PET is recommended for the staging of localized bladder cancer.
   (b) FDG-PET is recommended for T staging of the primary renal cancer.
   (c) FDG-PET is recommended for the staging of testicular cancer at presentation.
   (d) FDG-PET is not recommended for the detection of recurrence of bladder cancer.

2. In prostate cancer:
   (a) An increase in the choline/citrate ratio in spectroscopic examination is associated with a higher cancer grade.
   (b) Bone scan must be performed not less than 4 months after starting chemotherapy.
   (c) The most common cause of death is cardiovascular problems.
   (d) It has a 60% response rate to androgen withdrawal.

3. This radiopharmaceutical is considered to have clinical promise in prostate cancer:
   (a) ^{18}F-cis-4-L-proline, amino acid transport
   (b) ^{18}F-fluoride, hydroxyapatite crystal
   (c) ^{18}F-methylcholine, phospholipid synthesis
   (d) ^{11}C-acetate, fatty acid synthesis

4. It is a promising tracer for assessing the role of androgen receptor in metastatic prostate cancer:
   (a) ^{18}F-fluorodihydrotestosterone (FDHT)
   (b) 16α-[^{18}F]-fluoro-17β-estradiol (FES)
   (c) ^{11}C-acetate
   (d) 21-[^{18}F]fluoro-16 alpha-ethyl-19-norprogesterone

5. What is the most common site of metastasis of RCC?
   (a) Lung
   (b) Liver
   (c) Bone
   (d) Brain

6. A patient with prostate cancer and bone metastasis is subjected to treatment. What is the scan of choice for the evaluation of response to treatment?
   (a) ^{99m}Tc-PYP
   (b) ^{99m}Tc-MDP
   (c) ^{18}F-Flouride
   (d) ^{18}F-FDG

7. A 79-year-old man with urinary inconsistency is referred. Laboratory tests show a high level of PSA, and prostate biopsy indicates adenocarcinoma. Prostate immunoscintigraphy is performed for staging, and pelvis lymph nodes are NOT involved. Which item about this patient is correct?
   (a) A false-negative ProstaScint scan is possible.
   (b) Pelvis metastasis is ruled out.
   (c) FDG-PET is recommended for the evaluation of pelvis metastasis.
   (d) Clinical and radiographic studies are sufficient for staging, and further evaluation is NOT required.

8. Which of the following processes can be evaluated with ^{18}F-fluorocholine imaging?
   (a) Polyamine metabolism
   (b) Cell membrane synthesis
   (c) Protein synthesis
   (d) Cell proliferation

9. In prostate cancer:
   (a) FDG-PET is very sensitive for the staging of prostate cancer and other cancers.
   (b) If immunoscintigraphy is negative, staging lymphadenectomy will NOT be required.
   (c) Positive immunoscintigraphy is sufficient for the initiation of treatment.
   (d) Bone scan is more sensitive than immunoscintigraphy in the detection of metastasis.

10. All of the following statements regarding the role of PET in gynecologic tumors are true *except*:
   (a) PET is more useful in the estimation of prognosis than CA-125 in suspected recurrent ovarian cancer.
   (b) PET has a limited role as a primary modality in the evaluation of primary ovarian masses.
   (c) PET is useful in the staging of locally advanced untreated cervical carcinoma.
   (d) PET/CT is more sensitive than MRI for pelvic nodal metastases, but there is no difference in specificity.

11. About the role of PET in renal masses:
   (a) Diuresis is not important if PET is performed to evaluate a renal mass.
   (b) FDG uptake can help to differentiate benign or bland emboli from tumor thrombosis in RCC patients.
   (c) Primary renal tumors have a greater FDG uptake than metastatic renal tumors.
   (d) FDG-PET/CT has a more significant advantage in diagnosis and staging of RCC than the diagnostic CT.

12. What is the most appropriate modality for the staging of renal carcinoma?
    (a) MRI
    (b) CT scan
    (c) DTPA scintigraphy
    (d) DMSA scintigraphy

13. All of the following are routine components of patients with urethra cancers *except*:
    (a) Chest X-ray
    (b) Chest and abdomen CT scan
    (c) Bone scan
    (d) Lymphoscintigraphy

14. All of the following statements regarding RCC are correct *except*:
    (a) It accounts for 80% of all renal cancer in adults.
    (b) Treatment consists of surgery, resectioning of the capsule, and adrenalectomy in tumors greater than 3 cm.
    (c) It occurs more often in men than in women at ages 50–70.
    (d) RCC comprises 10% calcification, 10% bilateral, and 10% infiltrates to IVC.

15. In a 69-year-old patient with RCC, CT scan shows tumoral thrombosis and locoregional lymph node involvement. What is the stage of the disease?
    (a) Stage II
    (b) Stage IIIA
    (c) Stage IIIC
    (d) Stage IVA

16. All of the following statements regarding the application of PET for the evaluation of genitourinary tract (GUT) are correct *except*:
    (a) False-negative findings of PET in GUT cancers are NOT rare; therefore, negative PET does NOT exclude cancer.
    (b) FDG-PET is NOT valuable in the evaluation of prostate cancer.
    (c) FDG-PET in testis cancer is positive and has an important role in the evaluation of therapeutic efficiency.
    (d) PET is NOT indicated for the evaluation of GUT tumors because of renal uptake.

17. Regarding the role of PET/CT in renal cancers:
    (a) Change in FDG uptake is not a powerful index for evaluating the biological response to TKI.
    (b) A high SUVmax in patients with primary RCC is not correlated with a high likelihood of metastasis.
    (c) FDG-PET/CT has higher sensitivity and accuracy in detecting bone metastases in patients with RCC than bone scan.
    (d) FDG-PET/CT is currently recommended for the diagnosis and staging of RCC based on updated national and international guidelines.

18. What is the most appropriate definition of PSA velocity?
    (a) The ratio of PSA to prostate volume
    (b) The level of PSA with increasing age
    (c) The level of inactive PSA
    (d) Increase in PSA level over time

19. What is the most common extra-thoracic region of metastasis of primary mediastinal seminoma?
    (a) Liver
    (b) Bone
    (c) Brain
    (d) Pelvic lymph nodes

20. Which of the following statements regarding prostate cancer is NOT correct?
    (a) The higher the level of PSA is, the larger the tumor size.
    (b) The higher the grade of the tumor is, the higher the PSA density.
    (c) The higher the Gleason score is, the larger the tumor size.
    (d) The higher the PSA level and Gleason score are, the higher the probability of distant metastasis and lymphatic involvement.

21. A patient with localized prostate cancer is treated with radiotherapy only. PSA is 22 and 6 before and 6 months after treatment, respectively. What is the recommended intervention?
    (a) Repeat of PSA after 6 months
    (b) Repeat of prostate biopsy for the evaluation of residual tissue
    (c) Bone scan
    (d) PET scan and hormone therapy

1.24.1 Answer

	A	B	C	D
1			*	
2	*			
3				*
4	*			
5	*			
6				*
7	*			
8		*		
9				*
10	*			
11		*		
12		*		
13				*
14				*

	A	B	C	D
15			*	
16				*
17			*	
18				*
19			*	
20		*		
21	*			

1.25 Future Clinical Applications of PET: Amino Acid and Nucleoside Imaging

1. Methionine is uptaken in all of the following organs *except*:
   (a) Pancreas
   (b) Pituitary gland
   (c) Thyroid
   (d) Bone marrow

2. The clinical application of ^{18}F-FLT-PET is limited in:
   (a) Liver
   (b) Bone marrow
   (c) Brain
   (d) a and b

3. What is the best tracer for the assessment of cell proliferation?
   (a) Thymidine
   (b) α-Aminoisobutyric acid (AIB)
   (c) Methyl tyrosine
   (d) Leucine

4. Which of the following molecular imaging techniques can define the "poor prognosis" of cancer and the requirement for combined chemotherapy?
   (a) Hypoxia imaging with ATSM
   (b) Fatty acid metabolism with choline
   (c) Proliferation imaging with fluorothymidine
   (d) Apoptosis imaging with annexin

5. Which of the following anatomical regions is NOT observed in a normal PET scan with ^{11}C-epinephrine?
   (a) Salivary glands
   (b) Heart
   (c) Adrenal medulla
   (d) Liver

6. Which statement about the application of ^{18}F-FLT (fluorothymidine) in tumors is NOT correct?
   (a) The uptake of ^{18}F-FLT is greater than that of ^{18}F-FDG in most tumors because of its higher rate of proliferation.
   (b) ^{18}F-FLT accumulation in the liver and bone marrow increases the background.
   (c) ^{18}F-FLT is commonly used for the evaluation of brain tumors.
   (d) The uptake of ^{18}F-FLT is substantially related to tumor proliferation.

7. Which of the following radioactive agents is the most appropriate for the labeling of antibodies with positron-emitting radioisotopes?
   (a) ^{124}I
   (b) ^{15}O
   (c) ^{13}N
   (d) ^{18}F

8. Which of the following statements regarding the application of PET in the diagnosis of neuroendocrine tumors is NOT correct?
   (a) In contrast to primary reports, PET has NOT been helpful in the evaluation of therapeutic effects in neuroendocrine tumors.
   (b) Differentiated neuroendocrine cancers usually uptake ^{18}F-FDG.
   (c) ^{11}C-5HTP PET is more sensitive than anatomical methods, including MRI and CT, for the evaluation of metastatic tumors.
   (d) ^{68}Ga-octreotide PET is considered an alternative to ^{111}In-octreotide or HTP PET.

1.25.1 Answer

	A	B	C	D
1			*	
2				*
3	*			
4	*			
5			*	
6	*			
7	*			
8	*			

1.26 PET Imaging of Brain Tumors

1. The following are the primary tumors most commonly associated with cerebral metastases *except*:
   (a) Lung cancers
   (b) Kidney cancers
   (c) Liver cancers
   (d) Colon cancers

2. In PET imaging of brain tumors:
   (a) FDG uptake is evaluated qualitatively by comparing it with that in normal white matter.
   (b) Sedative/anesthetics may increase the normal gray matter glucose metabolism.
   (c) Supratentorial brain tumors reduce the FDG uptake in both cerebellums.
   (d) Corticosteroids may decrease the metabolism of normal gray matter glucose.

3. Crossed cerebellar diaschisis occurs as a result of the disruption of the:
   (a) Normal corticopontocerebellar pathway from thee cerebellar hemispheres to the contralateral cerebellar cortex
   (b) Normal corticopontocerebellar pathway from the cerebellar hemispheres to the ipsilateral cerebellar cortex
   (c) Normal corticopontocerebellar pathway from the cerebral hemispheres to the contralateral cerebellar cortex
   (d) Normal corticopontocerebellar pathway from the cerebral hemispheres to the ipsilateral cerebellar cortex

4. Which brain tumor is hypermetabolic in FDG-PET imaging?
   (a) Dysembryoplastic neuroepithelial tumors (DNETs)
   (b) Ganglioglioma
   (c) Gliomatosis
   (d) Primary CNS lymphoma

5. Which brain tumor shows either hypermetabolism or hypometabolism on FDG-PET imaging?
   (a) Pleomorphic xanthoastrocytoma
   (b) Ganglioglioma
   (c) Dysembryoplastic neuroepithelial tumors (DNETs)
   (d) Lymphoma

6. FDG uptake in meningioma is:
   (a) Less than that in gray matter
   (b) Equal to that in gray matter
   (c) Higher than that in gray matter
   (d) All of the above

7. Application of FDG-PET in brain tumors:
   (a) Hypermetabolic tumors have a higher FDG uptake than gray matter.
   (b) FDG canNOT detect the post-malignant degeneration of low-grade tumors.
   (c) Steroid treatment does NOT change the FDG uptake in tumors.
   (d) ^{11}C-methyl-methionine has limited efficacy in the grading of brain tumors.

8. A 69-year-old woman presents with multiple brain metastases of unknown origin. Which of the following regions are the most likely primary sites of involvement?
   (a) Prostate and colon
   (b) Prostate and lung
   (c) Lung and pancreas
   (d) Lung and colon

9. Brain PET scan of a patient shows a region of lower activity compared with white matter in the corresponding region of a tumoral lesion detected in MRI. Which tumor is the most probable?
   (a) Anaplastic astrocytoma
   (b) Oligodendroglioma
   (c) Glioblastoma multiforme
   (d) Lymphoma

10. Which of the following radiopharmaceuticals is characterized with high contrast images in the PET evaluation of brain tumors?
    (a) ^{18}F-Fluorodeoxyuridine
    (b) ^{18}F-FDG
    (c) ^{11}C-Methionine
    (d) ^{15}CO2

11. Application of PET in the evaluation of brain tumors:
    (a) FDG uptake is indirectly related to tumor grade.
    (b) PET is NOT useful in the estimation of prognosis.
    (c) After a period of chemotherapy, a temporary increase in glucose metabolism is observed in most brain tumors.
    (d) PET is NOT useful in the prediction of response to treatment.

12. Which item is NOT correct about brain tumors?
    (a) Approximately half of the intracranial tumors are glioma.
    (b) High-grade tumors are hypometabolic in FDG-PET study.
    (c) PET plays a key role in the grading of these tumors.
    (d) PET is important in the differentiation of tumor recurrence from necrosis after radiotherapy.

13. A 66-year-old man with a history of oligodendroglioma of the left hemisphere is under treatment with corticosteroids because of cerebral edema. What changes will be observed in the ^{18}F-FDG scan?
    (a) Increased ^{18}F-FDG uptake
    (b) Decreased ^{18}F-FDG uptake
    (c) The uptake is inversely related to the administered dose
    (d) No change in ^{18}F-FDG uptake

14. Age-related changes in PET images are seen in:
    (a) Basal ganglia
    (b) Visual cortices
    (c) Cerebellum
    (d) Frontal cortex

15. In which of the following categories of head and neck cancers is the clinical indication of FDG-PET well established and its value supported by a large amount of clinical experience and literature?
    (a) Cervical metastasis, unknown primary
    (b) Staging
    (c) Recurrence
    (d) Radiotherapy planning

16. Which of the following statements regarding oncologic radiotracers in brain tumors is NOT correct?
    (a) Target/background uptake for thallium in brain tumors is greater than that of ^{99m}Tc-MIBI.
    (b) ^{99m}Tc-MIBI is NOT helpful if the goal is to evaluate low-grade glioma.
    (c) ^{99m}Tc-MIBI is NOT helpful if the goal is to evaluate tumors near the choroid plexus.
    (d) ^{99m}Tc-MIBI and thallium can help in the evaluation of viability of tumors after radiotherapy.

17. Which of the following items about the application of PET in brain tumors is NOT correct?
    (a) Glioblastoma multiforme is a hypermetabolic tumor.
    (b) A high FDG uptake is associated with high-grade tumors.
    (c) The relative uptake in the tumor to that of gray matter is used for the quantitative evaluation of its metabolic activity.
    (d) ^{11}C-methionine is indicated for the determination of the tumor grade.

18. Which of the following statements regarding brain tumors is NOT correct?
    (a) FDG uptake in brain tumors is usually greater than that of white matter.
    (b) A minimal uptake in the choroid plexus is the main limitation of ^{99m}Tc-MIBI in the evaluation of brain tumors.
    (c) FDG uptake in brain tumors is NOT always greater than that of gray matter.
    (d) The tumor/background ratio of ^{201}Tl in brain tumors is high.

19. A patient with brain tumor is referred to your department. The biopsy report indicates it is metastatic in nature. It most likely originated from the:
    (a) Lung
    (b) Prostate
    (c) Stomach
    (d) Nasopharynx

20. Which of the following is NOT true in a patient who underwent surgery for brain tumor?
    (a) The first control MRI should be performed 72 h post-operation.
    (b) Any enhancing tissue on the first MRI indicates tumoral recurrence.
    (c) Granulation tissue develops in all patients post-operation.
    (d) The development of granulation tissue is seen after the first week of operation.

21. What is the order of uptake in high- and low-grade glioma in comparison with white and gray matter in PET scan?
    (a) High-grade glioma > gray matter > low-grade glioma > white matter
    (b) High-grade glioma > low-grade glioma > gray matter > white matter
    (c) High-grade glioma > white matter > low-grade glioma > gray matter
    (d) High-grade glioma > low-grade glioma > white matter > gray matter

22. What is the radiotracer of choice for the evaluation of low-grade brain tumors?
    (a) ^{18}F-fluorodeoxyuridine (FLT)
    (b) ^{67}Cu-PTSM
    (c) FDG
    (d) ^{11}C-thymidine

23. Which of the following radiotracers is normally uptaken in hypophysis?
    (a) ^{11}C-methionine
    (b) FDG
    (c) ^{11}C-thymidine
    (d) ^{67}Cu-PTSM

24. All of the following statements about FDG-PET are correct *except*:
    (a) The uptake in nonfunctional pituitary adenomas is greater than that of functional pituitary adenomas.
    (b) The FDG uptake in brain lymphoma is similar to that of low-grade glioma.
    (c) FDG-PET is valuable for the evaluation of brain metastases.
    (d) A higher FDG uptake in meningioma represents a more invasive form of the disease.

25. What are the recommended radiotracers for the presurgical localization of the functional cortex and for the identification of foci with high metabolic activity, respectively?
    (a) ^{11}C-methionine, ^{11}C-thymidine
    (b) $^{15}O\text{-}H_2O$, $^{15}O\text{-}H_2O$
    (c) ^{11}C-methionine, ^{18}F-fluorodeoxyuridine (FLT)
    (d) FDG-PET, ^{11}C-thymidine

26. The application of PET in the monitoring of brain tumors:
    (a) PET scan with FDG or ^{11}C-methionine is capable of identifying microscopic foci and low-grade glioma.
    (b) FDG uptake decreases after chemotherapy or radiotherapy.
    (c) A poor uptake of FDG after treatment denotes a successful treatment, whereas a high FDG uptake is due to tumor recurrence or residual.
    (d) A negative FDG uptake after treatment of the primary tumor excludes tumor recurrence or residual.

27. All of the following statements regarding the role of PET scan in brain cancers are correct *except*:
    (a) Hyper- or hypometabolic lesions are determined by comparing the metabolism of lesions with that of white matter.
    (b) Steroid therapy influences brain metabolism and interferes with the outcome of PET scan.
    (c) PET appears to be capable of distinguishing among various grades of tumors according to their metabolism.
    (d) The histology of a brain tumor can change over time, and PET can help in this aspect.

28. A patient underwent surgery for glioblastoma multiforme 9 months ago, followed by complete radiotherapy. She is now referred because of changes in her neurological state. Imaging demonstrates increased tumor size and enhancement. Which of the following methods is the most valuable for the differentiation of tumor recurrence from radiotherapy-induced necrosis?
    (a) CT scan with contrast
    (b) MRI with contrast
    (c) PET scan
    (d) Comparison of MRI with and without contrast

29. What is the most common primary brain tumor in adults?
    (a) High-grade glioma
    (b) Low-grade glioma
    (c) Meningioma
    (d) Ependymoma

30. PET imaging using radiolabeled amino acids provides high tumor-to-background imaging. The dynamic PET imaging of the following radiolabeled amino acids may further provide time-activity curves, which have been shown to give diagnostic information for tumor grading and evaluation of brain metastases following radiotherapy, *except*:
    (a) DOTATOC PET imaging
    (b) FET-PET imaging
    (c) FDOPA-PET imaging
    (d) MET-PET imaging

31. Which item about FDG-PET imaging is correct?
    (a) PET-MRI is a useful modality in the neuro-oncology field.
    (b) Whole-body imaging for tumor evaluation must be performed at least 30 min after injection.
    (c) Imaging for brain tumor evaluation must be performed at least 45 min after injection.
    (d) High blood sugar does NOT influence FDG uptake in malignant cells.

32. If the goal is to evaluate brain tumors, in which of the following items is FDG-PET the least valuable?
    (a) Diagnosis of tumor
    (b) Grading
    (c) Estimation of prognosis
    (d) Differentiation between relapse and necrosis after radiotherapy

33. Which item about brain tumors is NOT correct?
    (a) High-grade tumors are hypometabolic in FDG-PET study.
    (b) Half of intracranial tumors are glioma.
    (c) PET is valuable in tumor grading.
    (d) PET is indicated for the differentiation of a tumor relapse from necrosis.

34. About ^{18}F-FDG uptake and activity of malignant brain tumors:
    (a) Uptake is due to high glycolytic activity.
    (b) A positive correlation exists between malignancy and glycolytic activity.
    (c) FDG uptake is associated more with the proliferative activity of the tumor than with the number of viable tumoral cells.
    (d) Whole-body FDG scan is useful for distinguishing between primary and metastatic tumors.

35. Which of the following MRS findings is the most diagnostic for the differentiation of tumoral recurrence from radiation necrosis?
    (a) Increased ratio of choline (Cho) to creatine (Cr)
    (b) Increased ratio of NAA to creatine
    (c) Decreased absolute level of myoinositol level
    (d) Increased absolute level of alanine

36. What is the most common primary malignant brain tumor in adults?
    (a) Glioblastoma multiforme (GBM)
    (b) Medulloblastoma
    (c) Low-grade glioma
    (d) Lymphoma

1.26.1 Answer

	A	B	C	D
1			*	
2				*
3	*			
4				*
5	*			
6				*
7			*	
8			*	
9		*		
10	*			
11			*	
12		*		
13				*
14				*
15			*	
16	*			
17			*	
18		*		
19	*			
20				*
21	*			
22				*
23	*			
24		*		
25		*		
26			*	
27		*		
28			*	
29	*			
30		*		
31	*			
32	*			
33	*			
34			*	
35			*	
36	*			

1.27 Current and Future Directions in PET Technology

1. Lutetium oxyorthosilicate (LSO) and gadolinium oxyorthosilicate (GSO) scintillators in clinical PET scanners:
   (a) LSO has lower stopping power than GSO.
   (b) LSO has slower decay than GSO.
   (c) LSO has poorer energy resolution than GSO.
   (d) All of the above.

2. The choice of scintillation material for PET system should have the following features *except*:
   (a) Emission of a large number of scintillation photons
   (b) High density
   (c) High atomic number
   (d) Long scintillation light decay time

3. The benefits of using time of flight (TOF) in PET scanners include:
   (a) A significant reduction in the number of detected random coincidences
   (b) An improvement in the noise variance of reconstructed images
   (c) The ability to perform simultaneous emission and transmission imaging
   (d) All of the above

1.27.1 Answer

	A	B	C	D
1			*	
2				*
3				*

1.28 PET-MRI in Oncology

1. The following are advantages of PET-MRI over PET/CT *except*:
   (a) Improved lesion detection in the brain, breast, liver, and kidneys
   (b) Better demarcation of the T category in non-pulmonary soft tissues and bone
   (c) Improved outlining of lesion margins within the lung parenchyma
   (d) Better alignment of simultaneously acquired PET-MRI data

2. The following are potential advantages of PET/CT over PET-MRI *except*:
   (a) Not contraindicated in patients with pacemakers, aneurysm coils, etc.
   (b) Less susceptible to attenuation correction artifacts
   (c) Better conspicuity of benign bone lesions
   (d) Improved accuracy of local staging because of its superior soft tissue contrast

3. The following are potential advantages of PET-MRI over MRI *except*:
   (a) Ability to assess physiologic parameters such as glucose metabolism or tumor hypoxia
   (b) Identification of the malignant involvement of lymph nodes that are otherwise normal in size and morphology
   (c) Better anatomic delineation of gliomas
   (d) Not contraindicated in patients with pacemakers

4. The advantages of PET-MRI over PET/CT are seen in following primary malignancy(ies):
   (a) Better identification of high-grade prostate tumors
   (b) Superior T staging accuracy in gynecologic tumors
   (c) Greater sensitivity for liver metastases
   (d) All of the above

5. Superior T staging accuracy in PET-MRI versus PET/CT is seen in the following primary malignancies *except*:
   (a) Head and neck SCC
   (b) Breast
   (c) Gynecology
   (d) Lung

6. Which of the following statements correctly describes the role of PET imaging in head and neck cancer?
   (a) In patients with head and neck squamous cell carcinoma (HNSCC), FDG-PET-MRI does not improve lymph node metastasis detection in comparison with MRI.
   (b) FDG-PET/CT helps to improve initial staging, although its value in tumor recurrence detection is disputed.
   (c) PET-MRI allows for the combination of high hard tissue contrast and molecular information, which is promising in oncologic imaging.
   (d) PET-MRI is currently the most widely used modality in head and neck imaging.

7. The following are the important disadvantages of FDG-PET-MRI of the head and neck *except*:
   (a) Hypoglossal nerve palsy
   (b) Brown fat
   (c) Metal artifacts
   (d) Thyroid masses

8. The referring clinicians working in the head and neck field should know that:
   (a) FDG-PET-MRI is recommended for initial staging of HNSCC.
   (b) In patients with suspected HNSCC recurrence, FDG-PET-MRI is superior to stand-alone MRI.
   (c) FDG-PET-MRI is currently recommended for radiotherapy planning of HNSCC.
   (d) MRI has high accuracy for cervical lymph node metastases.

9. Which of the following statements correctly describes the role of PET-MRI in lymphoma?
   (a) FDG-PET-MRI is equivalent to FDG-PET/CT in the initial staging of lymphoma and has high sensitivity and specificity for nodal lymphoma involvement.
   (b) Currently, FDG-PET-MR is the imaging method of choice for FDG-avid lymphomas.
   (c) Initial results demonstrate that DWI is not a useful addition to FDG-PET-MRI.
   (d) In cases with suspected extranodal involvement, T1-weighted or contrast-enhanced MRI can be useful.

10. Typical PET-MRI pattern(s) in lymphoma:
   (a) Lymph nodes or focal lesions with a high FDG uptake
   (b) Multiple coalescing lymph nodes (bulky disease)
   (c) Lymph nodes or focal lesions with restricted diffusion
   (d) All of the above

11. Which of the following statements correctly describes the role of PET-MRI in breast cancer?
   (a) PET-MRI may potentially detect more distant metastases in breast cancer than PET/CT or MRI alone.
   (b) PET-MRI has the potential to guide breast biopsies because of its greater sensitivity than MRI.
   (c) Preliminary data suggest no synergy among SUV, DWI, and contrast-enhanced MRI parameters.
   (d) FDG-PET-MRI is the imaging method of choice for breast cancer.

12. Which of the following statements properly describes the role of PET-MRI in lung cancer?
    (a) PET-MRI has the potential to detect distant metastases of lung cancer with an even higher sensitivity than PET/CT or MRI alone.
    (b) PET-MRI systems will replace chest CT in detecting small primary lung tumors.
    (c) Metallic artifacts in the chest can result in the overestimation of SUV in chest wall lesions.
    (d) The misclassification of lung tissue as air can overestimate SUV in lung lesions.

13. Which of the following parameters regarding the clinical application of PET-MRI sequences in gynecologic cancers is true?
    (a) T1-weighted pre-contrast and post-contrast fat-suppressed images can help in tumor localization and extension.
    (b) T2-weighted high-resolution TSE images can assess myometrial and parametrial invasion.
    (c) Diffusion-weighted images can evaluate tumor cellularity.
    (d) All of the above.

14. Which of the following statements regarding the potential complementary role for PET-MRI in clinical indications is true?
    (a) Characterizes malignant tumor in breast cancer
    (b) Increases diagnostic accuracy and detects liver metastasis in colorectal cancer
    (c) Delineates structural change more clearly in bone metastasis
    (d) All of the above

15. In the following oncologic survey of cancers of the gastrointestinal tract, PET-MRI has the advantage over PET/CT in:
    (a) T staging of rectal carcinoma and characterization of liver lesions
    (b) Lymph node study in gastric cancers
    (c) Distant metastases in colorectal cancers
    (d) Response to treatment in esophageal cancers

16. PET-MRI may play an increasingly important role in clinical practice relative to PET/CT in the following organ malignancies *except*:
    (a) Brain
    (b) Breast
    (c) Prostate
    (d) Esophagus

1.28.1 Answer

	A	B	C	D
1			*	
2				*
3				*
4				*
5				*
6	*			
7				*
8		*		
9	*			
10				*
11	*			
12	*			
13				*
14				*
15	*			
16				*

1.29 Molecular Imaging and Precision Medicine

1. Which of the following statements regarding precision medicine (PM) is true?
   (a) PM is an emerging approach for disease treatment and prevention that takes into account the individual variabilities in genes, environment, and lifestyle of each person.
   (b) Radiomics using PET-MRI data may support the implementation of precision medicine in oncology.
   (c) HyperPET, the combination of hyperpolarized magnetic resonance spectroscopy and PET, may be valuable in cancer phenotyping.
   (d) All of the above.

2. The extraction and analysis of large amounts of advanced quantitative imaging features with high throughput from medical images is called:
   (a) Radiogenomics
   (b) Radiomics
   (c) Radiometabolomics
   (d) Transcriptomics

3. Which of the following statements regarding precision medicine in cancer is true?
   (a) Mutations introduced during primary tumor cell growth result in clonal heterogeneity.
   (b) In solid tumors, extensive heterogeneity within individuals and extensive heterogeneity between individuals are common.
   (c) Genomic analysis from single tumor biopsy specimens underestimates the mutational burden in such heterogeneous tumors.
   (d) All of the above.

4. What is the value of molecular imaging in the implementation of precision medicine in oncology?
   (a) Theranostics was successfully implemented in the field of nuclear medicine, and it has become a valid example of precision medicine.
   (b) Molecular imaging has high potential to validate the "treat what you see and see what you treat" concept.
   (c) Molecular imaging assists in the targeted imaging of tumor characterization, microenvironment, metabolism, angiogenesis, proliferation, apoptosis, receptor expression, and hypoxia, among others.
   (d) All of the above.

5. What are the specific advantages of functional PET assessment of the tumor in augmenting the concept of precision medicine?
   (a) Serves as a guide to multitargets in molecular-based therapy
   (b) Provides a dual-tracer PET imaging approach in individualizing therapy
   (c) Quantifies metabolic activity, metabolic tumor volume, and total lesion glycolysis as a disease prognosticator
   (d) All of the above

1.29.1 Answer

	A	B	C	D
1				*
2		*		
3				*
4				*
5				*

Suggested Readings

1. Ahmadzadehfar H, Biersack HJ, Freeman LM, Zuckier L. Clinical nuclear medicine. 2nd ed. Berlin: Springer; 2018.
2. Ell PJ, Gambhir SS. Nuclear medicine in clinical diagnosis and treatment. 3rd ed. Edinburgh, NY: Churchill Livingstone; 2004.
3. Sandler MP, Coleman RE, Patton JA, Wackers FJT, Gottschalk A. Diagnostic nuclear medicine. 4th ed. Philadelphia: Lippincott & Williams Wilkins; 2003.
4. Henkin RE. Nuclear medicine. 2nd ed. Philadelphia: Mosby Elsevier; 2006.
5. Rosenkrantz AB, Friedman K, Chandarana H, Melsaether A, Moy L, Ding YS, Jhaveri K, Beltran L, Jain R. Current status of hybrid PET/MRI in oncologic imaging. AJR Am J Roentgenol. 2016;206(1):162–72.
6. Fraum TJ, Fowler KJ, McConathy J. PET/MRI: emerging clinical applications in oncology. Acad Radiol. 2016;23(2):220–36.
7. Basu S, Alavi A. PET-lbased personalized management in clinical oncology: an unavoidable path for the foreseeable future. PET Clin. 2016;11(3):203–7.
8. Platzek I. (18)F-fluorodeoxyglucose PET/MR imaging in head and neck cancer. PET Clin. 2016;11(4):375–86.
9. Platzek I. 18F-Fluorodeoxyglucose PET/MR imaging in lymphoma. PET Clin. 2016;11(4):363–73.
10. Rice SL, Friedman KP. Clinical PET-MR imaging in breast cancer and lung cancer. PET Clin. 2016;11(4):387–402.
11. Ponisio MR, Fowler KJ, Dehdashti F. The Emerging role of PET/MR imaging in gynecologic cancers. PET Clin. 2016;11(4):425–40.
12. Kjær A, Torigian DA. Clinical PET/MR imaging in oncology future perspectives. PET Clin. 2016;11(4):489–93.
13. Kwon HW, Becker AK, Goo JM, Cheon GJ. FDG whole-body PET/MRI in oncology: a systematic review. Nucl Med Mol Imaging. 2017;51(1):22–31.
14. Paspulati RM, Gupta A. PET/MR imaging in cancers of the gastrointestinal tract. PET Clin. 2016;11(4):403–23.

2 Nuclear Medicine in Tumor Therapy

2.1 Principles of Radionuclide Therapy

1. All drugs may enhance uptake by altering the biokinetics of the radiopharmaceutical *except*:
   (a) β-Adrenergic blocking agents
   (b) Vasodilator drugs
   (c) Calcium channel-blocking drugs
   (d) Sympathomimetic agents
2. Which radionuclide does NOT emit alpha particles in targeting radiotherapy?
   (a) ^{213}Bi
   (b) ^{225}Ac
   (c) ^{211}At
   (d) ^{114m}In
3. Which of the palliative bone radionuclides has the lowest beta mean range?
   (a) ^{32}P
   (b) ^{188}Re
   (c) ^{153}Sm
   (d) ^{89}Sr
4. Which of the following radionuclides is considered group 1 "targeting therapy"?
   (a) ^{211}Astatine
   (b) ^{131}Cesium
   (c) ^{90}Yttrium
   (d) ^{67}Ga

2.1.1 Answer

	A	B	C	D
1				*
2				*
3			*	
4	*			

M. Assadi et al., *Principles of Nuclear Medicine*,
https://doi.org/10.1007/978-3-319-91701-6_2

2.2 Dosimetric and Radiobiological Considerations

1. What is the assignment of a radiation weighting factor for alpha particles?
   (a) 2
   (b) 12
   (c) 20
   (d) 40
2. Which one has the lowest tissue weighting factor for the calculation of an effective equivalent dose?
   (a) Red marrow
   (b) Lung
   (c) Thyroid
   (d) Breast

2.2.1 Answer

	A	B	C	D
1			*	
2			*	

2.3 Dosimetric and Radiobiological Considerations: Patient-Specific Dosimetry

1. Which technique is used for patient-specific 3D dosimetry?
   (a) Point kernel convolution
   (b) Marinelli method
   (c) MIRD
   (d) Quimby method

2.3.1 Answer

	A	B	C	D
1	*			

2.4 Benign Thyroid Disease

1. Which of the thyroid diseases is presented as hypoechoic on ultrasonography?
   (a) Grave's disease
   (b) Hashimoto's thyroiditis
   (c) Nontoxic goiter
   (d) a and b
2. Plaque-shaped calcifications occur in:
   (a) Follicular thyroid cancers
   (b) Papillary thyroid cancer
   (c) Medullary thyroid cancer
   (d) b and c
3. Follow-up examinations of thyroid nodules should be done:
   (a) Every 1–3 months
   (b) Every 2–4 months
   (c) Every 2–8 months
   (d) Every 3–12 months
4. Color Doppler ultrasonography should be used in:
   (a) Grave's disease
   (b) Hashimoto's thyroiditis
   (c) Amiodarone-induced thyrotoxicosis
   (d) Pendred syndrome
5. Which is NOT correct regarding the measurement of thyroid uptake?
   (a) Following contrast media application, uptake remains suppressed for about 6–8 weeks.
   (b) After amiodarone administration, it may be blocked for >1 year.
   (c) Nutritional intake significantly blocks thyroidal tracer uptake.
   (d) Excess intake of seafood significantly blocks thyroidal tracer uptake.
6. Before fine-needle biopsy, all medications should be withdrawn *except*:
   (a) PTU
   (b) Methimazole
   (c) Warfarin
   (d) Levothyroxine
7. Which of the following statements regarding laboratory testing in thyroid diseases is NOT correct?
   (a) The use of calcitonin and CEA is confirmed in the evaluation of suspicious nodules.
   (b) In iodine deficiency goiter, thyroglobulin levels (Tg) correlate with the amount of iodine deficiency.
   (c) In metastatic cases with unknown primary nodules, Tg > 1000 ng/ml increases the probability of primary DTC.
   (d) Tg measurement can be recommended as a routine tool in benign thyroid disease.

8. It is the development of one or more autonomous cell lines that hypersecrete T4 and T3:
   (a) Pendred syndrome
   (b) Plummer's disease
   (c) Marine–Lenhart syndrome
   (d) Grave's disease
9. What is the main indication of thyroid scintigraphy in thyroid nodule assessment?
   (a) All patients with functional changes and thyroid nodules with a diameter > 1 cm
   (b) Thyrotoxicosis without sonographically detected nodules
   (c) Patients with small nodules and signs of functional disorders
   (d) All of the above
10. What percentage of all patients with autonomy is euthyroid and would be overlooked if only in vivo parameters were measured?
   (a) About 80%
   (b) About 60%
   (c) About 40%
   (d) About 20%
11. The therapeutic effects of radioiodine in hyperthyroid disease depend on the following parameters *except*:
   (a) Patient age
   (b) Length of history
   (c) Initial volume
   (d) Cardiovascular problems
12. The risk for the development of Grave's disease after radioiodine therapy for goiter is:
   (a) 0%
   (b) <1%
   (c) <5%
   (d) <10%
13. In general, the thyroid depressant medication given for Grave's disease should not exceed:
   (a) 18 months
   (b) 12 months
   (c) 24 months
   (d) 10 months
14. All of the following patients can be expected to have a higher risk for persistence of Grave's disease *except*:
   (a) Large goiter
   (b) Young age
   (c) High antibody values
   (d) Lung problems

15. What is Marinelli's formula for dose calculation in radioiodine therapy?
    (a) (Target dose (Gy) × Target weight (g) × 24.67)/Maximal uptake (%) × Effective half-life (days)
    (b) (Target dose (Gy) × Effective half-life (days))/Maximal uptake (%) × Target weight (g)
    (c) (Target dose (Gy) × Maximal uptake (%) × 24.67)/Target weight (g) × Effective half-life (days)
    (d) (Target dose (Gy) × Target weight (g))/Maximal uptake (%) × Effective half-life (days)
16. In thyroid uptake assay, if the counting for thyroid is 7000, femur is 2000, iodide capsule phantom is 21,000, and background is 1000 after 24 h, what is the percentage of absorption in the thyroid?
    (a) 35
    (b) 10
    (c) 20
    (d) 25
17. Which of the following laboratory tests is NOT suitable for the diagnosis of corresponding thyroid disorders?
    (a) ESR: de Quervain's disease
    (b) Anti-TPO: Hashimoto's thyroiditis
    (c) CEA: medullary thyroid cancer
    (d) Anti-Tg: Grave's disease
18. Treatment for a patient with Grave's and ophthalmopathy:
    (a) The dose of radioactive iodine must be decreased.
    (b) Treatment with prednisolone for 4 weeks is effective.
    (c) Both.
    (d) None.
19. In perchlorate discharge test:
    (a) 300 mg of perchlorate is prescribed.
    (b) A reduction in activity of up to 20% is considered normal.
    (c) Both.
    (d) None.
20. In which of the following conditions is thyroid nodule malignancy the least probable?
    (a) Isoactive nodule in thyroid scintigraphy
    (b) Hyperactive nodule on scintigraphy
    (c) Enhanced uptake in thallium scan
    (d) Follicular proliferation in FNA
21. Which of the following studies is NOT necessary for the evaluation of a patient with Hashimoto's thyroiditis?
    (a) ESR
    (b) Biopsy
    (c) Anti-TPO
    (d) Sonography

22. Which of the following situations is considered a relative contraindication for the administration of ^{131}I in the treatment of Plummer disease?
    (a) Very large thyroid
    (b) Normal levels of T3 and T4
    (c) An autonomous node greater than 10 ml
    (d) Suppressed TSH
23. A 67-year-old hyperthyroid woman is a candidate for radioactive iodine therapy. Which of the following is necessary?
    (a) Pregnancy test before radiotherapy.
    (b) If hyperactivity is persistent after 2 months, radioactive iodine therapy should be repeated.
    (c) Antithyroid drugs must be discontinued 24 h before radioactive iodine therapy.
    (d) Drug treatment to make the patient euthyroid before iodine therapy.
24. Who can be a candidate for ^{131}I therapy?
    (a) A 12-year-old child with Grave's disease
    (b) A 21-year-old man with pain in the anterior neck, increased T4 levels, and decreased TSH
    (c) A 33-year-old woman with mild Grave's disease and a small goiter who has been under methimazole treatment for 6 months
    (d) All of the above
25. Which of the following diseases has the highest malignancy rate for a thyroid nodule?
    (a) Acute thyroiditis
    (b) Hashimoto's thyroiditis
    (c) Toxic nodular goiter
    (d) Grave's disease
26. Which of the following procedures has the highest priority for evaluating a thyroid nodule?
    (a) FNA
    (b) Thyroid scintigraphy
    (c) TSH measurement
    (d) Evaluation of iodine uptake in the thyroid
27. Which of the following drugs interacts with ^{123}I absorption in the thyroid?
    (a) Beta blockers
    (b) Amiodarone
    (c) Alpha blockers
    (d) Calcium channel blockers
28. About the treatment of Grave's disease with ^{131}I:
    (a) Capsules with standard doses are the most suitable considering exposure.
    (b) Pregnancy must be avoided for at least 12 months.
    (c) Beta blockers can be administered 5 days after radiation.
    (d) Ophthalmopathy may deteriorate after therapy.

29. Which of the following is recommended for the preparation of patients for radioiodine therapy?
    (a) Fasting
    (b) Previous administration of Lugol's solution
    (c) Bladder emptying before measurement
    (d) Discontinuation of caffeine-containing foods 24 h before measurement
30. FNA shows follicular neoplasia for a euthyroid patient with a single thyroid nodule. What is the next step?
    (a) Repeat of FNA after 6 months
    (b) Thyroid sonography
    (c) Thyroid scan
    (d) Surgery
31. Increased thyroid hormones and decreased TSH are found in a patient with symptoms of hyperthyroidism. A palpable nodule is found in the anterior neck upon physical examination. What is the next step?
    (a) FNA
    (b) Repeat of laboratory tests after 1 month
    (c) Thyroid scan
    (d) Thyroid sonography
32. Which of the following diseases is characterized by a low anti-TPO?
    (a) Hashimoto's disease
    (b) Addison's disease
    (c) Grave's disease
    (d) Lymphoma
33. Grave's ophthalmopathy:
    (a) It is completely improved with the treatment of thyrotoxicosis.
    (b) Prednisolone is prescribed 1 week before radioiodine therapy.
    (c) Prednisolone dose is 5 mg/kg/day.
    (d) Smoking cessation is necessary for a successful treatment.
34. The thyroid uptake percentage of which iodine reserve is measured in the radioactive iodine uptake method?
    (a) Extrathyroid organic iodine pool
    (b) Daily iodide uptake
    (c) Inorganic iodide pool
    (d) Whole-body iodine and iodide pools
35. Which statement is NOT correct?
    (a) Thyroid reserve is the largest iodine pool of the body.
    (b) GI absorption of iodide depends on its plasma level.
    (c) Food is usually the main source of inorganic iodide pool.
    (d) Thyroid hormone synthesis depends on the level of iodide in the gland.
36. Iodine uptake in the thyroid decreases in all of the following conditions *except*:
    (a) Hypothyroidism due to dyshormonogenesis
    (b) Atrophic thyroiditis
    (c) Heart failure
    (d) Renal failure

37. In which of the following conditions is T3 suppression NOT indicated?
    (a) Observation of suppressed tissue due to the overadministration of T4
    (b) Diagnosis of nodule autonomy
    (c) Grave's euthyroidism
    (d) A patient suspected to have Grave's disease with a high range but with normal hormone levels
38. In retrosternal goiter:
    (a) The absence of iodine uptake in the retrosternum excludes retrosternal goiter.
    (b) The accumulation of iodine in the thymus can cause false-positive results.
    (c) The rate of malignancy is high.
    (d) Spiral CT scan with contrast is NOT used for diagnosis.
39. About thyroid nodules:
    (a) Blood pool scintigraphy with ^{99m}Tc-MAA, in addition to sonography, is useful for the detection of cystic or solid thyroid nodules.
    (b) All cystic thyroid nodules are benign.
    (c) 201Tl washout is elongated in benign thyroid nodules in comparison with malignant nodules.
    (d) Thyroid scan is preferred to be conducted before FNA.
40. In ^{123}I thyroid scintigraphy:
    (a) ^{123}I does NOT produce the stunning phenomenon in cancerous cells or residual thyroid tissue.
    (b) Beta particles have low energy.
    (c) It is NOT indicated for the diagnosis of substernal goiters because of low energy.
    (d) Iodine uptake study is NOT possible with this tracer because of the multiple gamma photons.
41. What is the main advantage of a thyroid scan with a pinhole collimator?
    (a) Precise measurement
    (b) Observation of actual anatomy
    (c) High resolution
    (d) Appropriate geometric matching
42. Thyroid hormone tests show an increase in T3 resin uptake, decrease in total T4, and normal free T4 and T4 indices. What is the most probable diagnosis?
    (a) Hyperthyroidism
    (b) Hypothyroidism
    (c) Thyroxin-binding globulin (TBG) deficiency
    (d) Increase in thyroxin-binding globulin (TBG)
43. The thyroid hormone test for a patient suspected to have hyperthyroidism reveals an increase in T4, decrease in T3 resin uptake, and normal free T4 and free T4 indices. What is the most probable diagnosis?
    (a) TBG excess
    (b) Dysalbuminemia
    (c) Systemic disease
    (d) Hyperthyroidism

44. Which of the following hyperthyroxine conditions is considered euthyroid?
    (a) Grave's disease
    (b) Hyperthyroidism due to struma ovarii
    (c) Acute psychiatric attacks
    (d) Adenoma of hypophysis
45. What is the main disadvantage of pinhole collimators in a thyroid scan?
    (a) Inaccurate size and anatomy of the thyroid
    (b) Low resolution
    (c) Low uniformity
    (d) Scattering
46. Which variable is counted in sandwich immunometric assay?
    (a) Labeled ligand
    (b) Solid-phase antibody–ligand-labeled antibody
    (c) Ligand-labeled antibody
    (d) Labeled antibody
47. In which of the following diseases does the TSH stimulation test NOT increase iodine uptake?
    (a) Plummer's disease
    (b) Toxic nodule
    (c) Grave's disease
    (d) Subacute thyroiditis
48. The evaluation of umbilical cord blood of a newborn shows an increased level of serum TSH. Furthermore, sonography of the anterior neck reveals both lobes of the thyroid. What is the next step?
    (a) TRH stimulation test
    (b) Perchlorate discharge test
    (c) Thyroid scan by ^{99m}-Tc
    (d) Evaluation of the mother for Grave's disease
49. Thyroid weight is 85 g in a patient with Grave's disease, and any sign of ophthalmopathy is not found. What is the first therapeutic approach?
    (a) High-dose nonradioactive iodine
    (b) Dose ^{131}I
    (c) Subtotal thyroidectomy
    (d) Methimazole and PTU
50. In which of the following conditions does iodine uptake have the least application?
    (a) Evaluation of hypothyroidism
    (b) Suspicious subacute thyroiditis
    (c) Determination of ablation time in a patient with Jod–Basedow syndrome
    (d) Dose determination of radioactive iodine for the treatment of Grave's disease
51. Which item about in vitro thyroid tests is NOT correct?
    (a) The antibody is labeled in immunoradiometric assay (IRMA).
    (b) Ag is labeled in radioimmunoassay (RIA).
    (c) Non-isotopic labels require longer incubation time than isotopic labels.
    (d) Sandwich IRMA is a noncompetitive method.

52. Evaluation of thyroid function shows an increase in FT4I and TT4 with normal FT4 and T3RU. What is the most probable diagnosis?
    (a) Dysalbuminemia
    (b) TBG excess
    (c) TBG deficiency
    (d) Hypoalbuminemia
53. The Wolff–Chaikoff effect is:
    (a) Hyperthyroidism induced by excess iodine
    (b) Hyperthyroidism in multinodular goiter
    (c) Hypothyroidism in multinodular goiter
    (d) Hypothyroidism induced by excess iodine
54. The Jod–Basedow phenomenon is:
    (a) Hypothyroidism induced by excess iodine
    (b) Hyperthyroidism in multinodular goiter
    (c) Hyperthyroidism induced by excess iodine
    (d) Hypothyroidism in multinodular goiter
55. Plummer's disease is:
    (a) Hyperthyroidism in multinodular goiter
    (b) Hyperthyroidism induced by excess iodine
    (c) Hypothyroidism induced by excess iodine
    (d) Hypothyroidism in multinodular goiter
56. A 15-year-old girl complains about a menstrual disorder. Thyroid hormone assessment shows the following results: T4, 10.2 μg/dl; T3, 215 ng/dl; and TSH, 2 mIU/l. What is the choice of management?
    (a) Prescription of methimazole
    (b) Patient follow-up
    (c) Prescription of levothyroxine
    (d) Thyroid scan
57. In which of the following conditions is an increase in RAIU observed?
    (a) Chronic renal failure
    (b) Inflammatory bowel disease
    (c) Multi-hormonal contraceptives
    (d) Enriched dairy
58. Which item about hypertrophic nodule of the thyroid is NOT correct?
    (a) TSH dependency.
    (b) Warm or hot.
    (c) Increase in thyroid hormone levels.
    (d) It results from inflammatory or degenerative lesions of the thyroid.
59. In which group of neonatal hypothyroidism is reevaluation at age 3–4 years NOT required?
    (a) Ectopic
    (b) Dyshormonogenesis
    (c) Absence of thyroid in scan
    (d) Eutopic hypertrophic thyroid with increased uptake

60. Which of the following findings confirms the diagnosis of factitious thyrotoxicosis?
    (a) Normal thyroglobulin, high RAIU
    (b) High thyroglobulin, low RAIU
    (c) Low thyroglobulin, low RAIU
    (d) High thyroglobulin, high RAIU
61. Which item is NOT correct about thyroid scan with ^{99m}Tc-pertechnatate?
    (a) The maximum uptake is observed 10–20 min after radiopharmaceutical injection.
    (b) Esophageal activity is usually observed below the thyroid.
    (c) The radiopharmaceutical is trapped by the gland similar to ^{123}I.
    (d) The uptake in a normal thyroid gland is slightly lower than that of the salivary gland.
62. Which of the following drugs causes the inhibition of peripheral T4 to T3 conversion as well as hypophyseal inhibition?
    (a) Amiodarone
    (b) Glucocorticoids
    (c) Propranolol
    (d) Propylthiouracil (PTU)
63. In which of the following diseases is the anti-peroxidase antibody NOT detected?
    (a) Primary thyroid lymphoma
    (b) Medullary thyroid cancer
    (c) Hashimoto's disease
    (d) Grave's disease
64. Which item about Marine–Lenhart syndrome is NOT correct?
    (a) After radioiodine treatment, the nodular function is completely destroyed.
    (b) Higher rate of malignancy.
    (c) Cold node in diffused toxic goiter.
    (d) The node in the thyroid can be TSH dependent.
65. Radioiodine uptake (RAIU):
    (a) 24 h after iodine administration is the optimum time for diagnostic evaluation in a patient suspected to have thyrotoxicosis with a high turnover.
    (b) Chronic renal failure decreases RAIU.
    (c) The dose of radioactive iodine is at least 100 mCi.
    (d) Fasting is NOT required.
66. What is the choice hormone assessment for the diagnosis of thyroid dysfunction if you are allowed to do only one assessment?
    (a) T4
    (b) T3
    (c) TSH
    (d) FT3
67. In sick euthyroid syndrome (SUS):
    (a) High T3 is the major change in thyroid hormone evaluation.
    (b) rT3 increases.
    (c) Most of SUS patients show severe thyroid insufficiency.
    (d) TT4 decreases in progressed forms of the disease.

68. Which of the following conditions is considered a relative contraindication of radioactive iodine therapy in multinodular goiter?
    (a) Detection of a large cold nodule
    (b) Evidence of autonomy
    (c) The elderly
    (d) Relapse after surgery
69. In which of the following conditions is hypothyroidism the most common after iodine therapy?
    (a) Toxic adenoma
    (b) Multinodular goiter
    (c) Grave's disease
    (d) Plummer's disease
70. In which of the following conditions is thyroid scintigraphy NOT necessary?
    (a) Patients with a nodule and suppressed TSH
    (b) Hypothyroidism in an adult patient without a palpable nodule
    (c) Presence of small nodules with symptoms of malignancy
    (d) Follow-up of a patient with Grave's disease during treatment
71. A patient with goiter is evaluated. Increased levels of TT3, TT4, and FT4 are observed. Serum TSH is normal. There is no sign of thyrotoxicosis. What is the most probable diagnosis?
    (a) Generalized resistance to thyroid hormone
    (b) Sick euthyroid syndrome
    (c) TBG increase
    (d) TBG decrease
72. What is the best radiopharmaceutical for the evaluation of iodine metabolism and thyroid function?
    (a) ^{152}I
    (b) ^{123}I
    (c) ^{131}I
    (d) ^{99m}TcO4
73. A patient with thyrotoxicosis is subjected to radioiodine therapy. Three weeks later, laboratory tests show normal levels of FT4 and FT3 but suppressed TSH. What is the next step?
    (a) The patient must be prepared for a second dose of radioactive iodine.
    (b) Measurement of T3RU.
    (c) High-dose methimazole.
    (d) The follow-up study must be performed after a few weeks.
74. An 8-year-old child with symptoms of hyperthyroidism and dysphagia is evaluated. Sublingual thyroid is diagnosed through the thyroid scan. Which of the following items is the least risky?
    (a) Levothyroxine therapy
    (b) Radioiodine ablation and levothyroxine replacement
    (c) Surgical removal of the sublingual thyroid and levothyroxine replacement
    (d) Monthly follow-up of the patient

75. A woman with a cold nodule of the thyroid is evaluated. If she has a history of Hashimoto's thyroiditis, what will be the effect of Hashimoto's thyroiditis on the FNA results?
    (a) False positive.
    (b) False negative.
    (c) No effect.
    (d) FNA must be repeated with more probability.
76. A high technetium uptake and a low iodine uptake are reported for a patient. What is the most probable diagnosis?
    (a) Grave's disease
    (b) Plummer's disease
    (c) Hashimoto's thyroiditis
    (d) Autonomy nodule
77. In which of the following conditions is the pyramidal lobe most probably observed in a thyroid scan?
    (a) Existence of the TSH receptor antibody
    (b) Multinodular goiter
    (c) After the administration of antithyroid drugs
    (d) Subacute thyroiditis
78. In which of the following conditions is the stimulatory effect of iodine trapping observed?
    (a) SCN-
    (b) TcO4-
    (c) ClO4
    (d) TSH receptor antibody
79. In the RAIU test:
    (a) A decreased iodine uptake can be observed in heart failure.
    (b) The level of iodine pool in the body is directly related to the thyroid iodine uptake.
    (c) Amiodarone must be discontinued at least 6 weeks before the test.
    (d) A decreased iodine uptake is always associated with a decreased TcO4- uptake.
80. A 36-year-old woman is referred with an active nodule of the right upper pole in the technetium scan. TSH is normal, and iodine uptake is 30%. After T3 suppression, the scan is repeated: right lobe nodule is more obvious, but iodine uptake is reduced to 15%. Which item is correct?
    (a) Autonomicity of the nodule is ruled out because of the normal thyroid hormone levels.
    (b) Autonomy nodule in the right upper pole.
    (c) A TSH stimulation test is required for the final diagnosis.
    (d) Iodine scan is required for deciding on the autonomicity.

81. A 25-year-old woman is referred with symptoms of Grave's disease. She is planning for a pregnancy after next year. What is the recommended treatment for her?
    (a) Antithyroid drugs
    (b) Surgery
    (c) Radioactive iodine
    (d) Lugol's solution
82. Grave's ophthalmopathy:
    (a) After onset of the disease, it is improved in 3–6 months.
    (b) The possibility of ophthalmopathy is high in smokers but with minor complications.
    (c) It is not common and is observed only in 5% of cases.
    (d) The severe form of the disease is more common in men than in women.
83. A patient with TSH <0.01, T4:I4, and a history of amiodarone administration is referred. What is the recommended method for the differentiation of Jod–Basedow from drug-induced thyroiditis?
    (a) ^{123}I scan
    (b) Sonography
    (c) ^{99m}TcO4 scan
    (d) Fluorescent scan
84. FNA is performed for a thyroid nodule. In which of the following conditions is the probability of malignancy high?
    (a) Colloid adenoma
    (b) Hürthle cell adenoma
    (c) Microfollicular adenoma
    (d) Embryonal adenoma
85. Which sonography finding indicates the highest possibility of a benign thyroid nodule?
    (a) Hypoechoic nodule
    (b) Microcalcification
    (c) Egg-shaped calcification
    (d) Increased perfusion in Doppler sonography
86. A thyroid scan is requested for a neonate with congenital hypothyroidism. In which of the following conditions is a repeat of scan at age 3–4 years NOT necessary?
    (a) Observation of lingual thyroid
    (b) Absence of the thyroid gland
    (c) Observation of an enlarged and hot thyroid in a normal location
    (d) Observation of an enlarged thyroid with a reduced uptake in a normal location
87. A patient underwent ^{131}I therapy because of Grave's diseases 3 months ago. Clinical symptoms have improved, the patient has gained some weight, and thyroid size has notably decreased. However, laboratory tests still show hyperthyroidism. What is the best intervention?
    (a) Repeat of ^{131}I therapy with a higher dose
    (b) Patient referral for surgery
    (c) Drug therapy with methimazole and follow-up
    (d) Repeat of laboratory tests after 3 months without any medication

88. Serum T4, 3.5–4.00 μg/dl, and TSH, 22–28 mIU/l, are reported for a neonate in serial measurements. Furthermore, the thyroid does NOT appear in the ^{99m}Tc scan. What is the best intervention?
    (a) Levothyroxine treatment and reevaluation at age 3
    (b) Lifetime treatment with levothyroxine
    (c) Serum thyroid hormone evaluation of the mother before levothyroxine treatment
    (d) Levothyroxine therapy and genetic evaluation for dyshormonogenesis
89. In which group of patients is a higher level of TT3 considered normal?
    (a) Men over 40 years
    (b) Women over 40 years
    (c) Teens below 18 years
    (d) Women over 60 years
90. All of the following specific sonographic features of thyroid nodules indicate an increased incidence of malignancy *except*:
    (a) Spongiform nodules
    (b) Taller-than-wide shape
    (c) Hypoechogenicity
    (d) Microcalcifications
91. In which of the following conditions is thyroid scintigraphy NOT required?
    (a) Follow-up of a patient with Grave's disease under treatment
    (b) Thyroid nodule and suppressed TSH
    (c) Hypothyroidism in an adult without a palpable nodule
    (d) Small nodules with symptoms of malignancy
92. A 3-year-old child with a history of congenital hypothyroidism is referred for a thyroid scan. Diffused goiter is reported in the thyroid scan with ^{99m}TcO4. What is the next step?
    (a) Repeat of scan after the discontinuation of levothyroxine
    (b) Thyroid scan with ^{131}I
    (c) Measurement of serum thyroglobulin
    (d) Perchlorate test
93. Increased thyroid hormone levels, decreased TSH level, and decreased 24 h uptake of ^{131}I are observed. What is the most probable diagnosis?
    (a) Toxic metastasis
    (b) Plummer's disease
    (c) Grave's disease
    (d) TSH receptor mutation
94. In which of the following conditions is the thyroid uptake of iodine typically low?
    (a) Dyshormonogenesis
    (b) Chronic autoimmune thyroiditis
    (c) Struma ovarii
    (d) Iodine deficiency

95. Only one region with a minor increase in uptake in comparison with the thyroid cartilage is found in the thyroid scan of an infant with congenital hyperthyroidism. What is the next step?
    (a) Reevaluation at age 3 with discontinuation of levothyroxine
    (b) Lifetime levothyroxine therapy
    (c) Genetic consultation for dyshormonogenesis
    (d) Discontinuation of levothyroxine
96. A 33-year-old woman is subjected to a thyroid scan with two radioisotopes. A hot nodule in the right lobe is observed in the technetium scan, but it appears as a cold nodule in the scan with ^{131}I. Which item is correct?
    (a) This finding is indicative of malignancy with high specificity.
    (b) This finding is indicative of a defect in organification.
    (c) This finding rejects the presence of a follicular adenoma.
    (d) This finding rejects the presence of an adenomatous goiter.
97. In which type of goiter is delayed hypothyroidism the most common after ^{131}I radioiodine therapy?
    (a) Toxic diffuse goiter treated with 22 mCi of ^{131}I
    (b) Toxic nodular goiter treated with 22 mCi of ^{131}I
    (c) Toxic multinodular goiter treated with 5 mCi of ^{131}I
    (d) Toxic nodular goiter treated with 20 mCi of ^{131}I
98. In which of the following conditions is the patient euthyroid despite the high serum thyroxin?
    (a) Subacute thyroiditis
    (b) Factitious thyrotoxicosis
    (c) Peripheral resistance to thyroid hormone
    (d) Plummer's disease
99. Which of the following methods is NOT considered as a separation method in the RIA system?
    (a) Solid-phase method
    (b) Double-antibody method
    (c) Chromatography method
    (d) Chloramine-T method
100. Which item about immunoradiometric assay (IRMA) is NOT correct?
    (a) A low amount of the antigen is detectable in comparison with RIA.
    (b) Antibody is labeled with iodine instead of antigen.
    (c) The higher the level of the measured antigen is, the lower the level of counting.
    (d) Double-antibody methods can be used for separation.
101. A patient with pain in the anterior region of the neck and fever is referred. Laboratory examinations show an increase in sedimentation and a decrease in iodine uptake. What is the most probable diagnosis?
    (a) Subacute thyroiditis
    (b) Hashimoto's thyroiditis
    (c) Riedel's thyroiditis
    (d) Bacterial acute thyroiditis

102. Perchlorate discharge test is performed on a patient. A 15% decrease in iodine uptake is observed after termination of the test. All of the following diagnoses are possible *except*:
    (a) Chronic lymphocytic thyroiditis
    (b) Plummer's disease
    (c) Treatment with propylthiouracil
    (d) Pendred syndrome
103. A mediastinal mass with suspicious retrosternal thyroid is found in the radiography result of a patient. Which of the following radiopharmaceuticals is recommended for thyroid scintigraphy?
    (a) ^{123}I
    (b) ^{131}I
    (c) ^{201}Tl
    (d) ^{99m}Tc-MIBI
104. A patient suffering from chronic renal failure is routinely subjected to dialysis. What is the recommended treatment for hyperthyroidism for this patient?
    (a) Antithyroid drugs only
    (b) Administration of ^{131}I and dialysis the day after radioiodine
    (c) Administration of ^{131}I and dialysis 3 days after radioiodine
    (d) Surgery only
105. How is thyrotoxicosis factitia presented in scan and laboratory tests?
    (a) Decreased radioiodine uptake, decreased TSH
    (b) Increased radioiodine uptake, decreased TSH
    (c) Decreased radioiodine uptake, increased TSH
    (d) Normal radioiodine uptake, normal TSH
106. IRMA:
    (a) Antigen increases in this method.
    (b) There are two types of one and two sites.
    (c) The antigen is labeled.
    (d) The sensitivity of RIA is greater than that of IRMA.
107. What is the main adverse effect of hyperthyroidism treatment with radioactive iodine?
    (a) Impotency
    (b) Leukemia
    (c) Thyroid cancer
    (d) None of the above
108. Which of the following items is considered an advantage of RIA over ELISA?
    (a) Shorter shelf life
    (b) Higher sensitivity
    (c) Less radiation
    (d) Higher pipetting
109. What is the goal of the solid phase in radioimmunoassay?
    (a) Production of monoclonal antibody with hybridoma methods
    (b) Antigen labeling with ^{125}I
    (c) Separation of free antigen from bound antigen
    (d) Production of high-affinity antibody

110. What is the treatment of choice for a hot thyroid nodule with toxic symptoms in a 71-year-old woman?
    (a) Radioactive iodine after a short-term antithyroid treatment
    (b) Antithyroid + Lugol's solution
    (c) Antithyroid treatment
    (d) Surgery
111. After the treatment of hyperthyroidism with ^{131}I:
    (a) No long-term follow-up is required.
    (b) Therapeutic effects appear after 1–2 weeks.
    (c) Maximum therapeutic effect appears after 6 months.
    (d) About 80–90% of patients show improvement with one dose.
112. In which of the following conditions is the incidence of thyroid storm after ^{131}I therapy for hyperthyroidism lower?
    (a) Large goiter
    (b) Chronic hyperthyroidism
    (c) Administration of high doses
    (d) Toxic nodular goiter
113. In which of the following situations is thyrotoxicosis accompanied by an increased radioiodine uptake?
    (a) Trophoblastic tumor
    (b) Subacute thyroiditis
    (c) Factitious thyrotoxicosis
    (d) Higher intake of iodine
114. In which of the following conditions is thyrotoxicosis treatment with ^{131} iodine therapy indicated?
    (a) Increased hormone secretion from thyroid cancer metastases
    (b) Hypophysis adenoma with inappropriate TSH secretion
    (c) Jod–Basedow disease
    (d) Ovarian teratoma with a significant level of active thyroid tissue
115. What is the treatment of choice for hyperthyroidism in the third month of pregnancy?
    (a) Propylthiouracil
    (b) Radioactive iodine
    (c) Methimazole
    (d) Surgery
116. Congenital hypothyroidism:
    (a) It is a type of euthyroid hypothyroxinemia.
    (b) Blood sample for thyroid function tests must be obtained in the first 24–48 h after birth.
    (c) It does NOT need any specific treatment because this condition is transient.
    (d) Total T4 must be measured for the monitoring of treatment.
117. Which of the following drugs must be discontinued for a longer time before RAIU test?
    (a) Antithyroid drugs
    (b) Lugol's solution
    (c) Myelography contrasts
    (d) Thyroid hormones

118. Precipitation of bound antibodies in the double-antibody method is performed with centrifugation, but the pellet is suspended during the decanting of the test tube. What is the most appropriate intervention?
    (a) Application of bound antibody to the solid phase
    (b) Centrifugation at 37 °C
    (c) Refrigerated centrifugation
    (d) Prolongation of incubation
119. What is the most appropriate treatment for a patient with Grave's disease and a notable cold nodule on scintigraphy?
    (a) Antithyroid treatment + ^{131}I
    (b) Antithyroid treatment + surgery
    (c) Antithyroid treatment + beta blocker
    (d) Lugol's solution + beta blocker
120. About hyperthyroidism:
    (a) Antithyroid treatment has lesser side effects on children.
    (b) Large toxic nodules completely disappear after iodine therapy.
    (c) When the primary iodine therapy fails, the minimum interval for a repeat of iodine therapy is 3 months.
    (d) Thyroidectomy and iodine therapy are the best treatment for TSH-secreting hypophyseal tumors.
121. Fine-needle aspiration (FNA):
    (a) Hashimoto's thyroiditis is the common cause of a false-positive finding in the diagnosis of thyroid malignancies.
    (b) Its effective differentiation of follicular adenoma from follicular carcinoma is considered an advantage of this method.
    (c) The application of this method decreases the incidence of inappropriate thyroidectomy by 50%.
    (d) The incidence of cancer decreases in a patient who underwent surgery based on FNA outcome.
122. Which of the following reactants is labeled in IRMA?
    (a) Ligand
    (b) Analyte
    (c) Binder
    (d) Antigen
123. In perchlorate discharge test:
    (a) 24 h iodine uptake is the criterion of measurement.
    (b) More than 10% of the radioiodine is discharged from the thyroid in a normal subject.
    (c) The concentration of free iodine in patients with enzyme deficiency is less than that in normal subjects.
    (d) This test is performed for hypothyroid patients with suspected dyshormonogenesis.

124. Which of the following conditions can cause an increase in thyroid iodine uptake?
    (a) Pregnancy and lithium consumption
    (b) Hypothyroidism
    (c) Radiotherapy of the neck
    (d) Renal and heart failures
125. The 12 h iodine uptake is 80%, and the 24 h uptake is 10%. What is the most probable diagnosis?
    (a) Factitious thyrotoxicosis
    (b) Overdose
    (c) Thyroiditis
    (d) Thyrotoxicosis
126. In radioiodine therapy for hyperthyroidism:
    (a) The risk for thyroid cancer and leukemia increases.
    (b) Genetic disorders in offspring increase.
    (c) The administration of digoxin before radioiodine therapy is necessary for patients with atrial fibrillation.
    (d) Radioiodine administration is allowed for breastfeeding women.
127. What (mCi/g of thyroid tissue) is the recommended dose of ^{131}I for the treatment of Grave's disease?
    (a) 50–100
    (b) 100–120
    (c) 120–160
    (d) 160–200
128. Which of the following immunoassay methods is the most sensitive?
    (a) Chemiluminescent immunoassay
    (b) Enzyme-multiplied immunoassay technique
    (c) Fluorescent immunoassay
    (d) Radioimmunoassay
129. The concentration of radiolabeled antibody–antigen complex depends on which parameter in RIA?
    (a) Inverse relationship with the concentration of unlabeled antibody
    (b) Direct relationship with the concentration of labeled antibody
    (c) Inverse relationship with the concentration of unlabeled antigen
    (d) Direct relationship with the concentration of unlabeled antigen
130. All of the following items are considered diagnostic problems of thyroid FNA *except*:
    (a) Differential diagnosis of follicular adenoma and follicular carcinoma
    (b) Differential diagnosis of papillary adenoma and papillary carcinoma
    (c) False-positive findings in Hashimoto's thyroiditis
    (d) Requirement of an experienced cytopathologist

131. In the ^{131}I therapy of women with hyperthyroidism:
   (a) NO confirmed scientific evidence about the genetic disorders of their children has been found yet.
   (b) Their children will be born with genetic disorders.
   (c) The ovarian absorbed dose is greater than 1 Gy per 370 MBq (10 mCi) of the administered activity.
   (d) ^{131}I therapy is contraindicated in women of childbearing age and children.
132. In which of the following situations is the patient euthyroid despite hyperthyroxinemia?
   (a) Stroma ovarii
   (b) Silent thyroiditis
   (c) 5-Deiodinase genetic disorder
   (d) Factitious hyperthyroidism
133. A hot nodule in the thyroid technetium scan appears as a cold nodule in the radioactive iodine scan. Which of the following items is correct?
   (a) The incidence of malignancy in these nodules is 10%.
   (b) The incidence of malignancy in these nodules is 100%.
   (c) The incidence of malignancy in hot nodules is less than 1%.
   (d) About 45% of thyroid nodules show this inconsistency in scan results.
134. Which of the following methods is the most valuable for the differential diagnosis of hypertrophic nodules from autonomous nodules?
   (a) Thallium scan
   (b) Thyroid technetium scan with suppression test
   (c) MRI
   (d) Spiral CT scan
135. What is the method of choice for the diagnosis of anterior mediastinal tumors?
   (e) Thyroid scan with technetium
   (f) Thyroid scan with ^{131}I
   (g) MRI
   (h) Spiral CT with contrast
136. About the secretion and control of thyroid hormones:
   (a) TSH stimulates the secretion of T4 and T3 with a ratio of 1:10 (T3: tenfold of T4).
   (b) Among the plasma proteins, TBG has minimum affinity but maximum capacity for thyroid hormone binding.
   (c) A major part of T3 is secreted from follicular thyroid cells in response to TSH stimulation.
   (d) The negative feedback effect on anterior hypophysis is mainly mediated by T3.
137. Which of the following items does NOT describe the mechanism of amiodarone-induced thyroid dysfunction?
   (a) Increase in TBG
   (b) Wolff–Chaikoff effect
   (c) Jod–Basedow effect
   (d) Thyroiditis after tissue destruction

138. Which of the following statements about the thyroid gland is NOT correct?
   (a) Parafollicular cells originate from an ultimobranchial body in the embryonic period.
   (b) A 24 h iodine uptake test is sufficient for patients with thyrotoxicosis.
   (c) The pyramidal lobe is usually connected with the left thyroid lobe.
   (d) Fetal iodine uptake and thyroid hormone synthesis usually begin after the tenth gestational week.
139. A 39-year-old woman presents with symptoms of hyperthyroidism in the third trimester. Which parameter with a high level is predictive of a high probability of neonatal Grave's disease?
   (a) Thyroid-stimulating antibody
   (b) Thyroid-stimulating immunoglobulin (TSI)
   (c) TSH-binding inhibitor
   (d) Anti-TPO
140. What is the recommended hormonal test for a 90-year-old patient with poor general condition in the intensive care unit if the goal is to distinguish a thyroid from a non-thyroid illness?
   (a) T4 and T3RU
   (b) TSH and FT4
   (c) T3 and TT4
   (d) rT3 and FT4 index
141. What is the effect of lithium on the thyroid function?
   (a) Inhibition of the thyroid hormone secretion
   (b) Inhibition of the synthesis and release of thyroid hormones
   (c) Inhibition of tyrosine iodination and coupling
   (d) Inhibition of iodine organification
142. Which of the following outcomes is the most probable in patients with epilepsy under treatment with phenylhydantoin?
   (a) Increased T4, increased T4 RIA
   (b) Increased T4, normal T4 RIA
   (c) Decreased T4, increased T4 RIA
   (d) Normal free T4, decreased T4 RIA
143. Radioactive iodine uptake (RAIU) represents:
   (a) Iodine trapping
   (b) Iodine organification
   (c) All steps in the iodine turnover
   (d) Hormone release
144. About radioactive iodine uptake:
   (a) Discontinuation of interfering drugs before the test is NOT required.
   (b) The distance of the probe to patient's neck must be constant in each measurement.
   (c) Fasting does NOT change the results of the test.
   (d) 50–100 μCi of ^{131}I is required for each patient.

145. Which of the following radioisotopes is the most suitable for radioactive iodine uptake (RAIU)?
(a) ^{125}I
(b) ^{127}I
(c) ^{131}I
(d) ^{123}I
146. What is the main route of the excretion of iodine from the body?
(a) Renal
(b) Intestinal
(c) Salivary
(d) Perspiration
147. Radioactive iodine uptake (RAIU) is the most reliable for the:
(a) Diagnosis of hypothyroidism
(b) Diagnosis of hyperthyroidism
(c) Diagnosis of Hashimoto's thyroiditis
(d) Estimation of ^{131}I dose for thyroid ablation therapy
148. When is the preferred time for the discontinuation of methimazole before iodine therapy?
(a) 48–72 h
(b) 3–4 days
(c) 4–5 days
(d) 1 week
149. Choose the best item about the talk technique as a method of separating bound and free ligands.
(a) Less affinity, less potential to strip the Ab-bound ligand
(b) Greatest affinity, potential to strip the Ab-bound ligand
(c) No affinity, no stripping of the Ab-bound ligand
(d) Primary Ab bound to solid support and labeled secondary Ab
150. Choose the best item about the sandwich technique as a method of separating bound and free ligands.
(a) Greatest affinity, potential to strip the Ab-bound ligand
(b) Primary Ab bound to solid support and labeled secondary Ab
(c) No affinity, no stripping of the Ab-bound ligand
(d) Less affinity, less potential to strip the Ab-bound ligand
151. Choose the best item about the resin technique as a method of separating bound and free ligands.
(a) Greatest affinity, potential to strip the Ab-bound ligand
(b) Primary Ab bound to solid support and labeled secondary Ab
(c) No affinity, no stripping of the Ab-bound ligand
(d) Less affinity, less potential to strip the Ab-bound ligand

152. A 36-year-old woman with ophthalmopathy resulting from Grave's disease comes to your clinic, and you propose radiotherapy. What would be your radiotherapy plan for the patient?
    (a) Both orbits radiation via lateral opposing fields with 6–10 MV photons up to 5000 cGy
    (b) Both orbits radiation via lateral opposing fields with 6–10 MV photons up to 2400 cGy
    (c) Both orbits radiation via lateral opposing fields with 15–18 MV photons up to 5000 cGy
    (d) Both orbits radiation via lateral opposing fields with 15–18 MV photons up to 2400 cGy
153. All of the following properly describe thyroiditis (Riedel's struma) *except*:
    (a) Is a rare thyroid disorder that is more common in women than in men.
    (b) Its pattern is similar to that of anaplastic carcinoma.
    (c) Sonography can be used for the evaluation of extrathyroidal inflammation.
    (d) FNA can help in the diagnosis.
154. Which of the following rectus muscles has minimum involvement in thyroid ophthalmopathy?
    (a) Superior
    (b) Inferior
    (c) Medial
    (d) Lateral
155. What is the correct formula for the calculation of RAIU?
    (a) [(Neck counts – Background counts)/(Phantom counts – Thigh counts)] × 100
    (b) [(Neck counts – Thigh counts)/(Phantom counts – Background counts)] × 100
    (c) [(Neck counts – Phantom counts)/(Thigh counts – Background counts)] × 100
    (d) [(Neck counts – Thigh counts)/(Neck counts – Background counts)] × 100
156. What change is reported at the RAIU level in Hashimoto's thyroiditis?
    (a) Increase
    (b) Decrease
    (c) Normal
    (d) All of the above
157. What is the thyroid scan pattern for Hashimoto's thyroiditis?
    (a) 50% combination of hot and cold nodules, 30% nonhomogenous uptake, 20% normal
    (b) 50% normal, 30% nonhomogenous uptake, 20% combination of hot and cold nodules
    (c) 50% nonhomogenous uptake, 30% combination of hot and cold nodules, 20% normal
    (d) 50% combination of hot and cold nodules, 30% normal, 20% nonhomogenous uptake

158. Iodine reserve in the thyroid nodule to the normal thyroid tissue is 0.9. Which of the following items is correct?
   (a) The nodule is definitely benign.
   (b) The nodule is definitely malignant.
   (c) The nodule is malignant with high probability.
   (d) The nodule is benign with high probability.
159. Which of the following statements regarding the functional thyroid nodule is NOT correct?
   (a) Hypertrophic nodules are TSH dependent.
   (b) Autonomous adenoma is induced because of degeneration or inflammation.
   (c) Levothyroxine is indicated for the treatment of hypertrophic nodules.
   (d) Hypertrophic nodules demonstrate a normal or an increased level of TSH.
160. Graves's disease coexists with TSH-dependent cold thyroid nodules. What is this condition called?
   (a) Marine–Lenhart syndrome
   (b) Jod–Basedow phenomenon
   (c) Wolff–Chaikoff effect
   (d) Plummer's disease
161. A 15-year-old girl suffering from Grave's disease is subjected to methimazole treatment. Intermittent recovery and recurrence are observed 1 year after treatment. What is the recommended protocol for treatment?
   (a) Subtotal thyroidectomy
   (b) Replacement of methimazole with propylthiouracil
   (c) Emphasis on the regular administration of methimazole
   (d) Radioactive iodine therapy
162. What is the typical sign of Hashimoto's thyroiditis?
   (a) Thyroid is initially enlarged with a coarse echo.
   (b) Presence of small hypoechoic foci with irregular edges.
   (c) Thick and heteroechoic lesions.
   (d) Thick septa.
163. Which of the following statements regarding the sonography of a normal thyroid is NOT correct?
   (a) The right lobe is normally larger than the left lobe.
   (b) Thyroid vessels in the peripheral regions are hypoechoic.
   (c) The right posterior flexure of the capsule in the axial section may appear similar to hyperechoic nodules.
   (d) The color Doppler sonography of the thyroid overestimates the normal background flow.

2.4.1 Answer

	A	B	C	D		A	B	C	D		A	B	C	D
1				*	56		*			111				*
2				*	57		*			112		*		
3				*	58			*		113	*			
4			*		59	*				114			*	
5				*	60			*		115	*			
6				*	61				*	116				*
7	*				62	*				117			*	
8		*			63		*			118	*			
9				*	64	*				119		*		
10		*			65		*			120			*	
11				*	66			*		121	*			
12		*			67				*	122			*	
13		*			68	*				123				*
14				*	69			*		124	*			
15	*				70				*	125				*
16				*	71	*				126			*	
17				*	72		*			127		*		
18		*			73				*	128	*			
19	*				74		*			129			*	
20		*			75	*				130		*		
21		*			76			*		131	*			
22	*				77	*				132			*	
23				*	78				*	133	*			
24	*				79	*				134		*		
25				*	80		*			135				*
26			*		81			*		136				*
27		*			82				*	137	*			
28				*	83				*	138		*		
29	*				84				*	139	*			
30			*		85			*		140		*		
31			*		86	*				141	*			
32		*			87			*		142				*
33				*	88	*				143			*	
34			*		89			*		144		*		
35		*			90	*				145				*
36	*				91	*				146	*			
37	*				92				*	147				*
38		*			93	*				148				*
39				*	94			*		149	*			
40	*				95		*			150		*		

41			*		**96**		*			**151**			*	
42			*		**97**	*				**152**		*		
43	*				**98**			*		**153**	*			
44			*		**99**				*	**154**				*
45	*				**100**			*		**155**		*		
46		*			**101**	*				**156**				*
47			*		**102**		*			**157**			*	
48		*			**103**		*			**158**				*
49				*	**104**		*			**159**			*	
50	*				**105**	*				**160**	*			
51			*		**106**		*			**161**				*
52	*				**107**				*	**162**			*	
53				*	**108**		*			**163**				*
54			*		**109**			*						
55	*				**110**	*								

2.5 Radionuclide Therapy of the Thyroid: Treatment of Thyroid Malignancies

1. What is the most important prognostic factor in differentiated thyroid carcinoma?
   (a) Tumor features
   (b) Age
   (c) Sex
   (d) Elevated serum thyroglobulin >3 months after surgery
2. The fetal thyroid takes up iodine after the
   (a) 10th week of gestation
   (b) 12th week of gestation
   (c) 14th week of gestation
   (d) 8th week of gestation
3. Which one is categorized as an early side effect of ^{131}I therapy?
   (a) Anosmia
   (b) Azoospermia
   (c) Pulmonary fibrosis
   (d) Bone marrow aplasia
4. Choose the correct statement regarding thyroid cancers.
   (a) Papillary thyroid cancer is more prevalent in iodine-rich regions than in iodine-deprived regions.
   (b) After previous radiotherapy of the head and neck, follicular thyroid cancer is more prevalent than papillary thyroid cancer.
   (c) Both.
   (d) None.
5. Regarding the etiopathogenesis of thyroid cancer:
   (a) BRAF V600E is the most common alteration in sporadic follicular carcinoma.
   (b) Mutations in BRAF are the most recently identified MAPK effector in thyroid cancer.
   (c) BRAF and RET alterations represent a novel indicator of the progression and aggressiveness of thyroid carcinogenesis.
   (d) Promoter hypermethylation of multiple genes, especially TSHR, has been identified to play a role in thyroid cancers and particularly shows a close association with RAS mutational status.
6. If a pulmonary metastasis of thyroid cancer occurs after iodine therapy, the risk of pulmonary fibrosis will NOT be directly related to:
   (a) Age
   (b) Extent of pulmonary metastasis
   (c) Intensity of ^{131}I uptake
   (d) Frequency of ^{131}I administration

7. Which of the following complications is rare if a woman with papillary thyroid cancer and pulmonary micrometastasis is treated with 30 mCi of 131I?
   (a) Thyroid storm
   (b) Infertility
   (c) Sialadenitis
   (d) Pulmonary fibrosis
8. What is the most common delayed adverse effect of ^{131}I therapy for thyroid cancer?
   (a) Impotency
   (b) Leukemia
   (c) Salivary gland dysfunction
   (d) Bladder cancer
9. A 55-year-old patient with DTC and diffuse pulmonary metastasis is referred to your department. What is the required recommended ablative dose of radioiodine for this patient?
   (a) 30 mCi
   (b) 100 mCi
   (c) 150 mCi
   (d) 200 mCi
10. In the ^{131}I treatment of differentiated thyroid cancers:
    (a) A low-iodine food regimen must be discontinued 2 weeks after treatment.
    (b) Treatment with T4 is started 24 h after radioiodine therapy.
    (c) Co-treatment with T3 and T4 should be considered for patients with severe hypothyroidism.
    (d) T3 can be replaced by a T4 loading dose (three tablets of T4 for 3–5 days).
11. Which item does NOT increase the uptake of ^{131}I to improve its therapeutic effect?
    (a) Administration of exogenous TSH
    (b) T3 replacement therapy, 24 h after iodine therapy
    (c) Administration of diuretic before iodine therapy
    (d) Destruction of remnant normal thyroid
12. A 26-year-old man with thyroid cancer is twice subjected to ^{131}I (100 mCi for each time). The residual thyroid tissue is still observed on the whole-body scan. However, regional or distant metastasis is not observed in the scan, patient Tg is constantly low, and anti-Tg is negative. Which intervention is recommended?
    (a) Administration of 100 mCi of ^{131}I.
    (b) Administration of 150 mCi ^{131}I.
    (c) The patient must be referred for radioiodine therapy.
    (d) Follow-up only.
13. Differentiated thyroid cancer:
    (a) In most cases, treatment by external radiation is possible for one time only.
    (b) Multiple small metastatic pulmonary nodules, which are detectable in chest X-ray, are successfully treated with iodine.
    (c) Iodine therapy is NOT indicated for bone metastasis.
    (d) Radioactive iodine produces lower radiation exposure of the tumor compared with external radiation.

14. Which item is NOT effective for the reduction of exposure to radiation in radioiodine therapy in a patient with thyroid cancer?
    (a) NSAID
    (b) Omeprazole
    (c) Chewing gum
    (d) Water and fluids
15. Which item about papillary thyroid carcinoma is NOT correct?
    (a) When surgery is NOT possible, radioactive iodine is also ineffective.
    (b) Iodine therapy is NOT required when the tumor size is less than 1 cm.
    (c) Repeat of surgery is required when the 24 h iodine uptake after surgery is more than 20%.
    (d) Breastfeeding must be completely discontinued when a repeat of iodine therapy is necessary.
16. Which type of thyroid cancer demonstrates the best response to radioactive iodine therapy?
    (a) Anaplastic cancer
    (b) Hürthle cancer
    (c) Follicular cancer
    (d) Medullary cancer
17. A 36-year-old woman with papillary thyroid cancer is referred 8 weeks after thyroidectomy. A significant residual thyroid tissue (more than 2 g) is observed on the whole-body scan with radioiodine. What is the most appropriate intervention?
    (a) High-dose ^{131}I ablation for one time
    (b) High-dose ^{131}I ablation administered into three intervals
    (c) Levothyroxine administration and repeat of scan after 6 months
    (d) Repeat of surgery
18. A 29-year-old woman with a history of papillary thyroid cancer is subjected to 400 rad radiation with ^{131}I. What is the effect of radiation on future fertility?
    (a) Temporary infertility occurs for 2 years.
    (b) This amount of radiation has NO effect on fertility.
    (c) The risk of infertility increases to 50%.
    (d) Increase in the probability of high-risk pregnancy.
19. A patient is subjected to ^{131}I for several times because of thyroid cancer and bone metastasis. What is the radiation limit for blood exposure?
    (a) 500 rad
    (b) 400 rad
    (c) 300 rad
    (d) 200 rad

20. A patient with differentiated thyroid cancer is referred for follow-up evaluation after total thyroidectomy and replacement iodine therapy. Thyroglobulin test is also requested. Which item is correct?
    (a) If the whole-body scan with radioiodine is negative and there is an increase in anti-thyroglobulin antibody, the patient can be subjected to radioiodine treatment.
    (b) The positive predictive value of this test is less important than its negative predictive value for metastasis.
    (c) The diagnostic sensitivity of thyroglobulin test is 100%.
    (d) Recombinant TSH is required when the level of thyroglobulin is high despite the levothyroxine treatment.
21. A patient with differentiated thyroid cancer underwent complete surgical thyroidectomy and thyroid remnant ablation with ^{131}I. No abnormal tracer uptake is found on the whole-body scan with ^{131}I. Serum thyroglobulin is also undetectable. However, the TSH level still oscillates between 0.8 mIU/l and 1.5 mIU/l despite the increase in levothyroxine dose from 150 μg/day to 250 μg/day. Which of the following drugs can inhibit the suppression of TSH release?
    (a) Ketoconazole
    (b) Cholestyramine
    (c) Co-trimoxazole
    (d) Dopamine
22. In Hürthle cell lesion:
    (a) Pleomorphism is a feature of malignancy.
    (b) Capsule invasion or vascular invasion is not the criterion for malignancy.
    (c) Cytomorphological criteria can help to distinguish Hürthle cell carcinoma from adenoma.
    (d) Cytomorphological criteria can help to distinguish Hürthle cell neoplasm from Hürthle cell metaplasia.
23. In which of the following assays can anti-Tg autoantibodies overestimate the Tg levels?
    (a) IFMA
    (b) IEMA
    (c) IRMA
    (d) Hemagglutination
24. Which of the following metastatic lesions of differentiated thyroid cancer can better respond to ^{131}I ablation therapy?
    (a) Bone
    (b) Lung
    (c) Lymph nodes
    (d) Spread of metastatic lesions (in all body)
25. ^{123}I is preferred by some clinicians for the first thyroid scan after thyroidectomy of patients with differentiated thyroid cancer. What is the most important reason for this method?
    (a) Prevention of stunning
    (b) Inhibition of a higher uptake in the salivary glands
    (c) Decrease in radiation exposure of patients
    (d) Improvement of quality of images

26. What is the bone marrow dose in the treatment of thyroid cancers with ^{131}I (high activity)?
    (a) 5–10 CGy
    (b) 10–20 CGy
    (c) 50–100 CGy
    (d) 1000–5000 CGy
27. Which long-distance metastasis of differentiated thyroid cancer is usually resistant to ^{131}I and is therefore treated with surgery or radioiodine therapy?
    (a) Liver metastasis
    (b) Brain metastasis
    (c) Pulmonary metastasis
    (d) Bone metastasis
28. In which type of differentiated thyroid metastasis is the serum thyroglobulin level decreased?
    (a) Pulmonary
    (b) Lymph nodes
    (c) Bone
    (d) Liver
29. A patient with differentiated thyroid cancer underwent total thyroidectomy and ablation with 100 mCi of radioiodine. One year later, a palpable mass on the right side of the neck is reported in a follow-up study, and sonography shows an enlargement of the lymph nodes. What is the next step?
    (a) FNA biopsy
    (b) Thallium whole-body scan
    (c) 150 mCi of radioiodine
    (d) Iodine whole-body scan
30. Which of the following statements about differentiated thyroid cancer (DTC) is NOT correct?
    (a) Lithium increases the biologic half-life of radioiodine and radiation of tumoral tissue.
    (b) The maximum therapeutic effect of radioiodine is observed in the first 24 h; therefore, thyroid hormone replacement therapy after 24 h is recommended by some scientists.
    (c) A high level of TSH can increase the biologic half-life of radioiodine in some cases of DTC.
    (d) Avoidance of solid meal 4 h before radioactive iodine is recommended to decrease gastric radiation.
31. Which of the following statements about the measurement of Tg mRNA is NOT correct?
    (a) The sensitivity of this test is high for the identification of thyroid residual or metastasis.
    (b) Tg mRNA can be measured in peripheral blood by RT-PCR.
    (c) Discontinuation of medications is NOT required for the test.
    (d) The presence of antibodies does NOT interfere with the test.

32. What happens to the level of serum Tg when anti-Tg antibodies are positive in the blood?
    (a) RIA shows a false decrease in Tg level.
    (b) Both RIA and IMA show a false decrease in Tg level.
    (c) IMA shows a false decrease in Tg level.
    (d) Both RIA and IMA show a false increase in Tg level.
33. A 42-year-old woman with papillary thyroid cancer (stage T3N1M0) underwent surgery and then thyroid remnant ablation. One year later, Tg is 0.5 ng/ml after the discontinuation of medications. Physical examination and sonography are also negative. What is the probability of thyroid residual tissue or metastasis?
    (a) Less than 20%
    (b) Less than 10%
    (c) Less than 5%
    (d) Less than 1%
34. If bone marrow suppression is performed by 200 mCi of ^{131}I, which generation of blood cells shows the most rapid decrease, the most rapid recovery, and the least influence, respectively?
    (a) Platelets, WBC, RBC
    (b) Platelets, platelets, RBC
    (c) Platelets, WBC, WBC
    (d) Platelets, platelets, WBC
35. Which type of metastasis of differentiated thyroid cancer (DTC) expresses the highest level of Tg?
    (a) Pulmonary nodular metastasis
    (b) Diffuse pulmonary metastasis
    (c) Lymphatic metastasis
    (d) Bone metastasis
36. A 43-year-old woman is referred with a single nodule in the right lobe of the thyroid. History and clinical examination show only a mobile nodule 2 cm × 2 cm in size. Moreover, follicular neoplasm is reported in FNA. What is the most appropriate intervention?
    (a) Follow-up of the patient
    (b) Lobectomy of the right thyroid lobe
    (c) Total thyroidectomy
    (d) Surgery and frozen section analysis
37. In anaplastic thyroid cancer:
    (a) The average life expectancy is 2 to 3 years.
    (b) Extensive pulmonary metastasis and respiratory failure are the common causes of mortality.
    (c) Airway obstruction due to regional invasion is the common cause of death.
    (d) Total thyroidectomy followed by iodine therapy is indicated as the primary treatment.

38. In which of the following situations is discontinuation of thyroxin contraindicated for the induction of hypothyroidism required for thyroid scintigraphy or ^{131}I ablation therapy?
    (a) Hypopituitarism
    (b) Diabetes mellitus
    (c) Brain metastasis
    (d) Liver metastasis
39. In papillary thyroid cancer:
    (a) Hürthle cell tumor is a form of papillary thyroid cancer with poor prognosis.
    (b) Cervical lymph node metastasis is usually predictive of poor prognosis.
    (c) When the lesion size is smaller than 1 cm at the time of diagnosis, it is called papillary micro-adenocarcinoma.
    (d) The probability of involvement of the lymph nodes in papillary cancer is less than that in follicular cancer.
40. A 45-year-old woman is subjected to total thyroidectomy because of follicular thyroid carcinoma. If the concentration of serum thyroglobulin is 600 ng/ml before surgery, how long after surgery before the thyroglobulin level will be reduced to 1 ng/ml?
    (a) About 1 week
    (b) About 1 month
    (c) About 3 months
    (d) About 6 months
41. In which of the following situations is external radiotherapy indicated for the treatment of thyroid cancer?
    (a) Bone and brain metastases
    (b) Regional recurrent cancers regardless of their iodine uptake
    (c) Large and infiltrative cancers as preoperative treatment
    (d) All of the above

2.5.1 Answer

	A	B	C	D
1		*		
2		*		
3	*			
4	*			
5		*		
6	*			
7		*		
8			*	
9				*
10	*			

11		*		
12			*	
13	*			
14	*			
15	*			
16			*	
17				*
18		*		
19				*
20	*			
21		*		
22				*
23			*	
24			*	
25	*			
26			*	
27				*
28		*		
29				*
30			*	
31	*			
32			*	
33				*
34		*		
35				*
36		*		
37			*	
38			*	
39	*			
40			*	
41				*

2.6 Phosphorus-32 Therapy in Myeloproliferative Disease

1. ^{32}P therapy in the management of essential thrombocythemia should be considered especially in patients:
   (a) <45 years
   (b) >65 years
   (c) >50 years
   (d) <60 years
2. In which of the following diseases is the inconsistent distribution of reticuloendothelial and granulopoietic systems observed?
   (a) Bone radiotherapy
   (b) Polycythemia vera
   (c) Aplastic anemia
   (d) Idiopathic myelofibrosis
3. Which of the statements based on the following findings of the ^{99m}Tc-SC scan of a middle-aged man with anemia and thrombocytopenia is correct?
   Enlarged spleen and shifting of radiotracer, normal view of liver, mild pulmonary uptake, bone marrow does not appear.
   (a) Splenectomy is the treatment of choice for his thrombocytopenia.
   (b) Scan with ^{58}Fe should be performed for a conclusive diagnosis.
   (c) Polycythemia vera is one of the differentiated diagnoses.
   (d) Prescription of Fe tablet is the base of treatment.
4. Which of the following indices shows the most frequent oscillations in a normal subject?
   (a) Red blood cell volume (RCV)
   (b) Red blood cell mass (RCM)
   (c) Hematocrit (Hct)
   (d) Plasma volume (PV)
5. Which of the following diseases is characterized by a progressive increase in the spleen/liver uptake ratio over time in ^{51}Cr-RBC scan?
   (a) Splenomegaly
   (b) Splenic sequestration
   (c) Iron deficiency anemia
   (d) Thalassemia minor
6. Mismatch of the hematopoietic distribution and reticuloendothelial system is observed in which of the following blood disorders?
   (a) Aplastic anemia
   (b) Hemolytic anemia
   (c) Polycythemia vera
   (d) Leukemia

7. A remarkable increase in activity is observed in the vertebrae, ribs, hip, and upper and lower extremities in sulfur colloid scintigraphy. However, scan with 52-Fe does NOT show any increased activity in the peripheral, central bone marrow, or extramedullary. What is the most probable diagnosis?
   (a) Chemotherapy
   (b) Radiotherapy
   (c) Aplastic anemia
   (d) Myelofibrosis
8. A massive lesion is observed in the posterior mediastinum in the pulmonary radiography of a patient with thalassemia. 52-Fe scintigraphy shows a remarkable accumulation of the radiotracer in the same region. What is the most probable diagnosis?
   (a) Lymphoma
   (b) Thymoma
   (c) Extramedullary hematopoiesis
   (d) Retrosternal thyroid
9. Which of the following diseases results in an inappropriate increase in erythropoietin?
   (a) Polycythemia vera
   (b) Chronic pulmonary diseases
   (c) Hepatic carcinoma
   (d) High-altitude living
10. Which of the following conditions results in partial or apparent polycythemia?
   (a) Burning
   (b) Smoking
   (c) Renal carcinoma
   (d) Obesity
11. Extramedullary hematopoiesis is suggested by a hematologist for a 29-year-old thalassemia patient with a mass in the mediastinum. What is the radiopharmaceutical of choice for the scintigraphic evaluation of this suspicion?
   (a) ^{99m}Tc-NSAb
   (b) ^{52}Fe
   (c) ^{99m}Tc-SC
   (d) 111$^{\text{In-WBC}}$
12. About 32phosphorus:
   (a) ^{32}phosphorus is accumulated in the bone marrow in addition to bone.
   (b) It is a beta-specific radiating agent with a half-life of 7 days.
   (c) The range of bone penetration is 8 mm.
   (d) Much scientific evidence has indicated that the administration of androgens before treatment with phosphorus results in better clinical response.

13. Peripheral marrow expansion is observed in the bone marrow scan of a 53-year-old man with increased hematocrit. What is the most probable diagnosis?
    (a) Polycythemia vera resulting from myelofibrosis
    (b) Chronic myeloid leukemia
    (c) Polycythemia vera
    (d) Chronic lymphoid leukemia
14. In which of the following conditions is the possibility of leukemia after polycythemia vera the highest?
    (a) Chemotherapy with chlorambucil
    (b) No treatment
    (c) Treatment with ^{32}P
    (d) Phlebotomy
15. What is the protocol for a second dose of 32P if remission is NOT achieved with the first dose in the treatment of polycythemia vera?
    (a) After 1.5 months, 15% more than the first dose
    (b) After 6 months, 50% more than the first dose
    (c) After 1 year, 50% more than the first dose
    (d) After 3 months, 25% more than the first dose
16. Bone marrow expansion to the peripheral extremities is observed in the 99mTc-SC scan. In addition, only the liver and the spleen are observed in the 52Fe scan, which is performed for the evaluation of erythropoiesis. What is the most probable diagnosis?
    (a) Aplastic anemia
    (b) Sideroblastic anemia
    (c) Myelofibrosis
    (d) Myelodysplastic syndromes
17. What is the recommended scan for the evaluation of the severity of idiopathic myelofibrosis with bone marrow involvement and extramedullary hematopoiesis?
    (a) Tc-radiocolloid
    (b) 52Fe
    (c) NCA-95
    (d) In-chloride
18. Which of the radiopharmaceuticals for PET imaging the bone marrow targets proliferative activity?
    (a) 11C-choline
    (b) 11C-methionine
    (c) 18F-FLT
    (d) 11C-acetate

2.6.1 Answer

	A	B	C	D
1		*		
2			*	
3			*	
4				*
5		*		
6	*			
7			*	
8			*	
9			*	
10	*			
11		*		
12	*			
13			*	
14	*			
15				*
16			*	
17		*		
18			*	

2.7 Palliation of Bone Pain

1. Bone metastases are common in patients with the following primary carcinomas *except*:
   (a) Breast
   (b) Prostate
   (c) Colon
   (d) Lung
2. Which one is NOT a characteristic of an ideal radiopharmaceutical for palliative therapy in patients with bone metastases?
   (a) β particle: 0.8 MeV < Emax <2.0 MeV
   (b) Rapid clearance from the normal bone
   (c) Physical half-life smaller than or equal to the biologic half-life
   (d) Predictable from ^{99m}Tc-MDP bone images
3. Which one is NOT an absolute contraindication in radiopharmaceutical therapy of patients with bone metastasis?
   (a) Given before myelosuppressive chemotherapy
   (b) Platelet count <100,000
   (c) White count $<2.5 \times 10^6$/l
   (d) Rapidly decreasing blood counts
4. Which radiopharmaceutical produces γ photon for palliative therapy?
   (a) Sr-89
   (b) P-32
   (c) Sm-153
   (d) a and c
5. In which condition can radionuclide therapy be considered as an approach for the treatment of pain associated with bone metastasis?
   (a) Presence of disseminated intravascular coagulation (DIC)
   (b) Soft tissue metastasis
   (c) Spinal cord compression
   (d) History of radionuclide therapy
6. Which item should be reminded to the patient before the administration of strontium?
   (a) Patient must be isolated.
   (b) Life span is increased during pain relieving.
   (c) If the first dose is not effective in pain relieving, then second and third doses will be applied.
   (d) Pain is usually relieved after 2 weeks.
7. Which of the following radiopharmaceuticals is used for pain alleviation and is NOT a pure beta emitter?
   (a) ^{117}Sn
   (b) ^{89}Strontium
   (c) ^{153}Samarium
   (d) ^{186}Rubidium

8. About metastron (89 SrCl):
   (a) Scintigraphy is NOT possible because of the lack of gamma emission.
   (b) It produces a strong and stable complex with bones.
   (c) Renal toxicity is the limiting factor for application.
   (d) It reduces bone pain along with radiation of auger electron.
9. What is the treatment of choice for cord compression?
   (a) 153Sm-lexidronam
   (b) 186Re-etidronate
   (c) Teletherapy (radiotherapy)
   (d) 117mSn-pentetate
10. Which item about treatment with 89-Sr is NOT correct?
   (a) ^{89}Sr increases pain before therapeutic effects are achieved.
   (b) Strontium is an analog of calcium.
   (c) The biological distribution of strontium is similar to that of ^{99m}Tc-MDP.
   (d) ^{89}Sr has palliative and curative properties in the treatment of bone metastasis.
11. What is the most important limiting factor for the application of 89Sr?
   (a) Bone marrow toxicity
   (b) Cardiotoxicity
   (c) Nephrotoxicity
   (d) Hepatotoxicity
12. The distribution of 153Sm-EDTMP is performed on Saturdays. If you aim to inject 1.5 mCi/kg of the radiopharmaceutical for the palliative treatment of a 75 kg patient with cancer on Monday, how much of the radiopharmaceutical will be required on Saturday 16:00?
   (a) 100 mCi
   (b) 150 mCi
   (c) 300 mCi
   (d) 450 mCi
13. No improvement in pain has been noted after the first injection of 89Sr. What is the probability of pain alleviation after a second injection?
   (a) 5%
   (b) 25%
   (c) 50%
   (d) 90%
14. Arrhythmia and vasodilatation are observed after the rapid injection of which radiopharmaceutical?
   (a) ^{89}SrCl2
   (b) 153Sm-EDTMP
   (c) 156Re-HEDP
   (d) 117mSn-DTP

15. A patient with cancer is referred for palliative treatment with 153Sm-EDTMP. He received a bisphosphonate such as pamidronate on the previous day. What is the next step?
    (a) Radiopharmaceutical treatment should be postponed because of drug interaction.
    (b) 153Sm-EDTMP should be replaced by ^{89}SrCl2.
    (c) 153Sm-EDTMP should NOT be administered, and the patient must be referred for radiotherapy.
    (d) There is no contraindication, and the radiopharmaceutical can be readily administered.
16. You have been consulted about the radioisotope bone pain palliation of a patient with breast cancer. In which of the following conditions is this method recommended?
    (a) Singular lesion in the femur
    (b) Normal bone scan
    (c) Symptoms of cord compression in a region with a pathologic fracture of the lumbar vertebrae
    (d) History of radiotherapy for spinal cord lesions
17. Which of the following radiopharmaceuticals can be used as a free agent (without chelator) if the goal is to treat bone pains because of metastasis?
    (a) ^{186}Re
    (b) ^{153}Sm
    (c) ^{111m}Sn
    (d) ^{89}Sr
18. What is the mechanism of 117mSn-DTPA accumulation in bone tissue?
    (a) Formation of insoluble salts with bone
    (b) Chemical absorption on the surface of hydroxyapatite
    (c) Direct replacement with calcium in the bone
    (d) Direct replacement with phosphate in hydroxyapatite
19. 89SrCl2 is used for the palliative therapy for pain. Why can it NOT be used for imaging in the same patient?
    (a) Lack of gamma emission
    (b) Negligible energy of gamma emission
    (c) Distortion of imaging because of the high energy of the beta emission
    (d) Very low percentage of gamma emission
20. Which radioisotope requires relatively high doses for bone pain alleviation because of a short half-life?
    (a) ^{89}Sr
    (b) ^{188}Re
    (c) ^{117}mSn
    (d) ^{32}P
21. Which of the following complexes results in the flare phenomenon?
    (a) ^{89}SrCl2
    (b) ^{153}Sm-EDTMP
    (c) ^{32}P-orthophosphate
    (d) ^{32}P-orthophosphate + androgen

22. What is the reason behind the parathyroid hormone administration in palliation therapy with ^{32}P-orthophosphate?
    (a) Enhancement of the radiopharmaceutical uptake in bone
    (b) Elimination of the primary increase in pain due to the radiopharmaceutical
    (c) Prevention of nausea and vomiting
    (d) Prevention of cord compression
23. A 68-year-old man with bone metastasis of prostate cancer and bone pain is referred. 153Sm-lexidronam is requested for pain alleviation. Which item is NOT correct?
    (a) Pain alleviation appears in 14 days.
    (b) The drug is NOT secreted even with the second radiopharmaceutical administration; therefore, the kidneys do NOT appear in the scan.
    (c) Minor myelotoxicity occurs with the reduction of leucocytes and platelets, which improves in 6–8 weeks.
    (d) Kidneys do NOT appear in the scan because the radiopharmaceutical is NOT secreted from the kidneys.
24. Beta radiation with maximum tissue penetration is required for palliation therapy for bone metastasis. What is the radiopharmaceutical of choice for this purpose?
    (a) ^{188}Re
    (b) ^{32}P
    (c) ^{89}Sr
    (d) ^{117m}Sn
25. The hot lab report indicates that a vial containing 89-strontium was broken 500 days ago. The level of activity in this place is now 0.01 mCi. How much (mCi) of the radiopharmaceutical was present in the mentioned vial?
    (a) 0.01 × e−6.93
    (b) 0.01 × e+6.93
    (c) 0.01 × e−0.693
    (d) 0.01 × e+0.693
26. Which radiopharmaceutical emits gamma photons that are NOT suitable for imaging?
    (a) ^{32}P
    (b) ^{188}Re
    (c) ^{117m}Sn
    (d) ^{89}Sr
27. The instability of which radiopharmaceutical causes over-radiation of the thyroid in the body?
    (a) ^{153}Sm-EDTMP
    (b) 1^{17m}Sn-DTPA
    (c) ^{186}Re-HEDP
    (d) ^{89}Sr-chloride

28. Which of the following items is NOT required for the treatment of painful bone metastasis with unsealed beta emitters?
    (a) A time period of at least 6 months after chemotherapy
    (b) Presence of radiotracer uptake at the metastasis site in the bone scan
    (c) Leukocyte count of more than 4500
    (d) Platelet count of more than 100,000
29. In the radionuclide palliative therapy of bone pain due to metastasis:
    (a) 188Re-etidronate usually accumulates in the reactive bone around the tumor.
    (b) The half-life of ^{89}Sr is 7 days.
    (c) Higher doses of ^{89}Sr can be administered in comparison with 188Re-etidronate.
    (d) 188Re-etidronate has more therapeutic effects than 186Re-etidronate.
30. A 63-year-old patient with diffuse bone metastasis of prostate cancer is referred for treatment with strontium. Platelet count is 72,000, and WBC count is 6200. He only complains about fatigue, and tenderness is NOT observed in the physical examination. He does NOT take any other medication except antiandrogens. Which of the following methods is the most appropriate?
    (a) Platelet transfusion and then administration of ^{89}Sr
    (b) Whole-blood transfusion and administration of ^{89}Sr
    (c) Follow-up without administration of ^{89}Sr
    (d) Administration of ^{89}Sr and blood test after 1 week
31. Which of the following statements regarding hormone therapy in cancers is NOT true?
    (a) In patients with metastatic breast cancer, the therapeutic options include tamoxifen and aminoglutethimide.
    (b) Response is more common in estrogen receptor-positive breast cancer patients.
    (c) Pain relief in prostate cancer is commonly reported at 24 h.
    (d) Once the first-line hormone therapy fails, the second-line treatment is likely to give response rates significantly above 30%.
32. How long is the minimum time interval between the administrations of two doses of metastron?
    (a) 3 months
    (b) 6 months
    (c) 12 months
    (d) 18 months
33. Which group of patients with multiple myeloma responds appropriately to ^{89}Sr?
    (a) Patients with high alkaline phosphatase and WBC of more than 2400/μl
    (b) Patients with osteoblastic activity on bone scan
    (c) Patients with extensive and diffuse lesions in radiography
    (d) Patients with moderate to severe bone pain

34. Which item about painful bone metastases is NOT correct?
    (a) Radiotherapy has a minimum effect on palliative regional therapy.
    (b) The primary source is usually associated with prostate, breast, or pulmonary tumors.
    (c) Narcotics can cause nausea in these patients.
    (d) Radioisotopes such as ^{32}P can be used for palliative therapy.
35. About the application of unsealed source in the treatment of bone metastasis:
    (a) One day of hospitalization is required for patients treated with ^{32}P and ^{89}Sr.
    (b) The simultaneous administration of low-dose cisplatin increases the myelosuppressive effects.
    (c) The therapeutic effects on extensive metastasis are less than those in limited metastatic lesions.
    (d) It will NOT be effective if lytic lesion is observed in radiography.
36. Which of the following items is NOT important in patients candidated for the treatment of bone metastasis with an unsealed source?
    (a) Lesion number
    (b) Physical examination
    (c) Survival
    (d) Serum urea and creatinine levels
37. Which cancer causes over half of all pathologic fractures, while other carcinomas account for only 5–10% of the total cases?
    (a) Prostate
    (b) Breast
    (c) Lung
    (d) Renal
38. All radiotracers are gamma emitters *except*:
    (a) ^{89}Sr
    (b) ^{188}Re
    (c) ^{153}Sm
    (d) ^{32}P
39. Which radiotracer has the shortest half-life?
    (a) ^{188}Re
    (b) ^{89}Sr
    (c) ^{186}Re
    (d) ^{153}Sm
40. In the radiotherapy of painful bone metastasis:
    (a) Radionuclide administration is contraindicated when platelet count is below 100,000/μl
    (b) Cortone administration with radionuclide is recommended if cord compression is predicted
    (c) The rapid injection of ^{153}Sm EDTMP can cause flushing
    (d) The Foley catheter should remain in the bladder for 5 days if the patient experiences incontinence

2.7.1 Answer

	A	B	C
1			*
2			*
3			*
4			*
5			
6			
7	*		
8	*		
9			*
10			
11	*		
12			*
13			*
14	*		
15			
16			
17			
18	*		
19			
20		*	
21			
22	*		
23			
24	*		
25		*	
26			
27			*
28	*		
29	*		
30			*
31			
32	*		
33		*	
34	*		
35			*
36	*		
37		*	
38			
39	*		
40			

2.8 Therapeutic Use of Radiolabeled Antibodies: Hematopoietic Tumors

1. Which radionuclide of current interest in radioimmunotherapy (RIT) is an α emitter?
   (a) Bismuth-213
   (b) Copper-67
   (c) Yttrium-90
   (d) Rhenium-188
2. What is the most critical determining factor of the radiation dose in RIT?
   (a) Different antibody affinities
   (b) Biologic half-life of the antibody
   (c) Absolute tumor uptake of the radiolabel
   (d) Different antibody avidities
3. Which radiolabeled antibody is NOT studied in NHL?
   (a) ^{131}I-B1
   (b) ^{90}Y-2B8
   (c) ^{131}I-Lym-1
   (d) ^{213}Bi-M195
4. Which of the following radiopharmaceuticals is applied for the treatment of non-Hodgkin's lymphoma?
   (a) ^{90}Y-colloid
   (b) ^{131}I-tositumomab
   (c) ^{32}P-chromic phosphate
   (d) ^{153}Sm- PHYP
5. Zevalin:
   (a) It is an antibody against CD-20.
   (b) It is labeled as ^{131}I.
   (c) It is the choice treatment for lymphoma.
   (d) Its hematologic toxicity is transient.
6. ^{90}Y-Zevalin:
   (a) ^{111}In is used for scintigraphy because ^{90}Yttrium has no gamma emission.
   (b) Imaging at 48–72 h after radiotracer administration is enough.
   (c) Administration before rituximab can be neglected in patients with B-cell lymphoma.
   (d) The administered dose will be reduced to 0.3 mCi if the platelet count is below 100,000.
7. Which of the following statements about Zevalin is NOT correct?
   (a) The administration of nonradioactive rituximab before radiotracer administration on the same day of therapy is necessary.
   (b) It is an anti-CD20 on T-cells.
   (c) Myelosuppression occurs 8 weeks after the administration of Zevalin.
   (d) Weakness and malaise are among the non-hematologic adverse effects

8. Which of the following conditions is the most appropriate for radioimmunotherapy?
   (a) Radioactive iodine in comparison with radioactive metals
   (b) Intracellular antigens
   (c) Antigens in blood circulation
   (d) Extracellular antigens inseparable from cells
9. Which radiotracer requires a previous injection of Rituxan?
   (a) Quadromet
   (b) I-^{131}Bexxar
   (c) ^{90}Y-Zevalin
   (d) ^{111}In-Octreoscan
10. What is the most important side effect of ^{90}Y-Zevalin?
   (a) Hepatotoxicity
   (b) Cardiotoxicity
   (c) Nephrotoxicity
   (d) Myelotoxicity
11. What is the reason for the administration of ^{111}In-Zevalin before the therapeutic dose of ^{90}Y-Zevalin?
   (a) Evaluation of the grade and intensity of the disease
   (b) Saturation of the blood antigens
   (c) Saturation of the non-specific antibodies in the liver
   (d) Evaluation of the biodistribution of antibody
12. What is the primary radiotracer for the treatment of recently diagnosed NHL?
   (a) ^{131}I-tositumomab
   (b) Unlabeled anti-CD20
   (c) ^{123}I anti-CD20
   (d) ^{131}I CC49 antibody
13. What is the order of administration (left to right) of materials in immunotherapy with pre-targeting?
   (a) Avidin, biotinylated antibody, radiolabeled biotin
   (b) Radiolabeled biotin, avidin, biotinylated antibody
   (c) Biotinylated antibody, radiolabeled biotin, avidin
   (d) Biotinylated antibody, avidin, radiolabeled biotin
14. What is the reason for the administration of non-labeled (cold) antibody before the injection of radioisotope-labeled antibodies in radioimmunotherapy?
   (a) Prediction of biodistribution of the labeled antibody
   (b) Saturation of the antigenic sites in blood
   (c) Increase in stability of the labeled antibody in the body
   (d) Prediction of hypersensitivity to the radiopharmaceutical
15. Which of the following forms of antibodies has the highest molecular weight?
   (a) IgG
   (b) F(ab′)2
   (c) Fab′
   (d) scFv

16. Which item is considered a relative contraindication for radioimmunotherapy for lymphoma?
    (a) Platelet count of 100,000–150,000
    (b) Neutrophil count of 1500–2000
    (c) Bone cellularity of less than 25%
    (d) Bone marrow involvement of more than 25%
17. In which application of immunotherapy is the tumor supported by clinical evidence?
    (a) B-cell Hodgkin's lymphoma
    (b) Acute myeloid lymphoma
    (c) B-cell non-Hodgkin's lymphoma
    (d) T-cell non-Hodgkin's lymphoma
18. A 38-year-old woman with enlarged cervical lymph nodes and a diagnosis of low-grade non-Hodgkin's lymphoma is referred. She has NOT received any treatment for lymphoma. What is your radioimmunotherapy recommendation for this patient?
    (a) Hospitalization and treatment with ^{131}I-tositumomab
    (b) Standard chemotherapy
    (c) Hospitalization and treatment with ^{90}Y-ibritumomab
    (d) Treatment with ^{90}Y-ibritumomab without hospitalization
19. ^{90}Y-ibritumomab tiuxetan is indicated for the refractory form of which of the following lymphomas?
    (a) Follicular lymphoma
    (b) Low-grade non-Hodgkin's lymphoma
    (c) Transformed B-cell non-Hodgkin's lymphoma
    (d) Nodular sclerosing Hodgkin's lymphoma
20. False-negative findings on radiocolloid bone marrow scintigraphy (BMS) are usually found in the early stages of:
    (a) ALL
    (b) AML
    (c) CLL
    (d) CML
21. Which of the following is the primary organ for blood reserve?
    (a) Liver
    (b) Kidney
    (c) Bone marrow
    (d) Spleen

2.8.1 Answer

	A	B	C	D
1	*			
2			*	
3				*
4		*		
5	*			
6	*			
7		*		
8				*
9			*	
10				*
11				*
12	*			
13				*
14		*		
15	*			
16				*
17			*	
18		*		
19				*
20			*	
21				*

2.9 Therapeutic Use of Radiolabeled Antibodies: Hematopoietic Tumors (Solid Tumors)

1. The radioimmunotherapy (RIT) of solid tumors has been studied with encouraging results in the following cancers *except*:
   (a) Renal cell carcinoma
   (b) Breast cancer
   (c) Glioma
   (d) Osteosarcoma
2. Which radionuclide has the highest energy and tissue range?
   (a) Y-90
   (b) I-131
   (c) Re-186
   (d) P-33
3. Toxicity of radioimmunotherapy:
   (a) Patients with tumoral involvement of the marrow experience more toxicity than others
   (b) Radiosensitivity of a tissue is identical in all patients
   (c) A correlation exists between toxicity and radiation-absorbed dose
   (d) A positive correlation exists between the number of radioactive molecules and toxicity
4. What is DOTA in radioimmunotherapy?
   (a) A radiometal
   (b) A chelator
   (c) An antibody
   (d) A halogen
5. What are the most commonly used radioisotopes in radioimmunotherapy?
   (a) ^{90}Y, ^{33}P
   (b) ^{125}I, ^{131}I
   (c) ^{131}I, ^{90}Y
   (d) ^{211}At, ^{177}Lu
6. A ^{111}In-capromab pendetide scan is requested for a patient. What is the suspected tumor?
   (a) Colon cancer
   (b) Prostate cancer
   (c) Hodgkin's lymphoma
   (d) Non-Hodgkin's lymphoma
7. CT scan of a 59-year-old woman reveals a large abdominal mass with poor vascularization. What is the radiopharmaceutical of choice for radioimmunotherapy?
   (a) ^{90}Y-ibritumomab
   (b) ^{131}I-tositumomab
   (c) ^{90}Y rituximab
   (d) ^{90}Y satumomab

8. Which item canNOT cause failure of immunotherapy?
   (a) Small size of the tumor
   (b) Low-level antibody
   (c) Inappropriate vascularization of the tumor
   (d) Inadequate antigen expression on the tumor surface

2.9.1 Answer

	A	B	C	D
1				*
2	*			
3	*			
4		*		
5			*	
6		*		
7	*			
8	*			

2.10 MIBG Therapy

1. ^{131}I-MIBG scintigraphy has the least sensitivity in:
   (a) Neuroblastoma
   (b) Medullary thyroid carcinoma
   (c) Carcinoid
   (d) Pheochromocytoma
2. Which statement regarding ^{131}I-MIBG therapy is NOT true?
   (a) It provides valuable palliation.
   (b) It improves quality of life.
   (c) It is well tolerated compared with chemotherapy.
   (d) A correlation exists between whole-body absorbed dose and tumor response.
3. In pheochromocytoma:
   (a) The incidence of malignancy increases in tumors arising in adults.
   (b) The brain is a common site of distant metastasis of this tumor.
   (c) High dopamine excretion is regarded as a good prognosis.
   (d) Plasma chromogranin a may be of prognostic value.
4. In ^{131}I-MIBG therapy for malignant pheochromocytoma:
   (a) The drugs interfering with MIBG uptake must be discontinued 2 weeks before treatment.
   (b) Thyroid blockade must be performed 24 h before the treatment and continued for 4 weeks.
   (c) Weekly full blood count is recommended for at least 6 weeks.
   (d) ^{131}I-MIBG infusion for 10 min is indicated by monitoring blood pressure.
5. In the ^{131}I-MIBG therapy of medullary thyroid carcinoma:
   (a) Nearly 90% of MTC focuses on MIBG.
   (b) A complete response is rare.
   (c) Partial response is reported in >90%.
   (d) The best response seems to be obtained after the third treatment.
6. A 40-year-old woman undergoes left adrenalectomy for pheochromocytoma. All investigations at that time are within normal ranges. Six years later, she develops shoulder pain, and workup shows multiple bone metastases and elevated plasma-free normetanephrine. Both MIBG and octreoscan scan show multiple areas of uptake in the bones. What do you suggest for her treatment?
   (a) Long-acting octreotide
   (b) MIBG therapy
   (c) Local radiotherapy and systemic chemotherapy
   (d) a and b
7. Which of the following drugs is indicated for the increase in ^{131}I-MIBG retention if the goal is to treat malignant pheochromocytoma?
   (a) Nifedipine
   (b) Reserpine
   (c) Labetalol
   (d) Imipramine

8. Which of the following statements about the therapeutic application of ^{131}I-MIBG is NOT correct?
   (a) The therapeutic dose is 100–300 mCi, which is infused in 1–4 h.
   (b) The minimum interval between treatments is 4 and 6 months for children and adults, respectively, and the treatment is scheduled according to the platelet count.
   (c) Uptake-reducing drugs must be discontinued 1 week before the treatment.
   (d) The maximum exposure rate of bone marrow is 20 Gy.
9. In which of the following tumors is treatment with ^{131}I-MIBG the most effective?
   (a) Medullary thyroid cancer
   (b) Carcinoid
   (c) Neuroblastoma
   (d) Pheochromocytoma

2.10.1 Answer

	A	B	C	D
1		*		
2				*
3				*
4			*	
5		*		
6				*
7	*			
8				*
9			*	

2.11 Receptor-Targeted Radiopeptide Therapy

1. Regarding ^{111}In-/^{90}Y-lanreotide:
   (a) Its lipophilicity is greater than that of DOTA-Tyr3-octreotide.
   (b) It has a higher kidney dose than DOTA-Tyr3-octreotide.
   (c) It has high affinity for sst1.
   (d) It has a lower whole-body dose than DOTA-Tyr3-octreotide.
2. The affinity of ^{177}LU-TATE for … is sevenfold that of DOTA-Tyr3-octreotide.
   (a) sst1
   (b) sst2
   (c) sst3
   (d) sst4
3. Which of the following radiopharmaceuticals is indicated for the treatment of tumors that express the somatostatin receptor?
   (a) ^{111}Indium-DTPA-octreotide
   (b) ^{177}Lutetium-DOTA-octreotide
   (c) ^{90}Iterium-DOTA-iridium
   (d) ^{111}Indium-DOTA-octreotide
4. A 40-year-old woman underwent treatment with ^{90}Y-DOTATOC for carcinoid metastasis to the liver. Co-treatment with which drug is indicated for the prevention of radiopharmaceutical-induced nephrotoxicity?
   (a) Normal saline
   (b) Furosemide
   (c) Arginine
   (d) Dextrose
5. Which of the following radiopharmaceuticals is indicated for the treatment of renal cancer?
   (a) ^{131}I-A33
   (b) ^{90}Y-G250
   (c) ^{90}Y-M195
   (d) ^{131}I-3F8
6. Which of the following interventions is recommended for the reduction of radiation exposure, especially to kidneys, in peptide receptor radionuclide therapy (PRRT)?
   (a) Hydration
   (b) Diuretics
   (c) Unlabeled octreotide before treatment
   (d) Simultaneous infusion of positively charged amino acids
7. What is the target antigen of rituximab for the treatment of B-cell lymphoma?
   (a) CD21
   (b) CD22
   (c) CD20
   (d) CD37

8. Which of the following radiotracers is the most effective for peptide receptor radionuclide therapy (PRRT)?
   (a) [^{111}In-DTPA] octreotide
   (b) [^{177}Lu-DOTA] octreotate
   (c) [^{90}Y-DOTA] octreotide
   (d) [^{131}I] octreotate
9. Which of the following radioisotopes is used for antibody labeling and requires thyroid blocking with perchlorate?
   (a) ^{90}Y
   (b) ^{213}Bi
   (c) ^{177}Lu
   (d) ^{188}Re
10. Which of the following statements regarding 177 Lu-PSMA radioligand therapy for prostate cancer is false?
    (a) The degree of PSMA expression positively correlates with tumor stage and early recurrence.
    (b) Small intestine, renal tubules, and salivary glands also demonstrate low levels of PSMA expression.
    (c) PSMA is a type II transmembrane protein with one monomer and an extracellular domain only.
    (d) Currently, two PSMA ligands are predominantly reported for clinical 177Lu-based RLT.
11. 177Lu-PSMA RLT may be considered in patients with:
    (a) mCRPC, progressive after exhaustion of approved therapies
    (b) Confirmed PSMA expression of tumor and metastases
    (c) Serum creatinine of less than two times the upper limit of normal
    (d) All of the above
12. Most sites perform repeat RLT at which intervals:
    (a) 8 weeks
    (b) 10 weeks
    (c) 12 weeks
    (d) 6 weeks
13. A clinical examination and blood tests following RLT should be performed at which intervals for the evaluation of toxicity and response:
    (a) 6–8 weeks
    (b) 2–4 weeks
    (c) 4–6 weeks
    (d) 8–10 weeks
14. Alpha therapy such as 225Ac-labeled PSMA617 may be useful in which of the following cases?
    (a) Patients with disease progression under 177Lu-PSMA
    (b) Patients with diffuse bone marrow involvement
    (c) Patients who do NOT discontinue myelosuppressive therapy before RLT
    (d) a and b

15. The nephrotoxicity of radiolabeled peptides during PRRT in neuroendocrine tumors (NET) may be reduced by:
    (a) Radioprotectors
    (b) Dose fractionation
    (c) Mitigating agent
    (d) All of the above
16. The carrier molecules for targeted therapy should have the following criteria *except*:
    (a) The carrier molecule has binding affinity to a variety of radionuclides.
    (b) The carrier molecule is resistant to self-radiolysis.
    (c) The carrier molecule should not be toxic or immunogenic.
    (d) The carrier molecule must possess high affinity and specificity for the target.

2.11.1 Answer

	A	B	C	D
1	*			
2		*		
3		*		
4			*	
5		*		
6				*
7			*	
8		*		
9				*
10			*	
11				*
12	*			
13		*		
14				*
15				*
16		*		

2.12 Use of Labeled Lipiodol in the Treatment of Hepatic Tumors

1. In ^{131}I-lipiodol therapy:
   (a) The response rate is greater than 90%.
   (b) The response rate is higher for multinodular HCC than for nodular HCC.
   (c) The response rate increases with the decrease in the size of HCC.
   (d) The assessment of therapeutic response based on tumor size is optimal.
2. Which of the following complications is a rare side effect of ^{131}I-lipiodol therapy?
   (a) Increased temperature
   (b) Asthenia
   (c) Hepatalgia
   (d) Digestive hemorrhage
3. In inoperable HCC:
   (a) ^{131}I-lipiodol therapy and chemoembolization have the same effectiveness, but ^{131}I-lipiodol therapy is better tolerated.
   (b) ^{131}I-lipiodol therapy and chemoembolization have the same effectiveness, but chemoembolization is better tolerated.
   (c) ^{131}I-lipiodol therapy and chemoembolization have the same effectiveness and tolerance.
   (d) ^{131}I-lipiodol therapy is more effective than chemoembolization, but chemoembolization is better tolerated.
4. Which of the following situations is a proven indication of ^{131}I-lipiodol therapy?
   (a) Adjuvant treatment close to surgical resection
   (b) Neoadjuvant treatment before hepatic transplantation
   (c) Treatment of certain HCCs that are too large to be operated on at the outset
   (d) Curative treatment for small-sized HCCs inaccessible to local treatment
5. ^{131}I-lipiodol therapy is NOT contraindicated in patients with:
   (a) Iodine allergy
   (b) Distant metastases
   (c) Thrombopenia ($<100 \times 10^9$/l)
   (d) Evolved cirrhosis
6. A patient with colon cancer metastasis to the liver is a candidate for the embolization of hepatic artery. An intrahepatic shunt was evaluated before treatment. Which item is correct regarding this study?
   (a) It is evaluated by Tc-SC.
   (b) Ulceration after surgery is possible when activity is observed in the stomach.
   (c) Radionuclide is administered intraperitoneally (IP).
   (d) The treatment is contraindicated if more than 5% of the activity is accumulated in the lungs.

7. The hepatic arterial administration of drugs is used for the selective chemotherapy of liver tumors. Which of the following variables do NOT increase the efficiency of ^{131}I-lipiodol for the treatment of liver tumors?
   (a) Hypothermia
   (b) Different drug emulsions
   (c) Angiotensin II
   (d) Vasodilators

2.12.1 Answer

	A	B	C	D
1			*	
2				*
3	*			
4	*			
5			*	
6		*		
7	*			

2.13 Alternative Approaches to Targeting Therapy

1. Conventional radiotherapy is limited to approximately 60 Gy. However, by intracavitary administration of radiolabeled agents, the application of additional radiation up to … Gy is possible.
   (a) 100 Gy
   (b) 50 Gy
   (c) 200 Gy
   (d) 1000 Gy
2. All of the following radionuclides have been shown to prevent fluid reaccumulation in cystic lesions *except*:
   (a) ^{90}Y
   (b) ^{186}Re
   (c) ^{32}P
   (d) ^{153}Sm
3. Patients with ovarian cancer without any response to chemotherapy can be treated intraperitoneally with:
   (a) ^{177}Lu-CC49MAb
   (b) ^{188}Re-C595 antibody
   (c) ^{186}Re colloid
   (d) ^{198}Au
4. Which radionuclide is indicated for dermal/epidermal contact therapy?
   (a) ^{186}Re-colloid
   (b) ^{198}Au
   (c) ^{166}Ho
   (d) ^{32}P
5. Regarding intracoronary application in radionuclide therapy:
   (a) Radiation of the dilated wall has an antiproliferative effect on the target cells.
   (b) The use of radioactive stents can be recommended without restriction.
   (c) Low-dose radiation (11 Gy) significantly prevents neointima.
   (d) ^{188}Re-perrhenate is a more suitable candidate for brachytherapy with liquid-filled balloons than ^{188}Re-MAG3.

2.13.1 Answer

	A	B	C	D
1				*
2				*
3	*			
4			*	
5	*			

Suggested Readings

1. Ahmadzadehfar H, Biersack HJ, Freeman LM, Zuckier L. Clinical nuclear medicine. 2nd ed. Berlin: Springer; 2018.
2. Ell PJ, Gambhir SS. Nuclear medicine in clinical diagnosis and treatment. 3rd ed. Edinburgh, NY: Churchill Livingstone; 2004.
3. Sandler MP, Coleman RE, Patton JA, Wackers FJT, Gottschalk A. Diagnostic nuclear medicine. 4th ed. Philadelphia: Lippincott & Williams Wilkins; 2003.
4. Henkin RE. Nuclear medicine. 2nd ed. Philadelphia: Mosby Elsevier; 2006.

Nuclear Medicine in Bone and Joint Disorders

3

3.1 Bone Scintigraphy: Procedure and Interpretation

1. Which of the following radiopharmaceuticals has been proposed as an agent that reduces the required interval between injection and scan?
   (a) ^{99m} Tc-dicarboxypropane-diphosphonate (DPD)
   (b) ^{99m}Tc-dimethyl-amino-diphosphonate (DMAD)
   (c) ^{99m}Tc-aminomethylenediphosphonic acid (AMDP)
   (d) ^{99m}Tc-EC-AMDP
2. Which radiopharmaceutical can detect equivocal lesions observed on the ^{99m}Tc-MDP scan in a symptomatic patient?
   (a) ^{99m} Tc-dicarboxypropane-diphosphonate (DPD)
   (b) ^{99m}Tc-dimethyl-amino-diphosphonate (DMAD)
   (c) ^{99m}Tc-aminomethylenediphosphonic acid (AMDP)
   (d) ^{99m}Tc-hydroxymethylene-diphosphonate (HMDP)
3. How long is the shelf life of ^{99m}Tc-medronate?
   (a) 12 h
   (b) 10 h
   (c) 8 h
   (d) 5 h
4. In the SPECT imaging of the knee, the most important information can be obtained from:
   (a) Sagittal images
   (b) Transaxial images
   (c) Coronal images
   (d) All views produce the same information

M. Assadi et al., *Principles of Nuclear Medicine*,
https://doi.org/10.1007/978-3-319-91701-6_3

5. In the bone scan of a patient with Blount's disease:
   (a) The medial half of the femoral physis has greater activity than the lateral half.
   (b) The lateral half of the femoral physis has greater activity than the medial half.
   (c) The lateral half of the tibial physis has greater activity than the medial half.
   (d) The medial half of the tibial physis has greater activity than the lateral half.
6. On bone scan:
   (a) An improperly set photopeak produces a false-negative bone scan.
   (b) Uptake by the thyroid alone has been reported in metastatic visceral calcification.
   (c) The clearance of retained urine following frusemide administration is not helpful in identifying patients with obstruction.
   (d) Gastric air bubble is especially observed in the elderly.
7. Regarding the alteration of the biodistribution of bone tracer following radiotherapy:
   (a) It does not have any effect on the nonirradiated bone.
   (b) The most important effect is the decrease in areas of increased uptake.
   (c) No lesion occurs 2 months following radiotherapy.
   (d) All lesions resolve in 1 year.
8. Hot kidneys on bone scan are NOT seen in:
   (a) Hyperparathyroidism
   (b) Amphotericin B therapy
   (c) Myoglobinuria
   (d) Nephrocalcinosis
9. Focal myocardial accumulation on bone scan is seen in:
   (a) Kawasaki disease
   (b) Amyloidosis
   (c) Acute myocardial necrosis
   (d) Hypercalcemia
10. Regarding the uptake in soft tissue tumors on bone scan:
   (a) All malignant and 50% of benign soft tissue tumors accumulate the bone agents.
   (b) Approximately 70% malignant and benign soft tissue tumors accumulate the bone agents.
   (c) Approximately 50% of malignant and benign soft tissue tumors accumulate the bone agents.
   (d) Nearly all malignant and benign soft tissue tumors accumulate the bone agents.

11. In which of the following conditions is pelvic diastasis observed on bone scan?
    (a) Pregnant women
    (b) Gait disorder
    (c) Obese subjects
    (d) Advanced osteoporosis
12. A symmetric circular lesion with distinct edges is observed in the mid-lower sternum on the bone scan of a 35-year-old patient suspected to have femoral osteomyelitis. What is the most probable diagnosis?
    (a) Simple bone cyst
    (b) Establishment of infection in the sternum (multifocal osteomyelitis)
    (c) Sternal foramen (natural variation)
    (d) Destructive metastasis
13. Bone scan in a patient with pulmonary cancer reveals a generalized increase in cortical uptake in both tibias as well as an enhanced focal uptake in the periarticular regions of the knee. What is the most possible diagnosis?
    (a) Reflex sympathetic dystrophy (RSD)
    (b) Shin splint
    (c) Bone metastasis
    (d) Hypertrophic pulmonary osteoarthropathy (HPO)
14. Which of the following changes in the bone scan of elderly patients is unusual and must be taken seriously?
    (a) Observation of femoral arteries
    (b) Nonhomogenous increase in uptake in large joints
    (c) Focal increase in activity in the ribs
    (d) Observation of thyroid cartilage
15. What is the most common cause of diffusely increased uptake in visceral organs on bone scan?
    (a) Infectious/inflammatory process
    (b) Metabolic bone disease
    (c) Traumatic lesions
    (d) Metastatic visceral calcification
16. Which of the following items has the greatest "bone marrow expansion"?
    (a) Sickle thalassemia (Hb S-Thal)
    (b) Aplastic anemia
    (c) Alpha trait thalassemia
    (d) Sickle cell anemia (Hb S/S)
17. Which of the following statements regarding hypertrophic osteoarthropathy and bone scan findings is correct?
    (a) Hypertrophic osteoarthropathy results from renal failure.
    (b) The activity of long bones increases from epiphysis.
    (c) An increased focal uptake is found in the long bones, fingers, scapula, and clavicle.
    (d) Radiography is superior to bone scan in identifying lesions.

18. Which item has NO effect on the radiopharmaceutical uptake in radiotherapy of bone?
    (a) Type of bone tissue
    (b) Dose and intensity of the radiotracer
    (c) Extent of the surrounding soft tissue
    (d) Interval between radiation and scan
19. Which modality is the most sensitive for the detection of rhabdomyolysis?
    (a) Simple radiography
    (b) CT scan
    (c) MRI
    (d) Bone scan
20. Which of the following findings on bone scan demonstrates the concurrent administration of the hematopoietic growth factor along with radiotherapy?
    (a) Generalized increase in skeletal uptake
    (b) Increase in cranial uptake
    (c) Generalized decrease in vertebral uptake
    (d) Decrease in organ uptake
21. In which of the following conditions is bone scan recommended?
    (a) Screening for histiocytosis X
    (b) Evaluation of the progression of bone lesions in multiple myeloma
    (c) Negative radiographic findings in a multiple myeloma patient with bone pain
    (d) Evaluation of the whole skeleton in a patient with a unicameral bone cyst in the calcaneus
22. Which of the following findings is considered a normal variant on bone scan?
    (a) Noticeable cranial sutures in adults
    (b) Increased uptake in the spinous process in the C2 vertebra
    (c) Absence of growth plates in an 11-year-old girl
    (d) Increased uptake in the patella
23. Flare phenomenon:
    (a) The appearance of new lesions excludes the flare phenomenon.
    (b) It indicates the improvement of metastasis after radiotherapy.
    (c) It is commonly observed in bone metastasis of prostate cancer.
    (d) It appears as an increased SUV in FDG-PET.
24. Which organ exhibits the highest uptake of ^{99m}Tc-MDP on bone scan?
    (a) Bone
    (b) Bone marrow
    (c) Kidney
    (d) Bladder
25. Bone scan is performed on a 28-year-old patient. An aligned increase in uptake is observed in the bilateral ribs in the posterior view. What is the most probable diagnosis?
    (a) Metastasis
    (b) Shine-through of the costochondral junction
    (c) Previous traumatism
    (d) Calcification of muscle attachment sites

26. An increased uptake is observed at the base of the cranium on the bone scan of a 4-month-old baby. What is the most probable diagnosis?
    (a) Osteomyelitis
    (b) Pituitary tumor
    (c) Normal finding
    (d) Fracture of the cranial base
27. Which region is NOT involved in hypertrophic osteoarthropathy?
    (a) Long bones
    (b) Hip
    (c) Vertebrae
    (d) Scapula
28. The bone scan of a patient with low back pain reveals an increased focal activity on both sides of the L4–L5. What is the most probable diagnosis?
    (a) Primary tumor
    (b) Spondylolisthesis
    (c) Metastasis
    (d) Osteomyelitis
29. In which of the following conditions is the watershed effect reported on bone scan?
    (a) Osteomyelitis
    (b) Infection of soft tissue
    (c) Bone metastasis
    (d) Bone fracture
30. Which of the following findings is reported in a patient with chronic reflex sympathetic dystrophy?
    (a) Increased activity in all three phases
    (b) Increased activity in angiography and blood pool, normal pattern in the static phase
    (c) Increased activity in angiography and blood pool, decreased activity in the static phase
    (d) Decreased activity in all three phases
31. Which statement about hypertrophic osteoarthropathy and bone scan is NOT correct?
    (a) Increased cortical uptake in the distal regions of long bones.
    (b) Small bones of the foot and hand are usually involved.
    (c) Nonhomogenous and irregular increase in activity is indicative of the ruling out of the disease.
    (d) Abnormal scan findings are reversible after treatment of the underlying disease.
32. What changes are expected on the bone scan after treatment with primary therapeutic doses of bisphosphonates?
    (a) Decreased bone uptake, increased soft tissue uptake
    (b) Increased bone uptake, decreased soft tissue uptake
    (c) Increased bone and soft tissue uptake
    (d) No change in bone uptake, increased soft tissue uptake

33. Which statement about hypertrophic osteoarthropathy is NOT correct?
    (a) A tramline sign can be found in long bones.
    (b) Normal bone scan is obtained at least 6 months after a successful treatment.
    (c) It is NOT observed in the vertebra.
    (d) It is commonly observed in pulmonary cancer.
34. The thinning of which cranial bone as a region of reduced uptake on bone scan is demonstrated?
    (a) Temporal
    (b) Parietal
    (c) Occipital
    (d) Frontal
35. The increased uptake of labeled MDP in which cranial region is observed in renal osteodystrophy?
    (a) Frontal
    (b) Parietal
    (c) Temporal
    (d) Suture
36. A decreased uptake of radiopharmaceutical in bones and an increased activity in soft tissue are reported on bone scan. What is the most probable diagnosis?
    (a) Active acromegaly
    (b) Severe thyrotoxicosis
    (c) Aluminum-induced osteomalacia
    (d) Hypervitaminosis D
37. What is the most common site of the symmetrical increase in MDP uptake in hypertrophic pulmonary osteoarthropathy (HPO)?
    (a) Tibia
    (b) Scapula
    (c) Clavicle
    (d) Rib
38. What is the most appropriate position for the spot scintigraphy of the lumbar vertebrae in the posterior view?
    (a) Sitting with bended back
    (b) Prone
    (c) Upright
    (d) Supine
39. Symphysis pubis evaluation in the anterior view of bone scan is not possible because of a full bladder. What is the alternative view?
    (a) Cephalad
    (b) Posterior
    (c) Lateral
    (d) Caudal

40. Which bone is the most common site of a single malignant lesion with an increased uptake of MDP in a patient with a history of breast cancer?
    (a) Tibia
    (b) Radius
    (c) Sternum
    (d) Rib
41. Bone scan shows an increased focal uptake near the fourth and fifth proximal metacarpal bones of the wrist. In which bone is the mentioned focus located?
    (a) Trapezoid
    (b) Hamate
    (c) Lunate
    (d) Scaphoid
42. An increased uptake is observed in one of the lumbar vertebrae on the bone scan of a 67-year-old woman with breast cancer. SPECT investigation shows an increased uptake in the anterior margin of L3. What is the most probable cause of this finding?
    (a) Infection
    (b) Degeneration
    (c) Metastasis
    (d) Fracture
43. Bone scan is requested to evaluate the metastasis of breast cancer in a patient who received intravenous bisphosphonate yesterday. How long should the bone scan be postponed?
    (a) 1 week
    (b) 2 weeks
    (c) 3 weeks
    (d) 4 weeks
44. A 56-year-old man recently diagnosed with small-cell carcinoma of the right lung underwent chemotherapy 3 years ago. Bone scan is performed to identify the cause of acute joint pains in the lower extremities. A dissymmetric increase in uptake is observed in the hip, knee, and ankle joints, whereas the other parts of the skeleton show a normal uptake. No noticeable finding is found in the radiography of the mentioned regions. What is the most probable diagnosis?
    (a) Paraneoplastic polyarthritis
    (b) Metastatic arthropathy
    (c) Pulmonary hypertrophic osteoarthropathy
    (d) Reaction to bone marrow suppression secondary to chemotherapy
45. In which of the following conditions does bone scan have the highest paraclinical value for the diagnosis of a suspected lesion?
    (a) A 67-year-old woman with hip pain after a fall 3 years ago; normal radiography.
    (b) A 32-year-old man with back pain; radiography shows bone lesion in the neural arch of L4.
    (c) A 27-year-old football player with chronic pain of the knee; for the evaluation of the cause of pain.
    (d) A 49-year-old woman with rheumatoid arthritis; for therapeutic monitoring.

46. Bone scan is performed on a young patient with pain in the vertebral column without a history of any disease. Only a minor diffuse and a homogenous uptake are observed in the liver and spleen. No abnormal uptake in bones or other parts can be seen. What is the most probable diagnosis?
    (a) Diffuse metastasis of the liver due to a malignancy
    (b) Higher free technetium in the administered radiopharmaceutical
    (c) Colloid formation during the preparation of the radiopharmaceutical
    (d) Acute hepatitis with diffuse necrosis
47. A diffuse uptake in the liver is observed on the bone scan of a 49-year-old patient with back pain. Which diagnosis is NOT possible?
    (a) Amyloidosis
    (b) Hepatic necrosis
    (c) Colorectal metastasis
    (d) Aluminum increase
48. A reduced activity is observed around a brown tumor on the bone scan of a patient with hyperparathyroidism. A repeat of the bone scan 2 months later shows an increased activity in this region. What is the reason for the change in activity over time?
    (a) Parathyroidectomy
    (b) Normal pattern of the disease
    (c) Drug treatment
    (d) Contamination
49. A 74-year-old woman with a history of mastectomy is referred for bone scan. An increased activity is observed in the T12 aside from the sternum and ribs. Furthermore, SPECT shows an increased activity in the vertebral body and pedicle of this vertebra. What is the most probable cause of this increased activity?
    (a) Metastasis
    (b) Degenerative lesions
    (c) Trauma
    (d) Infection
50. Bone scan of the knee is performed because of edema after trauma. An increased activity in all three phases of angiography, blood pool, and delayed is observed only in the femoral parts near the knee. Which of the following conditions is indicated?
    (a) Septic arthritis
    (b) Arthritis
    (c) Osteomyelitis
    (d) Adjacent soft tissue infection
51. In which cranial region is an increased uptake of the labeled MDP radiotracer observed in renal osteodystrophy?
    (a) Frontal
    (b) Parietal
    (c) Temporal
    (d) Suture

52. Which of the following disorders is characterized by a decrease in radiotracer uptake in bones and an increase in soft tissue activity on bone scan?
    (a) Active acromegaly
    (b) Severe thyrotoxicosis
    (c) Aluminum-induced osteomalacia
    (d) Hypervitaminosis D
53. A 56-year-old patient with pain in the lower extremities that began last year is referred for bone scan. Atrophic changes are observed in the physical examination. Furthermore, decreased perfusion and blood pool and a periarticular increased uptake in the left leg are observed on bone scan. What is the most probable diagnosis?
    (a) Degenerative changes
    (b) Inflammation and infection
    (c) Trauma
    (d) Reflex sympathetic dystrophy
54. Focal uptake in the L5 interarticularis region is found on the bone scan and SPECT of a 12-year-old girl, who is referred because of back pain. What is the most probable diagnosis?
    (a) Spondylolysis
    (b) Spondylolisthesis
    (c) Facet joint arthropathy
    (d) Traverse sacral articulation
55. What is the cause of a tramline on a bone allograft scan?
    (a) Ossification
    (b) Fracture
    (c) Tumor relapse
    (d) Osteomyelitis
56. Which statement is correct?
    (a) Bone scan with ^{99m}Tc-MDP has better quality in infants than in adults.
    (b) Bone scan with ^{99m}Tc-HDP has better quality in infants than in adults.
    (c) Bone scan with ^{99m}Tc-MDP has better quality in adults than in infants.
    (d) Bone scan with ^{99m}Tc-HDP has better quality in adults than in infants.
57. Which method is NOT indicated for the diagnosis of Osgood–Schlatter?
    (a) Bone scan
    (b) Radiography
    (c) Clinical examination
    (d) CT scan
58. An 8-year-old child with flank pain is referred for bone scan. Bone scan only shows an increase in uptake in L2, and the rest is normal. No lesion is observed in radiography. What is the next appropriate step?
    (a) Lumbar MRI
    (b) Lumbar CT scan
    (c) ^{99m}Tc-WBC scan
    (d) Repeat of bone scan after 3 months

59. Effects of radiotherapy on bone scan:
    (a) Bone uptake decreases until 5 years after radiotherapy.
    (b) This effect has NO defined threshold.
    (c) An increased bone uptake can be observed immediately after radiotherapy.
    (d) The induction of bone necrosis is the mechanism of this effect.
60. Which of the following items is the least responsible for the diffuse hepatic uptake in bone scintigraphy with ^{99m}Tc-MDP?
    (a) Presence of free technetium in the radiopharmaceutical
    (b) Increase in aluminum in the eluted technetium generator
    (c) Formation of colloidal molecules in the prepared radiopharmaceutical
    (d) Presence of diffuse hepatic calcification
61. The spleen is NOT observed in hepatosplenic scintigraphy, but a diffuse uptake in the spleen is seen on bone scan. What is the most probable diagnosis?
    (a) Budd–Chiari syndrome
    (b) Cirrhosis
    (c) Malignant melanoma
    (d) Sickle cell anemia
62. Hot skull:
    (a) It is indicative of metastasis in patients suffering from cancer.
    (b) It is observed in patients suffering from lung and breast cancer but is NOT indicative of metastasis.
    (c) It is observed in renal osteoarthropathy.
    (d) b and c.
63. A child who was healthy until yesterday is referred for bone scan because of bone pain. A multifocal increase in uptake is observed on the scan. What is the most probable diagnosis?
    (a) Multiple bone metastases
    (b) Hematogenous osteomyelitis
    (c) Battered child
    (d) Multiple bone infarcts due to sickle cell anemia
64. Radiotracer uptake is observed in the stomach, lungs, and kidneys in addition to bones in the whole-body bone scan with ^{99m}Tc-MDP. What is the most probable diagnosis?
    (a) Histiocytosis
    (b) Myelofibrosis
    (c) Hyperparathyroidism
    (d) Hyperthyroidism

65. What is the flare phenomenon?
    (a) Improvement of scan pattern with a completely normal pattern of bone scan
    (b) Improvement of bone scan pattern with reduced number or intensity of regions with an increased uptake
    (c) Deterioration of bone scan pattern with the diffused involvement of the skeleton, with more concentration in the extremities, and the absence of kidneys
    (d) Deterioration of bone scan pattern with increased number or intensity of regions with an increased uptake
66. Which of the following conditions is NOT associated with the increase in bone turnover?
    (a) Hyperparathyroidism
    (b) Increase in growth hormone
    (c) Hypothyroidism
    (d) Increase in cortisol
67. In hypertrophic pulmonary osteoarthropathy (HPOA):
    (a) The symptoms disappear after treatment of the underlying disease.
    (b) The symptoms are always accompanied by the underlying disease.
    (c) Involvement of the bone marrow is the main pathologic finding.
    (d) A diffuse increase in uptake in the long bones is reported on the bone scan.
68. In the quantitative evaluation of the sacroiliac joint on bone scan:
    (a) The specificity of this test is high.
    (b) The accuracy of the test decreases if there is a concurrent involvement of the sacrum and sacroiliac joints.
    (c) The sensitivity of the test increases with the progression of the inflammatory lesions of the sacroiliac joints.
    (d) The relative activity of the sacroiliac joints to the sacrum joints normally increases with age.
69. Which item about the flare phenomenon is NOT correct?
    (a) It happens in the early months after the treatment of bone metastasis.
    (b) It usually occurs in hematological tumors.
    (c) Repeat of scan after 4–6 months shows improvement of lesions.
    (d) Clinical improvement is observed at this time.
70. Which of the following bone scan findings is associated with Tietze syndrome?
    (a) Increase in costochondral uptake
    (b) Decease in anterolateral costal uptake
    (c) Increase in costovertebral uptake
    (d) Decrease in costovertebral uptake

71. Hypertrophic osteoarthropathy (HOA):
    (a) Sarcoidosis and tuberculosis can be accompanied by HOA.
    (b) Involvement of the axial bones is reported.
    (c) It is observed only in abdominal and pulmonary malignant lesions.
    (d) The primary and idiopathic forms are more common in those aged >50 years.
72. Which of the following bone regions has the maximum radiotracer retention in those aged <15 months?
    (a) Physeal–metaphyseal region
    (b) Diaphyseal region
    (c) Metaphyseal region
    (d) Epiphyseal region
73. Bone SPECT scan:
    (a) It is valuable for the evaluation of cranial lesions and growth plate in children.
    (b) A full bladder can cause a false-positive increase in uptake in the hip and femoral head bones.
    (c) A significant uptake in the C1 cranial vertebrae is a normal variation.
    (d) The thoracic vertebrae have a lower uptake than the lumbar vertebrae.
74. In which of the following diseases is a four-phase bone scan indicated?
    (a) Malignant bone tumor
    (b) Sudeck's atrophy
    (c) Bone fracture
    (d) Diabetic foot
75. What is the most common cause of appearance of cranial sutures on the bone scan of an adult subject?
    (a) Renal osteodystrophy
    (b) Paget's disease
    (c) Fibrous dysplasia
    (d) Hyperparathyroidism
76. What are the bone scan and bone marrow scan patterns on the day after bone marrow infarction, respectively?
    (a) Decreased uptake, increased uptake
    (b) Increased uptake, decreased uptake
    (c) Decreased uptake, decreased uptake
    (d) Increased uptake, increased uptake
77. Which component of hydroxyapatite is replaced by ^{18}F in the PET imaging of bones?
    (a) Calcium
    (b) Phosphate
    (c) Oxygen
    (d) Hydroxyl

78. A remarkable decrease in bone uptake is found on the bone scan. Which of the following diseases is NOT possible?
    (a) Aluminum toxicity in chronic renal failure
    (b) Osteoporosis
    (c) Treatment with etidronate disodium (EHTP)
    (d) Cirrhosis
79. Which of the following regions demonstrates an uptake on the bone scan due to recent chemotherapy?
    (a) Periarticular zone
    (b) Kidneys
    (c) Lungs
    (d) Liver
80. Which of the following regions demonstrates an uptake on the bone scan due to heterotopic calcification?
    (a) Liver
    (b) Periarticular zone
    (c) Lungs
    (d) Kidneys
81. Which of the following regions demonstrates an uptake on the bone scan due to vitamin D toxicity?
    (a) Periarticular zone
    (b) Kidneys
    (c) Lungs
    (d) Liver
82. Which of the following diseases is associated with the Mickey Mouse sign?
    (a) Renal osteodystrophy
    (b) Paget's disease
    (c) Pulmonary hypertrophic osteoarthropathy
    (d) Humeral traumatic periostitis
83. Which of the following diseases is associated with Ringman's lesion?
    (a) Renal osteodystrophy
    (b) Paget's disease
    (c) Pulmonary hypertrophic osteoarthropathy
    (d) Humeral traumatic periostitis
84. Which of the following diseases is associated with the Lone Ranger sign?
    (a) Renal osteodystrophy
    (b) Paget's disease
    (c) Pulmonary hypertrophic osteoarthropathy
    (d) Humeral traumatic periostitis
85. Which of the following diseases is associated with the tramline sign?
    (a) Renal osteodystrophy
    (b) Paget's disease
    (c) Pulmonary hypertrophic osteoarthropathy
    (d) Humeral traumatic periostitis

86. All the following items regarding ^{18}F-FDG-PET of bones are correct *except*:
    (a) Normal bones show a low uptake of ^{18}F-FDG.
    (b) ^{18}F-FDG uptake in the vertebral body and the proximal femoral shaft is greater than that of other bones.
    (c) The uptake of ^{18}f-FDG is directly related to MDP uptake.
    (d) Bone shaft and bone marrow uptake are equal.
87. In which of the following conditions is the diffuse increase in uptake in the calvarium NOT evident on bone scan?
    (a) Chemotherapy
    (b) Metabolic disorders
    (c) Elderly patients
    (d) Treatment with bisphosphonates
88. About vertebral tumors:
    (a) If the goal is to detect malignancy, the positive predictive value of an increased vertebral body uptake on bone SPECT scan is 43–50%.
    (b) An increased uptake in the posterolateral and anterolateral regions of the vertebral body is associated with the resolution of the vertebral body on the SPECT bone scan due to malignancy.
    (c) MRI is NOT a useful method for the detection of metastasis and epidural tumors with paravertebral involvement.
    (d) Vertebral hemangioma with a diameter of 3 cm can be observed as a decrease or an increase in uptake in SPECT.
89. In which of the following situations is a faint kidney sign observed on the ^{99m}Tc-MDP bone scan?
    (a) Renal obstructive disease
    (b) Diffuse bone metastasis
    (c) Diffuse osteoporosis
    (d) Pulmonary osteoarthropathy
90. What is the role of leptin in bone growth?
    (a) Stimulation of sympathetic activity and inhibition of osteoblastic activity with a central mechanism
    (b) Inhibition of ossification with a peripheral effect on growth cartilage
    (c) Decrease in bone growth with a decrease in thickness of the growth plate
    (d) Stimulation of the pre-osteoclastic activity and bone resorption
91. What is the main weakness of a bone scan?
    (a) High-radiation exposure when the patient is dehydrated
    (b) Hepatosplenic uptake if the MDP kit is exposed to oxygen
    (c) Low sensitivity
    (d) Non-specific
92. A bone scan is requested for a 49-year-old woman with a history of sarcoidosis to rule out the possible involvement of bone. Which bony regions are more likely to be involved?
    (a) Humerus
    (b) Phalanx bones of the feet and hands
    (c) Femurs
    (d) Ribs

93. What is the most common cause of skull sclerosis?
    (a) Paget's disease
    (b) Hyperostosis frontalis interna (HFI)
    (c) Histiocytosis x
    (d) Craniopharyngioma
94. Which of the following conditions is associated with the pseudo-Charcot joint?
    (a) Hemochromatosis
    (b) Tabes dorsalis
    (c) Hemophilia
    (d) Calcium pyrophosphate deposition disease (CPPD)
95. A patient with a history of cirrhosis is presented with pain in the upper limb. Bone scintigraphy shows increased activity in the distal third of the radius and ulna bones. The patient's radiograph also reveals a linear periosteal reaction in the same region. What is the most likely diagnosis?
    (a) Hypertrophic osteoarthropathy
    (b) Melorheostosis
    (c) Avascular necrosis
    (d) Venous stasis
96. Which of the following diseases is associated with osteoblastic changes?
    (a) Systemic mastocytosis
    (b) Whipple disease
    (c) Amyloidosis
    (d) Eosinophilic gastroenteropathy
97. A skeletal survey by scintigraphy is better than X-ray in all of the following diseases *except*:
    (a) Metastasis
    (b) Multiple myeloma
    (c) Stress fractures
    (d) Non-Hodgkin's lymphomas (NHLs)
98. A focal cardiac uptake of the radiotracer on the bone scan is reported in all of the following situations *except*:
    (a) Hypercalcemia
    (b) Unstable angina
    (c) Pericarditis
    (d) Kawasaki disease
99. All of the following statements regarding the whole-body bone scan (WBBS) in amyloidosis are correct *except*:
    (a) WBBS is valuable in primary amyloidosis in plasma cell disorders.
    (b) ^{99m}Tc-pyrophosphate is preferred over Tc-MDP.
    (c) Kidneys are observed in the WBBS of patients with amyloidosis.
    (d) Tc-MDP uptake may be observed in cardiac amyloidosis.

100. Which of the following complexes is capable of detecting lesions that do NOT appear on the MDP scan and demonstrates a very low uptake in normal bone and a highly intense uptake in lesions?
   (a) Dimethyl-amino-diphosphonate (DMAD)
   (b) Aminomethylenediphosphonic acid (AMDP)
   (c) Hydroxyethylidene diphosphonate (HEDP)
   (d) Hydroxymethylene diphosphonate (HMDP)
101. What is the most reliable method for the evaluation of bone tumors (especially size and therapeutic monitoring)?
   (a) Bone scan
   (b) Gallium scan
   (c) Thallium scan
   (d) MIBI scan
102. Which of the following items are advantages of hybrid PET/MRI in musculoskeletal malignancies?
   (a) High soft tissue contrast.
   (b) May reduce the overall imaging time ("one-stop shop").
   (c) Advanced MRI sequences are suitable for multiparametric lesion characterization.
   (d) All of the above.
103. Which of the following statements about bone scan imaging is NOT correct?
   (a) Bone uptake generally reaches its peak in 2 h.
   (b) Upright position or sitting with bended spine is the best position for acquiring data on the lumbar spine.
   (c) The quantitative evaluation of activity has gained clinical acceptance for the evaluation of hip avascular necrosis or arthritis (ratio of the involved region to diaphysis).
   (d) The key point of the accumulation of the radiotracer in bone extracellular fluid is definitely the occlusion of the opening of microvascular pathways.
104. In which of the following regions is the pinhole collimator recommended for bone scan?
   (a) Frog-leg hip
   (b) Maximal internal rotation hip
   (c) Tarsal bones
   (d) All of the above
105. In which of the following items are the mechanisms of intraosseous and extraosseous uptake of the radiotracer similar?
   (a) Binding to tissue receptors
   (b) Precipitation of the calcium salts of the radiotracer in amorphous calcium phosphate (ACP)
   (c) Precipitation of the calcium salts of the radiotracer in myofibrils
   (d) Binding to collagen

106. Which part of the growth plate uptakes the bone radiotracer?
    (a) Resting
    (b) Proliferative
    (c) Hypertrophic
    (d) All of the above
107. In which of the following situations is the asymmetric uptake in growth plate or even the delayed appearance of the radiotracer in ossific centers reported?
    (a) Chronic renal failure
    (b) Long-term corton therapy
    (c) Radiotherapy
    (d) All of the above
108. Regarding the interpretation of a bone scan:
    (a) Medial femoral physis shows higher activity than lateral physis, and vice versa, for proximal tibial physis.
    (b) The bone scan pattern in a type V Salter–Harris fractures is an increased activity.
    (c) The intense accumulation of activity in sternoclavicular and acromioclavicular joints in adults is pathologic.
    (d) The prominence of the C1 vertebrae is a normal variant.
109. The differential diagnosis of a diffuse uptake along the entire calvarium includes:
    (a) Aging
    (b) Extensive chemotherapy
    (c) Metabolic disorders
    (d) All of the above
110. The differential diagnosis of thyroid uptake includes all of the following conditions *except*:
    (a) Poor labeling
    (b) Papillary thyroid cancer
    (c) Hyperthyroid state
    (d) Visceral metastatic calcification
111. What is the most identified and specific pattern of visceral metastatic calcification?
    (a) Gastric uptake
    (b) Lung uptake
    (c) Thyroid uptake
    (d) Colon uptake
112. The differential diagnosis of a hot kidney in a bone scan includes all of the following conditions *except*:
    (a) Administration of amphotericin B
    (b) Hyperkalemia
    (c) Myoglobinuria
    (d) Cirrhosis

113. What is the bone scan pattern in patients being treated with etidronate disodium (EHDP)?
    (a) Appearance of spleen on the bone scan
    (b) Hot kidney on the bone scan
    (c) Marked decrease of bone uptake
    (d) Marked increase of uptake of cranial sutures
114. Which of the following statements about radiotherapy and bone scan is NOT correct?
    (a) Regions of decreased uptake due to radiotherapy are the most common iatrogenic changes on bone scan.
    (b) Bone scan rarely shows decreased activity in regions receiving less than 30 Gy of radiation.
    (c) Decreased activity on bone scan appears 4–6 months after radiotherapy.
    (d) Decreased activity on bone scan may remain for 1.5 years.
115. Which of the following statements about radiotracer retention in the pyelocaliceal system on bone scan is NOT correct?
    (a) Pyelocaliceal retention is observed in more than 20% of cases of bone scans.
    (b) Pyelocaliceal retention in the supine position is NOT important.
    (c) In one study, only 2.1% of cases with pyelocaliceal retention have shown obstructive uropathy.
    (d) Furosemide administration can help in the diagnosis.
116. All of the following situations are included in the differential diagnosis of the focal renal uptake (often linear) on bone scan *except*:
    (a) Urinary retention
    (b) Administration of iron dextran V
    (c) Adrenal uptake of the radiotracer
    (d) Costal uptake of the radiotracer
117. All of the following findings are reported in limb paralysis *except*:
    (a) Marked increase in the axial skeleton uptake on bone scan
    (b) Increased uptake in the paralyzed zone on bone scan
    (c) Increased osteogenesis and bone resorption
    (d) Decreased osteogenesis and bone absorption
118. All of the following statements regarding the presentation of blood disorders on bone scan are correct *except*:
    (a) Femoral vein thrombosis can cause an extensive femoral uptake on bone scan.
    (b) Chronic vein insufficiency commonly causes a marked uptake on bone scan.
    (c) The appearance of the spleen on the bone scan of all patients suffering from sickle cell anemia is indicative of functional asplenia.
    (d) Only half of the patients suffering from sickle cell anemia in whom the spleen does NOT appear on bone scan demonstrate functional asplenia.

119. All of the following statements regarding the presentation of visceral metastatic calcification on bone scan are correct *except*:
    (a) A diffuse increase in uptake in different organs is commonly due to visceral metastatic calcification, which is usually associated with hypercalcemia.
    (b) Hypercalcemia may be due to hyperparathyroidism, and the severity of disorders in the primary form of the disease is greater than that in the secondary forms.
    (c) Different carcinomas, such as lymphoma and multiple myeloma, can become the primary pathologies.
    (d) It may be observed in the lungs, myocardium, kidneys, thyroid, liver, and spleen.
120. All of the following statements regarding breast uptake on bone scan are correct *except*:
    (a) 90% of benign breast lesions are associated with the bilateral uptake of the bone radiotracer.
    (b) 25% of malignant breast lesions are associated with the bilateral uptake of the bone radiotracer.
    (c) Further workup is required only for the unilateral breast uptake.
    (d) Further workup is required for both the unilateral and the bilateral breast uptake.
121. Which of the following types of metastasis is best demonstrated in FDG-PET?
    (a) Osteolytic lesion.
    (b) Osteoblastic lesion.
    (c) Both items are equally demonstrated.
    (d) Mostly osteoblastic lesion.

3.1.1 Answer

	A	B	C	D		A	B	C	D
1				*	62				*
2		*			63			*	
3			*		64			*	
4		*			65				*
5				*	66				*
6			*		67	*			
7		*			68		*		
8	*				69		*		
9			*		70	*			
10	*				71	*			
11	*				72	*			
12			*		73	*			
13				*	74		*		
14			*		75	*			
15				*	76			*	
16				*	77				*
17			*		78				*
18			*		79		*		
19				*	80		*		
20	*				81			*	
21			*		82		*		
22		*			83				*
23				*	84	*			
24				*	85			*	
25		*			86				*
26			*		87				*
27			*		88				*
28		*			89		*		
29		*			90	*			
30				*	91				*
31			*		92		*		
32	*				93		*		
33		*			94				*
34		*			95	*			
35	*				96	*			
36			*		97		*		
37	*				98	*			
38	*				99		*		
39				*	100	*			
40			*		101			*	

	A	B	C	D		A	B	C	D
41		*			102				*
42		*			103			*	
43			*		104				*
44	*				105				*
45	*				106			*	
46			*		107			*	
47			*		108	*			
48	*				109				*
49	*				110		*		
50			*		111	*			
51				*	112		*		
52			*		113			*	
53				*	114		*		
54	*				115				*
55	*				116		*		
56		*			117		*		
57	*				118		*		
58	*				119		*		
59			*		120				*
60	*				121	*			
61				*					

3.2 Evaluation of Primary Bone Tumors

1. Bone marrow scintigraphy is found to be of particular value in:
   (a) Paget's disease
   (b) Hemangiosarcoma
   (c) Malignant fibrous histiocytoma
   (d) Ewing sarcoma
2. Radiographically, it is usually eccentric with sharply marginated and sclerotic edges and is confined within the cortex with displacement of the medullary bone. The scintigraphic appearance is of a mild increase in uptake in the delayed study only or of no increase in uptake.
   (a) Non-ossifying fibroma (NOF)
   (b) Fibrous cortical lesion
   (c) Cortical desmoids
   (d) All of the above
3. Radiographically, lesions are lucent with an expanded cortex and a thin rim of surrounding bone. It may have a soap-bubble appearance. The scintigraphic pattern is of hypervascularity and a ring-like appearance.
   (a) Giant-cell tumor (GCT)
   (b) Aneurysmal bone cyst (ABC)
   (c) Enchondroma
   (d) Unicameral bone cyst
4. Radiographically, the lesions are small, ill-defined lytic areas that may have a bull's eye sclerotic regional centrally. The early phase of scintigraphy may show intense activity, but a delayed phase usually shows a centrally reduced uptake.
   (a) Ewing sarcoma
   (b) Langerhans cell histiocytosis (LCH)
   (c) Osteogenic sarcoma
   (d) Chondroblastoma
5. What is the most prevalent malignant primary tumor of the bone?
   (a) Multiple myeloma
   (b) Osteogenic sarcoma
   (c) Chondrosarcoma
   (d) Ewing sarcoma
6. A slight increase in uptake in the metaphysis of the second metacarpus of the right hand is observed on bone scan. The patient reports only slight pain, and radiography reveals a focal radiolucent region with distinct edges. What is the most probable diagnosis?
   (a) Bone aneurysmal cyst
   (b) Bone island
   (c) Enchondroma
   (d) Osteosarcoma

7. What is the most suitable tracer for the discrimination of a real tumor relapse from bone healing in the flare phenomenon?
   (a) ^{18}F-FDG
   (b) ^{99m}Tc-MDP
   (c) ^{18}F-Fluoride Ion
   (d) ^{89}Sr
8. A three-phase bone scan reveals a focal region in the proximal femur with a markedly enhanced uptake in all three phases in a 16-year-old girl with severe bone pain. Radiography shows a small calcified region with a sclerotic margin in this area. What is the most probable diagnosis?
   (a) Epidermoid cyst
   (b) Fibrous cortical lesion
   (c) Hemangioma
   (d) Osteoid osteoma
9. What is the main advantage of SPECT bone scan?
   (a) Uniform energy resolution
   (b) Enhanced contrast resolution
   (c) Better field of uniformity
   (d) Improved image linearity
10. Which of the following variables has NO effect on the abnormal increase in the ^{99m}Tc-MDP uptake in soft tissue tumors?
    (a) Calcification
    (b) Radiation
    (c) Tissue necrosis
    (d) Tumor size
11. The doughnut sign is observed on the bone scan of all the following bone lesions *except*:
    (a) Bone cyst
    (b) Osteoclastoma
    (c) Aneurysmal bone cyst
    (d) Enchondroma
12. What is the most common bone scan finding when a patient with Paget's disease is further challenged with osteosarcoma?
    (a) Appearance of a photopenic region in bone
    (b) Increased uptake in soft tissue
    (c) Generalized increased uptake in bone
    (d) Positive results in all three phases of bone scan
13. The following changes are observed on the three-phase bone scan of a 14-year-old child with bone pain in the knee: highly increased perfusion and blood pool in the knee and highly increased and nonhomogenous uptake of ^{99m}Tc-MDP in the metaphysis of the distal femur. What is the most probable diagnosis?
    (a) Neuroblastoma
    (b) Osteogenic sarcoma
    (c) Ewing sarcoma
    (d) Lymphoma

14. Which of the following procedures is used for the diagnosis of "recall reaction" in children with a suppressed immune system?
    (a) Bone scan
    (b) ^{99m}Tc-RBC scintigraphy
    (c) ^{99m}Tc-Sulfur colloid scan
    (d) Pulmonary scintigraphy
15. Bone scan in neuroblastoma:
    (a) Renal blood-pool and serial images of the first 15 min must be obtained from children with an abdominal tumor.
    (b) All observed lesions on bone scan usually appear in simple radiography.
    (c) Primary tumors do NOT uptake ^{99m}Tc-MDP.
    (d) Bone scan is not a good choice for the evaluation of bone involvement in neuroblastoma.
16. Osteoma is a benign tumor with a remarkable uptake of the radiotracer. Which bone is NOT commonly involved?
    (a) Calvarium
    (b) Hip
    (c) Mandibular
    (d) Paranasal sinus
17. An 18-year-old girl with confirmed lymphoma is recently suffering from sporadic bone pains. Multifocal lesions in the ribs with different uptake intensities are found on the bone scan. What is the most probable diagnosis?
    (a) Multiple bone infections
    (b) Metastasis
    (c) Osteomalacia
    (d) Flare phenomenon in the context of treatment
18. On a whole-body scan with ^{201}Tl:
    (a) It does NOT clearly show the tumor activity.
    (b) It has limited precision for the therapeutic monitoring of chemotherapy.
    (c) The scan pattern is NOT affected by bone healing.
    (d) It is the scan of choice for the staging of malignant tumors.
19. Bone scan and simple radiography have high sensitivity in Langerhans histiocytosis of children. In which of the following regions is the sensitivity of radiography higher than that of bone scan?
    (a) Ribs
    (b) Skull
    (c) Vertebrae
    (d) Hip
20. Which statement about pediatric and juvenile osteosarcoma is NOT correct?
    (a) It is the most common primary malignant tumor of bone in children and juveniles.
    (b) The liver is the most common site of metastasis.
    (c) Bone scan is very sensitive for the localization of the primary tumor and bone metastasis.
    (d) MRI is more sensitive than bone scan for the precise localization of amputation in the organ with osteosarcoma.

21. In which of the following tumors does gallium and thallium scintigraphy NOT show an increased uptake?
    (a) Chondrosarcoma
    (b) Osteosarcoma
    (c) Ewing sarcoma
    (d) Giant-cell tumor
22. In which of the following bone disorders are doughnut lesions the least possible?
    (a) Osteoblastoma
    (b) ABC
    (c) Chondromyxoid fibroma
    (d) Giant-cell tumor
23. Which statement about bone island is NOT correct?
    (a) The lesions may become larger after adolescence.
    (b) They can be observed as cold zones on bone scan.
    (c) These lesions are usually benign.
    (d) They consist of lamellar and mature bone regions.
24. Which statement is NOT correct about the evaluation of bone tumors?
    (a) Gallium scan is preferred over the ^{99m}Tc-MDP scan for the evaluation of tumor size.
    (b) MRI is the best modality for the evaluation of bone marrow.
    (c) The involvement of bone marrow and bone metastasis are more common in Ewing sarcoma than in osteosarcoma.
    (d) The size of osteosarcoma is underestimated on bone scan.
25. In which of the following disorders is a cold lesion NOT found on bone scan?
    (a) Osteomyelitis
    (b) Sickle cell crisis
    (c) Legg–Perthes disease
    (d) Osteoid osteoma
26. In which type of leukemia is bone involvement the most common?
    (a) CLL
    (b) AML
    (c) CML
    (d) ALL
27. A large radiolucent lesion in the mid-tibia is found in radiography with an intermediate uptake on the labeled MDP bone scan. What is the most probable diagnosis?
    (a) Aneurysmal bone cyst
    (b) Adamantinoma
    (c) Bone island
    (d) Enchondroma

28. A lytic expansile lesion on the proximal end of the fibula is observed in radiography with doughnut sign on the labeled ^{99m}Tc-MDP bone scan. What is the most probable diagnosis?
    (a) Aneurysmal bone cyst
    (b) Adamantinoma
    (c) Bone island
    (d) Enchondroma
29. A lytic lesion in the second metaphysis of the hand is observed in radiography with a minor increased uptake on the labeled MDP bone scan. What is the most probable diagnosis?
    (a) Aneurysmal bone cyst
    (b) Adamantinoma
    (c) Bone island
    (d) Enchondroma
30. An ovoid sclerotic lesion with a diameter of 2 cm is accidentally found in mandibular radiography. This region shows an increased uptake on bone scan. What is the most probable diagnosis?
    (a) Osteoid osteoma
    (b) Osteoblastoma
    (c) Osteoma
    (d) Osteochondroma
31. Bone scan is performed for a 17-year-old patient with trauma of the left wrist. A minor focal increase in uptake with distinct edges is observed in the metaphysis of the second metacarpus of the right hand. No signs of redness, tenderness, or extra appendage are found. What is the most probable diagnosis?
    (a) Osteoid osteoma
    (b) Enchondroma
    (c) Chondroblastoma
    (d) Osteochondroma
32. A 13-year-old child with fever and tenderness of the pelvis is subjected to bone scan. A severe increase in uptake in the ileum is found in all three phases. The increased uptake in this region is homogenous in the delayed phase, and the soft tissue of the pelvis does NOT show an abnormal uptake. In addition, radiography reveals keratinization in this region. What is the most probable diagnosis?
    (a) Osteosarcoma
    (b) Hemangiosarcoma
    (c) Ewing sarcoma
    (d) Chondrosarcoma
33. In which of the following conditions is bone scan the most valuable for the evaluation of metastasis in a child with neuroblastoma and bone pain?
    (a) Detection of bone metastasis near the knee
    (b) Evaluation of the viability of bone metastatic lesions after chemotherapy
    (c) Detection of extraosseous metastasis
    (d) Evaluation of bone metastasis in a patient with normal MIBG scintigraphy

34. Bone scan is performed for a child with a history of retinoblastoma of the right eye, recent enucleation, and radiotherapy for 1 month. An increased uptake is found in the right periorbital (A) and calvarium (B). What is the most probable cause of the increased uptake in the A and B regions, respectively?
    (a) Tumor relapse; metastasis
    (b) Tumor relapse; benign reactive hyperemia
    (c) Benign reactive bone growth; metastasis
    (d) Benign reactive bone growth; benign reactive hyperemia
35. A lytic lesion without reactive ossification in the mandible is found in the radiography of a 15-year-old child. Bone scan reveals a photopenic lesion in the corresponding region. What is the most probable diagnosis?
    (a) Ewing sarcoma
    (b) Osteomyelitis
    (c) Multiple myeloma
    (d) Histiocytosis
36. Enucleation of the right eye and radiotherapy was performed for a child with retinoblastoma 2 years ago. An increased uptake in the right periorbital region is observed on scan for the evaluation of metastasis. What is the most probable cause of this finding?
    (a) Bone growth due to the absence of the globe of the eye globe.
    (b) Tumor relapse and periorbital metastasis.
    (c) This finding is non-specific, and MRI must be performed.
    (d) Secondary neoplasm after radiotherapy.
37. MRI is performed for a child with a 14-day history of rhinorrhea and epistaxis. A massive tumor is found in the paranasal region, which shows an increased uptake on bone scan. What is the most common diagnosis?
    (a) Lymphoepithelioma
    (b) Neurofibrosarcoma
    (c) Rhabdomyosarcoma
    (d) Hodgkin's lymphoma
38. About the uptake pattern of bone scan and bone metastasis of neuroblastoma:
    (a) Bone metastasis with poor localization usually contributes to neuroblastoma.
    (b) Bone metastasis of neuroblastoma is detectable in the metaphysis.
    (c) It is a good method for the therapeutic monitoring of metastasis.
    (d) An increased uptake in neuroblastoma metastasis is inversely related to prognosis.
39. How does an aneurysmal bone cyst appear in different imaging methods?
    (a) Hypoactive on bone scan
    (b) Sclerotic region in X-ray
    (c) Doughnut pattern in angioscintigraphy
    (d) Multiple cavernous spaces containing fluid in MRI

40. Which of the following bone lesions is usually observed as an active lesion with an increased uptake on bone scan?
    (a) Osteoblastoma
    (b) Osteoma
    (c) Osteochondroma
    (d) Bone island
41. Bone scan is performed 1 month after radiotherapy of a primary Ewing sarcoma. No significant decrease in activity in comparison with the pre-therapy scan is found. Which of the following statements is correct about this patient?
    (a) Scan must be repeated after 2–3 months.
    (b) This finding indicates the lack of improvement of the disease.
    (c) Chemotherapy must be considered.
    (d) Surgical removal of the tumor is indicated.
42. Which of the following diseases is characterized by a lytic expansile lesion on the proximal end of the fibula in radiography and by a doughnut sign on the labeled MDP bone scan?
    (a) Aneurysmal bone cyst
    (b) Adamantinoma
    (c) Bone island
    (d) Enchondroma
43. Osteochondroma:
    (a) It is the most common form of benign bone tumor.
    (b) A normal uptake on a scan excludes the possibility of malignancy.
    (c) It is more common in boys than in girls.
    (d) All of the above.
44. Histiocytosis X:
    (a) Long bones are the most common site of involvement.
    (b) Bone scan is more sensitive than radiography in detecting skull lesions.
    (c) Radiography is more sensitive than bone scan in detecting lesions in the vertebral column and hip.
    (d) Bone involvement is the most common clinical presentation.
45. A child with a pathologic diagnosis of Langerhans cell histiocytosis is referred for the evaluation of bone metastasis to the spine. What is the recommended imaging method for the evaluation?
    (a) Whole-body bone scan
    (b) CT scan
    (c) MRI
    (d) Whole-body bone scan with conventional radiography
46. Langerhans cell histiocytosis:
    (a) Long bones are the most common site of involvement of the diaphysis.
    (b) Pedicles are the most common site of vertebral involvement.
    (c) Radiography is more sensitive than a scan for the evaluation of hip involvement.
    (d) Radiography alone is sufficient for the evaluation of bone involvement.

47. A 4-year-old boy with a lesion in the distal femoral metaphysis and a possible diagnosis of osteochondroma is referred for bone scan. An increased uptake is observed in cartilage cap of the lesion. Which item is correct?
    (a) An increased uptake indicates malignant deformations.
    (b) An increased uptake is normally observed in immature skeleton.
    (c) If the uptake is equal to that of the adjacent bone, the possibility of malignancy is completely rejected.
    (d) Bone scan has no application in the evaluation of this patient.
48. In osteosarcoma, bone scan is NOT indicated for:
    (a) Evaluation of primary bone lesion
    (b) Evaluation of bone metastasis
    (c) Accidental uptake in pulmonary metastasis
    (d) Determination of the margins of the primary tumor for surgery
49. A 19-year-old boy is referred with nocturnal tibial pain, which is alleviated with aspirin. Radiography shows a lucent lesion with sclerotic margins in the tibia, and significant uptake is observed in bone scintigraphy. What is the most probable diagnosis?
    (a) Aneurysmal bone cyst
    (b) Osteoid osteoma
    (c) Fibrous dysplasia
    (d) Bone cysts
50. A 14-year-old boy is referred with fever and hip pain. Lytic and blastic lesions in the left iliac wing are found in hip radiography. A nonhomogenous uptake is found in the same region in on bone scan. What is the most probable diagnosis?
    (a) Osteosarcoma
    (b) Ewing sarcoma
    (c) Bone lymphoma
    (d) Neuroblastoma
51. A doughnut sign in the left distal femur is found on the bone scan of a patient with pain in the left leg. What is the most probable diagnosis?
    (a) Giant-cell tumor
    (b) Enchondroma
    (c) Osteoblastoma
    (d) Hemangioma
52. An increased uptake is detected in the vertebral body of one lumbar vertebra on the FDG-PET scan. Which of the following lesions is NOT possible?
    (a) Simple bone cyst
    (b) Malignant tumor
    (c) Osteomyelitis
    (d) Compression fracture
53. Which of the following tumors is characterized by multicentric lesions with metastasis to the bone and arteriovenous shunt?
    (a) Ewing sarcoma
    (b) Rhabdomyosarcoma
    (c) Neuroblastoma
    (d) Osteosarcoma

54. Bone scan is performed on a patient complaining of pain in the lower extremities. A region of increased uptake in the right proximal tibia is found in the angiography and blood-pool phases, and it is represented by a doughnut sign in the delayed images. What is the most probable diagnosis?
    (a) Giant-cell tumor, fibrous cortical lesion
    (b) Enchondroma, adamantinoma
    (c) Aneurysmal bone cyst, chondromyxoid fibroma
    (d) Hemangiosarcoma, osteoid osteoma
55. A cold region in the upper humerus is observed on the bone scan of a 29-year-old man. What is the most probable diagnosis?
    (a) Osteosarcoma
    (b) Osteomyelitis
    (c) Simple bone cyst
    (d) Ewing sarcoma
56. Bone scan is performed on a patient with suspected histiocytosis X. Which item is correct?
    (a) An increased uptake is common.
    (b) A normal uptake is common.
    (c) A decreased uptake is common.
    (d) Regions with an increased and a decreased uptake are commonly reported.
57. Bone scan is performed on a 19-year-old boy with painful edema of the posterior part of the upper left tibia. An increased uptake limited to the tibial epiphysis is reported. What is the most probable diagnosis?
    (a) Giant-cell tumor
    (b) Hemangioma
    (c) Adamantinoma
    (d) Chondroblastoma
58. What is the best diagnostic method for osteochondroma?
    (a) Doppler sonography
    (b) CT scan
    (c) MRI
    (d) Bone scan
59. All of the following statements regarding histiocytosis X are correct *except*:
    (a) About 80% of patients have lytic lesions.
    (b) Trauma can be an underlying factor.
    (c) Bone scan is a reliable diagnostic method.
    (d) Bone scan is valuable for the diagnosis of tumor recurrence.
60. The precise determination of the borders of the primary tumor and bone malignancy is critical for surgery and radiotherapy. Which of the following methods is recommended for such a purpose?
    (a) Conventional bone scan
    (b) SPECT bone scan
    (c) MRI
    (d) Gallium scan

61. What is the most appropriate radiotracer for the evaluation of metastasis or recurrence of malignant fibrous histiocytoma?
    (a) ^{99m}Tc-MDP
    (b) ^{67}Gallium
    (c) ^{201}Thallium
    (d) ^{99m}Tc-MIBI
62. A 47-year-old patient with Ollier's disease (familial multiple osteochondroma) is referred with pain and edema of the right proximal humerus. Bone scan shows an intermediate increase in uptake in the right proximal humerus with a markedly focal increase in uptake and well margins in some regions. What is the most probable diagnosis?
    (a) Osteosarcoma
    (b) Chondroblastoma
    (c) Chondrosarcoma
    (d) Ewing sarcoma
63. Bone scan of a 59-year-old woman with history of back pain for a few months shows a decreased activity in one of the lumbar vertebrae. An obvious trabeculation is observed in radiography. What is the most probable diagnosis?
    (a) Metastasis
    (b) Hemangioma
    (c) Osteoblastoma
    (d) Fibrous dysplasia
64. A 13-year-old boy is presented with pain in the right thigh. His radiography shows a well-defined lytic lesion in the diaphysis of the right femur. The bone scan also demonstrates an increased activity in the same region. Which of the following statements is true?
    (a) He needs to be evaluated for metastasis.
    (b) Osteoid osteoma cannot be excluded.
    (c) It is a benign lesion accompanied by fracture.
    (d) Biopsy should be performed to rule out a malignant process.
65. What is the most important differential diagnosis of aneurysmal bone cyst (ABC)?
    (a) Giant-cell tumor
    (b) Fibrosarcoma
    (c) Eosinophilic granuloma
    (d) Osteoid osteoma
66. On the X-ray of a 13-year-old boy following trauma, an eccentric lucent lesion with a thinned cortex and a sclerotic margin is observed in the distal diaphysis of the right tibia. On the CT scan, a cortical lesion with a disruption of the cortex is seen in the same site. Bone scan also shows a minimally increased 99 Tc-MDP uptake in the same region. What is the most likely diagnosis?
    (a) Aneurysmal bone cyst (ABC)
    (b) Osteomyelitis
    (c) Eosinophilic granuloma (EG)
    (d) Non-ossifying fibroma (NOF)

67. Which of the following bone tumors develops a bony sequestrum?
    (a) Fibrosarcoma
    (b) Chondrosarcoma
    (c) Osteosarcoma
    (d) Osteoblastoma
68. All of the following cancers may cause multiple blastic lesions in a 53-year-old man *except*:
    (a) Bronchogenic carcinoma
    (b) Renal cell carcinoma
    (c) Colon cancer
    (d) Thyroid cancer
69. On the X-ray of a 26-year-old, a cystic lesion with sclerosis in its inferior margin in the right iliac wing is observed. However, there is no evidence of a periosteal reaction, soft tissue mass, and calcification. All of the following are a possible diagnosis *except*:
    (a) Giant-cell tumor
    (b) Enchondroma
    (c) Fibrous dysplasia
    (d) Chondromyxoid fibroma (CMF)
70. Which of the following conditions is not associated with an eccentric bony lesion?
    (a) Simple bone cyst
    (b) Eosinophilic granuloma
    (c) Brown tumor
    (d) GCT
71. All of the following statements regarding non-ossifying fibroma are true *except*:
    (a) A biopsy is required if it enlarges.
    (b) Cortical disruption is commonly seen on the CT scan.
    (c) The most common site is around the knee.
    (d) Periostitis is not observed.
72. What is the most important finding in distinguishing benign from malignant bony lesions?
    (a) Presence of activity in bone scintigraphy
    (b) Widening of the transitional zone of the lesion
    (c) Periostitis
    (d) Cortical disruption
73. Which of the following statement about osteosarcoma is not true?
    (a) It usually occurs in those aged 30 years and below.
    (b) It is usually found on the distal ends of long bones.
    (c) The lesions are commonly associated with cortical disruption.
    (d) The lesions exhibit no sclerotic change.

74. A cortical thickening with a central lucency in the right tibia is observed on the radiography of a 16-year-old boy. What is the next best modality?
    (a) MRI
    (b) CT scan
    (c) Bone scan
    (d) Sonography
75. A lytic eccentric lesion in the subarticular region of the proximal right tibia is found on X-ray. What is the most likely diagnosis?
    (a) Chondroblastoma
    (b) Simple bone cyst
    (c) Giant-cell tumor
    (d) Aneurysmal bone cyst
76. A patient with leg pain is presented. His radiograph shows an expansile and lytic lesion accompanied by cartilage calcification. What is the best next step?
    (a) Radiography after 6 months
    (b) MRI
    (c) Surgery
    (d) CT scan
77. A cortical irregularity with periosteal reaction in the posteromedial epicondyle of the right femur is observed on the radiography of a 16-year-old boy with a history of recent trauma. What is the diagnosis?
    (a) Cortical desmoid
    (b) Avulsion fracture
    (c) Osteosarcoma
    (d) Osteochondritis
78. A 36-year-old man with low back pain is presented. His CT and radiographic images show a mixed lytic and expansile lesion containing a calcified matrix in the pedicle and spinous process of the T12 vertebra. All of the following can cause this pathology *except*:
    (a) Osteoblastoma
    (b) TB
    (c) ABC
    (d) Giant-cell tumor
79. All of the following skeletal lesions can have multiplicity *except*:
    (a) Osteoid osteoma
    (b) Fibrous dysplasia
    (c) Enchondroma
    (d) Eosinophilic granuloma
80. Which of the following bone tumors is rarely seen in the calcaneus bone?
    (a) Simple bone cyst
    (b) Chondroblastoma
    (c) Giant-cell tumor
    (d) Aneurysmal bone cyst

81. A 66-year-old man with bone pain is presented. A fusiform, lucent lesion with scalloping of the inner cortex and periosteal reaction is observed on plain radiograph. Extension into the soft tissue is also reported. What is the typical finding in bone scintigraphy?
    (a) Patchy areas of moderately increased activity
    (b) High focal uptake
    (c) Diffuse and homogenous areas of intensely increased activity
    (d) a and b
82. Which of the following statements about Ewing sarcoma is NOT correct?
    (a) It is commonly observed in children and young adults.
    (b) It is common in the pelvis or femur.
    (c) Uptake of a primary Ewing sarcoma decreases 6–9 months after radiotherapy.
    (d) Lack of decrease in the tumor uptake after radiotherapy indicates tumor recurrence or fracture.
83. What is the first method performed for the evaluation of skeletal involvement in multiple myeloma?
    (a) X-ray
    (b) MRI
    (c) Bone scan
    (d) FDG-PET
84. What is the bone scan pattern in osteosarcoma secondary to Paget's disease?
    (a) Intense and expanded uptake in photopenic areas
    (b) A photopenic lesion surrounded by diffusely increased activity
    (c) Diffuse and homogenous areas of intensely increased activity
    (d) a and b
85. All of the following benign bone pathologies are presented by an intense radiotracer uptake *except*:
    (a) Aneurysmal bone cyst
    (b) Fibrous dysplasia
    (c) Giant-cell tumor
    (d) Enchondroma
86. Which of the following tumors is always presented by an increased uptake on bone scan?
    (a) Chondroblastoma
    (b) Desmoplastic fibroma
    (c) Enchondroma
    (d) Epidermoid cyst
87. The doughnut sign on bone scan is observed in all of the following tumors *except*:
    (a) Giant-cell tumor (GCT)
    (b) Aneurysmal bone cyst(ABC)
    (c) Osteosarcoma
    (d) Osteoid Osteoma

88. What is the pattern of adamantinoma (ameloblastoma) on bone scan?
    (a) Mostly exhibits as intense uptake
    (b) Moderate uptake
    (c) Normal or mildly increased uptake
    (d) Markedly intense
89. On bone scintigraphy, a lesion exhibits increased activity in the angiography phase and decreased activity in the delayed views. What is the most likely diagnosis?
    (a) Fibrous cortical lesion
    (b) Giant-cell tumor
    (c) Osteochondroma
    (d) Hemangioma
90. What is the most benign tumor of the sacrum?
    (a) Giant-cell tumor
    (b) Aneurysmal bone cyst
    (c) Hemangioma
    (d) Eosinophilic granuloma
91. A 17-year-old man began experiencing spinal pain 5 months ago. Only tenderness of the L2 vertebrae is observed in the physical examination, and radiography shows a tumoral lesion in the posterior elements of L2. Which of the following tumors is the least probable?
    (a) Osteoid osteoma
    (b) Osteoblastoma
    (c) Aneurysmal bone cyst
    (d) Histiocytosis
92. What is the best diagnostic modality for the identification of a nidus in osteoid osteoma?
    (a) Plain radiography
    (b) CT scan
    (c) MRI
    (d) Bone scan
93. What is the most probable diagnosis for a bony lesion in the T9 vertebral body of a 17-year-old patient?
    (a) Giant-cell tumor
    (b) Aneurysmal bone cyst
    (c) Osteoid osteoma
    (d) Histiocytosis
94. A patient is evaluated for a tumor in the distal posterior femoral bone. She mentions a history of trauma in the same region. On the CT scan, a lobulated mass is attached to the posterior femoral condyles with surrounding tissues displacement. Peripheral ossification is more intense and mature than ossification in the central regions. What is the most probable diagnosis?
    (a) Periosteal osteosarcoma
    (b) Parosteal osteosarcoma
    (c) Osteochondroma
    (d) Myositis ossificans

95. Which of the following radiographic parameters in the plain film of bone disorders is the most important for the differentiation of benign and malignant lesions?
    (a) Periostitis
    (b) Orientation
    (c) Cortical destruction
    (d) Zone of transition
96. Which of the following benign tumors or lesions demonstrate a pattern the most similar to malignant lesions?
    (a) Non-ossifying Fibroma
    (b) Fibrous dysplasia
    (c) Eosinophilic granuloma
    (d) Aneurysmal bone cyst
97. Which of the following bone tumors is associated with a high incidence of regional recurrence and malignant transformation?
    (a) Osteochondroma
    (b) Chondromyxoid fibroma
    (c) Giant-cell tumor
    (d) Desmoplastic fibroma
98. Which of the following studies is NOT required for the identification of metastasis of Ewing sarcoma?
    (a) Bone scan
    (b) Bone marrow sampling
    (c) Pulmonary CT scan
    (d) Abdominal CT scan
99. PET imaging with which radiotracer has been reported in malignant fibrous histiocytoma?
    (a) ^{13}N-glutamate
    (b) ^{11}C-methionin
    (c) ^{11}C-α-aminoisobutyric acid
    (d) alpha-[^{11}C]methyl-L-tryptophan
100. Which of the following benign tumors is the differential diagnosis of permeative lesions?
    (a) Giant-cell tumor (GCT)
    (b) Eosinophilic granuloma (EG)
    (c) Aneurysmal bone cyst (ABC)
    (d) Non-ossifying fibroma (NOF)

3.2.1 Answer

	A	B	C	D		A	B	C	D
1				*	51	*			
2				*	52	*			
3		*			53				*
4		*			54			*	
5		*			55			*	
6			*		56				*
7	*				57				*
8				*	58			*	
9		*			59			*	
10				*	60			*	
11				*	61			*	
12	*				62		*		
13		*			63		*		
14			*		64			*	
15	*				65	*			
16		*			66				*
17			*		67	*			
18			*		68		*		
19		*			69		*		
20		*			70	*			
21	*				71	*			
22	*				72		*		
23		*			73				*
24				*	74			*	
25				*	75			*	
26				*	76			*	
27		*			77	*			
28	*				78				*
29				*	79	*			
30			*		80				*
31		*			81				*
32			*		82			*	
33				*	83	*			
34			*		84		*		
35				*	85				*
36			*		86		*		
37			*		87				*
38	*				88	*			
39				*	89				*
40	*				90	*			
41	*				91				*
42	*				92		*		
43				*	93				*
44				*	94				*
45				*	95				*
46	*				96			*	
47		*			97			*	
48				*	98				*
49		*			99			*	
50		*			100		*		

3.3 Evaluation of Malignancy: Metastatic Bone Disease

1. About bone scan in breast cancer:
   (a) Routine bone scan is not indicated preoperatively.
   (b) Women with stage II or higher should have a postoperative study as the baseline.
   (c) Staging bone scan is NOT indicated for patients with a primary tumor less than 2 cm in diameter.
   (d) All of the above.
2. In metastatic bony lesions:
   (a) MRI detects more lesions than bone scan in the spine, pelvis, and femur.
   (b) Bone scan detects more lesions than bone scan in the ribs and skull.
   (c) The overall detection of metastases by MRI is equivalent to that by bone scan.
   (d) All of the above.
3. In a patient with a confirmed malignant tumor, the observation of a single metastatic lesion in which region is highly indicative of bone metastasis?
   (a) Vertebrae
   (b) Ribs
   (c) Cranium
   (d) Femur
4. What is the metastatic probability of a singular lesion in the manubrium on the bone scan of a patient with breast cancer?
   (a) Very low
   (b) Low
   (c) Intermediate
   (d) Very high
5. In which group of prostate cancer patients is bone scan the least necessary?
   (a) Patients with a high PSA growth rate
   (b) Patients with a high LDH
   (c) Patients undergoing hormone therapy
   (d) Patients with bone pain
6. What region of solitary lesion is the most common in a patient with malignant breast cancer?
   (a) Cranium
   (b) Sternum
   (c) Vertebrae
   (d) Pelvis
7. Whole-body bone scan is conducted 3 h after the administration of ^{99m}Tc-MDP on a 65-year-old man with prostate cancer. No noticeable uptake in bones is observed, and only blood-pool activity is noted. What is the best diagnosis?
   (a) Advanced osteoporosis
   (b) Treatment with amphotericin B
   (c) Cirrhosis
   (d) IV administration of iron dextran

8. Bone scan is recommended in which of the following prostate cancer conditions?
   (a) A patient with newly identified prostate cancer and low PSA
   (b) A patient with confirmed prostate cancer for 10 years and low PSA
   (c) A patient with bone pain and low PSA
   (d) All of the above
9. The sunburst view is the most common in bone metastasis with the origin of:
   (a) Prostate
   (b) Breast
   (c) Pulmonary
   (d) Neuroblastoma
10. Which item is NOT correct about bone metastasis?
    (a) ^{99m}Tc-MDP uptake is directly related to the invasiveness of the tumor.
    (b) Sclerotic lesions appear earlier in X-ray than lytic lesions.
    (c) Bone scan may be normal if metastasis is confined to the bone marrow.
    (d) Approximately 55% of singular lesions of bone have a neuroblastic origin.
11. What is the radiopharmaceutical of choice for the therapeutic monitoring of skeletal tumors?
    (a) ^{18}F-FDG-PET
    (b) ^{99m}Tc-MIBI
    (c) ^{201}Tl
    (d) ^{67}Ga
12. Which item is NOT correct about the evaluation of bone metastasis and response to treatment?
    (a) The flare phenomenon is observed in most cases of breast cancer.
    (b) Superscan is common in prostate cancer.
    (c) Osteoblastic response to treatment indicates poor prognosis.
    (d) For the proper evaluation of treatment, bone scan must be performed 6 months after treatment.
13. Radical prostatectomy was performed 3 months ago for a patient with prostate cancer. He is now under treatment with antiandrogens, and the level of serum PSA in last week's laboratory report is 5 ng/mL. The patient has experienced diffuse sporadic bone pains since 2 weeks ago. What is the method of choice for further evaluation?
    (a) Bone scan
    (b) Repeat of PSA test
    (c) Radiography of pain zone
    (d) FDG-PET scan
14. Chemotherapy is conducted on a patient with breast cancer. How long after chemotherapy is bone scan indicated?
    (a) 7 months
    (b) 3 months
    (c) 9 months
    (d) 1 month

15. In which of the following malignancies is the probability of metastasis to the distal humerus and femur the highest?
    (a) Kidney
    (b) Colon
    (c) Hepatoma
    (d) Pancreas
16. ^{99m}Tc-MIBI scan is performed on a 72-year-old man with multiple myeloma. Bone marrow washout is faster than 1 h. Which statement is correct?
    (a) Lack of Pgp expression.
    (b) This patient possibly demonstrates resistance to multiple drugs.
    (c) Bone scan is a sensitive method for the evaluation of bone involvement.
    (d) ^{99m}Tc-MIBI scan findings have NO relationship with Pgp expression.
17. A 46-year-old woman with a history of breast cancer presents with a painful right knee. She has not yet received any medication. Which type of periarticular changes is expected?
    (a) Metastatic arthropathy
    (b) Polyarthritis carcinoma
    (c) Hypertrophic osteoarthropathy
    (d) Osteonecrosis in the healing phase
18. The reduced uptake of L2 is observed on the bone scan of a 49-year-old woman with renal cell carcinoma. She mentions a history of radiotherapy of 19 Gy about a month ago. What is the most probable diagnosis for L2 lesion?
    (a) Metastasis
    (b) Necrosis after radiotherapy
    (c) Bone tumor
    (d) Artifact
19. A 55-year-old woman with right breast cancer underwent mastectomy last year. A focal increased uptake on the left side of the sternal body is found on bone scan. What is the most probable diagnosis?
    (a) Metastasis
    (b) Trauma during surgery
    (c) Normal variation (cartilage ossification)
    (d) New trauma
20. What is the main benefit of bone scan in patients with pulmonary cancer?
    (a) Early diagnosis of metastasis
    (b) Prevention of pathologic fractures
    (c) Prevention of unnecessary surgery
    (d) Staging of cancer
21. Total prostatectomy is recently performed on a 75-year-old patient with prostate cancer. PSA before and after surgery is reported at 100 and 8 ng/mL, respectively. The patient has NOT received anti-androgen therapy. Which study is recommended for the evaluation of bone metastasis?
    (a) Bone scan is indicated if tumor size is greater than 1 cm.
    (b) Whole-body bone scan is NOT indicated.
    (c) Bone scan is required if the lymph nodes of the pelvis are involved.
    (d) Bone scan is required if the PSA level after 1 week is greater than 10.

22. In which of the following situations is metastatic involvement of the peripheral bones the most common?
    (a) Renal cell carcinoma
    (b) Breast cancer
    (c) Prostate cancer
    (d) Lymphoma
23. A 49-year-old man with prostate cancer underwent surgery. Initial PSA was 0.4 ng/mL, and it reached 2.4 ng/mL after surgery. Which of the following interventions is the most appropriate?
    (a) Bone scan
    (b) Pulmonary CT scan
    (c) MRI of lumbar vertebrae
    (d) Follow-up
24. A 59-year-old man with prostate cancer and diffuse bone metastasis underwent orchiectomy. Bone scan shows multiple focal uptakes 2 months after surgery, and PSA has increased from 82 ng/mL to 141 ng/mL. What is the most probable diagnosis?
    (a) Progression of the disease
    (b) Flare phenomenon
    (c) Imaging artifact
    (d) Response to treatment
25. A 59-year-old man underwent surgery 7 months ago because of prostate cancer. He now complains about back pain, and his PSA level is 2 ng/mL. What is the next step?
    (a) Bone scan
    (b) Thoracic MRI
    (c) Thoracic CT scan
    (d) Thoracolumbar radiography
26. What is the most common bone marrow metastasizing tumor in children?
    (a) Ewing sarcoma
    (b) Wilms' tumor
    (c) Pulmonary tumors
    (d) Soft tissue tumors
27. Which of the following statements about the diagnosis of bone metastasis is NOT correct?
    (a) Most bone metastatic lesions initially appear in the bone marrow.
    (b) In neuroblastoma, MIBG scan can be used for a more accurate diagnosis of metastatic lesions found on bone scan.
    (c) Bone metastasis of pulmonary tumors indicates very poor prognosis.
    (d) MRI and FDG-PET can differentiate metastatic lesions from changes after radiation.

28. A singular bone lesion in the … most likely indicates metastasis in a patient with identified soft tissue malignancy.
    (a) Pelvis
    (b) Cranium
    (c) Femur
    (d) Humerus
29. Which of the following findings in vertebral SPECT is favorable to metastasis?
    (a) Focal increase in uptake in the spinous of C2
    (b) Increased uptake in the body and lamina of L2
    (c) Increased uptake in the anterior body of L2
    (d) Increased uptake in the body of T11 extended to the pedicle
30. Multiple bone lesions in the axial skeleton and extremities are reported on bone scan. What is the most probable primary tumor?
    (a) Lung cancer
    (b) Prostate cancer
    (c) Breast cancer
    (d) Lymphoma
31. All of the following statements regarding the application of PET and bone scan in bone malignancy are true *except*:
    (a) The positive predictive value (PPV) of PET/CT for bone malignancy is 98% when the PET and CT results are concordant.
    (b) Bone lesions that are positive on CT but negative on PET have a PPV of 17% for malignancy.
    (c) The sensitivity of PET is substantially superior to that of bone scan for lesions that are invisible on CT.
    (d) Previous chemotherapy decreases the PPV of PET and CT in bone metastases.
32. The presence of calcification in … is most likely due to a malignant process.
    (a) Kidney
    (b) Mediastinum
    (c) Lung
    (d) Breast
33. In which of the following tumors is metastasis not common?
    (a) Chondrosarcoma
    (b) Giant-cell tumor
    (c) Ewing sarcoma
    (d) Osteosarcoma

34. What are the most likely origins of a metastatic sclerotic lesion in a 63-year-old woman and a mixed sclerotic and lytic lesion in a 65-year-old woman on their radiographs?
    (a) Breast–lung
    (b) Breast–breast
    (c) Colon–lymphoma
    (d) Colon–breast
35. In which metastatic bone lesions are periosteal reactions commonly seen?
    (a) Breast
    (b) Prostate
    (c) Neuroblastoma
    (d) Nephroblastoma
36. What is the most appropriate modality for the assessment of multiple myelomas?
    (a) MRI
    (b) ^{99m} Tc-MIBI
    (c) PET/CT
    (d) Bone scan
37. Multiple bilateral periosteal reactions in the radial and metacarpal bones of a 73-year-old patient are observed on radiography. What is the next reasonable step to undertake for this patient?
    (a) Bone scan
    (b) Measurement of calcium and alkaline phosphates levels
    (c) CXR
    (d) MRI
38. What are the most accurate diagnostic tests for the evaluation of metastasis and lymphoma of the vertebrae?
    (a) CT scan, MRI
    (b) MRI, bone scan
    (c) Bone scan, MRI
    (d) MRI, MRI
39. What is the most sensitive method for the evaluation of the pulmonary metastasis of osteosarcoma?
    (a) CXR
    (b) ^{201}Tl scan
    (c) Bone scan
    (d) CT scan
40. How long before X-ray and bone scan show positive findings in breast cancer?
    (a) 1 year
    (b) 2–3 months
    (c) 4–6 months
    (d) 6–9 months

41. Bone scan in breast cancer:
    (a) For a breast tumor smaller than 3 cm, bone scan is NOT necessary unless the patient is symptomatic.
    (b) For a breast tumor smaller than 3 cm, bone scan is NOT necessary unless there are suspicious findings in laboratory tests.
    (c) Bone scan is usually required in stages II–IV.
    (d) Patients with known breast cancer with an isolated sternal lesion have a very high likelihood (approximately 70%) of metastatic origin of the lesion.
42. All of the following statements regarding the application of bone scan in different cancers are correct *except*:
    (a) Bone scintigraphy is not required as a routine preoperative test for the management of patients with newly diagnosed lung cancer because of its relatively low efficacy.
    (b) Patients with Hodgkin's disease have more frequent extremity lesions and fewer axial lesions than those with non-Hodgkin's lymphoma.
    (c) Lung tumors that metastasize through the arterial route can be detected as isolated solitary lesions in the distal aspects of the extremities.
    (d) The sensitivity of MIBG scan in neuroblastoma is 10% lower than that of bone scan for bone and bone marrow metastasis.
43. If the goal is to stage known neuroblastoma, which of the following tests can provide the most information?
    (a) Bone scan
    (b) CT scan
    (c) MIBG
    (d) MRI
44. Which of the following items does NOT describe the advantages of MIBG over bone scan for the evaluation of neuroblastoma tumors?
    (a) Higher intra-observer consistency
    (b) Possibility of a postoperative evaluation of tumor viability
    (c) Possibility of the evaluation of extraosseous involvement
    (d) Lower sensitivity but higher specificity
45. What is (are) the indication(s) of bone scan in prostate cancer?
    (a) Elevation of PSA level
    (b) Patients who have symptoms
    (c) Patients who have been hormonally treated
    (d) All of the above
46. A patient with identified primary malignancy (bone or soft tissue) is evaluated. What is the probability of malignancy of a solitary lesion in the mentioned regions?
    (a) Hip and skull: 70–80%
    (b) Vertebrae: 40–50%
    (c) Extremities: 40–50%
    (d) Ribs: 30%

47. Which of the following statements about the application of bone scan in bone cancers is NOT correct?
    (a) The evaluation of a pathological fracture is required for a patient with primary malignancy and a focal increase in uptake in a region with a history of trauma.
    (b) The bladder is usually seen by using a superscan with modern gamma cameras.
    (c) The intensity of a lesion on bone scan is predicative of the histopathologic outcome.
    (d) The increased intensity in old lesions or even the appearance of new lesions is reported in the flare phenomenon.
48. The flare phenomenon is observed in 20% of cases and is associated with all of the following variables *except*:
    (a) Tumor type
    (b) Treatment protocol
    (c) Time interval between treatment and bone scan
    (d) Tumor staging
49. Early stages of the metastasis are limited to bone marrow, and NO lesion is found in the skeleton. This finding is the most common in … cancer with incidence of 25%.
    (a) Prostate
    (b) Thyroid
    (c) Breast
    (d) Lung
50. Which of the following bone pathologies show thallium uptake on the scan?
    (a) Fibrous dysplasia
    (b) Osteochondroma
    (c) Recent fracture
    (d) None of the above
51. What is the first recommended imaging method for a patient with primary malignancy and recent back pain or change in the pattern of back pain?
    (a) X-ray
    (b) MRI
    (c) Bone scan
    (d) CT scan
52. All of the following statements regarding the role of bone scan in prostate cancer are correct *except*:
    (a) Abnormal bone scan at the time of clinical diagnosis is common.
    (b) The grade of prostate cancer is related to the superscan pattern on bone scan.
    (c) Serial bone scan is definitely valuable after the treatment of prostate cancer.
    (d) The serum PSA level is always reliable for the evaluation of the probability of bone metastasis.

53. In which type of pulmonary cancer is bone metastasis the most common?
    (a) Squamous cell lung carcinoma
    (b) Adenocarcinoma
    (c) Large-cell lung carcinoma
    (d) Small-cell lung carcinoma (SCLC)
54. The probability of the appearance of cold lesions on bone scan is most common in … tumors.
    (a) Renal
    (b) Prostate
    (c) Brain
    (d) Breast
55. In which type of eosinophilic granuloma (EG) is scintigraphy valuable?
    (a) Unifocal eosinophilic granuloma
    (b) Multifocal EG
    (c) Both
    (d) None
56. Which scan can help in the primary evaluation, staging, and follow-up of histiocytosis?
    (a) ^{99m}Tc-MIBI scan
    (b) Thallium scan
    (c) Gallium scan
    (d) Bone scan
57. Although simultaneous bone and gallium scan is NOT valuable for the evaluation of metastatic bone lesions, it provides helpful information on:
    (a) Rhabdomyosarcoma
    (b) Retinoblastoma
    (c) Hepatoblastoma
    (d) Diffuse anaplastic Wilms' tumor
58. Imaging demonstrates a synovial sarcoma for a 28-year-old woman with a history of pain and edema of the right arm. CBC, LFT, and RFT are normal, and NO other specific symptom is found. Which of the following studies is critical for staging?
    (a) Chest X-ray
    (b) Plain radiography of the extremity
    (c) Bone scan
    (d) Brain MRI
59. Biopsy demonstrates a high-grade sarcoma for a 34-year-old man with a history of left thigh mass. In addition, MRI shows a tumor with the size of 11 × 7 cm in the left lateral thigh. The patient is subjected to neo-adjuvant chemotherapy. Which of the following therapeutic monitoring studies provides the most prognostic information?
    (a) CT scan of the extremity
    (b) MRI of the extremity
    (c) PET scan
    (d) None of the above

60. A 67-year-old man with a history of lung cancer from 1 year ago complains of thigh pain. Tenderness of the right femoral shaft is observed in the physical examination. What is the next diagnostic intervention?
    (a) Radiography of the right femur
    (b) Whole-body bone scan
    (c) Chest CT scan
    (d) Measurement of serum alkaline phosphatase
61. Which of the following prognostic factors is the least important in the regional recurrence of breast cancer?
    (a) Age
    (b) Pattern of tumor margin
    (c) Systemic treatment
    (d) Tumor location
62. A 66-year-old man with PSA of 4 ng/mL and prostate carcinoma (score: 3 + 4), but NO clinical problem was found in radical prostatectomy. What is the recommended method for the evaluation of metastasis?
    (a) Bone scan
    (b) CT scan
    (c) MRI
    (d) None of the above
63. A patient with prostate cancer and metastasis to the hip and spine is subjected to hormone therapy. He mentions pain in the neck starting from 4 months ago and a progressive paresis of the right fourth and fifth fingers. What is the recommended method for the evaluation of cord compression?
    (a) Plain radiography of the neck
    (b) MRI of the cervical vertebrae
    (c) Bone scan
    (d) MRI of the whole vertebral column

3.3.1 Answer

	A	B	C	D
1				*
2				*
3	*			
4				*
5		*		
6			*	
7				*
8			*	
9	*			
10	*			
11	*			
12			*	
13	*			
14		*		
15	*			
16		*		
17	*			
18	*			
19	*			
20			*	
21		*		
22	*			
23	*			
24	*			
25	*			
26	*			
27				*
28	*			
29				*
30	*			
31				*
32	*			
33		*		
34		*		
35			*	
36	*			
37			*	
38				*
39				*
40			*	

	A	B	C	D
41			*	
42				*
43			*	
44				*
45				*
46			*	
47			*	
48				*
49			*	
50				*
51		*		
52				*
53				*
54	*			
55	*			
56			*	
57				*
58	*			
59			*	
60	*			
61				*
62				*
63				*

3.4 Assessment of Infection

1. What is the most common primary route of contamination of bone and joint structures?
   (a) Hematogenous spread
   (b) Contiguous sources
   (c) Implantation
   (d) Lymphatic spread
2. What is the earliest sign of acute osteomyelitis on ultrasonography?
   (a) Periosteal thickening
   (b) Cortical erosions
   (c) Subperiosteal collections
   (d) Deep soft tissue swelling
3. Regarding chronic recurrent multifocal osteomyelitis:
   (a) The most common organism is *Staphylococcus aureus*.
   (b) Pelvis is the most common site of the disease.
   (c) Treatment with antibiotics alters the course of the disease.
   (d) The bone scan appearance is distinguishable from that of SAPHO (synovitis, acne, pustulosis, hyperostosis, and osteitis) syndrome.
4. In which of the following conditions is osteomyelitis the easiest to be revealed on bone scan?
   (a) Early stages of osteomyelitis in pediatrics
   (b) Painful swelling of the tibia in adults
   (c) Regional tenderness of the vertebrae among geriatrics
   (d) Fever and immobility of the lower extremities in a newborn
5. What is the bone scan pattern in septic arthritis?
   (a) Increased uptake in phases 1 and 2 confined to soft tissue; diffusely increased uptake in joints in phase 3
   (b) Abnormal uptake in phases 1 and 2; normal uptake in joints in phase 3
   (c) Normal uptake in phases 1 and 2; increased uptake in joints in phase 3
   (d) Normal uptake in phase 1; increased uptake in phases 2 and 3
6. The ^{99m}Tc-MDP bone scan reveals a high uptake, whereas the radionuclide bone marrow scan shows a normal uptake in the same region in a patient with sickle cell anemia, who is currently experiencing acute bone pain. What is the most possible diagnosis?
   (a) Acute bone infarction
   (b) Metastasis
   (c) Osteomyelitis
   (d) Chronic infarction of bone

7. A 44-year-old man with fever of unknown origin (FUO) is subjected to ^{111}In-WBC scan. Primary images show a radiotracer uptake in both lungs, whereas delayed images reveal a decreased pulmonary activity and an increased hepatic uptake of the radiopharmaceutical. What is the diagnosis?
   (a) Extensive pulmonary vasculitis possibly due to Wegener's granulomatosis
   (b) Drug-induced cholangitis
   (c) Systemic cytomegalovirus infection
   (d) Degradation of WBC during radiopharmaceutical preparation
8. Which of the following factors distinguishes ^{99m}Tc-HMPAO-WBC from ^{111}In-WBC scan?
   (a) Splenic uptake of the radiodrug
   (b) Pattern of distribution in the bone marrow
   (c) Higher background radioactivity
   (d) Hepatic clearance of Tc
9. In which case does vascular permeability play a negligible role in the accumulation of the radiotracer in an infectious region?
   (a) ^{67}Ga- Citrate
   (b) ^{99m}Tc-HMPAO-WBC
   (c) Radiolabeled monoclonal antigranulocyte antibody
   (d) ^{111}In-IgG
10. In which condition is gallium scan preferred over labeled leukocyte scan for the detection of infection?
   (a) Suspected vertebral tuberculous osteomyelitis
   (b) A pediatric case with major thalassemia and recent fever
   (c) Fever in a patient with a history of renal transplantation and dialysis last year
   (d) Fever in a patient who underwent laparotomy for pancreatitis a week ago
11. Painful swelling of the right knee is found in a 14-year-old child with sickle cell anemia. Bone scan reveals a homogenous increased uptake in this knee. On the bone marrow scan, a region of photon deficiency is found in the distal metaphysis of the right femur. What is the most probable diagnosis?
   (a) Osteomyelitis followed by septic arteritis
   (b) Hemarthrosis
   (c) Reactive arthritis to infarction of bone marrow
   (d) Intra-articular fracture of femur
12. A child with sickle cell anemia is presented to the emergency room with sever bone pain. Bone marrow scintigraphy reveals lesions in the painful zones, but bone scan is normal. What is the most probable diagnosis?
   (a) Ischemia
   (b) Osteomyelitis
   (c) Osteonecrosis
   (d) Post-ischemic healing

13. A sickle cell anemia patient is referred to the emergency room with acute bone pain and fever. Bone scan is normal in the painful zone, but the bone marrow scan reveals a marrow dysfunction. Which statement is correct?
    (a) This is an osteomyelitis case, and gallium scan is not necessary.
    (b) Osteomyelitis cannot be excluded; therefore, gallium scan is recommended.
    (c) The patient is experiencing an ischemic crisis, and gallium scan is not required.
    (d) Neither osteomyelitis nor ischemic crisis is correct, and gallium scan is required.
14. Bone marrow scan with ^{99}mTc-sulfur colloid is performed on a 12-year-old girl with sickle cell anemia and pain below the knee, which shows reduced activity in the left upper third of the tibia. Reduced activity in this region is also observed on bone scan. What is the best diagnosis?
    (a) Osteomyelitis
    (b) Infarction
    (c) Normal tissue
    (d) Cellulitis
15. Bone scan is performed on a 34-year-old man with a history of a painful medial femoral shaft for 4 weeks. An increased activity is observed in this region in all three phases. An increased uptake is also found on the labeled leucocyte scan. What is the most probable diagnosis?
    (a) Osteogenic sarcoma
    (b) Osteoid osteoma
    (c) Acute osteomyelitis
    (d) Buccal fracture of the bone
16. Charcot joint in diabetic patients:
    (a) It is observed in 30% of diabetic patients.
    (b) It is common in fourth and fifth decade.
    (c) The most common region is the metatarsophalangeal joint.
    (d) Swelling is a common finding.
17. What is the scan of choice for the evaluation of infection in a diabetic foot?
    (a) Four-phase bone scan
    (b) Labeled leucocyte
    (c) Labeled polyclonal IgG
    (d) Labeled ciprofloxacin
18. In which of the following groups is cold osteomyelitis most commonly reported?
    (a) Sickle cell anemia
    (b) Infants
    (c) Elderly
    (d) After trauma

19. The diagnosis of chronic active osteomyelitis:
    (a) The specificity and sensitivity of radiography are high.
    (b) The sensitivity of bone scan is low.
    (c) Bone scan becomes normal shortly after the improvement of osteomyelitis.
    (d) A normal bone scan is indicative of the ruling out of this disease.
20. What is the usual region of initiation of vertebral osteomyelitis in children?
    (a) Disk space
    (b) Vertebral pedicle
    (c) Vertebral body
    (d) Vertebra posterior accessories
21. Which item about bone scan and osteomyelitis is NOT correct?
    (a) A normal scan does NOT exclude osteomyelitis in neonates.
    (b) A bone scan has high sensitivity and low specificity for the violated bone.
    (c) Serial scans are a good criterion for therapeutic monitoring.
    (d) A four-phase bone scan increases the accuracy of diagnosis.
22. A 16-year-old boy with confirmed acute osteomyelitis of the left tibia has reexperienced ambiguous pain in the past 6 months. Hyperflow, hyperemia, and increased focal uptake are observed in the three-phase bone scan. What is the most probable diagnosis?
    (a) Chronic healing phase
    (b) Chronic active osteomyelitis
    (c) Cortical fracture due to osteonecrosis
    (d) Post-infectious focal osteoporosis change
23. If the goal is to diagnose osteomyelitis in a diabetic foot, which of the following pairs of scans is recommended?
    (a) Three-phase bone scan, ^{111}In-WBC scan
    (b) Three-phase bone scan, ^{67}Ga scan
    (c) ^{111}In-WBC scan, ^{99m}Tc-antigranulocyte antibody scan
    (d) ^{111}In-WBC scan, ^{67}Ga Scan
24. Which statement regarding the application of bone scan in pediatric osteomyelitis is NOT correct?
    (a) The clinical diagnosis of osteomyelitis in children is problematic.
    (b) A simple radiography of the hip and vertebrae is more sensitive than bone scan for the detection of osteomyelitis.
    (c) Bone scan is usually positive 72 h after clinical presentation.
    (d) Bone infections in infants younger than 6 weeks are usually invasive and destructive.
25. Which item is NOT correct about osteomyelitis?
    (a) Patients with sickle cell anemia are prone to salmonella osteomyelitis.
    (b) Osteomyelitis is common in children.
    (c) The peak of incidence of osteomyelitis is in children below 1 year or between 9 and 11 years old.
    (d) Imaging must be performed with a constant count frame.

26. Which item about granulomatous osteomyelitis is NOT correct?
    (a) Tuberculosis (TB) is the most common cause.
    (b) Multifocal involvement is common.
    (c) Spondylitis is the most severe and prevalent form of the disease in TB.
    (d) Involvement of the extremities is common in brucellosis.
27. What is the method of choice for the evaluation of osteomyelitis associated with bedsores?
    (a) FNA
    (b) ^{111}In-WBC
    (c) Gallium
    (d) Three-phase scan
28. Bone scan is performed on a 15-year-old boy with gluteal pain and minor fever who is not capable of walking. An increased uptake is observed on the end plate of the L2 and L3 vertebrae. What is the most probable diagnosis?
    (a) Tumoral involvement
    (b) Osteomyelitis
    (c) Fracture
    (d) Diskitis
29. Bone scan is performed for the diagnosis of soft tissue infection on a diabetic patient with an extensive wound on the right sole. An increased uptake is observed on the anterior right foot in the perfusion and blood-pool phases. A diffusely increased uptake is also observed in the metatarsal bones and phalanx of the same foot in the 3 h delayed images. What is the next step?
    (a) Diagnosis of extensive osteomyelitis of the right metatarsal and toes
    (b) 6–8 h delayed imaging of the foot
    (c) Repeat of foot imaging with a higher zoom immediately after the 3 h images
    (d) Gallium scan after 1 week
30. In which group of patients is bone scan the most valuable for the diagnosis of bone infection?
    (a) A neonate with suspected acute bone infection and fever in less than 1 week
    (b) Patients with a peripheral vascular disease, body wound, and suspected bone infection
    (c) Young patients with a suspected chronic infection of prosthesis
    (d) A middle-aged patient with the onset of clinical presentation last week and normal radiography
31. An old diabetic patient with acute pain of the vertebral column is subjected to bone and gallium scans for the diagnosis of infection. An increased uptake in the same region on both scans but with different extensiveness is found. What is the most probable diagnosis?
    (a) Fracture healing
    (b) Diabetic neuroarthropathy
    (c) Bone infection
    (d) Sterile inflammation of the intervertebral disk

32. What is the radiopharmaceutical of choice for bone marrow study?
    (a) ^{99m}Tc-NSAb
    (b) 52Fe
    (c) ^{111}In-WBC
    (d) ^{99m}Tc-WBC
33. A patient with sickle cell anemia is presented with acute pain of the mid-spine. What is the radiopharmaceutical of choice for the diagnosis of the cause of pain?
    (a) ^{99m}Tc-SC
    (b) ^{99m}Tc-MDP
    (c) ^{67}Ga
    (d) ^{99m}Tc-NSAb
34. On radiography, rupture of the articular surfaces, bone fragmentation, and sclerosis in the ankle is found in a diabetic patient with wound. An increased uptake is also observed in all three phases of bone scan. What is the next step according to the possible diagnosis?
    (a) Gallium scan
    (b) ^{111}In-WBC scan
    (c) ^{99m}Tc-SC scan
    (d) CT scan
35. What is the method of choice for the therapeutic monitoring of a patient with chronic osteomyelitis?
    (a) Gallium scan
    (b) Bone scan
    (c) Radiography
    (d) MRI
36. A 54-year-old patient with diabetic neuropathy is referred with toe ulcer. Which scan provides the most specificity for the diagnosis of osteomyelitis?
    (a) Three-phase bone scan
    (b) Gallium scan
    (c) Gallium scan + three-phase bone scan
    (d) Three-phase bone scan + ^{111}In-WBC scan
37. Cold osteomyelitis is found on bone scan. Which item is the most common?
    (a) A neonate with reduced activity of the involved bone on scan
    (b) A 5-year-old with increased activity of the involved bone on scan
    (c) A neonate with silent osteomyelitis and a good prognosis
    (d) A 5-year-old with silent osteomyelitis and a poor prognosis
38. A child with effusion of the hip joint and suspected septic arthritis is referred for bone scan. A reduced activity of the involved joint is observed in all three phases of the scan. What is the most common cause of this finding?
    (a) Inadequate dose of the administered radiopharmaceutical
    (b) Hip apophyseal avulsion
    (c) Antibiotic therapy
    (d) Ischemia due to intra-capsular vascular tamponade

39. What is the recommended intervention for a 54-year-old diabetic man with a right foot ulcer and exposed tarsus bone?
    (a) Three-phase bone scan
    (b) ^{111}In-labeled leukocyte scan
    (c) Treatment without any further diagnostic procedure
    (d) Technetium-labeled antigranulocyte antibody scan
40. An 8-month-old infant with a history of fever and agitation was hospitalized 4 days ago. Normal CBC and sedimentation as well as a negative blood culture are reported, and osteomyelitis of the right femur is suspected. What is the diagnostic method of choice?
    (a) Gallium citrate scan
    (b) ^{111}In-labeled leukocyte scan
    (c) MRI
    (d) Three-phase bone scan
41. Bone scan is performed on a 12-year-old boy with pain in the buttocks and mild fever who is unable to walk. An increased uptake is found on the end plate of second and third lumbar vertebrae. What is the most probable diagnosis?
    (a) Tumoral involvement
    (b) Osteomyelitis
    (c) Fracture
    (d) Diskitis
42. What is the most common cause of vertebral osteomyelitis in a 54-year-old man?
    (a) *Staphylococcus aureus*
    (b) *Streptococcus*
    (c) *Escherichia coli*
    (d) *Klebsiella pneumoniae*
43. A 6-year-old child with a history of falling down 12 days ago, progressive limping, and mild fever is evaluated. Blood culture is negative, and a linear increased uptake between L3 and L4 is observed on bone scan. What is the most probable diagnosis?
    (a) AVN
    (b) Spondylitis
    (c) Compression fracture
    (d) Metastasis
44. Which item about cold osteomyelitis is NOT correct?
    (a) It has poor prognosis compared with cases with a higher uptake.
    (b) It is common in neonates.
    (c) It is due to interosseous infection.
    (d) None of the above.
45. Chronic recurrent multifocal osteomyelitis (CRMO syndrome):
    (a) *Staphylococcus aureus* is the most common cause of the disease.
    (b) It is common in children aged 7–10 years.
    (c) The prevalence in girls is twice of that in boys.
    (d) The most common site of involvement is the diaphysis of the long bones.

46. A 13-year-old teenager with pain in the right proximal tibia is referred following mild trauma, redness, and edema 3 days ago. What is the first diagnostic approach?
    (a) MRI of the tibia
    (b) X-ray of the tibia
    (c) Three-phase bone scan
    (d) FDG-PET
47. An 8-year-old child diagnosed with hematogenous osteomyelitis of the femoral head is hospitalized and has received intravenous antibiotic therapy. Clinical symptoms are deteriorating, and there has been no sign of improvement. Which of the following methods is recommended for the diagnosis?
    (a) MRI
    (b) Three-phase bone scan
    (c) Gallium scan
    (d) CT scan
48. A four-phase bone scan is conducted on a diabetic man with a history of pain, erythema, and wound in the right foot from 3 weeks ago. A radiotracer uptake is reported in the angiographic, blood pool, and 3 h delayed images, but the 24 h delayed images are normal. What is the most probable diagnosis?
    (a) Cellulitis
    (b) Osteomyelitis
    (c) Thrombophlebitis
    (d) Vascular insufficiency
49. Which of the following radiopharmaceuticals is the least valuable if the goal is the therapeutic monitoring of acute osteomyelitis?
    (a) ^{99m}Tc-MDP
    (b) ^{111}In-labeled WBC
    (c) ^{67}Ga-citrate
    (d) ^{99m}Tc-labeled WBC
50. Which of the following methods is the most sensitive for the detection of osteomyelitis in a diabetic foot?
    (a) ^{67} gallium scan
    (b) MRI
    (c) ^{111}In-labeled leukocyte
    (d) Three-phase bone scan
51. Which of the following methods is considered safe and is the method of choice for the diagnosis of neonatal osteomyelitis?
    (a) Three- or four-phase bone scan with ^{99m}Tc-MDP
    (b) MRI
    (c) ^{99m}Tc-WBC scan
    (d) CT scan

52. Osteomyelitis:
    (a) Bone scan is always positive in acute infantile osteomyelitis.
    (b) Gallium scan is sensitive for the detection of acute osteomyelitis and can discriminate bone lesion from articular lesion.
    (c) The sensitivity and specificity of gallium scan for the diagnosis of acute and chronic osteomyelitis are similar.
    (d) Bone radiography is required for interpreting the gallium scan of a patient with suspected chronic osteomyelitis.
53. Which of the following statements about osteomyelitis in infants younger than 6 weeks is NOT correct?
    (a) Multiple bone involvement is common in osteomyelitis.
    (b) Bone involvement is usually destructive.
    (c) Radiography is usually abnormal at the time of clinical presentation.
    (d) Bone scan usually shows an increased activity in the involved region.
54. Which of the following bone scan findings excludes acute osteomyelitis?
    (a) Normal perfusion in the involved site
    (b) Hyperperfusion in the involved site
    (c) Increased radiotracer uptake in delayed imaging
    (d) Decreased radiotracer uptake in delayed imaging
55. A 9-year-old boy is referred with back pain and fever. Bone scan shows an increased uptake in the L2 and L3 vertebrae, and blood culture is positive for *Staphylococcus aureus*. What is the next appropriate intervention?
    (a) L2 and L3 aspiration.
    (b) Lumbar MRI.
    (c) Lumbar CT scan.
    (d) No further diagnostic workup is required.
56. Regarding the evaluation of acute osteomyelitis, bone scan is the least effective in:
    (a) Early diagnosis
    (b) Positioning of biopsy
    (c) Therapeutic monitoring
    (d) Differential diagnosis from cellulitis
57. What is the modality of choice for the assessment of osteomyelitis?
    (a) MRI
    (b) Three-phase bone scan
    (c) CT scan
    (d) Ultrasonography
58. What is the best modality for the assessment of disease activity in chronic osteomyelitis?
    (a) Three-phase bone scan
    (b) ^{111}In-WBC scan
    (c) MRI
    (d) Serial CT scan

59. What region of osteomyelitis is the most common in sickle cell anemia?
    (a) Diaphysis
    (b) Metaphysis
    (c) Epiphysis
    (d) Physis
60. If the goal is to diagnose osteomyelitis, the bone scan of which region of the foot is the most accurate?
    (a) Forefoot
    (b) Midfoot
    (c) Hindfoot
    (d) The accuracy of the scan is equal in all three regions
61. For evaluating the infection of a neuropathic foot, CT is conducted prior to MRI in all of the following situations *except*:
    (a) Cortical destruction
    (b) Sequestration
    (c) Intraosseous gas
    (d) Periosteal new bone
62. What is the second-line diagnostic method for osteomyelitis (especially acute infections) after bone scan?
    (a) ^{67}Ga scan
    (b) ^{111}In-chloride scan
    (c) ^{111}In-WBC scan
    (d) ^{99m}Tc-HMPAO scan
63. All statements about the sensitivity and specificity of Tc-labeled nanocolloid are correct *except*:
    (a) Tc-labeled nanocolloid is more sensitive than ^{67}Ga for the evaluation of peripheral osteomyelitis.
    (b) The sensitivity of Tc-labeled nanocolloid for the evaluation of peripheral osteomyelitis is equal to that of Tc-labeled WBC.
    (c) Tc-labeled nanocolloid is more sensitive and specific than ^{99m}Tc-MDP for the evaluation of vertebral osteomyelitis.
    (d) Tc-labeled nanocolloid is less sensitive and specific than ^{99m}Tc-MDP for the evaluation of septic arthritis.
64. Which of the following statements about bone infection is NOT correct?
    (a) The main advantage of a perfusion study is its high negative predictive value (NPV) in the acute inflammatory process.
    (b) Multifocal abnormal sites can be seen when osteomyelitis is caused by organisms such as *Staphylococcus aureus* or viruses.
    (c) The sensitivity and specificity of labeled leukocytes are NOT equal in acute and chronic infection.
    (d) The sensitivity and specificity of labeled leukocytes decrease with previous antibiotics or steroid therapy.

65. Which of the following items does NOT describe the advantages of ^{99m}Tc-HMPAO-labeled leukocyte scan over ^{111}In-WBC scan?
    (a) Higher sensitivity and specificity
    (b) Possibility of SPECT imaging
    (c) Higher rate of labeling
    (d) Availability
66. In which of the following studies is the production of human anti-mouse antibody (HAMA) the most probable?
    (a) ^{99m}Tc-antigranulocyte antibody
    (b) ^{111}In-white blood cell (WBC(
    (c) ^{99m}Tc-HMPAO-labeled leukocyte
    (d) ^{99m}Tc-nanocolloid scan
67. Which of the following statements regarding the application of ^{111}In-white blood cell (WBC) scan for the evaluation of bone infection is NOT correct?
    (a) Indeed, 10–30% of infected vertebral bodies may appear as a photon-deficient lesion on a leukocyte scan
    (b) The demonstration of an incongruent leukocyte and a colloid image with increased leukocyte activity and decreased colloid uptake has a high diagnostic value for vertebral infection
    (c) ^{67}Ga or ^{111}In-WBC scans are helpful when the differentiation of osteomyelitis from septic arthritis is problematic with bone scan
    (d) ^{99m}Tc-MDP and ^{67}Ga scan are less specific than Tc-MDP and In-WBC when the goal is to discriminate between osteomyelitis and septic arthritis
68. Which of the following scans is NOT indicated for therapeutic monitoring?
    (a) ^{99m}Tc-WBC
    (b) ^{99m}Tc-MDP
    (c) 111In-WBC
    (d) Gallium
69. A patient suffering from sickle cell anemia is referred with bone pain that began 2 days ago. ^{99m}Tc-colloid scintigraphy and ^{99m}Tc-MDP bone scan show a decreased and an increased uptake in the involved region, respectively. What is the most probable diagnosis?
    (a) Infarct.
    (b) Osteomyelitis.
    (c) ^{111}In-WBC scintigraphy is required for the diagnosis.
    (d) Tumor.
70. Which of the following arteries is mainly responsible for the perfusion of a hip joint in an 8-year-old subject?
    (a) Metaphyseal artery
    (b) Lateral metaphyseal artery
    (c) Round ligament artery
    (d) Ligamentum teres artery

71. What is the main source of the spread of infection that causes septic arthritis?
    (a) Osteomyelitis of the adjacent joint
    (b) Wound in the adjacent joint
    (c) Hematogen
    (d) Iatrogenic
72. At what age is multifocal osteomyelitis common?
    (a) Neonates
    (b) 4–5 years old
    (c) 20–30 years old
    (d) 50–60 years old
73. What is the responsible organism for pediatric diskitis?
    (a) *Staphylococcus aureus*
    (b) *Escherichia coli*
    (c) *Staphylococcus epidermidis*
    (d) None of the above
74. A butterfly pattern of the vertebral uptake is reported on gallium scan. What is the most probable diagnosis?
    (a) Osteomyelitis
    (b) Soft tissue abscess
    (c) Septic arthritis
    (d) Diskitis
75. A child suffering from sickle cell anemia is referred because of pain. Bone marrow and bone scans are abnormal in the painful zone, but gallium scan is normal. What is the most probable diagnosis?
    (a) Osteomyelitis
    (b) Ischemia
    (c) Post-ischemic healing
    (d) Infarction
76. What region of skeletal involvement in bone tuberculosis is the most common?
    (a) Upper cervical vertebrae
    (b) Lower thoracic vertebrae
    (c) Large weight-bearing joints in lower extremities
    (d) Small joints in upper extremities
77. When do radiologic changes in simple bone infection appear in plain radiography?
    (a) 24 h
    (b) 48 h
    (c) 7–10 days
    (d) 10–14 days

3.4.1 Answer

	A	B	C	D
1	*			
2				*
3		*		
4		*		
5	*			
6			*	
7				*
8				*
9		*		
10	*			
11			*	
12	*			
13			*	
14		*		
15			*	
16				*
17				*
18		*		
19				*
20	*			
21			*	
22		*		
23	*			
24		*		
25				*
26				*
27	*			
28				*
29		*		
30				*
31			*	
32	*			
33				*
34		*		
35	*			
36				*
37	*			
38		*		
39			*	
40				*

	A	B	C	D
41				*
42	*			
43		*		
44				*
45			*	
46		*		
47	*			
48	*			
49	*			
50			*	
51			*	
52				*
53				*
54	*			
55		*		
56			*	
57	*			
58			*	
59	*			
60	*			
61				*
62			*	
63			*	
64		*		
65	*			
66	*			
67				*
68		*		
69		*		
70				*
71			*	
72	*			
73				*
74		*		
75			*	
76		*		
77				*

3.5 Radionuclide Assessment of a Painful Joint Prosthesis

1. The overall accuracy of radionuclide bone imaging for the evaluation of a prosthetic joint is about:
   (a) 80–90%
   (b) 90–100%
   (c) 70–80%
   (d) 50–70%
2. Which of the sequential bone/gallium images is interpreted as positive for infection?
   (a) When gallium is normal regardless of bone scan
   (b) When the spatial distribution of two tracers is congruent
   (c) When the spatial distribution of two tracers is incongruent
   (d) When the relative intensity of uptake of the tracers are similar
3. Which of the following studies is most suited for the monitoring bone graft perfusion?
   (a) MRI
   (b) CT
   (c) Bone scan
   (d) Radiography
4. Bone scan is requested for a patient who underwent joint prosthesis surgery 1 year ago, and it demonstrates no clinical problem. Which prosthesis is most likely to exhibit normal periarticular activity?
   (a) Porous hip prosthesis
   (b) Cemented hip prosthesis
   (c) Femoral part of the knee prosthesis
   (d) Tibial part of the knee prosthesis
5. Which of the following complications is the least common in a knee prosthesis?
   (a) Fracture
   (b) Infection
   (c) Dislocation
   (d) Osteonecrosis
6. All of the following can produce a photopenic view of a hip joint on bone scan *except*:
   (a) Septic arthritis
   (b) Joint needle aspiration
   (c) Transient synovitis
   (d) Arthrography with contrast media
7. What is the method of choice for the screening of prosthesis loosening?
   (a) Bone scan
   (b) Nuclear arthrography
   (c) Radiologic arthrography
   (d) Leukocyte scan

8. Which modality is recommended for the evaluation of prosthesis loosening in a patient who underwent surgery last year?
   (a) Concurrent bone scan and radionuclide arthrography
   (b) ^{99m}Tc-sulfur colloid scan
   (c) ^{99m}Tc-medronate scan
   (d) Bone scan
9. About femoral head prosthesis:
   (a) Mild increase of uptake in bone scan 6 months after arthroplasty indicates loosening.
   (b) Loosening can be because of mechanical lesion or secondary to infection.
   (c) More than 50% of prostheses show loosening in 5 years after application.
   (d) Infection is more prevalent than loosening.
10. All of the following statements regarding loosening are correct *except*:
   (a) Gallium scan is more effective than bone scan in diagnosing infection.
   (b) ^{99m}Tc-MDP uptake around the prosthesis is observed for 9–12 months.
   (c) A three-phase bone scan is indicated for the detection of infection.
   (d) Bone scan can help to detect the loosening of a knee prosthesis.
11. What is the recommended method for the detection of infection in a painful knee prosthesis?
   (a) Leukocyte–marrow imaging
   (b) Three-phase bone scan
   (c) Leukocyte–bone imaging
   (d) Leukocyte imaging
12. About the loosening of a femoral joint prosthesis:
   (a) The pattern of isotopic arthrogram is completely different from that of contrast arthrography.
   (b) The diagnostic accuracy of transmission emission is similar to that of dual tracer.
   (c) The diagnostic accuracy of isotopic arthrography with MDP and indium colloid is NOT better than that of contrast arthrography.
   (d) The diagnostic accuracy of isotopic arthrography for the acetabular component is similar to that of contrast arthrography.
13. Bone scan is performed for the evaluation of graft perfusion 3 days after bone graft from the fibula to the right humerus. A diffusely increased uptake is observed in the whole graft. Which is the correct interpretation of the scan?
   (a) This finding is due to surgical trauma, and bone scan must be repeated 8 weeks later.
   (b) This finding indicates the viability of the graft.
   (c) A bone marrow scan is also required to determine viability.
   (d) This finding indicates graft infection.

14. Which of the following statements regarding the evaluation of joint prosthesis by bone scan is NOT correct?
    (a) Diffuse uptake around a hip prosthesis is usually indicative of infection.
    (b) A normal bone scan does NOT necessarily exclude the existence of lesions in a painful prosthesis.
    (c) Low specificity is the main limitation of bone scan for the evaluation of a painful prosthesis.
    (d) Continuous uptake after 1 year is more common in a cemented hip prosthesis than in a cementless prosthesis.
15. What is the main reason for the controversial results of a prosthesis evaluation with labeled WBC?
    (a) The nature of acute infection
    (b) The lack of a satisfactory method for data interpretation
    (c) The variable distribution of bone marrow in the population
    (d) The nature of chronic infection
16. What is the difference in sensitivity and specificity between radionuclide and contrast arthrography if the goal is to detect loosening in the acetabular portion (AP) and femoral portion (FP)?
    (a) Radionuclide arthrography is more specific and sensitive than contrast arthrography in FP.
    (b) Contrast arthrography is more specific and sensitive than radionuclide arthrography in AP.
    (c) Radionuclide arthrography is more sensitive but less specific than contrast arthrography in FP.
    (d) Contrast arthrography is more sensitive but less specific than radionuclide arthrography in AP.

3.5.1 Answer

	A	B	C	D
1				*
2			*	
3			*	
4		*		
5		*		
6		*		
7	*			
8	*			
9		*		
10				*
11	*			
12		*		
13		*		
14				*
15		*		
16		*		

3.6 Vascular Manifestations

1. Kohler's disease is the avascular necrosis (AVN) of the:
   (a) Second metatarsal head
   (b) Lunate
   (c) Navicular
   (d) Scaphoid
2. The most common site of secondary osteonecrosis is:
   (a). Femoral heads
   (b). Knees
   (c). Humeral heads
   (d). Elbows
3. Regarding osteochondritis dissecans (OCD):
   (a) It generally affects children, usually girls, aged 8–12 years.
   (b) The lateral condyle of the knee is the most commonly affected (79%).
   (c) The vascular phase images do not appear particularly predictive.
   (d) The focal hyperemia on blood-pool images is not a strong indicator of fragment loosening.
4. Bone scan in Legg–Calve–Perthes disease (LCPD):
   (a) The abnormality is clearly shown by pinhole imaging.
   (b) The SPECT is likely to be required.
   (c) Quantification in blood flow in the femoral head has proven advantages.
   (d) The abnormality is particularly shown with the hip in the maximum lateral rotation.
5. Regarding transient osteoporosis:
   (a) It is due to vascular infarction.
   (b) A history of trauma is rare.
   (c) The most commonly affected joints are the knees.
   (d) Spontaneous resolution generally does not occur.
6. In complex regional pain syndrome (CRPS):
   (a) All patients exhibit sympathetic disturbance.
   (b) Bone scan is utilized in the diagnosis.
   (c) Abnormality in all three phases of bone scan is noted in all patients with clinical syndrome.
   (d) Blood-pool images are useful to differentiate CRPS from the effects of disuse.
7. Bone scan findings in a patient with reflex sympathetic dystrophy (RSD):
   (a) Normal perfusion and blood pool is observed in the involved organ.
   (b) An enhanced periarticular uptake is observed in the static phase in the involved organ.
   (c) Normal activity is observed all over the long bones of the compromised organ.
   (d) A direct relationship exists between the intensity of activity and the duration of disease.

8. In the evaluation of transplanted bone:
   (a) Allograft transplantation can withstand photopenic surgery.
   (b) CT is more sensitive than scan for the detection of vascularization.
   (c) An increase in uptake begins from the central parts and develops toward the surroundings of the allograph transplantation.
   (d) Enhanced perfusion is NOT observed until the microvascularization of autograft.
9. Spontaneous osteonecrosis of the femoral head:
   (a) It is common in women.
   (b) It is unilateral.
   (c) It is usually observed in individuals below 40 years old.
   (d) Bone scan pattern is similar to that of Legg–Perthes.
10. Bone scan is performed on a 9-year-old child with limping and groin pain. The femoral head does NOT appear in the scan. Which diagnosis is the least likely?
   (a) Legg–Calve–Perthes
   (b) Toxic synovitis
   (c) Septic arthritis
   (d) Maltreated developmental dysplasia
11. Which item describes the findings of a three-phase bone scan in the first 6 months of idiopathic knee necrosis?
   (a) Decreased activity in the angiography and blood-pool phases, increased activity in the static phase
   (b) Increased activity in the angiography and blood-pool phases, decreased activity in the static phase
   (c) Decreased activity in all three phases
   (d) Increased activity in all three phases
12. A 77-year-old man with osteoarthritis of both knees experienced severe focal pain in the right knee 3 weeks ago. Radiography shows non-specific degenerative lesions. Bone scan exhibits an increased uptake in the internal right knee joint in the first two phases. A nonhomogenous increase in uptake on both sides of the knee joint and a focal zone of a much higher uptake in the internal condyle of the right femur are observed in the delayed phase. What is the most probable diagnosis?
   (a) Aggravation of osteoarthritis
   (b) Spontaneous osteonecrosis
   (c) Secondary infection
   (d) Pathologic fracture
13. A patient is presented with a localized severe pain of the left knee that started 1 month ago. He mentions no history of any specific disease. Radiography of the knee is normal. Bone scan shows a markedly increased uptake in the medial femoral condyle in all three phases. What is the most probable diagnosis?
   (a) Trauma
   (b) Idiopathic osteonecrosis of the knee
   (c) Severe arthritis
   (d) Osteoid osteoma

14. Bone scan is performed on a child with sickle cell anemia and pain of the lower extremities. A decreased uptake in both distal tibias is found on the sulfur colloid scan. Which findings in the bone scan (B) and gallium scan (G) are indicative of post-ischemic healing?
    (a) Normal B, normal G
    (b) Abnormal B, abnormal G
    (c) Abnormal B, normal G
    (d) Normal B, abnormal G
15. Which of the following diseases has a scan view similar to that of Legg–Calve–Perthes disease?
    (a) Septic arthritis
    (b) Dislocation of the hip
    (c) Slipped capital femoral epiphysis
    (d) Transient arthritis
16. Which statement about Perthes' disease (avascular necrosis of the femoral head) is NOT correct?
    (a) It is common in boys.
    (b) Subcortical radiolucent changes are the first radiologic findings.
    (c) Abnormalities on bone scan appear 6 weeks earlier than in radiography.
    (d) Perfusion with neovascularization has better prognosis than recanalization.
17. An 8-year-old child is presented with right hip pain and limping. Radiography as well as articular aspiration and culture are normal. Bone scan is performed 2 days later and shows a small area of decreased uptake in the femoral head. What is the most probable diagnosis?
    (a) Avascular necrosis
    (b) Osteomyelitis
    (c) Arthritis
    (d) Decrease in uptake due to articular aspiration
18. Which phase of bone scan is critical and determinative for the diagnosis of reflex sympathetic dystrophy?
    (a) Arterial phase of angiography
    (b) Delayed phase
    (c) Venous phase of angiography
    (d) Blood-pool phase
19. A photopenic region in the femoral head is detected on the bone scan of an 8-year-old child with intermittent limping. Which diagnosis is the least probable?
    (a) Avascular necrosis
    (b) Transient synovitis
    (c) Septic arthritis
    (d) Intra-capsular hemorrhage due to trauma

20. Which statement best describes avascular necrosis (AVN) of the femoral head?
    (a) MDP uptake is normal during the first 48 h.
    (b) Changes in the bone marrow scan appear earlier than those in bone scan.
    (c) Regions of increased uptake are reported on the first day, and they subsequently transform into cold lesions.
    (d) Improvement occurs in 2–3 months after the manifestation of AVN.
21. In which of the following situations is bone infarction not observed?
    (a) Caisson disease
    (b) Medullar infarction resulting from radiotherapy
    (c) Sickle cell disease
    (d) Aneurysmal bone cyst (ABC)
22. A 13-year-old boy with Henoch–Schonlein purpura (HSP) develops acute pain in the right hip joint. Physical examination reveals limitation of movement especially in internal rotation. His bone scan shows intense activity in the right hip region. His X-ray survey demonstrates sclerosis and fragmentation of the right femoral head with intact joint space. What is the most likely diagnosis?
    (a) Osteoarthritis (OA)
    (b) Avascular necrosis
    (c) Developmental dysplasia of the hip (DDH)
    (d) Slipped capital femoral epiphysis
23. What is the diagnostic test of choice for avascular necrosis?
    (a) CT scan
    (b) Bone scan
    (c) MRI
    (d) Simple X-ray
24. Avascular necrosis can be developed in all of the following situations *except*:
    (a) Radiotherapy
    (b) Caisson disease
    (c) Tunnel workers
    (d) Treatment with NSAIDS
25. What is the most common involved joint in osteochondritis dissecans (OCD)?
    (a) Ankle
    (b) Wrist
    (c) Hip
    (d) Shoulder
26. A 16-year-old obese boy complains of right hip pain with radiation to the right knee during heavy exercise. What is the most likely diagnosis?
    (a) Osteitis condensans ilii
    (b) Developmental dysplasia of the hip (DDH)
    (c) Slipped capital femoral epiphysis
    (d) Osteochondritis dissecans (OCD)

27. A patient with a soft tissue mass in the posterior thigh is referred to your department. Radiograph shows a soft tissue mass with suspected calcification in the same region. What is the most appropriate modality for the evaluation of myositis ossificans?
    (a) CT scan
    (b) Biopsy
    (c) Bone scan
    (d) MRI
28. Which of the following statements regarding the evaluation of osteonecrosis by bone scan is NOT correct?
    (a) Bone scan is more valuable than bone marrow scan for the evaluation of avascular necrosis (AVN) in adults.
    (b) In idiopathic osteonecrosis or Legg–Calve–Perthes disease, the earliest sign is the absence of activity in the superolateral portion of the femur.
    (c) A diffusely increased activity is observed in the third stage of Legg–Calve–Perthes disease.
    (d) Spontaneous osteonecrosis of the knee in the elderly is common in the medial femoral condyle, and the scan pattern is an abnormal decreased uptake.
29. Which of the following statements about the presentation of lesions in avascular necrosis (AVN) is NOT correct?
    (a) Whereas bone scan shows lesions in early stages of AVN, MRI is normal.
    (b) Improvement of lesions begins from the peripheral zones *except* bone metaphysis.
    (c) Distinguishing bone infarct from osteomyelitis in bone physis is difficult.
    (d) The common feature of all causes of osteonecrosis is the rapid death of osteocytes (even in 12 h).
30. Which of the following statements about avascular necrosis (AVN) of the femoral head is NOT correct?
    (a) The diagnostic sensitivity of SPECT is greater than that of planar imaging.
    (b) Radiocolloid scan is conducted prior to bone scan in determining the femoral head viability in the first 24 h.
    (c) Myeloid cells die more rapidly than osteocytes.
    (d) A bone marrow scan is well accepted for the evaluation of AVN.
31. What is the difference in sensitivity and specificity between MRI and bone scan for the evaluation of avascular necrosis of the scaphoid?
    (a) Bone scan is more sensitive, and MRI is more specific.
    (b) Bone scan is more sensitive and specific.
    (c) MRI is more sensitive and specific.
    (d) Bone scan is more specific, and MRI is more specific.

32. Which of the following statements about glucocorticoid-induced osteonecrosis is NOT correct?
    (a) The prevalence of the disease is about 2–4%, with a maximum rate of 25%.
    (b) Determining the patients who will experience avascular necrosis after corticosteroid therapy is difficult.
    (c) The risk of osteoporosis increases with dose and long-term treatment, but NO definite relationship exists between them.
    (d) Corticosteroid therapy decreases the size of lipocytes in the bone marrow, thereby increasing resistance in the arterial or venous blood flow.
33. Which of the following diseases commonly exhibits large lesions on bone scan consistent with the obstruction of large vessels (especially in the juxta-articular regions)?
    (a) Caisson disease
    (b) Gaucher's disease
    (c) Glucocorticoid-induced osteonecrosis
    (d) Spontaneous osteonecrosis
34. Spontaneous osteonecrosis:
    (a) In the acute phase of the disease, bone scan shows a decreased uptake in flow and delayed views.
    (b) It usually occurs in the external compartment of the knee.
    (c) Although bone scan is the most sensitive method for the early diagnosis of micro-fractures, it is NOT helpful in distinguishing spontaneous osteonecrosis in the medial tibial plateau from an internal meniscus tear.
    (d) In the acute phase of the disease, bone scan becomes normal in 6 months, but most cases experience a subacute phase.
35. Which of the following statements about Legg–Calve–Perthes disease (LCPD) is NOT correct?
    (a) Lateral epiphyseal vessels, which connect to the lateral side of the femoral head, are the only route of perfusion in children aged 3–12 years old.
    (b) A scan is indicated for staging of the disease until complete radiological improvement, which normally occurs 11 ± 8 months after normal scan.
    (c) The pattern of disease on bone scan is exhibited as a photopenic lesion in the proximal femoral epiphysis, which can be demonstrated by pinhole collimators WITHOUT the need for SPECT, although a quantitative evaluation is useful.
    (d) The pattern of improvement of avascular necrosis of the femoral head on bone scan is exhibited as a strip activity along the lateral epiphysis of the femoral head.

36. What is referred to as the avascular necrosis of the second metatarsal head?
    (a) Freiberg's disease
    (b) Kohler's disease
    (c) Panner's disease
    (d) Kienbock's disease
37. Which of the following parameters demonstrate the highest diagnostic accuracy for reflex sympathetic dystrophy syndrome (RSDS)?
    (a) Increased activity in the blood pool
    (b) Diffused activity in the carpus or tarsus
    (c) Periarticular uptake in small joints
    (d) All of the above
38. Which of the following statements about reflex sympathetic dystrophy syndrome (RSDS) is NOT correct?
    (a) Decreased blood-pool activity in disuse osteoporosis is used for distinguishing from RSDS.
    (b) Normal or decreased activity in the acute phase of RSDS is reported in adults.
    (c) Patellofemoral surgery more commonly causes knee RSDS than trauma.
    (d) Sudeck's atrophy and shoulder–hand syndrome are the most common variations of RSDS.
39. In which phase of avascular necrosis (AVN) of the femoral head is a crescent sign observed?
    (a) Stage I
    (b) Stage II
    (c) Stage III
    (d) Stage IV
40. What is the most valuable imaging modality for the evaluation of avascular necrosis?
    (a) Plain radiography
    (b) CT scan
    (c) Isotopic scan
    (d) MRI

3.6.1 Answer

	A	B	C	D
1			*	
2	*			
3			*	
4	*			
5		*		
6				*
7		*		
8	*			
9				*
10				*
11				*
12		*		
13		*		
14		*		
15			*	
16				*
17	*			
18		*		
19		*		
20		*		
21				*
22		*		
23			*	
24				*
25	*			
26			*	
27	*			
28				*
29		*		
30				*
31	*			
32				*
33	*			
34				*
35			*	
36	*			
37				*
38		*		
39		*		
40				*

3.7 Bone Scintigraphy in Trauma

1. In thermal injury:
   (a) Psychiatric illness is not the main risk factor for cold injury.
   (b) The pathophysiology of frostbite is related more to the absolute temperature than to the length of cold exposure.
   (c) Bone scan cannot determine the need for amputation.
   (d) Pertechnetate scan is a valuable tool for the assessment of frostbite injury.
2. Bone scan of a patient with tibial pain reveals a single focal spindle-like lesion along the cortex of the medial tibia. What is the most probable diagnosis?
   (a) Tibial stress fracture
   (b) Shin splint
   (c) Myositis ossificans
   (d) Soft tissue injury
3. When is the most appropriate time for the surgical resection of myositis ossificans?
   (a) When bone scan reveals a marked increase in uptake.
   (b) When bone scan shows a decreased uptake.
   (c) When an increased perfusion and a decreased uptake occur.
   (d) The intensity of bone uptake does not affect the outcome of surgery.
4. Which of the following patterns on bone scan has the best prognosis when the non-union fracture of the tibial shaft is confirmed in radiography?
   (a) Photon deficiency of the fracture zone
   (b) Intense uptake on both sides of the fracture
   (c) Diffuse nonhomogenous uptake along the shaft
   (d) Extra-osseous uptake around the fracture
5. Which bone is exposed to stress fracture during marching?
   (a) Fibula
   (b) Metatarsus
   (c) Calcaneus
   (d) Femur
6. Acquired heterotopic ossification:
   (a) Fever is reported in the early stages.
   (b) Joint ankylosis is common.
   (c) Radiography is usually abnormal 1 week after bone scan.
   (d) Bone scan usually becomes normal in 12 weeks.
7. In which of the following conditions is stress fracture not considered as insufficient fracture?
   (a) Professional runner
   (b) Hyperparathyroidism
   (c) Osteomalacia
   (d) Hyperthyroidism

8. What is the hallmark of toddler's fracture?
   (a) Mild linear increase in activity along the tibia
   (b) Multiple spots of increased activity in the ribs
   (c) Spontaneous fracture in a simple cyst in the humerus
   (d) Slipped capital femoral epiphysis
9. Bone scan is used for the evaluation of maturation of myositis ossificans. Which of the following findings is suggestive of maturity?
   (a) A similar uptake in normal bone in the static phase
   (b) Increased uptake in the static phase
   (c) Hyperflow in the angiography phase
   (d) Higher blood pool
10. Bone scan is used for the estimation of prognosis in fracture healing. Which of the following findings predicts the best prognosis?
   (a) Reduced activity
   (b) Isoactivity
   (c) Mild increase in activity
   (d) Significant increase in activity
11. A patient mentions pain at the fracture site 1 month after tibial fracture. Bone callus is not clearly observed at the fracture site, two parts are aligned, and the fracture surface is smooth. Which finding on scintigraphy predicts the best prognosis?
   (a) Homogenous increase in ^{99m}Tc-MDP uptake at the fracture site in the blood-pool and delayed phases
   (b) Reduced uptake of ^{99m}Tc-MDP and increased uptake of ^{67}Ga at the fracture site
   (c) Increased uptake of ^{99m}Tc-MDP in both parts of the fracture as well as reduced uptake between the two parts and the homogenous uptake of ^{67}Ga
   (d) Isoactive uptake of ^{99m}Tc-MDP and ^{67}Ga at the fracture site
12. What is the common site of a toddler's fracture?
   (a) Tibia
   (b) Fibula
   (c) Femur
   (d) Second metatarsus
13. Non-accidental traumas of children (child abuse):
   (a) Bone trauma is common in children aged 1–3 years.
   (b) Bone fracture is usually singular.
   (c) The sensitivity of bone scan for the detection of bone lesions is less than that of whole-body plain radiography.
   (d) Bone scan is not sensitive for the detection of hairline fracture of the skull.

14. In which of the following regions is the abnormal ^{99m}Tc-MDP uptake observed in forearm splints?
    (a) Distal end of the humerus
    (b) Radius
    (c) Epicondyle
    (d) Ulna
15. Bone scan is performed on a 9-year-old boy with a history of right knee trauma. Hyperemia and increased uptake are observed in the medial femoral condyle. What is the most probable diagnosis?
    (a) Osteochondritis dissecans
    (b) Anterior cruciate ligament (ACL) injury
    (c) Meniscal Tear
    (d) Posterior cruciate ligament (PCL) injury
16. A young patient is presented with a history of severe trauma of the lower extremities a few months ago. A region of heterotopic calcification in soft tissue around the left hip is reported, and it shows a marked uptake in all three phases of bone scan. What is the most important clinical application of bone scan in this patient?
    (a) Determination of the necessity for antibiotic therapy
    (b) Time planning for surgical treatment
    (c) Evaluation of the possible existence of similar lesions in other parts of the body
    (d) Early detection of malignancy
17. A 36-year-old man with a history of right femoral fracture 8 months ago complains about pain in the same region. A decreased uptake is observed in this region on bone scan. Which item is correct?
    (a) Delayed union.
    (b) Reactive non-union.
    (c) Scan finding is indicative of a poor prognosis.
    (d) Hypertrophic non-union.
18. A 25-year-old athlete with leg pain is presented. Bone scan is performed for suspected stress fracture. Which finding is NOT indicative of the diagnoses of stress fracture?
    (a) Mild diffuse uptake in the diaphysis
    (b) Linear peripheral uptake parallel to the periosteum
    (c) Focal band of the increased uptake in the diaphysis
    (d) Marked uptake with bone enlargement
19. A 3-year-old child is referred from the department of forensic medicine because of child abuse that occurred last night. A mild diffuse increase in activity along the lower two-thirds of the right tibia is observed in the anterior, posterior, and lateral views of bone scan. What is the most probable diagnosis?
    (a) Periosteal injury
    (b) Toddler's fracture
    (c) Stress fracture
    (d) Osteonecrosis

20. A 19-year-old boy is presented with pelvis pain and a good general condition. A focal increase in uptake with distinct margins is observed in the right supero-lateral iliac crest. What is the most probable diagnosis?
    (a) Exocytosis
    (b) Avulsion fracture
    (c) Ewing sarcoma
    (d) Enchondroma
21. Spondylolysis is suggested for a child according to the radiography of the vertebral column. An increased uptake in which region on bone SPECT scan is indicative of the need for spiral CT scan?
    (a) Articular facet of the region with spondylolysis
    (b) Bilateral articular facet
    (c) Articular facet of the opposite side of spondylolysis
    (d) Central neural arch
22. Hyperemia and increased uptake in the medial femoral condyle are detected on the bone scan of a 12-year-old boy with a history of trauma to the right knee. What is the most probable diagnosis?
    (a) Osteochondritis dissecans
    (b) Anterior cruciate ligament (ACL) injury
    (c) Meniscal tear
    (d) Posterior cruciate ligament (PCL) injury
23. What are the most common sites of a non-union fracture (left to right)?
    (a) Tibia, femur, humerus
    (b) Femur, tibia, humerus
    (c) Humerus, femur, tibia
    (d) Tibia, humerus, femur
24. Fracture of the sacral bone is common in osteoporosis. What is the most common pattern of this fracture on bone scan?
    (a) Dissymmetric uptake in the sacral ala
    (b) H-like pattern
    (c) Increase in linear activity in the sacral latitude
    (d) None of the above
25. Which of the following injuries is described as the Jones fracture?
    (a) Fragmentation of the tibial and fibular sesamoid bones
    (b) Osteochondral fracture of the patella
    (c) Stress fracture in the fifth metatarsal
    (d) Stress fracture in the femoral neck
26. Which item about bone non-union is NOT correct?
    (a) It is possible if a satisfactory improvement is NOT observed after 6 months.
    (b) The reactive form of a non-union canNOT be differentiated from a delayed union.
    (c) An increased perfusion indicates better prognosis.
    (d) The humerus is the most common site of involvement.

27. Stress fracture:
    (a) Blood-pool and angiography phases are abnormal in first 8–12 weeks.
    (b) Blood-pool and angiography phases become normal during primary improvement in contrast to shin splints.
    (c) The posterior upper third of the tibia is the most common site in children.
    (d) In 50% of cases, uptake in the delayed phase becomes normal in 2 years.
28. Which of the following items corresponds to the pattern of a shin splint on bone scan?
    (a) Increase in tibial uptake only in the angiography and blood-pool phases
    (b) A spindle-like marked increase in uptake in the fibula
    (c) Increase in linear uptake in the posteromedial tibia
    (d) A transverse increase in uptake vertical to the bone axis
29. What is the common pattern of a classic toddler's fracture?
    (a) Focal lesion in the femur
    (b) Focal lesion in the calcaneus
    (c) Spiral lesion in the tibial mid-shaft
    (d) Epiphyseal separation in the distal femoral growth plate
30. Which of the following statements about the scaphoid bone fracture is NOT correct?
    (a) It may remain undetected in radiography 2–3 weeks after fracture.
    (b) MRI is NOT conducted prior to scintigraphy for diagnosis.
    (c) Scintigraphy in the first 48 h is recommended for a differential diagnosis from traumatic hyperemia and synovitis.
    (d) In contrast to bone scintigraphy, MRI canNOT detect other accompanying complications such as carpal instability.
31. A patient with a right tibial fracture underwent surgery but still experiences pain and edema 6 months after surgery. A remarkable increase in uptake is observed on the three-phase bone scan. What is the most important applied finding of the scan?
    (a) Specific pattern of a reactive non-union fracture.
    (b) Typical pattern of a delayed union fracture.
    (c) Scan outcome is indicative of a good prognosis.
    (d) Emergency orthopedic surgery is required.
32. Suspected fractures in the C2–C3 vertebrae are observed on CXR following head trauma. What is next best diagnostic test?
    (a) Cervical MRI
    (b) Bone scan
    (c) Cervical CT scan
    (d) PET
33. What is the most common region of insufficiency fracture?
    (a) Sacrum
    (b) Spine
    (c) Pubis
    (d) Femoral neck

34. Which scan is helpful for the therapeutic monitoring of myositis ossificant and juxta-articular ossification other than bone scan?
    (a) ^{67}Ga
    (b) ^{201}Tl
    (c) ^{99m}Tc-MIBI
    (d) ^{111}In-octreotide
35. Which of the following statements about bone marrow edema is NOT correct?
    (a) History of edema is present in most cases.
    (b) Sudden pain (usually in the hips) is the common symptom of bone marrow edema.
    (c) In most cases, it improves spontaneously in 4–10 months.
    (d) Typical transient osteoporotic lesions demonstrate an increased uptake in all three phases.
36. Muscular stretching and compression cause stress fracture in … and … , respectively.
    (a) Epiphysis, metaphysis
    (b) Diaphysis, physis
    (c) Metaphysis, epiphysis
    (d) Metaphysis, diaphysis
37. Which of the following statements about shin splint is NOT correct?
    (a) Shin splint occurs because of muscular overuse.
    (b) It is characterized by stress at the muscle insertion site, with changes in the metabolism of this region and induction of rapid periosteal reaction, osteoblastic activity, and vascular growth.
    (c) It is the same as localized stress reaction at the insertion site of enthuses.
    (d) Extreme activity in children and young adults can induce exostosis.
38. What is the pattern of the different phases of fracture on bone scan?
    (a) Acute phase (first 2–4 weeks): diffusely increased uptake
    (b) Subacute phase (first 8–12 weeks): diffusely increased uptake
    (c) Recovery phase (first 2–4 weeks): diffusely increased uptake
    (d) Subacute phase (first 4–8 weeks): linear increased uptake
39. What percentage of cases with fracture can be demonstrated by bone scan on the first day and in the first week, respectively?
    (a) 85%, 100%
    (b) 90%, 95%
    (c) 80%, 95%
    (d) 95%, 100%
40. How long after fracture does bone scan become completely (100%) normal?
    (a) 2 years
    (b) 3 years
    (c) 1 year
    (d) 1.5 years

41. Disuse osteoporosis after fracture:
    (a) Ten days of immobility can cause an increased uptake in the surrounding region of the bone damage.
    (b) This change may last for 3 months.
    (c) It is distinguished from RSDS by normal vascular phases.
    (d) All of the above.
42. How long does it take for scaphoid bone fractures to completely (100%) appear on bone scan, and how long is the most appropriate time interval for a repeat scan after a primary equivocal scan?
    (a) 72 h, 1 week
    (b) 48 h, 2 weeks
    (c) 48 h, 3 weeks
    (d) 24 h, 2 weeks
43. What is the difference in size and intensity of lesions between a stress fracture and a traumatic fracture?
    (a) Similar size but higher intensity of the lesions in a traumatic fracture
    (b) Similar intensity but a larger size of the lesions in a traumatic fracture
    (c) Similar intensity but a larger size of the lesions in a stress fracture
    (d) Similar size but higher intensity of the lesions in a stress fracture
44. Which grade of stress fracture is demonstrated by an ovoid or spindle-like lesion with intense activity and involvement of the whole bone shaft?
    (a) Grade I
    (b) Grade II
    (c) Grade III
    (d) Grade IV
45. Which of the following statements is NOT correct about the presentation of stress fracture on bone scan?
    (a) The pattern of the three-phase bone scan is that of a local hyperemia and an increased uptake in the delayed phase.
    (b) Increased activity in the angiography phase and blood pool is observed in 2–4 weeks.
    (c) The angiography phase and then the blood-pool phase normalize during recovery.
    (d) An increased uptake in the delayed phase becomes normal 3–6 months after stress fracture.
46. Which of the following statements about the presentation of a pediatric fracture on bone scan is NOT correct?
    (a) Epiphyseal fracture always increases metabolic activity and induces a marked increase in uptake.
    (b) Metaphyseal corner fracture is observed in child abuse.
    (c) Oblique mid-shaft abnormality is a typical finding in toddler's fracture.
    (d) A generalized increase in uptake along the whole injured bone may be observed in hidden toddler's or infantile femoral or tibial fracture.

47. What is the recommended method for the evaluation of patients with a suspected femoral neck fracture and a sub-optimal pattern of standard imaging?
    (a) 5 h and 24 h delayed imaging, scan with a pinhole collimator
    (b) 5 h delayed imaging, repeat of scan on succeeding days
    (c) 5 h and 24 h delayed imaging, repeat of scan on succeeding days
    (d) 24 h delayed imaging, scan with a pinhole collimator
48. About the application of bone scan in scaphoid bone fracture:
    (a) MRI is more sensitive than bone scan.
    (b) The longer the time interval after the fracture is, the better the presentation of the fracture on bone scan.
    (c) 48 h after trauma is the most appropriate time for a bone scan.
    (d) The diagnosis of a scaphoid fracture by X-ray is problematic even 2–3 weeks after trauma.
49. A 35-year-old golfer is referred for bone scan. The fracture of which of the following bones is expected?
    (a) Ulna
    (b) Navicular
    (c) Lunate
    (d) Hamate
50. What is the pattern of an intraosseous ganglion in a three-phase bone scan, and what is the most common pathological error of diagnosis?
    (a) Increased uptake in all three phases, osteoid osteoma
    (b) Increased uptake in all three phases, enchondroma
    (c) Increased uptake in the delayed phase, chondroblastoma
    (d) Increased uptake in the delayed phase, chondromyxoid fibroma (CMF)
51. All of the following bones are the common sites of fracture in child abuse *except*:
    (a) First rib
    (b) Metaphyseal corner
    (c) Tibial diaphysis
    (d) Scapula
52. X-ray is more reliable than bone scan for the evaluation of fracture in:
    (a) Tibia
    (b) Skull
    (c) Ribs
    (d) Calcaneus
53. About the presentation of insufficiency and fatigue fractures on bone scan:
    (a) Insufficiency fracture is due to extreme muscular activity.
    (b) Fatigue fracture is due to weight burden.
    (c) Resolution of bone scan for fatigue fracture is low.
    (d) The bone scan pattern is similar for both fractures.

54. Which statement about the presentation of vertebral lesions on bone scan is correct?
    (a) About 83% of lesions in the vertebral body and pedicles appearing on vertebral SPECT are benign.
    (b) The vertebral body and posterior ligaments are simultaneously involved in malignant lesions, but the pedicles are intact.
    (c) An intact disk does NOT necessarily exclude the possibility of diskitis.
    (d) Lesions with involvement of the vertebral body are usually benign, and propagation from the body is the typical finding of osteophyte.
55. What is the recommended protocol for differentiating pars interarticularis fracture from facet arthritis?
    (a) Oblique-angle SPECT
    (b) 3D volume-rendered display
    (c) Horizontal-angle SPECT
    (d) a and b
56. Serial bone scan can help to monitor the improvement of lesions in spondylolysis. How long is the required time for a confident recovery?
    (a) 1 month
    (b) 3 months
    (c) 6 months
    (d) 1 year
57. Femoral stress fracture:
    (a) Superior femoral neck fracture is common in young athletes.
    (b) Inferior femoral neck fracture is common in the elderly and is induced by compression.
    (c) Superior femoral neck fracture is mainly due to tension.
    (d) Inferior femoral neck fracture is mainly due to tension.
58. What is the most common site of femoral shaft stress fracture?
    (a) Middle one-third, medial side
    (b) Upper one-third, medial side
    (c) Lower one-third, lateral side
    (d) Lower one-third, medial side
59. All of the following statements regarding the presentation of lower limb stress fracture on bone scan are correct *except*:
    (a) The second and third metatarsals are the most common sites of stress fracture in metatarsals.
    (b) Although the tibia is the most common site of stress fracture, the most common tibial site of fracture has not reached a consensus.
    (c) Stress fracture of the navicular bone usually occurs in the lower one-third.
    (d) The frog-leg view better localizes bone lesions in a femoral stress fracture.

60. An increased uptake in the bipartite patella, which leads to unstable synchondrosis, commonly occurs in the .... part of the patella.
    (a) Medial
    (b) Lateral
    (c) Inferior
    (d) Superior
61. What is the most important indication for the scintigraphic evaluation of the knee?
    (a) Chronic knee pain
    (b) Acute knee pain
    (c) Meniscus tear
    (d) Sinding–Larsen syndrome
62. Which of the following statements about the application of bone scan in knee trauma is NOT correct?
    (a) A focal increased activity in the avulsion is due to the medial collateral ligament in the Pellegrini–Stieda lesion.
    (b) SPECT is valuable for the localization and determination of the extent of meniscus tear or injury with accuracy of more than 90%.
    (c) Normal SPECT indicates NO need for arthroscopy.
    (d) The sensitivity of SPECT for the diagnosis of cruciate ligament tears is greater than that of MRI.
63. In which phase of slipped capital femoral epiphysis (SCFE) does the avascular necrosis of the femoral neck occur?
    (a) Phase II
    (b) Phase III
    (c) Phase IV
    (d) Phase V
64. Trochanteric bursitis usually occurs in ... subjects and is associated with trauma in ... of cases.
    (a) Young and thin, 80%
    (b) Old and overweight, 90%
    (c) Old and overweight, 25%
    (d) Young and thin, 75%
65. The bone scan pattern in the healing phase of fractures:
    (a) Decreased uptake in the atrophic non-union and lack of uptake in the reactive non-union.
    (b) The scan pattern in atrophic non-union and that in delayed union is similar.
    (c) False-positive outcomes are observed on bone scan 3 months after grafting because of creeping substitution.
    (d) Serial scans or SPECT have NOT been successful in decreasing the incidence of false-positive findings of bone scan in bone grafting.

66. If the goal is to evaluate the hydroxyapatite ocular implant, a scan is contraindicated earlier than … after surgery.
    (a) 6 months
    (b) 1 month
    (c) 1 year
    (d) 3 months
67. Which of the following statements about non-accidental trauma is NOT correct?
    (a) A true stress fracture occurs as a result of repeated severe trauma and involves at least 50% of the cortex.
    (b) Bone scan and radiographic skeletal survey are required for a definite diagnosis.
    (c) Bone scan is NOT capable of identifying the type, expansion, and age of the lesion.
    (d) ^{99m}Tc-MDP uptake in the lesion is observed even in severe malnutrition.
68. Which of the following studies is required in the approach for a long-bone non-union?
    (a) Whole-body bone scan
    (b) MRI without regional injection
    (c) Culture and antibiogram from the non-union region
    (d) Tomography of the non-union region
69. Which of the following methods provides the most useful information on the viability of deep tissues in frostbite?
    (a) Bone scan
    (b) MRI
    (c) CT scan
    (d) Angiography
70. What is the most common region of the distal femoral involvement in osteochondritis dissecans?
    (a) Lateral aspect of the medial femoral condyle
    (b) Medial aspect of the medial femoral condyle
    (c) Lateral aspect of the lateral femoral condyle
    (d) Medial aspect of the lateral femoral condyle

3.7.1 Answer

	A	B	C	D
1			*	
2	*			
3		*		
4		*		
5		*		
6	*			
7	*			
8	*			
9	*			
10				*
11	*			
12	*			
13				*
14				*
15			*	
16		*		
17			*	
18				*
19		*		
20		*		
21				*
22	*			
23	*			
24		*		
25			*	
26				*
27			*	
28			*	
29			*	
30				*
31			*	
32			*	
33		*		
34		*		
35	*			
36	*			
37			*	
38	*			
39				*
40		*		

	A	B	C	D
41				*
42	*			
43		*		
44				*
45				*
46	*			
47			*	
48				*
49				*
50	*			
51				*
52		*		
53				*
54				*
55				*
56			*	
57			*	
58	*			
59			*	
60		*		
61		*		
62				*
63			*	
64			*	
65	*			
66				*
67				*
68			*	
69	*			
70	*			

3.8 Bone Scintigraphy in Sports Medicine

1. Regarding stress-related injuries:
   (a) The relative incidence of stress fractures increases with age.
   (b) The most common sites among pediatrics and adults are different.
   (c) The least common site in pediatrics is the pars interarticularis.
   (d) About 5% of fractures are bilateral.
2. The osteochondroses of the inferior pole of the patella and the capitellum are called:
   (a) Panner's disease, Sinding–Larsen–Johansson disease
   (b) Sinding–Larsen–Johansson disease, Panner's disease
   (c) Osgood–Schlatter disease, Panner's disease
   (d) Sever's disease, Sinding–Larsen–Johansson disease
3. Posterolateral ankle pain is due to the following causes *except*:
   (a) Posterior impingement syndrome
   (b) Shepherd's fracture
   (c) Cedell fracture
   (d) Impingement of the os trigonum
4. This injury is commonly associated with a fracture of the proximal fibula (Maisonneuve fracture), and imaging should include this region:
   (a) Stress fracture of the talus
   (b) Acute fractures of the plafond and interosseous membranes
   (c) Acute calcaneal fracture
   (d) Navicular fracture
5. What is the most common fracture in sports medicine?
   (a) Femur
   (b) Tibia
   (c) Fibula
   (d) Humerus
6. A 29-year-old runner complains about femoral pain than began 6 weeks ago. Radiography is normal. Which of the following patterns in the three-phase bone scan is suggestive of shin splints?
   (a) Increased activity in the angiography and blood-pool phases; increased activity along the upper one-third of the medial femur in the delayed phase
   (b) Decreased activity in the angiography and blood-pool phases; diffusely increased activity in less than one-fifth of the femur in the delayed phase
   (c) Normal activity in the angiography and blood-pool phases; increased activity along the upper one-third of the medial border of the femur in the delayed phase
   (d) Focal increased activity in the angiography and blood-pool phases and in the upper part of the femur in the delayed phase
7. What is the diagnostic test of choice for meniscal tears?
   (a) CT scan
   (b) Arthroscopy
   (c) Bone SPECT
   (d) MRI

3.8.1 Answer

	A	B	C	D
1	*			
2		*		
3			*	
4		*		
5		*		
6			*	
7				*

3.9 Growth and Metabolic Disorders

1. An asymmetrical cortical activity that may cross joints to involve contiguous bones:
   (a) Engelmann's disease
   (b) Ribbing disease
   (c) Caffey disease
   (d) Melorheostosis disease
2. Normal bone scintigraphy is observed in:
   (a) Osteopathia striata
   (b) Osteopoikilosis
   (c) Osteopetrosis
   (d) a and b
3. Sclerotic lesions in fibrous dysplasia are seen in the:
   (a) Ribs
   (b) Skull
   (c) Femur
   (d) Sternum
4. What is the gold standard for the definitive diagnosis of metabolic bone disorders?
   (a) MRI
   (b) CT
   (c) Bone histomorphometry
   (d) Bone scintigraphy
5. In Paget's disease:
   (a) Activity crosses the joint margins.
   (b) The normal bone anatomy is not preserved.
   (c) SPECT is not widely considered as of major value.
   (d) Serial scintigraphy is easy to justify in clinical remission.
6. Paget's disease:
   (a) It is usually polyostotic, but it can be monostotic in 20–30% of cases.
   (b) Reduced activity is observed in the initial osteolytic stages.
   (c) Extremities are not involved in the abnormal organ uptake.
   (d) Bone expansion is observed only when the ribs and clavicle are involved.
7. Which of the following is highly suggestive of sarcomatous degeneration in Paget's disease?
   (a) Increased serum alkaline phosphatase and a focal intense hyperactivity in the involved bone
   (b) Increased urinary hydroxyproline and an enhanced uptake of gallium in the involved bone
   (c) Reduced uptake of ^{99m}Tc-SC in the involved bone
   (d) Reduced focal uptake of ^{99m}Tc-MDP in the involved bone

8. Which item is considered a WHO criterion for osteoporosis?
   (a) T-scores equal to or less than −2.5.
   (b) Z-scores equal to or less than −2.0.
   (c) Z-scores equal to or less than −1.5.
   (d) T-scores equal to or less than −2.0.
9. Bone scan is performed on a 55-year-old woman who takes etidronate for osteoporosis. A diffusely increased uptake in the bones is found, but the kidneys do not appear. What is the most probable diagnosis?
   (a) Effects of etidronate on bone metabolism
   (b) Metabolic disease of bone
   (c) Etidronate-induced renal failure
   (d) Osteoporosis
10. In which of the following diseases is a lytic flame-shaped lesion observed in the long bones?
    (a) Paget's disease
    (b) Fibrous dysplasia
    (c) Eosinophilic granuloma
    (d) Brown tumor
11. Bone mineral density (BMD) measurement is NOT indicated for:
    (a) Diagnosis of osteoporosis
    (b) Predicting fracture risk
    (c) Therapy monitoring
    (d) Bone loss screening
12. Which region displays an increased uptake on the bone scan of a 9-year-old child with Blount's disease (tibia vara)?
    (a) Lateral femoral physis
    (b) Medial tibial physis
    (c) Medial femoral physis
    (d) Lateral tibial physis
13. A T-score of −2.3 and a Z-score of −2.9 are determined by the bone mineral density of the lumbar vertebrae. What is the diagnosis according to the WHO criteria?
    (a) Osteopenia
    (b) Osteoporosis
    (c) Normal
    (d) Severe osteoporosis
14. A young woman with generalized bone pain, muscular weakness, and a waddling gate is referred. Which bone scan finding is in contrast to the diagnosis of osteomalacia?
    (a) Increase in the relative uptake in soft tissue in comparison with that in bone
    (b) Decreased uptake in the kidneys and bladder
    (c) Asymmetric focal increase in the uptake in the pubis and interior parts of both femurs
    (d) A diffusely increased uptake in the cranium and mandible

15. The bone mineral density of a 57-year-old woman with fracture of the distal radius is determined and shows a T-score of −2.7. What is the most probable diagnosis?
    (a) Normal
    (b) Osteoporosis
    (c) Osteopenia
    (d) Established osteoporosis
16. A patient complains about diffuse bone pain. An increased uptake in the sternum, acromioclavicular joint, and around the large joints is detected on bone scan. What is the most probable diagnosis?
    (a) Fibrous dysplasia
    (b) Paget's disease
    (c) Hyperparathyroidism
    (d) Metastatic arthropathy
17. What is the region of interest (ROI) in the bone densitometry of a 6-year-old child?
    (a) Total body
    (b) Spine
    (c) Hip
    (d) Distal forearm
18. Which item is indicated by a 1–2% reduction of bone mineral density in each year after menopause?
    (a) Osteoporosis.
    (b) Osteopenia.
    (c) It commonly happens.
    (d) It is primary to a metabolic disease.
19. BMD is requested for a fracture risk assessment of a 76-year-old woman. Compression fracture of L1 is noted in her documents. Which of the following items is correct regarding this finding?
    (a) The fracture risk is more than 60%.
    (b) L1 should be omitted in the calculation of the BMD.
    (c) Severe osteoporosis should be emphasized in the report.
    (d) Severe osteopenia should be emphasized in the report.
20. A 12-year-old girl is presented with pain in the right lower limb, and she looks like a 19-year-old girl. A high level of growth hormone is reported in the laboratory tests, and a marked increase in uptake is observed in the whole femur, tibia, and right pubis. What is the most probable diagnosis?
    (a) Paget's disease
    (b) Metastasis
    (c) Osteomyelitis
    (d) McCune–Albright syndrome

21. A 68-year-old woman diagnosed with osteoporosis is subjected to treatment with bisphosphonate and sodium fluoride. A focal increase in uptake in the long bones and periarticular area is observed on bone scan, and she complains about leg pain. What is the recommended intervention?
    (a) Increase in bisphosphonate dose
    (b) Discontinuation of bisphosphonate
    (c) Discontinuation of NaF
    (d) Administration of calcium carbonate
22. The Z-score is −2 in the BMD of a 64-year-old man. How many times is the risk of fracture compared with the age-matched group?
    (a) Twice
    (b) 1.5 times
    (c) 4 times
    (d) 8 times
23. A significant diffuse increase in uptake is found around the right hip on the bone scan of a 67-year-old patient who complains about hip pain. PSA is normal, and he mentions no history of trauma. What is the most probable diagnosis?
    (a) Metastasis
    (b) Multiple myeloma
    (c) Paget's disease
    (d) Chondrosarcoma
24. The following data are reported in the bone mineral density of a 48-year-old woman: patient's BMD, 782 mg/cm^2; young adult mean BMD, 992 mg/cm^2; young adult SD, 100 mg/cm^2; age-matched mean BMD, 912; and age-matched SD, 120 mg/cm^2. Which item is correct?
    (a) T-score, −2.10; Z-score, −0.98
    (b) T-score, −2.32; Z-score, −0.86
    (c) T-score, −1.80; Z-score, −1.30
    (d) T-score, −2.70; Z-score, −1.43
25. What is the meaning of a T-score of −2 in the bone mineral density (BMD) of a 68-year-old woman?
    (a) Patient's BMD is 2 SD (standard deviation) lower than that of the age- and sex-matched normal group.
    (b) Patient's BMD is 2 SD lower than that of young women.
    (c) Patient's BMD is 1.2 SD lower than that of an age- and sex-matched normal group.
    (d) Patient's BMD is 1.2 SD lower than that of young women.
26. Which method of bone marrow densitometry is the most accurate?
    (a) Single-photon absorptiometry (SPA)
    (b) Dual-photon absorptiometry (DPA)
    (c) Dual X-ray absorptiometry (DXA)
    (d) Quantitative computerized tomography (QCT)

27. Which BMD method gives more radiation to the patient?
    (a) Single-photon absorptiometry
    (b) Dual-photon absorptiometry
    (c) Dual-energy X-ray absorptiometry
    (d) Quantitative computerized tomography
28. A patient with Paget's disease is under treatment with bisphosphonate. What is the recommended scan for therapeutic monitoring?
    (a) Angiography phase of bone scan
    (b) Gallium scan
    (c) Bone marrow scan
    (d) In-WBC
29. A new region of decreased uptake in the femur is reported in the last serial bone scan of a patient with identified Paget's disease and involvement of the vertebrae, ribs, and femur. What is the most probable diagnosis?
    (a) Osteogenic sarcoma
    (b) Appropriate response to treatment with EHDP
    (c) Osteolytic phase (circumscripta)
    (d) Bone infarction
30. Which of the following bone scan findings is the least specific for the diagnosis of metabolic disease?
    (a) Increased periorbital uptake
    (b) Increased uptake in the maxilla and the mandible
    (c) Hot patella sign
    (d) Rosary beads in the ribs
31. The following findings are reported in the bone mineral densitometry of a woman. The Z-score is −1.5, and the BMD is 1.5 SD less than mean. What is the recommended intervention?
    (a) Hip BMD for a more accurate diagnosis
    (b) Follow-up after 1–2 years without any intervention
    (c) Complete workup and annual BMD
    (d) Treatment with estrogen, calcium, and calcitonin
32. Paget's disease:
    (a) Absence of articular involvement.
    (b) Burn-out lesions are observed as lytic regions in radiography.
    (c) A whole-body evaluation must be considered because this disease is always polyostotic.
    (d) The steal phenomenon from intra-cerebral blood flow causes the symptoms of cerebrovascular insufficiency in the flow phase of bone scan.
33. Which of the following statements regarding the scan pattern in hyperparathyroidism is NOT correct?
    (a) Decreased renal and soft tissue uptake
    (b) Extensive increase in bone uptake
    (c) Decreased sternal and mandibular uptake
    (d) Increased osteoblastic activity in bones

34. In which of the following bones is a solitary lesion the least common in fibrous dysplasia?
    (a) Femur
    (b) Vertebrae
    (c) Rib
    (d) Cranium
35. Which of the following radiotracers does NOT show an uptake in Paget's disease?
    (a) ^{67}Ga-citrate
    (b) ^{111}In-pentetreotide
    (c) ^{99m}Tc (V) DMSA
    (d) ^{111}In-leukocyte
36. Which of the following parameters is best examined by dual-energy X-ray absorptiometry?
    (a) Bone strength
    (b) Bone structure
    (c) Bone mass
    (d) Bone marrow
37. Looser's zone and triradiate pelvic findings are seen in:
    (a) Osteosarcoma, rickets
    (b) Osteomalacia, osteosarcoma
    (c) Osteosarcoma, osteomalacia
    (d) Osteomalacia, osteomalacia
38. The bone scan of a 64-year-old man shows an increased activity in the spine. Spine radiography exhibits an increased density in the upper and lower zones of the vertebral body with a striated appearance. What is the most likely diagnosis?
    (a) Hyperparathyroidism
    (b) Renal osteodystrophy
    (c) Osteomalacia
    (d) Vertebral tuberculosis
39. An 87-year-old man is presented with severe back pain and a marked increased activity in the pelvis, femur, and calvarium on bone scan. His spine radiograph shows a pathologic fracture accompanied with a marked cortical thickening and trabecular coarsening. Evidence of a lytic lesion is not found. The thickening of the calvarium is also seen in his skull X-ray. The patient is precipitated to which of the following malignancies?
    (a) Fibrosarcoma
    (b) Chondrosarcoma
    (c) Ewing sarcoma
    (d) Osteosarcoma
40. All of the following statements regarding Paget's disease are true *except*:
    (a) Pathological fracture is a complication of this disease.
    (b) Sclerotic changes occur later in the disease process.
    (c) Bone scan can easily differentiate this disease from tumors.
    (d) Cotton wool spots seen on plain films are a characteristic of this disease.

41. What is the most common radiographic finding in the skeletal system of patients with renal osteodystrophy?
    (a) Osteopenia
    (b) Subperiosteal resorption
    (c) Looser's zone
    (d) Osteosclerosis
42. Which criterion is the most accurate for evaluating the activity of Paget's disease?
    (a) Alkaline phosphatase
    (b) Perfusion images
    (c) Blood-pool images
    (d) Static images
43. Paget's disease:
    (a) All bone lesions have similar intensity in whole skeleton.
    (b) Bone scan and bone radiography show different patterns of expansion of bone lesions.
    (c) Involvement of whole bone with deformation at the edges is the common pattern of Paget disease.
    (d) ^{18}F-FDG is capable of distinguishing Paget's disease from metastatic lesions.
44. Bone lesions are commonly observed in polyostotic fibrous dysplasia (which is a form of the McCune–Albright syndrome) in all of the following regions *except*:
    (a) Facial
    (b) Spine
    (c) Skull
    (d) Legs
45. Which radiotracer shows an intense uptake in fibrous dysplasia?
    (a) ^{67} Gallium
    (b) ^{111}In-WBC
    (c) ^{201}Tl
    (d) FDG
46. Paget's disease:
    (a) More than 50% of patients are symptomatic.
    (b) The probability of experiencing headache is high.
    (c) It is polyostotic in 10–25% of cases.
    (d) X-ray is normal, whereas bone scan is abnormal in the initial stages of the disease.
47. The presentation of Paget's disease on bone scan:
    (a) The distribution of lesions on bone scan is different from that in radiography.
    (b) The avidity of multiple Paget's disease lesions is equal.
    (c) Osteoporosis circumscripta is common in the scapula.
    (d) The burn-out lesions of Paget's disease are commonly observed on bone scan.

48. Regarding the follow-up of patients with Paget's disease:
    (a) Bone scan can differentiate the therapeutic effects from the recurrence of a bone lesion.
    (b) The evaluation of vascularity is more reliable than serial bone scan for therapeutic monitoring.
    (c) Paget's disease lesions usually present an FDG uptake.
    (d) Although a scapular giant-cell tumor is rarely connected with Paget's disease, the diagnosis of the disease is critical because of its poor prognosis.
49. Which of the following diseases is presented by the Mickey Mouse sign?
    (a) Paget's disease
    (b) Metastasis
    (c) Osteosarcoma
    (d) a and b
50. Which of the following statements about the application of radiotracers in Paget's disease is NOT correct?
    (a) ^{67}Ga more accurately displays biochemical changes than ^{99m}Tc-MDP.
    (b) The role of ^{201}Tl is NOT definite.
    (c) A ^{111}In-WBC uptake is reported in regions with a positive uptake of gallium and bone radiotracer.
    (d) Measurement of the 24 h whole-body retention of ^{99m}Tc-phosphate is indicated for therapeutic monitoring.
51. Which drug changes the dominant pattern of a homogenous uptake of Paget's disease to a focal lesion, which can be mistaken for metastasis?
    (a) Calcitonin
    (b) Ethane-1-hydroxy-1, 1-diphosphonic acid (EHDP)
    (c) Pamidronate
    (d) Alendronate
52. Which of the following statements about fibrous dysplasia is NOT correct?
    (a) In contrast to Paget's disease, bone borders are NOT conserved in fibrous dysplasia.
    (b) Mandibular lesions of cherubism can be easily observed.
    (c) Bone scan is necessary for cranial fibrous dysplasia.
    (d) Monostotic fibrous dysplasia is a form of the McCune–Albright syndrome.
53. What are the patterns of uptake of gallium and thallium in fibrous dysplasia?
    (a) Increased uptake of both radiotracers
    (b) Decreased uptake of both radiotracers
    (c) Increased uptake of gallium and decreased uptake of thallium
    (d) Decreased uptake of gallium and increased uptake of thallium
54. The distribution pattern of lesions in polyostotic and idiopathic fibrous dysplasia is similar in all of the following regions *except*:
    (a) Skull
    (b) Face
    (c) Scapula
    (d) Legs

55. Which of the following bone disorders exhibits lesions similar to the pattern of fibrous dysplasia (FD)?
    (a) Amyloidosis
    (b) Sarcoidosis
    (c) Metastases
    (d) Paget's disease
56. Which imaging modality shows more lesions in fibrous dysplasia (FD)?
    (a) X-ray
    (b) Bone scan
    (c) Gallium scan
    (d) Thallium scan
57. Pseudo-osteomyelitis in Gaucher's disease is distinguished from osteomyelitis on bone scan according to:
    (a) Decreased uptake in the initial days
    (b) Increased activity in the initial days
    (c) Decreased uptake after the first week
    (d) Increased uptake after the first week
58. In which of the following diseases does osteochondroma occur?
    (a) Neurofibromatosis
    (b) Ribbing disease
    (c) Diaphyseal aclasis
    (d) Engelmann's disease
59. Which of the following diseases exhibits a bone scan pattern similar to that of osteopetrosis as the radiotracer accumulated in the metaphysis of long bones?
    (a) Erdheim–Chester disease
    (b) Engelmann's disease
    (c) Schmidt's metaphyseal dysplasia
    (d) Diaphyseal aclasis
60. What is the recommended method for the therapeutic monitoring of osteopetrosis?
    (a) Bone densitometry
    (b) Bone scan
    (c) CT scan
    (d) a and b
61. The differential diagnosis of ribbing disease includes all of the following situations *except*:
    (a) Child abuse
    (b) Congenital measles
    (c) Scurvy
    (d) Engelmann's disease
62. Which of the following bone diseases is characterized by multiple benign enostoses and by bone islands that are typically clustered around joints?
    (a) Engelmann's disease
    (b) Osteopathia striata
    (c) Melorheostosis
    (d) Osteopoikilosis

63. Which of the following diseases exhibit a normal pattern on bone scan?
    (a) Chronic familial hyperphosphatemia
    (b) Craniotubular dysplasia
    (c) Caffey's disease
    (d) Osteopoikilosis
64. Which of the followings statements regarding the application of bone scan in metabolic disorders is NOT correct?
    (a) A generalized increase in uptake is the common finding of all metabolic disorders on bone scan.
    (b) An increase in whole-body retention of radiotracers is the diagnostic and specific finding of an accelerated turnover.
    (c) An increase in whole-body retention of radiotracers is indicated for the estimation of the severity of primary hyperparathyroidism as well as the therapeutic monitoring and ruling out of bone metabolic disorders such as osteomalacia.
    (d) This method is only reliable when serum creatinine is normal and is NOT indicated for osteodystrophy.
65. What is the pathognomonic sign of renal osteodystrophy?
    (a) Hot patella
    (b) Rosary beads
    (c) Lone Ranger sign
    (d) Striped tie sign
66. Which of the following statements regarding renal osteodystrophy is NOT correct?
    (a) Bone scan overestimates the metabolic index scoring compared with normal condition.
    (b) Visceral calcification is reported in this disease.
    (c) Periarticular amyloid deposits may be observed in patients undergoing dialysis.
    (d) Brown tumor is a rare disease that is due to an intense increase in osteoblastic activity.
67. The Looser's zone lesions of osteomalacia exhibit … pattern on bone scan and are commonly reported in …
    (a) Asymmetric, skull
    (b) Symmetric, ribs
    (c) Asymmetric, pelvis
    (d) Symmetric spine
68. … hyperparathyroidism is demonstrated by a much intense uptake and common bone metabolic disorders, whereas the … form is characterized by a superscan.
    (a) Primary, secondary
    (b) Primary, primary
    (c) Secondary, secondary
    (d) Secondary, primary

69. In which of the following diseases is the quantitative measurement of calcium metabolism indicated?
    (a) Active acromegaly
    (b) Primary hyperparathyroidism
    (c) Severe thyrotoxicosis
    (d) Primary hypothyroidism
70. Which of the following diseases is demonstrated by a marked periarticular accumulation on bone scan?
    (a) Milk–alkali syndrome
    (b) Menkes' kinky hair syndrome
    (c) Congenital lipodystrophy
    (d) Congenital syphilis
71. The bone scan pattern is similar in all of the following diseases *except*:
    (a) Hypervitaminosis A
    (b) Hypervitaminosis D
    (c) Scurvy
    (d) Severe hyperthyroidism
72. The measurement of bone density with single-photon absorptiometry (SPA) is reliable in the:
    (a) Femoral neck
    (b) Calcaneus
    (c) Spine
    (d) a and c
73. Dual-energy X-ray absorptiometry (DEXA):
    (a) DEXA overestimates the BMD of the lumbar spine.
    (b) DEXA measures the volumetric density (g/cm^3) of bone.
    (c) The differences in bone depth are considered in DEXA among patients.
    (d) The lateral view in DEXA is less accurate than the anterior–posterior (AP) view.
74. Which of the following studies requires the longest postponing of DEXA?
    (a) Intravenous pyelogram (IVP)
    (b) Bone scintigraphy
    (c) GI survey
    (d) CT angiography
75. Which of the following variables is NOT considered for matching a patient in the Z-score?
    (a) Age
    (b) Race
    (c) Weight
    (d) Sex

76. All of the following items regarding bone loss are correct *except*:
    (a) The rate of femoral neck bone loss in men decreases with age in contrast to that in women.
    (b) Early bone loss in the axial skeleton is greater than that in the peripheral skeleton in a patient who has recently undergone oophorectomy.
    (c) The systematic measurement of BMD can be used for identifying the necessity of treatment.
    (d) Osteopenia appears in radiography only when there is more than 30% loss of bone minerals.
77. What level of changes in the femoral neck and spine is considered clinically important in serial BMD?
    (a) Changes exceeding 5% in the femoral neck and 1% in the spine
    (b) Changes exceeding 2.8% in the femoral neck and 1% in the spine
    (c) Changes exceeding 7% in the femoral neck and 3% in the spine
    (d) Changes exceeding 8% in the femoral neck and 7% in the spine
78. All of the following statements regarding the interpretation of the BMD are correct *except*:
    (a) Standard deviation (SD) is about 10% of the mean.
    (b) A Z-score of +1 indicates that a patient's BMD is 10% higher than the average BMD of the population.
    (c) A 1 SD decrease in BMD increases the probability of fracture by two times.
    (d) The WHO guidelines define osteoporosis as a BMD of less than −2.5 SD in normal young women; this value can also be extrapolated for children.
79. What is the recommended time interval for serial BMD in the menopausal state?
    (a) 1–2 years
    (b) 2–3 years
    (c) 2–4 years
    (d) 3–5 years
80. Osteoporotic fracture is common in all of the following bones *except*:
    (a) Hip
    (b) Wrist
    (c) Spine
    (d) Calcaneus
81. What is the current treatment of choice for osteoporosis?
    (a) Hormone replacement therapy (HRT)
    (b) Bisphosphonates (BPs)
    (c) Parathyroid hormone (PTH)
    (d) Selective estrogen receptor modulators (SERMs)
82. Which of the following treatments for osteoporosis is identified by a large increase in bone density as well as a marked reduction in the incidence of vertebral and other fractures in comparison with other methods?
    (a) Hormone replacement therapy (HRT)
    (b) Bisphosphonates (BPs)
    (c) Parathyroid hormone (PTH)
    (d) Selective estrogen receptor modulators (SERMs)

83. Which of the following tracers or radiation is used in dual-photon absorptiometry (DPA)?
    (a) X-ray
    (b) ^{153}gadolinium
    (c) ^{89}strontium
    (d) ^{32}phosphorus
84. All of the following items are considered advantages of dual-energy X-ray absorptiometry (DXA) *except*:
    (a) High precision
    (b) Short scan times
    (c) Low radiation dose
    (d) Unstable calibration
85. All of the following statements regarding T-score and Z-score are correct *except*:
    (a) The Z-score can NOT be used to diagnose osteoporosis.
    (b) The Z-score indicates the difference between the patient's measured BMD with that of healthy young adults matched for sex and ethnic group.
    (c) The T-score indicates the difference between the patient's measured BMD and the ideal peak bone mean achieved by a young adult.
    (d) The Z-score is compared with the mean BMD expected for the patient's peers, e.g., for a healthy normal subject matched for age, sex, and ethnic origin.
86. Every reduction of 1 SD in the BMD is equal to an approximately … increase in the likelihood of a fracture.
    (a) Twofold
    (b) Threefold
    (c) Fourfold
    (d) Fivefold
87. What is the optimal parameter if the goal is the therapeutic monitoring of osteoporosis?
    (a) T-score of the hip
    (b) Z-score of the calcaneus
    (c) Z-score of the spine
    (d) T-score of the forearm
88. What is the absorbed dose of radiation in dual-energy X-ray absorptiometry (DXA)?
    (a) 10–100 μSv
    (b) 10–20 μSv
    (c) 1–10 μSv
    (d) 50–100 μSv

89. How far is the recommended distance for the staff to maintain when they work with dual-energy X-ray absorptiometry (DXA), especially the one with a fan-beam system?
    (a) 1–2 m
    (b) 0.5–1 m
    (c) 2–3 m
    (d) 3–4 m
90. All of the following variables are lower in the dual-energy quantitative computed tomography (QCT) than in the single QCT *except*:
    (a) Accuracy error
    (b) Precision
    (c) Radiation dose
    (d) Artifact
91. Which of the following statements regarding quantitative computed tomography (QCT) is NOT correct?
    (a) Data acquisition by volumetric bone density is the advantage of QCT over areal bone density in DXA.
    (b) The radiation exposure in QCT is greater than that in a standard CT.
    (c) High responsiveness of the vertebral trabecular bone to aging and disease is the advantage of spinal QCT.
    (d) This method is currently NOT commonly used.
92. All of the following factors describe the advantages of peripheral quantitative computed tomography (PQCT) in the forearm over pDXA *except*:
    (a) Small footprint of the devices
    (b) Low cost
    (c) Low effective dose (0.1 μSv)
    (d) High radiation
93. Which of the following statements about the estimation of BMD by the quantitative ultrasound (QUS) method is NOT correct?
    (a) QUS is used to estimate the BMD in the peripheral skeleton.
    (b) The speed of sound (SOS) decreases in osteoporosis.
    (c) Broadband ultrasonic attenuation (BUA) increases in osteoporosis.
    (d) The addition of BUA and SOS is equal to QUS.
94. What is the definition of established osteoporosis?
    (a) BMD T-score < -2.5
    (b) BMD T-score between -2.5 and -3.5
    (c) BMD T-score < -2.5 with at least one osteoporotic fracture
    (d) BMD T-score between -2.5 and -3.5 in menopause

3.9.1 Answer

	A	B	C	D		A	B	C	D
1				*	48	*			
2				*	49				*
3		*			50			*	
4			*		51			*	
5			*		52				*
6	*				53			*	
7				*	54			*	
8	*				55		*		
9		*			56		*		
10	*				57	*			
11				*	58			*	
12		*			59	*			
13	*				60				*
14	*				61		*		
15				*	62				*
16			*		63				*
17	*				64		*		
18			*		65			*	
19		*			66	*			
20				*	67		*		
21			*		68			*	
22			*		69		*		
23			*		70			*	
24	*				71				*
25		*			72		*		
26			*		73				*
27				*	74			*	
28		*			75			*	
29	*				76			*	
30			*		77			*	
31			*		78				*
32				*	79			*	
33			*		80				*
34		*			81		*		
35				*	82			*	
36			*		83		*		
37				*	84				*
38		*			85		*		
39				*	86	*			
40			*		87			*	
41	*				88			*	
42		*			89			*	
43		*			90			*	
44		*			91		*		
45	*				92				*
46				*	93			*	
47	*				94			*	

3.10 Arthritis: Current Status of Scintigraphy and Future Trends

1. Regarding bone scan in rheumatoid arthritis:
   (a) A negative bone scan accurately excludes active arthritis.
   (b) Bone scan can differentiate the different degrees of arthritis in RA.
   (c) An increased activity in the talocalcaneonavicular is observed in Reiter's syndrome.
   (d) Bone scan cannot differentiate between early non-erosive and SLE.
2. ^{99m}Tc-HMPAO-labeled lymphocyte scintigraphy in RA patients shows a good correlation between intensity of uptake and all of the following factors *except*:
   (a) Joint swelling
   (b) Joint pain score
   (c) Radiological score
   (d) a and c
3. All the following statements regarding the role of ^{99m}Tc-IgG in RA are correct *except*:
   (a) It is a more specific method for detecting synovitis.
   (b) It can distinguish different degrees of arthritis activity.
   (c) It has higher sensitivity than clinical and laboratory measurements.
   (d) It is routinely used as a diagnostic tool.
4. Which radiopharmaceutical is capable of monitoring a systemic therapeutic intervention in RA patients?
   (a) ^{67}Ga
   (b) ^{99m}Tc-MDP
   (c) ^{99m}Tc-pyrophosphate
   (d) b and c
5. Which item about patients with rheumatoid arthritis and a normal bone scan is NOT correct?
   (a) Their osseous articular erosion is low.
   (b) They have a good prognosis.
   (c) Response to drug treatment is weak.
   (d) They do not have synovitis.
6. Rheumatoid arthritis is diagnosed for a patient. Bone scan is normal, and abnormal activity is NOT observed in the joints. Which item is correct?
   (a) Scan findings exclude rheumatoid arthritis.
   (b) It is highly probable that this patient will NOT suffer from articular changes in the future.
   (c) Polyclonal IgG scan is recommended for a better diagnosis.
   (d) Treatment can be postponed.

3.10.1 Answer

	A	B	C	D
1	*			
2			*	
3				*
4			*	
5			*	
6		*		

3.11 Radiation Synovectomy

1. Which radionuclide is recommended for the radiation synovectomy of finger joints?
   (a) ^{90}Y
   (b) ^{169}Er
   (c) ^{186}Re
   (d) ^{32}P
2. Hematologic malignancy has been reported following radiation synovectomy with:
   (a) ^{198}Au
   (b) ^{186}Re
   (c) ^{169}Er
   (d) ^{165}Dy
3. Maneuvers reducing the extra-articular spread of activity include all of the following items *except*:
   (a) Post-procedure joint splinting
   (b) Bed rest
   (c) Joint immobilization
   (d) Pre-injection of intra-articular heparin
4. The radionuclide carrier causing synovitis the most immediately after joint injection:
   (a) ^{90}Y resin colloid
   (b) ^{165}Dy-FHMA
   (c) ^{153}Sm-PHYP
   (d) b and c
5. All joints are recommended to be immobilized after injection of radiocolloids for:
   (a) 72 h
   (b) 48 h
   (c) 24 h
   (d) 1 week
6. What is the best radiopharmaceutical for metacarpal synovectomy?
   (a) ^{198}Au
   (b) ^{90}Y
   (c) ^{169}Er
   (d) ^{186}Re
7. In the treatment of painful metastasis of bone, which radionuclide does NOT produce gamma emission?
   (a) ^{32}Phosphorus
   (b) ^{89}Strantium
   (c) ^{186}Robidium
   (d) ^{188}Robidium

8. Which radionuclide is the most suitable for synovectomy of the shoulder joint?
   (a) ^{186}Re
   (b) ^{90}Y
   (c) ^{32}P
   (d) ^{153}Sm
9. Which one is considered a disadvantage of radionuclide synovectomy of the knee?
   (a) Immobilization of the patient
   (b) Administration of steroids
   (c) Incidence of neoplasm in adjacent bones
   (d) Radiation of other tissues in case of a radionuclide scape
10. A patient is a candidate for radiosynovectomy because of resistant arthritis in the finger joint. What is the most suitable management?
   (a) Y-190citrate is the radionuclide of choice.
   (b) Radiotracer should be administered at 10–20 mCi.
   (c) The joint must be immobilized for 3 days.
   (d) Hospitalization is required after radiation.
11. A woman diagnosed with pigmented villonodular synovitis of the knee joint is evaluated. You are consulted for an alternative therapy because of problematic surgery. Which one is the preferred radioactive agent?
   (a) ^{90}Y
   (b) ^{32}P
   (c) ^{153}Sm
   (d) ^{198}Au
12. Which complex is commonly used for the preparation of ^{32}P-labeled colloidal particles for radiosynovectomy?
   (a) Sodium silicate
   (b) Albumin
   (c) Chromium
   (d) Resin

3.11.1 Answer

	A	B	C	D
1		*		
2	*			
3				*
4	*			
5		*		
6			*	
7	*			
8	*			
9				*
10			*	
11	*			
12			*	

Suggested Readings

1. Ahmadzadehfar H, Biersack HJ, Freeman LM, Zuckier L. Clinical nuclear medicine. 2nd ed. Berlin: Springer; 2018.
2. Ell PJ, Gambhir SS. Nuclear medicine in clinical diagnosis and treatment. 3rd ed. Edinburgh, NY: Churchill Livingstone; 2004.
3. Sandler MP, Coleman RE, Patton JA, Wackers FJT, Gottschalk A. Diagnostic nuclear medicine. 4th ed. Philadelphia: Lippincott & Williams Wilkins; 2003.
4. Henkin RE. Nuclear medicine. 2nd ed. Philadelphia: Mosby Elsevier; 2006.

Nuclear Medicine in Gastrointestinal Function

4

4.1 Salivary Gland Disorders

1. Early stages of sialadenitis on scintigraphy are characterized by:
   (a) Prolonged T max, shortened E5%
   (b) Shortened T max, prolonged E5%
   (c) Shortened T max, normal E5%
   (d) Prolonged T max, normal E5%
2. Which of the following statements about sialoscintigraphy is NOT correct?
   (a) It can exclude space-occupying lesions.
   (b) It is the most reliable index of the recovery of salivary glands after antibiotic therapy.
   (c) It can support a correct clinical diagnosis.
   (d) It is the most sensitive index of the recovery of salivary glands after anti-inflammatory therapy.
3. Salivary gland dysfunction is NOT seen in:
   (a) Chronic pancreatitis
   (b) Amyotrophic lateral sclerosis
   (c) Autoimmune thyroiditis
   (d) Hepatitis
4. Which salivary gland tumor is NOT cold on scintigraphy?
   (a) Warthin's tumor
   (b) Papillary cystadenoma
   (c) Oncocytoma
   (d) All of the above

M. Assadi et al., *Principles of Nuclear Medicine*,
https://doi.org/10.1007/978-3-319-91701-6_4

5. Which technique is preferred for the primary diagnosis of salivary gland tumors?
   (a) PET
   (b) MRI
   (c) Dual-isotope SPECT
   (d) ^{67}Ga
6. Which of the following lesions appear as a cold spot in the salivary gland scan with ^{99m}Tc-pertechnetate?
   (a) Papillary cystadenoma
   (b) Oncocytoma
   (c) Oxyphilic adenoma
   (d) Pleomorphic adenoma
7. Which one is recommended for the follow-up of Sjogren's syndrome?
   (a) Sialoscintigraphy with Tc
   (b) Biopsy of lips
   (c) Dacryoscintigraphy
   (d) ^{67}Ga scan
8. In sialoscintigraphy:
   (a) Parenchymal involvement occurs in the initial stage of chronic inflammation.
   (b) Excretion is compromised in the early stage of Sjogren's syndrome.
   (c) Parenchymal absorption is disturbed in a short time after radioiodine therapy.
   (d) Papillary cystadenoma has a minor radiotracer uptake.
9. Sialoscintigraphy is performed on a patient with edema of the salivary glands. A symmetric bilateral uptake is observed in the parotid glands with reduced T max and normal E5%. The scan of the submandibular glands is also normal. What is the most probable diagnosis?
   (a) Acute viral sialadenitis
   (b) Sjogren's syndrome
   (c) Bilateral parotid sialolithiasis
   (d) Bilateral facial nerve paralysis
10. Sialoscintigraphy in Sjogren's syndrome:
    (a) Sialoscintigraphy alone canNOT differentiate a simple chronic inflammation from Sjogren's syndrome.
    (b) In Sjogren's syndrome, the submandibular glands show a higher uptake and a lower secretory response to stimulation than the parotid glands.
    (c) The level of oral radioactivity is NOT correlated with the severity of disease.
    (d) ^{67}Ga scintigraphy is NOT helpful for the detection of recurrence.

11. Sialoscintigraphy with technetium is performed on a 44-year-old woman. The salivary glands and oral cavity appear at the 15th and 30th min after tracer injection, respectively. The activity of the parotid glands is homogenous and lower than that of the thyroid. What is the most probable diagnosis?
    (a) Papillary cystadenoma
    (b) Sjogren's syndrome
    (c) Cystic hygroma
    (d) Sialolithiasis
12. Sialoscintigraphy with technetium is performed on 5-year-old child. A lesion in the right parotid gland is observed in the 5th min of imaging, which shows a small retention after lemon stimulation. What is the most probable diagnosis?
    (a) Papillary cystadenoma
    (b) Sjogren's syndrome
    (c) Cystic hygroma
    (d) Sialolithiasis
13. Sialoscintigraphy of a 55-year-old man shows an increased regional uptake in the right parathyroid gland, which is intensified after lemon administration. What is the most probable diagnosis?
    (a) Sialadenitis
    (b) Papillary cystadenoma
    (c) Abscess
    (d) Acute parotitis
14. Scintigraphy of Sjogren's syndrome:
    (a) Sialoscintigraphy is valuable for the diagnosis of the early stage of the disease.
    (b) ^{67}Ga scan is indicated for the diagnosis.
    (c) A rapid and diffuse uptake is the common scan pattern.
    (d) It has NO value in follow-up after treatment.
15. In sialoscintigraphy:
    (a) Radiotherapy increases the diffuse uptake in the salivary glands.
    (b) Uptake in the salivary glands decreases in acute parotiditis.
    (c) Warthin's tumor is detected as a photopenic lesion.
    (d) Uptake in the salivary gland is normally equal or higher than that of the thyroid.
16. Sialoscintigraphy is indicated for the evaluation of:
    (a) Reiter's syndrome and steal disease
    (b) Ankylosing spondylitis and brucellosis
    (c) Lupus and rheumatoid arthritis
    (d) Behcet's syndrome and Felty's syndrome

17. Sialoscintigraphy is performed on a 59-year-old man. An increased activity of the rim sign around the sensitive parotid is observed in the angiography phase, but no uptake is demonstrated in images at the 40th min. What is the most probable diagnosis?
    (a) Acute inflammation
    (b) Abscess
    (c) Adenoma cystitis
    (d) Mixed cell tumor
18. A 57-year-old woman with a history of nasopharynx cancer is referred with a dry mouth after completion of the treatment. She also reports a history of radiotherapy. The patient is subjected to sialoscintigraphy with ^{99m}Tc-pertechnetate and gallium scan. What is the expected scan pattern for the salivary glands?
    (a) Sialoscintigraphy, reduced uptake; gallium scan, reduced uptake
    (b) Sialoscintigraphy, increased uptake; gallium scan, increased uptake
    (c) Sialoscintigraphy, reduced uptake; gallium scan, increased uptake
    (d) Sialoscintigraphy. increased uptake; gallium scan, reduced uptake
19. The parotid glands appear at the 5th min of sialoscintigraphy with technetium, and oral accumulation of activity is observed at the 25th min. What is the grade of the disease based on the intensity of involvement of the salivary glands?
    (a) Grade 1
    (b) Grade 2
    (c) Grade 3
    (d) Grade 4
20. Which of the following findings is common in the sialoscintigraphy of a patient with Warthin's tumor?
    (a) Increased parotid uptake, which decreases after lemon stimulation
    (b) Decreased parotid uptake, which increases after lemon stimulation
    (c) Increased parotid uptake, which enhances after lemon stimulation
    (d) Lack of radiotracer uptake before and after lemon stimulation
21. A focal increase in uptake is observed in sialoscintigraphy. What is the most probable diagnosis?
    (a) Sjogren's syndrome
    (b) Abscess
    (c) Warthin's tumor
    (d) Cyst
22. Sialoscintigraphy with technetium:
    (a) This scan is NOT indicated for the evaluation of graft versus host disease.
    (b) Papillary cystadenoma shows an increased uptake.
    (c) This scan is NOT indicated for Bell's palsy.
    (d) Scan pattern does NOT depend on the stage of sialadenitis.

23. Which of the following diseases demonstrates a diffusely decreased activity on scintigraphy with technetium?
    (a) Sterile acute parotitis
    (b) Sialolithiasis
    (c) Abscess
    (d) Warthin's tumor
24. A diffusely decreased technetium uptake and an increased gallium uptake are reported on sialoscintigraphy. What is the most probable diagnosis?
    (a) Sterile acute parotitis
    (b) Warthin's tumor
    (c) Radiotherapy
    (d) Recurrence of chronic parotitis
25. Which of the following statements about Sjogren's syndrome is NOT correct?
    (a) Sialoscintigraphy alone canNOT discriminate a simple inflammatory process from Sjogren's syndrome.
    (b) An increased salivary and a decreased lacrimal uptake in gallium scan are pathognomonic for this syndrome.
    (c) A higher technetium uptake in the submandibular glands and lower a secretory response to stimulation in comparison with the parotid glands indicates Sjogren's syndrome.
    (d) Gallium is indicated for therapeutic monitoring.
26. Which of the following statements regarding the study of salivary gland function is NOT correct?
    (a) It is performed with 4 mCi of technetium pertechnetate.
    (b) Dynamic images are obtained for 40 min.
    (c) E5% is the count of salivary gland 5 min after radiotracer injection.
    (d) Submandibular and parotid gland function can be examined through this method.
27. What is the most common salivary gland tumor?
    (a) Pleomorphic adenoma
    (b) Warthin's tumor
    (c) Cystadenocarcinoma
    (d) Oncocytoma
28. Which tumor of the salivary glands is malignant?
    (a) Godwin's tumor
    (b) Acinic cell tumor
    (c) Pleomorphic adenoma
    (d) Oncocytoma

4.1.1 Answer

	A	B	C	D
1			*	
2	*			
3				*
4				*
5			*	
6				*
7				*
8		*		
9	*			
10		*		
11		*		
12			*	
13		*		
14		*		
15				*
16			*	
17		*		
18			*	
19		*		
20			*	
21			*	
22		*		
23		*		
24			*	
25		*		
26			*	
27	*			
28		*		

4.2 Esophageal Function (Transport and Motility)

1. Which drug increases the contraction amplitude, duration, velocity, and propagation time of the esophagus?
   (a) Cisapride
   (b) Domperidone
   (c) Glucagon
   (d) Metoclopramide
2. Regarding esophageal scintigraphy:
   (a) It shows a normal local bolus transport in Barrett's esophagus.
   (b) It shows an abnormal clearance in Barrett's esophagus.
   (c) The relationship between gastric emptying rate and gastric esophageal reflux is confirmed.
   (d) Reflux of gastric content may not be the sole mechanism in esophagitis.
3. In esophageal scintigraphy:
   (a) Fasting is not required.
   (b) Solid bolus food is the most physiologic product.
   (c) Tc-pertechnetate is the radiopharmaceutical of choice.
   (d) Supine position is the preferred position after esophageal surgery.
4. For the radioisotopic evaluation of esophageal reflux:
   (a) The test is performed in a sitting position.
   (b) 1 mCi of Tc-99m is administered.
   (c) 24 h images are useful.
   (d) Fasting is not required.
5. What is the radiopharmaceutical of choice for the rapid and sequential scintigraphy of the esophagus?
   (a) ^{99m}Tc
   (b) ^{81m}Kr
   (c) ^{111}In
   (d) ^{67}Ga
6. A radioactive retention in the upper segment is found on esophageal transit scintigraphy. What is the most probable diagnosis?
   (a) Diffuse esophageal spasm
   (b) Nutcracker esophagus
   (c) Zenker's diverticulum
   (d) Cervical vertebropathy
7. Prolonged transit and retention of activity in the distal segment with reflux to the medial esophagus are found on esophageal transit scintigraphy. What is the most probable diagnosis?
   (a) Diffuse esophageal spasm
   (b) Nutcracker esophagus
   (c) Zenker's diverticulum
   (d) Cervical vertebropathy

8. Prolonged transit and decreased and segmental emptying with radiopharmaceutical fragmentation are found on esophageal transit scintigraphy. What is the most probable diagnosis?
   (a) Diffuse esophageal spasm
   (b) Nutcracker esophagus
   (c) Zenker's diverticulum
   (d) Cervical vertebropathy
9. A condensed image method is performed in which of the following scans?
   (a) Hepatobiliary scan
   (b) Liver and spleen scan
   (c) Gastric emptying study
   (d) Esophageal transit study
10. In which of the following studies is supine position in front of the gamma camera the most suitable?
    (a) Esophageal transit study for the therapeutic monitoring of achalasia
    (b) Gastroesophageal reflux study
    (c) Gastric emptying scan for a patient with suspected diabetic gastroparesis
    (d) Gastric emptying scan for a patient with suspected Zollinger–Ellison syndrome
11. Gastroesophageal reflux scintigraphy:
    (a) It is the method of choice for the evaluation of reflux in adults.
    (b) Scan is performed in a sitting position.
    (c) Reflux of more than 10% is considered abnormal.
    (d) Drinking a mixture of orange juice and HCl in a sitting position is recommended for the scan.
12. Segmental evaluation of esophageal transit scintigraphy in the proximal, distal, and gastric fundus is presented. How long is the esophageal transit time (ETT) and the esophagogastric transit time (GETT), respectively?
    (a) 0.35 s and 0.75 s
    (b) 0.05 s and 0.25 s
    (c) 0.25 s and 0.75 s
    (d) 0.35 s and 1.25 s

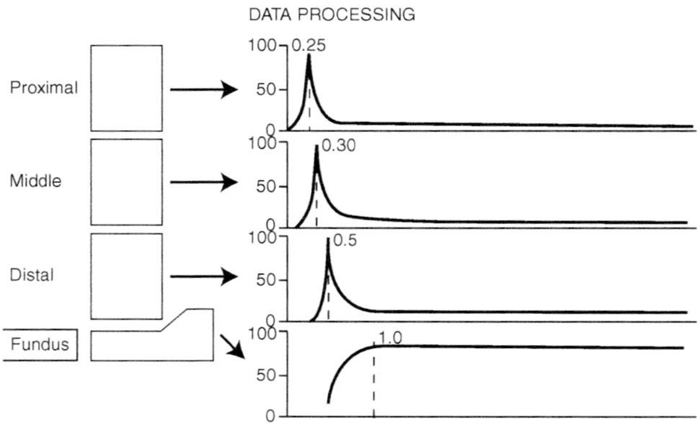

13. A 49-year-old woman with identified hiatal hernia complains about heartburn but does NOT experience dysphagia or odynophagia. After esophageal scintigraphy and washing with 120 cc of water, a significant activity remains in all segments of the esophagus. What is the most probable diagnosis?
    (a) Gastroesophageal reflux disease (GERD) and extensive esophagitis
    (b) Achalasia
    (c) Diffuse esophageal spasm
    (d) Normal finding
14. Which of the following statements about esophageal reflux is NOT correct?
    (a) Abdominal compression even up to 100 mmHg does NOT induce reflux in normal subjects.
    (b) If reflux is equal or more than 4%, it is considered an abnormal finding.
    (c) The scan sensitivity is greater than 85%.
    (d) Acidic materials decrease the sensitivity of the test.
15. What is the recommended view for imaging suspected upper esophageal dyskinesia?
    (a) Anterior in the upright position
    (b) Anterior in the supine position
    (c) Posterior
    (d) Lateral
16. Which of the following items increases lower esophageal sphincter (LES) pressure?
    (a) Cholecystokinin
    (b) Prostaglandin E1
    (c) Prostaglandin E2
    (d) Prostaglandin F2-alpha
17. What is the meaning of the deglutitive inhibition phenomenon on esophageal scintigraphy, and how long does it take?
    (a) Inhibition of the primary peristaltic wave, 10–20 s
    (b) Inhibition of secondary peristaltic wave, 20–30 s
    (c) Inhibition of tertiary peristaltic wave, 10–20 s
    (d) Complete inhibition of the previous contraction when a newly swallowing-induced contraction is formed, 20–30 s
18. Which of the following indices on esophageal scintigraphy denotes the time interval between the entrance of bolus activity to the esophagus and the decrease of more than 90% of esophageal activity?
    (a) Esophageal transit times
    (b) Segmental emptying time
    (c) Global esophageal emptying time
    (d) Esophagogastric transit time

19. Which of the following diseases is demonstrated by the following findings on esophageal scintigraphy? "The marked and prolonged retention of radioactive bolus in the distal segment; very little activity in the stomach; chaotic movement of the activity in condensed images."
    (a) Achalasia
    (b) Diffuse esophageal spasm
    (c) Nutcracker esophagus
    (d) Progressive systemic sclerosis
20. Which of the following diseases is demonstrated by the following findings on esophageal scintigraphy? "Prolonged transit time; decreased segmental esophageal emptying; periods of esophageal retrograde movement; fragmentation of the radioactive bolus; multiple peaks of activity in all segments in the time–activity curves."
    (a) Non-specific motility disorders
    (b) Diffuse esophageal spasm
    (c) Nutcracker esophagus
    (d) Progressive systemic sclerosis
21. Prolonged retention of activity in the distal esophagus and in the mid-distal to mid-esophagus as well as esophageal reflux are reported on esophageal scintigraphy. What is the most probable diagnosis?
    (a) Non-specific motility disorders
    (b) Diffuse esophageal spasm
    (c) Nutcracker esophagus
    (d) Progressive systemic sclerosis
22. Prolonged esophageal transit time with an uncoordinated pattern is reported on esophageal scintigraphy. What is the most probable diagnosis?
    (a) Non-specific motility disorders
    (b) Diffuse esophageal spasm
    (c) Nutcracker esophagus
    (d) Progressive systemic sclerosis
23. Which of the following diseases is demonstrated by the stagnation of bolus in the lower two-thirds of the esophagus?
    (a) Achalasia
    (b) Diffuse esophageal spasm
    (c) Nutcracker esophagus
    (d) Progressive systemic sclerosis
24. Esophageal scintigraphy shows an ovoid or spherical area of persistent esophageal retention of radioactivity in the upper segment. What is the most probable diagnosis?
    (a) Achalasia
    (b) Zenker diverticulum
    (c) Nutcracker esophagus
    (d) Progressive systemic sclerosis

25. What is the best quantitative method for the pre- and postoperative evaluation of hiatal hernia and gastroesophageal reflux disease (GERD)?
    (a) Scintigraphy
    (b) Manometry
    (c) Barium swallow
    (d) Upper GI endoscopy

4.2.1 Answer

	A	B	C	D
1				*
2				*
3		*		
4			*	
5		*		
6			*	
7		*		
8	*			
9				*
10		*		
11				*
12			*	
13	*			
14				*
15				*
16				*
17				*
18			*	
19	*			
20		*		
21			*	
22	*			
23				*
24		*		
25	*			

4.3 Gastric Motility

1. What is the effect of caffeine on the gastric emptying rate?
   (a) No significant effect
   (b) Hastens
   (c) Slows
   (d) b and c
2. Which of the following factors may hasten gastric emptying?
   (a) Erythromycin
   (b) Cigarette smoking
   (c) Chronic doses of alcohol
   (d) Small doses of morphine
3. All of the followings statements regarding gastric emptying in pediatrics are true *except*:
   (a) Children with delayed emptying problems are common.
   (b) Children with intestinal pseudo-obstruction commonly demonstrate delayed gastric clearance.
   (c) Solid gastric emptying results are more reliable than liquid in predicting postoperative drainage after fundoplication.
   (d) In long-term diabetic children, the relationship between symptoms and gastric emptying is poor.
4. On gastric emptying scintigraphy with a solid meal:
   (a) Bulk meals reduce the gastric emptying rate.
   (b) High-calorie meals reduce the gastric emptying rate.
   (c) High-calorie meals do NOT decrease the lag time.
   (d) The physical property of the meal does NOT influence the lag time.
5. What is the most appropriate time for emptying half of the activity in the solid phase of stomach emptying scintigraphy?
   (a) 25 min
   (b) 40 min
   (c) 90 min
   (d) 180 min
6. A woman with a history of diabetes for 12 years complains about abdominal discomfort after meals. She is under insulin treatment. Delayed gastric emptying is reported on the scan with solid food. Which item is NOT an interfering or misleading factor?
   (a) Discontinuation of insulin
   (b) Overadminstration of fats in solid meal preparation
   (c) Activity of the small intestine in ROI
   (d) Problems in the labeling of solid meals

7. A sigmoid curve is observed on the gastric emptying scan with solid food. All items influence the emptying rate and lag phase *except*:
   (a) Physical properties of the food
   (b) Contraction of stomach antrum
   (c) Pyloroduodenal coordination
   (d) Antroduodenal coordination
8. Which radiopharmaceutical is NOT used for gastric emptying scintigraphy?
   (a) ^{14}C-lactose
   (b) ^{67}Ga-EDTA
   (c) ^{14}C-octanoic acid
   (d) ^{14}C-glycine
9. Which of the following drugs accelerates gastric emptying?
   (a) Loperamide
   (b) Omeprazole
   (c) Cimetidine
   (d) L-Dopa
10. Which of the following diseases is characterized by the rapid emptying of fluid and solid food on the scan?
    (a) Anorexia nervosa
    (b) Pernicious anemia
    (c) Zollinger–Ellison syndrome
    (d) Patients with HIV
11. Gastric scintigraphy is performed on a 24-year-old woman with microcytic anemia and BMI of 16.8. Emptying of a solid meal is delayed, but liquid emptying is normal. What is the most probable diagnosis?
    (a) Anorexia nervosa
    (b) Zollinger–Ellison syndrome
    (c) Atrophic gastritis
    (d) Advanced diabetic gastroparesis
12. Which scintigraphy test is recommended for the evaluation of a patient with dysphagia and suspected gastric accommodation?
    (a) Liquid emptying scintigraphy with In-labeled DTPA
    (b) Gastric volume change study with Tc-pertechnetate simultaneous with the solid meal emptying test
    (c) Solid meal emptying scintigraphy with Tc-labeled sulfur colloid
    (d) Simultaneous solid meal and liquid emptying test with two radiopharmaceuticals
13. Which organ is exposed to greater radiation if the ^{99m}Tc-sulfur colloid-labeled egg is administered on a healthy subject?
    (a) Esophagus
    (b) Stomach
    (c) Small intestine
    (d) Lower segment of the large intestine

14. Gastric emptying scintigraphy is requested for a patient. Which of the following items is recommended for the preparation of a solid meal?
    (a) Addition of 500 μCi of Tc-SC to mixed yolk and albumen before cooking and then cooking until congealing
    (b) Addition of 100 μCi of In-DTPA to mixed yolk and albumen before cooking and then cooking without salt
    (c) Addition of 500 μCi of Tc-SC to yolk before cooking and then cooking with separated yolk and albumen
    (d) Addition of 100 μCi of In–oxine to a large cooked egg with mixed yolk and albumen
15. On gastric emptying scan:
    (a) The intrathoracic stomach emptying rate is faster than that of a normal esophagus.
    (b) The intrathoracic stomach shows a slow primary phase of emptying, which occurs in the first 10 min.
    (c) The amount of reflux in the intrathoracic stomach is high.
    (d) The scan 6 months after gastric vagotomy shows a rapid emptying rate.
16. A gastric emptying scan is requested for a patient with a history of gastric surgery. A rapid emptying rate of fluids and a delayed emptying of a solid meal are seen on the scan. This view is observed in which of the following surgeries?
    (a) Distal gastrostomy
    (b) Distal gastrostomy + truncal vagotomy
    (c) Subtotal gastrostomy + truncal vagotomy
    (d) Roux-en-Y diversion + vagotomy
17. Gastric emptying graphy of a solid meal is presented. What is the reason for this scan pattern?
    (a) Distal gastrostomy
    (b) Truncal vagotomy
    (c) Roux-en-Y surgery
    (d) Lupus

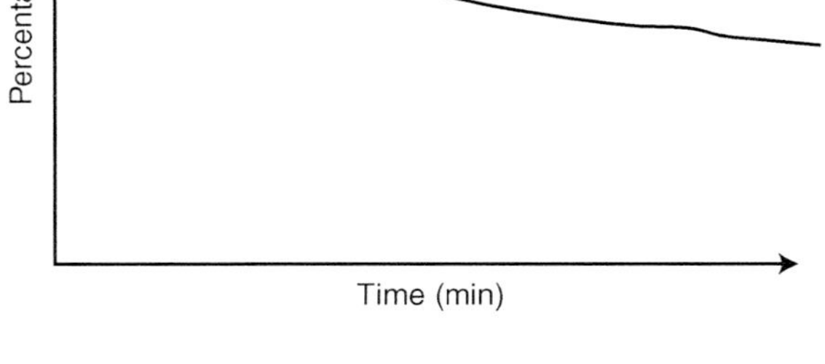

18. A diabetic patient who has been undergoing treatment with insulin for 10 years is subjected to gastric emptying scintigraphy. What is the expected scan pattern?
    (a) Delay in emptying of fluids with normal or delayed emptying of a solid meal
    (b) Normal emptying of fluids and a solid meal
    (c) Delay in emptying of a solid meal with normal or delayed empting of fluids
    (d) Delay in emptying of fluids in the early stage with delayed and protracted emptying of solid meal
19. What is the normal pattern of gastric emptying for a solid meal?
    (a) Rapid emptying followed by a slower rate (exponential)
    (b) Lag phase followed by a linear phase and finally slow emptying (sigmoid)
    (c) Emptying with a constant rate (linear)
    (d) Emptying with a different and irregular rate (irregular and with indentations)
20. Which of the following findings on gastric emptying scintigraphy is associated with atrophic gastritis?
    (a) Stasis of solid meal and fluids
    (b) Delayed liquid emptying and normal emptying of solid meals
    (c) Rapid emptying rate of fluids and solid meals
    (d) Rapid emptying rate of fluids and normal emptying of solid meals
21. What are the patterns of gastric emptying of liquid and solid meals in patients with chronic gastritis, respectively?
    (a) Slow, rapid
    (b) Normal, slow
    (c) Rapid, slow
    (d) Slow, normal
22. Which of the following factors has the least effect on gastric emptying?
    (a) Obesity
    (b) Food temperature
    (c) Food calorie
    (d) Food volume
23. Which of the following drugs or situations decreases the gastric emptying rate?
    (a) Domperidone
    (b) Renal failure
    (c) Vagotomy
    (d) Duodenal ulcer
24. Which of the following disease is presented by delayed solid and liquid gastric emptying?
    (a) Chronic gastritis
    (b) Atrophic gastritis
    (c) Pernicious anemia
    (d) Anorexia nervosa

25. Which phase of gastric emptying is influenced by diabetes?
    (a) Lag phase
    (b) Proximal stomach function
    (c) Antral motor activity
    (d) All of the above
26. Gastric emptying scintigraphy is requested for a patient with bloating and early stomach fullness after feeding. Based on the following gastric emptying curve on semisolid food, what is the most probable diagnosis?

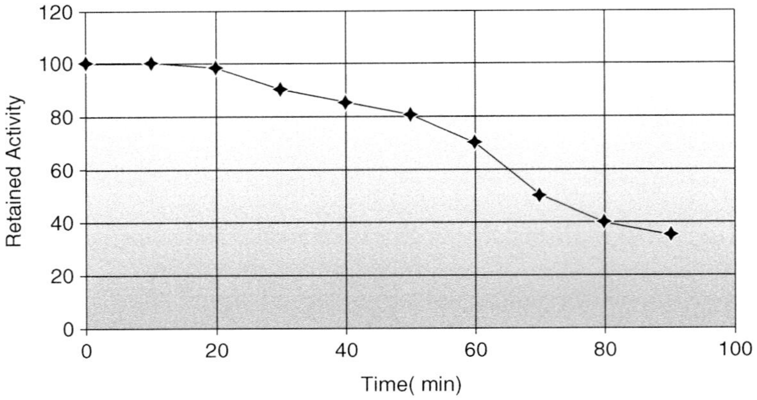

    (a) The findings are completely normal.
    (b) Gastric emptying is abnormal only in the second phase.
    (c) The findings are indicative of truncal vagotomy.
    (d) The findings are indicative of Zollinger–Ellison syndrome.

4.3.1 Answer

	A	B	C	D
1	*			
2	*			
3				*
4	*			
5			*	
6				*
7			*	
8	*			
9	*			
10			*	
11	*			
12		*		
13			*	
14	*			
15			*	
16		*		
17			*	
18			*	
19		*		
20	*			
21		*		
22	*			
23		*		
24		*		
25				*
26	*			

4.4 Intestine: Evaluation of Absorption

1. Which compound is used to assess fat malabsorption in children with cystic fibrosis?
   (a) ^{14}C-triolein
   (b) ^{13}C-MTG breath test
   (c) ^{14}C-trioctanoin
   (d) ^{14}C-tripalmitin
2. What is the amount of activity in the ^{14}C-urea breath test?
   (a) 40 kBq
   (b) 400 MBq
   (c) 40 MBq
   (d) 4 kBq
3. Intestinal permeability using 51C-EDTA is normal in:
   (a) Alcoholics
   (b) Crohn's disease
   (c) Ulcerative colitis
   (d) Celiac disease
4. The accuracy of the ^{14}C-urea breath test is:
   (a) >90%
   (b) 80–90%
   (c) 70–80%
   (d) 60–70%
5. Which of the following radiopharmaceuticals is indicated for the "permeability" study of small intestine?
   (a) ^{51}Cr-EDTA
   (b) ^{14}C-glycocholic acid
   (c) ^{99m}Tc-DTPA
   (d) ^{14}C-lactolose
6. In the urea breathing test:
   (a) 1 mg of C-11-labeled urea is administered
   (b) Fasting is required
   (c) Omeprazole must be discontinued 72 h before the test
   (d) Higher than 18 dpm/mmol in a 10 min breath sample is considered positive
7. Increased intestinal permeability using ^{51}Cr-EDTA is observed in all the following conditions *except*:
   (a) Crohn's colitis
   (b) Ulcerative colitis
   (c) Celiac disease
   (d) Alcoholics

8. An indeterminate outcome is found in the radioactive urea breath test. What is the next step?
   (a) More hyamine should be added to the breathing vial until a positive or a negative result is confirmed.
   (b) Fresh scintillation solution should be added to the breathing vial to overcome the indeterminate outcome.
   (c) More exaltation samples should be added to the breathing vial until a positive or a negative outcome is obtained.
   (d) The sample should be counted after few hours, and the test must be re-conducted if the indeterminate outcome is repeated.
9. Which of the following conditions causes false-positive results in the radioactive urea breath test?
   (a) Antibiotic therapy in the recent 30 days
   (b) Bismuth administration in the recent 1 month
   (c) Pantoprazole administration in the recent 2 weeks
   (d) Gastric resection
10. What is the formula for calculating the dpm in the urea breath test?
    (a) (Sample dpm − blank dpm)/machine efficiency
    (b) (Sample dpm − blank dpm)/machine efficiency
    (c) (Sample dpm − machine efficiency)/blank dpm
    (d) (Sample dpm − machine efficiency)/blank dpm
11. Which item causes a false-normal level of cobalamin in a patient with a low cobalamin level?
    (a) Myeloma
    (b) Liver parenchymal disease
    (c) Pregnancy
    (d) OCP
12. The ^{14}C labeling of … for the breath test provides similar information to that on gastric emptying test with a ^{99m}Tc-sulfur colloid-labeled egg.
    (a) Glycine
    (b) Galactose
    (c) Xylose
    (d) Octanoic acid
13. What is the reason for the intramuscular injection of 1 mg non-radioactive B12 in the Schilling test?
    (a) Decreased liver radiation due to the administration of radiocobalt cobalamin
    (b) Increased tubular secretion of labeled cobalamin from the kidney
    (c) Saturation of binding sites in the plasma and tissues
    (d) Increased binding of labeled cobalamin to the internal factor

14. The Schilling test is performed for a patient with megaloblastic anemia. Labeled B12 in the urine is less than 5% in the primary step and normal in the second phase (administration of labeled B12 with an internal factor). What is the most probable diagnosis?
    (a) Pernicious anemia
    (b) Malabsorption
    (c) Bacterial overgrowth syndrome
    (d) Pancreas insufficiency
15. The first step of the Schilling test of a patient is abnormal. After the administration of radioactive B12 + internal actor, urinary excretion is greater than 90%. Which item is correct?
    (a) Decreased vitamin B12 intake
    (b) Internal factor-dependent B12 malabsorption
    (c) No specific disease is identified
    (d) Internal factor-independent B12 malabsorption
16. The Schilling test is performed with the co-administration of ^{58}Co-B12 and internal factor + ^{58}Co-B12. Which of the following items is correct?
    (a) The diagnosis of pernicious anemia is confirmed if the ratio of urinary excretion of IF + ^{58}Co-B12 to that of ^{58}Co-B12 is greater than 1.4.
    (b) Internal factor deficiency is possible if the urinary excretion of labeled B12 in both tests is less than 7%.
    (c) Pernicious anemia is possible if the urinary excretion of labeled B12 in both tests is equal and greater than 9%.
    (d) Internal factor deficiency is possible if urinary excretion of labeled B12 is greater than 9% and that of IF + labeled B12 is less than 7%.
17. Which of the following items can cause false-positive findings in the urea breath test?
    (a) Achlorhydria
    (b) Tetracycline
    (c) Bismuth
    (d) Hiatal hernia
18. Schilling test:
    (a) Daily injection (IV) of vitamin B12 three days before the test
    (b) Fasting from the previous day until the oral administration of vitamin B12
    (c) Intravenous injection of unlabeled vitamin B12 six hours after oral administration
    (d) Collection of 72 h urine for all patients
19. In the ^{14}C-glycocholic acid breath test:
    (a) The carbon of urea is converted into CO_2 in this test.
    (b) It is used to detect bile salt malabsorption.
    (c) The peak CO_2 appears after 1 h in *Staphylococcus* cholangitis.
    (d) This test is indicated for the evaluation of the therapeutic effects of antibiotics for peptic ulcer.

20. Diagnosis of intestinal bacterial overgrowth:
   (a) The ^{14}C-glycocholic acid test is only indicated for patients with bile salt malabsorption.
   (b) ^{14}C-D-xylose is catabolized by anaerobic bacteria in the intestine.
   (c) ^{14}C-xylose is mainly uptaken in the large intestine.
   (d) Increased fecal excretion of ^{14}C is observed in patients with bile salt malabsorption.
21. For the diagnosis of *Helicobacter pylori*:
   (a) ^{14}C-D-xylose is used for evaluating *H. pylori* infection.
   (b) ^{13}C and liquid scintillation are also indicated for the evaluation of *H. pylori* infection.
   (c) About 1 mmol hyamine hydroxide traps 1 mmol CO_2.
   (d) The presence of thymolphthalein in the solution causes the change in color to orange after blowing.
22. In which of the following conditions is the level of cobalamin falsely normal?
   (a) Folate deficiency
   (b) Aplastic anemia
   (c) Pregnancy
   (d) Liver disease
23. Which of the following variables is the least important in the assessment of B12 absorption?
   (a) Patient's weight and height
   (b) Renal function
   (c) Fasting
   (d) History of hypersensitivity to B12 injection
24. In which of the following situations is the decrease in the serum level of cobalamin factual?
   (a) Pregnancy
   (b) Aplastic anemia
   (c) Tapeworm (cestode) infection
   (d) Folate deficiency
25. What is the reason for the utilization of alkaline solutions, such as hyamine, in the ^{14}C-urea breath test?
   (a) Hydrolysis of radioactive urea to radioactive CO_2
   (b) Amplification of emitted photons from the scintillation solution
   (c) Elimination of the chemiluminescent effect
   (d) Trapping of radioactive CO_2 in exhalation
26. Which of the following radiotracers is the most specific if the goal is to examine fat malabsorption?
   (a) ^{14}C-tripalmitin
   (b) ^{14}C-triolein
   (c) ^{14}C-trioctanoin
   (d) ^{14}C-mixed TG

27. Which of the following items is NOT an indication for the urea breath test (UBT) with ^{14}C?
    (a) Primary diagnosis of *H. pylori* in duodenal ulcer
    (b) Primary diagnosis of *H. pylori* in gastric ulcer
    (c) Confirmation of the eradication of *H. pylori* in duodenal ulcer
    (d) Confirmation of the eradication of *H. pylori* in gastric ulcer
28. How long after the eradication of *H. pylori* is the urea breath test (UBT) recommended?
    (a) 1 week
    (b) 2 weeks
    (c) 3 weeks
    (d) 4 weeks
29. All of the following medications must be discontinued 30 days before the urea breath test (UBT) *except*:
    (a) Sucralfate
    (b) Bismuth
    (c) Azithromycin
    (d) Amoxicillin

4.4.1 Answer

	A	B	C	D
1		*		
2	*			
3			*	
4	*			
5	*			
6		*		
7		*		
8				*
9				*
10		*		
11		*		
12				*
13			*	
14	*			
15		*		
16	*			
17	*			
18			*	
19		*		
20				*

21			*	
22				*
23				*
24			*	
25				*
26			*	
27	*			
28				*
29	*			

4.5 Studies on Small Bowel and Colonic Transit

1. Regarding total colonic transit time:
   (a) It is about 70 h.
   (b) Segmental transit time for the right colon is more than rectosigmoid.
   (c) Segmental transit time for the left colon is more than rectosigmoid.
   (d) Men have a significantly shorter transit time for the whole colon than women.
2. Which radiopharmaceutical is not used in colon scintigraphy?
   (a) ^{111}In-DTPA
   (b) ^{67}Ga
   (c) ^{131}I-cellulose
   (d) ^{99m}Tc-glycocholic acid
3. Before colon scintigraphy:
   (a) Ask to cease medications prescribed for constipation for 5 days.
   (b) No dietary modification is required.
   (c) It is not recommended within a 6-week period following colonoscopy.
   (d) a and b.
4. Which drug is effective in patients with constipation-predominant irritable bowel syndrome?
   (a) Cisapride
   (b) Prucalopride
   (c) Tegaserod
   (d) Metoclopramide
5. In which of the following conditions is defecoscintigraph indicated?
   (a) Colon cancer
   (b) Severe constipation
   (c) Megacolon
   (d) Hemorrhoids
6. Nuclear medicine procedures are NOT helpful for the diagnosis of:
   (a) Steatorrhea
   (b) Intestinal obstruction
   (c) Lactase deficiency
   (d) Protein-losing enteropathy
7. A patient with a history of chronic constipation comes to your department. Colonic transit scintigraphy with ^{67}Ga-citrate shows a slow transit throughout the colon without a significant segmental retention of the activity. The pattern of scintigraphy in this patient indicates:
   (a) Functional rectosigmoid obstruction (FRSO)
   (b) Colonic inertia
   (c) Normal pattern
   (d) Obstruction

4.5.1 Answer

	A	B	C	D
1				*
2				*
3		*		
4			*	
5		*		
6		*		
7		*		

4.6 Hepatobiliary Function

1. Which drug tends to reduce bile formation?
   (a) Corticosteroids
   (b) Gastrin
   (c) Insulin
   (d) Chlorpromazine
2. Which iminodiacetic acid derivative used on scintigraphy has the lowest liver T1/2 and the highest liver uptake?
   (a) HIDA
   (b) DISIDA
   (c) Mebrofenin
   (d) BIDA
3. Regarding the effects of drugs on the sphincter of Oddi function:
   (a) The effect of morphine is reversed by atropine.
   (b) Diazepam does not influence the sphincter of Oddi function.
   (c) The effect of morphine is not reversed by CCK.
   (d) Sphincter relaxation is caused by erythromycin.
4. Pulmonary uptake is observed on hepatosplenic scintigraphy. Which one is NOT probable?
   (a) Progressed cirrhosis
   (b) Error in the preparation of the radiotracer
   (c) Biliary tuberculosis
   (d) Administration of antacid
5. A patient with a recent history of cholecystectomy is complaining about cholic pain after meals. Which item regarding the possibility of the sphincter of Oddi dysfunction is NOT correct?
   (a) Measurement of liver enzymes and biliary sonography are required.
   (b) Endoscopic retrograde cholangiopancreatography (ERCP) must be replaced with MR cholangiopancreatectomy for the diagnosis of cholelithiasis.
   (c) Manometry of the sphincter of Oddi is NOT technically successful in 20% of cases.
   (d) Endoscopic sphincterotomy is one of the therapeutic approaches.
6. What is the mechanism of morphine-induced rapid filling of the gallbladder on hepatobiliary scan?
   (a) More hepatic secretion of the radiotracer
   (b) Increased tonicity of the sphincter of Oddi
   (c) Contraction of the gallbladder
   (d) Dilatation of the cystic duct

7. Which of the following hematological diseases is presented by a small spleen in hepatosplenic scintigraphy?
   (a) Polycythemia vera
   (b) Leukemia
   (c) Anemia or iron deficiency
   (d) Hypoblastic anemia
8. An increased activity in the caudate lobe is observed on the hepatosplenic scan with sulfur colloid of a 65-year-old man. What is the most probable diagnosis?
   (a) Focal nodular hyperplasia
   (b) Thrombosis of the inferior vena cava
   (c) Thrombosis of the superior vena cava
   (d) Thrombosis of hepatic veins
9. A 56-year-old man with pain and tenderness in the RUQ is presented to the emergency room. Rim sign is observed on hepatobiliary scan. What is the most probable diagnosis?
   (a) Chronic cholecystitis
   (b) Cystic duct syndrome
   (c) Acute cholecystitis
   (d) Dyskinesia of the gallbladder
10. A nubbin focal accumulation of activity near the CBD and medial to the gallbladder cavity persisting for 4 h is found on hepatobiliary scan. What is the most probable diagnosis?
   (a) Biliary tumor
   (b) Dilatation of the cystic duct
   (c) Chronic cholecystitis
   (d) Obstruction of CBD
11. A normal scan is reported for a patient highly suspected of having acute acalculous cholecystitis. Which of the following tests has the least diagnostic value?
   (a) ^{111}In-WBC scan
   (b) Hepatobiliary scan with morphine injection
   (c) CT scan of the liver and bile ducts
   (d) Sonography of the gallbladder and bile ducts
12. A 59-year-old woman experiences pain in the RUQ without fever 7 days after cholecystectomy. Hepatobiliary scan shows a region of increased uptake out of the biliary system. What is the most probable diagnosis?
   (a) Biliary obstruction
   (b) Abscess
   (c) Biliary leakage
   (d) Cholangitis

13. A hepatobiliary scan is requested for a 59-year-old woman with pain in the epigastric region and in the RUQ. She has been fasting for 7 h, and the gallbladder does NOT appear in first hour of the scan. What is the next step?
    (a) CCK administration and continuation of imaging
    (b) Morphine administration and continuation of imaging
    (c) Final interpretation of the scan with the diagnosis of acute cholecystitis
    (d) Continuation of imaging after a fatty meal
14. A hepatobiliary scan with ^{99m}Tc-BrIDA is requested to rule out acute cholecystitis in a 47-year-old patient. The gallbladder and the common bile duct are clearly observed in the first hour, but the transit of activity into the intestine is detected in the 150th min. Which item is the least likely to justify this finding?
    (a) CCK administration before scan
    (b) Gallbladder dyskinesia
    (c) Ampulla of Vater
    (d) Sphincter of Oddi dyskinesia
15. Biliary diversion surgery is performed because of biliary obstruction. The diameter of the bile ducts is reported to be normal in the postoperative evaluations, and abnormal air in the bile ducts is NOT observed. What is the recommended method for patients' follow-up?
    (a) Cholescintigraphy
    (b) Percutaneous transhepatic cholangiography
    (c) Sonography
    (d) Magnetic resonance cholangiopancreatography (MRCP)
16. Which of the following items is NOT correct about gallbladder ejection fraction?
    (a) Normal ejection fraction is greater than 50%.
    (b) Cholecystokinin must be infused during the 15th–20th min.
    (c) The decreased size of the gallbladder following cholecystokinin administration denotes the ejection fraction.
    (d) Morphine increases the internal pressure of the bile duct and moves the activity toward the cystic duct.
17. What is the recommended radiopharmaceutical for the delayed (24 h) biliary scintigraphy of patients with a bilirubin level higher than 10?
    (a) ^{99m}Tc-EDTA
    (b) ^{99m}Tc-HIDA
    (c) ^{99m}Tc-DISIDA
    (d) ^{99m}Tc-Br-IDA
18. On hepatobiliary scintigraphy:
    (a) Gallbladder secretion decreases with cholecystokinin infusion during the 15th–20th min instead of 1–2 min.
    (b) Biliary dilatation may remain after the occlusion removal.
    (c) A delay in the radiotracer entrance into the intestine is a specific finding for biliary occlusion.
    (d) This scan is NOT helpful post-cholecystectomy.

19. HIDA scan is performed on a child with suspected caroli disease. Which of the following patterns is NOT typically observed?
    (a) Photopenic regions that are gradually filled with bile
    (b) Dilatation of intrahepatic bile ducts
    (c) Prolongation of the hepatointestinal transit
    (d) Low uptake in the liver
20. Intestines appear earlier than the gallbladder on biliary scintigraphy with mebrofenin. What is the most probable diagnosis?
    (a) CBD dilatation
    (b) Morphine administration
    (c) Chronic cholecystitis
    (d) Acute acalculous cholecystitis
21. Which of the following factors does NOT influence biliary kinetics?
    (a) Total parenteral nutrition
    (b) Corticosteroids
    (c) Morphine
    (d) Cholecystectomy
22. Which of the following statements about the diagnosis of patients who experience biliary cholic after cholecystectomy is NOT correct?
    (a) Endoscopic retrograde cholangiopancreatography (ERCP) is NOT valuable for diagnosis.
    (b) ERCP is normal or non-specific for patients with type 2 or 3 sphincter of Oddi dysfunction (SOD).
    (c) Biliary scintigraphy is NOT valuable for patients with type 1 SOD who underwent endoscopic sphincterotomy.
    (d) Biliary scintigraphy before manometry is NOT helpful for the diagnosis of SOD in patients with suspected type 2 or 3 SOD.
23. In chronic cholecystitis:
    (a) Routine cholescintigraphy has low sensitivity but high specificity for diagnosis.
    (b) Sonography is the method of choice for diagnosis.
    (c) Gallbladder response to a fatty meal is abnormal in more than 80% of patients with cholelithiasis.
    (d) Rim sign around the gallbladder is a common finding.
24. Which of the following statements about hepatobiliary imaging is NOT correct?
    (a) Acute cholecystitis is accompanied by cholelithiasis in more than 90% of cases.
    (b) Real-time ultrasound is the screening method of choice for cholelithiasis.
    (c) Sludge in the gallbladder can be echogenic on sonography and cause acoustic shadows.
    (d) The prognosis of acute acalculous cholecystitis is usually worse.

25. Which of the following statements about chronic acalculous cholecystitis is NOT correct?
    (a) Evaluation of gallbladder contractility is the best diagnostic method.
    (b) It is equivalent to dyskinesia or gallbladder spasm in the literature.
    (c) CCK stimulation is more accurate and practical than fatty food technique.
    (d) The bolus injection of CCK must be performed if CCK is used for stimulation.
26. An increased hepatic uptake on liver-colloid imaging is seen in:
    (a) Gaucher's disease
    (b) Fatty liver disease
    (c) Interferon therapy
    (d) Sarcoidosis
27. A small liver on liver-colloid imaging is suggestive of:
    (a) Cirrhosis
    (b) Being due to schistosomiasis
    (c) Being due to collagen vascular disease
    (d) All of the above
28. When is the most appropriate time for the evaluation of liver function on hepatobiliary scan?
    (a) 2 min after radiotracer administration
    (b) 5 min after radiotracer administration
    (c) 10 min after radiotracer administration
    (d) 15 min after radiotracer administration

4.6.1 Answer

	A	B	C	D
1				*
2			*	
3		*		
4			*	
5		*		
6		*		
7				*
8				*
9			*	
10		*		
11		*		
12			*	
13		*		
14		*		
15			*	

16			*	
17				*
18		*		
19				*
20			*	
21		*		
22		*		
23		*		
24			*	
25				*
26			*	
27				*
28			*	

4.7 Scintigraphic Measurement of Hepatic Function

1. Which radiopharmaceutical is used in functional hepatic mass:
   (a) ^{99m}Tc-IDA
   (b) ^{99m}Tc-albumin
   (c) ^{131}I-rose bengal
   (d) ^{11}C-hyaluronan
2. Regarding the complications of liver transplantation:
   (a) The incidence of graft rejection is 70%.
   (b) The most common cause of death is biliary leakage and peritonitis.
   (c) Scintigraphic pattern of graft rejection is similar to that of intrahepatic cholangitis.
   (d) The core complication is portal vein thrombosis.
3. Which of the following findings in hepatosplenic scintigraphy indicates a poor prognosis for parenchymal liver disease?
   (a) Ascite
   (b) Atrophy of liver
   (c) Massive splenomegaly
   (d) Pulmonary uptake
4. Hepatobiliary scintigraphy is performed for a patient with a history of liver transplantation. Liver uptake is normal, but the extrahepatic biliary ducts appear with delay. Moreover, parenchymal radiotracer retention is observed. What is the most probable diagnosis?
   (a) Rejection
   (b) Infection
   (c) Hepatic artery thrombosis
   (d) Thrombosis of the suprahepatic veins
5. A patient with a history of liver transplantation is presented with necrosis of the common bile duct and sepsis. Which of the complications of transplantation is predicted, and what is the recommended method for diagnosis?
   (a) Rejection, hepatobiliary scintigraphy
   (b) Obstruction and biliary leakage, sonography
   (c) Hepatic artery stenosis, hepatobiliary scintigraphy
   (d) Hepatic artery thrombosis, Doppler sonography
6. What is the radiopharmaceutical of choice for the evaluation of liver transplantation?
   (a) ^{99m}Tc-sulfur colloid
   (b) ^{99m}Tc-disida
   (c) ^{111}In-chloride
   (d) ^{131}I-IgG

7. What is the most common cause of allograft liver dysfunction after liver transplantation?
   (a) Rejection
   (b) Biliary disorders
   (c) Vascular disorders
   (d) Infection
8. The ^{99m}Tc-labeling of … is helpful for hepatogram and for the determination of hepatic extraction fraction.
   (a) Sulfur colloid
   (b) Erythrocyte
   (c) Galacrosil serum albumin
   (d) Mebrofenin
9. Scintigraphic evaluation of a rejected liver transplant:
   (a) An abnormal ^{99m}Tc-IDA scan is NOT a specific finding.
   (b) Scintigraphic findings are specific.
   (c) A sequential study is NOT helpful for therapeutic monitoring.
   (d) Cholestasis is one of the symptoms of rejection.
10. What is the most common radiopharmaceutical for the evaluation and imaging of pancreas transplantation?
   (a) ^{99m}Tc-sestamibi
   (b) ^{111}In-labeled platelets
   (c) ^{99m}Tc-HMPAO
   (d) ^{99m}Tc-MAG3

4.7.1 Answer

	A	B	C	D
1		*		
2			*	
3				*
4	*			
5				*
6		*		
7	*			
8				*
9	*			
10	*			

Suggested Readings

1. Ahmadzadehfar H, Biersack HJ, Freeman LM, Zuckier L. Clinical nuclear medicine, 2, Springer Heidelberg;2018
2. Ell PJ, Gambhir SS. Nuclear medicine in clinical diagnosis and treatment. 3rd ed. Edinburgh: Churchill Livingstone; 2004.
3. Sandler MP, Coleman RE, Patton JA, Th Wackers FJ, Gottschalk A. Diagnostic nuclear medicine. 4th ed. Philadelphia: Lippincott & Williams Wilkins; 2003.
4. Henkin RE. Nuclear medicine. 2nd ed. Philadelphia: Mosby Elsevier; 2006.

Nuclear Medicine in Acute Care

5

5.1 Nuclear Cardiology and Cardiac Transplantation

1. What is the gold standard diagnostic test for cardiac transplant rejection?
   (a) PET
   (b) ^{123}I-IPPA
   (c) MRI
   (d) Endomyocardial biopsy
2. All of the following radionuclide imaging methods are examined for the diagnosis of cardiac transplant rejection *except*:
   (a) ^{99m}Tc-annexin V
   (b) Radiolabeled somatostatin analog
   (c) ^{111}In-antimyosin
   (d) ^{11}C-MQNB

5.1.1 Answer

	A	B	C	D
1				*
2				*

M. Assadi et al., *Principles of Nuclear Medicine*,
https://doi.org/10.1007/978-3-319-91701-6_5

5.2 Cardiovascular Conditions: Venous Thrombosis

1. Regarding radionuclide venography (RNV):
   (a) The negative RNV cannot exclude the presence of deep vein thrombosis (DVT).
   (b) It can be used as a screening test.
   (c) In ascending dynamic RNV, the injection is performed antecubitally.
   (d) In static RNV, the administration of radiopharmaceutical is usually performed in the pedal veins.
2. Impedance plethysmography (IPG):
   (a) IPG can detect most calf thrombi.
   (b) IPG is unable to detect thrombi that produce obstruction in the thigh.
   (c) Congestive heart failure can lead to false-negative results.
   (d) Peripheral arterial disease can reduce the accuracy of the test.
3. All of the following statements regarding Doppler ultrasonography are true *except*:
   (a) It has high accuracy in patients with initial episodes of DVT.
   (b) False-positive results are generally related to incompressibility of the iliac and femoral veins.
   (c) It fails to distinguish between recent and chronic thrombi.
   (d) Collateral formations, which are best seen on RNV, are also visualized on ultrasonography.
4. What is the most common site of bilateral DVT and its rate?
   (a) Femoro–saphenous junction, 30%
   (b) External–internal iliac junction, 40%
   (c) Ilio–femoral junction, 18%
   (d) Iliac–IVC junction, 20%
5. Which of the following findings on static RNV is the most indicative of acute DVT?
   (a) A focal hot spot with a network of collaterals on ^{111}In-platelet scan
   (b) A segmental hot spot with a network of collaterals on ^{111}In-platelet scan
   (c) A focal hot spot without a network of collaterals on ^{111}In-platelet scan
   (d) A segmental hot spot without a network of collaterals on ^{111}In-platelet scan
6. What is the mechanism of ^{111}In-platelet accumulation in regions of active thrombosis?
   (a) Chemisorption
   (b) Compartmental localization
   (c) Cell sequestration
   (d) Capillary blockade

7. Which item is NOT correct about ^{99m}Tc-apcitide scan?
   (a) It is a synthetic peptide.
   (b) It binds to glycoprotein IIa and IIIb receptors on the surface of the platelets.
   (c) It has high sensitivity for distinguishing acute and chronic thrombosis.
   (d) Aspirin and heparin increase the incidence of false-negative results.
8. What is the dilution effect in venography?
   (a) It represents the complete vascular occlusion where dilution occurs.
   (b) A normal condition indicating the perfusion of organs with drainage to the corresponding vessels.
   (c) It indicates hemangioma in the corresponding vessels.
   (d) This condition is observed in vascular grafts and indicates a partial occlusion.
9. A patient with a history of deep vein thrombosis underwent thrombolytic therapy. On radionuclide venography 9 months after the base scan, the involved vein is thinner than the opposite site and has less activity. In addition, collaterals are also observed. Which item is the most probable?
   (a) The findings represent a deficiency in resolving the thrombosis.
   (b) Thrombosis is progressing.
   (c) Thrombosis is resolving.
   (d) Venography is NOT indicated for follow-up.
10. On radionuclide venography:
    (a) The frog leg position is helpful for the differentiation of superficial and deep veins.
    (b) A high volume of pertechnetate significantly decreases the image quality especially in post-phlebitic syndrome.
    (c) A tourniquet can help to increase the radiotracer entrance into the superficial veins.
    (d) A hot spot pattern is the pathognomonic sign of deep vein thrombosis.
11. Which of the following statements regarding ascending dynamic radionuclide venography is NOT correct?
    (a) Obstruction of popliteal vessels is usually associated with frequent collaterals.
    (b) Obstruction of iliac vessels is usually associated with frequent collaterals.
    (c) The extent of collateral network depends on grade, size, and age of vein thrombosis.
    (d) The absence of the observation of a vein is NOT indicative of an obstruction in the entire length of the vein.
12. Which of the following statements about the diagnosis of deep vein thrombosis (DVT) is NOT correct?
    (a) Sonography of regions inferior to the knee is less valuable.
    (b) ^{99m}Tc-apcitide is valuable for the diagnosis of acute DVT.
    (c) If the patient is overweight, ^{99m}Tc-apcitide is less valuable.
    (d) ^{99m}Tc-apcitide can also be used for the diagnosis of DVT in the upper limbs.

13. All of the following veins can be evaluated properly by ultrasonography *except*:
    (a) Iliac vein
    (b) Popliteal vein
    (c) Femoral vein
    (d) Posterior tibial vein
14. All of the following statements regarding the sonographic assessment of the lower limb veins are correct *except*:
    (a) Compressability assessment has sensitivity of 90–95%.
    (b) Non-visibility of thrombosis in the proximal veins does NOT exclude thrombosis in the system.
    (c) A duplicated deep vein causes a false-positive result.
    (d) The value of sonography in addition to the detection of thrombosis is the diagnosis of underlying conditions.
15. What is the next step for the evaluation of a patient with signs and symptoms suggestive of acute DVT if Doppler ultrasonography is normal?
    (a) CT scan
    (b) Contrast venography
    (c) ^{99m}Tc-apcitide
    (d) MRI
16. ^{99m}Tc-apcitide and contrast venography are the most consistent in:
    (a) DVT of the calf.
    (b) DVT of the knee.
    (c) DVT of the thigh.
    (d) Consistency is equal for all three regions.
17. What is the main effect of anticoagulant administration on the outcome of ^{99m}Tc-apcitide scan?
    (a) Increase in the incidence of false-negative outcomes
    (b) Increase in the incidence of false-positive outcomes
    (c) Decrease in the incidence of false-negative outcomes
    (d) No effect
18. What is the target organ of the ^{99m}Tc-apcitide scan?
    (a) Bladder
    (b) Gallbladder
    (c) Lungs
    (d) Liver
19. Deep vein thrombosis (DVT):
    (a) Most patients with pulmonary emboli do NOT exhibit DVT.
    (b) Sonography is recommended for screening high-risk asymptomatic patients.
    (c) The accuracy of MRI for the detection of DVT is low.
    (d) The accuracy of CT scan for the detection of DVT is low.

5.2.1 Answer

	A	B	C	D
1		*		
2				*
3				*
4			*	
5		*		
6	*			
7				*
8		*		
9			*	
10	*			
11	*			
12			*	
13				*
14			*	
15			*	
16			*	
17				*
18	*			
19	*			

5.3 Pulmonary Embolism

1. In pulmonary embolism (PE):
   (a) A low false-positive rate of the D-dimer test enables it to be used as a screening tool.
   (b) In a high clinical suspicion, a normal D-dimer assay should preclude imaging to ascertain PE.
   (c) Ultrasound has replaced conventional venography in detecting thrombus above the knee.
   (d) Postmortem studies have shown that 20% of hospitalized patients have PE.
2. Which sign of PE on plain chest radiography is rare?
   (a) Westermark's sign
   (b) Fleischner sign
   (c) Hampton's hump sign
   (d) Cavitation
3. What is the gold standard for examining PE?
   (a) CT pulmonary angiography
   (b) MR angiography
   (c) Pulmonary angiography
   (d) Ventilation/perfusion scan
4. The absorbed radiation dose attributable to CT pulmonary angiography is approximately equivalent to:
   (a) 40 chest radiographs
   (b) 140 chest radiographs
   (c) 400 chest radiographs
   (d) 240 chest radiographs
5. The accuracy of a single-slice CTPA for the detection of subsegmental PE is …, and the rate of pure subsegmental PE is ….
   (a) <10%, 50%
   (b) <25%, 30%
   (c) <10%, 30%
   (d) <25%, 50%
6. Complete matching on the V/Q scan is seen in:
   (a) Pleural effusion
   (b) Lobar pneumonia
   (c) Bronchial asthma
   (d) Gross cardiomegaly
7. Which pulmonary vasculitis disease affects medium-sized and large arteries of the pulmonary vasculature and gives V/Q scans indistinguishable from PE?
   (a) Systemic lupus erythematosus (SLE)
   (b) Polyarteritis nodosa
   (c) Wegener's granulomatosis
   (d) Takayasu's arteritis

8. What is the technique of choice for the demonstration of chronic thromboembolic pulmonary hypertension (CTEPH)?
   (a) MR angiography
   (b) V/Q scan
   (c) CT angiography
   (d) V/Q scan + chest radiograph
9. Compared with CTPA, V/Q scan is considered the initial examination for patients with:
   (a) Cardiorespiratory diseases
   (b) A consolidation on chest radiograph
   (c) Objective risk factor
   (d) Normal chest radiograph
10. What is the best radiologic method for the detection of pulmonary emboli?
   (a) CT with contrast
   (b) CT angiography
   (c) MRI
   (d) MRI angiography
11. What is the most suitable radiopharmaceutical for a pulmonary ventilation scan in a pregnant woman with suspected emboli?
   (a) ^{99m}Tc-DTPA aerosol
   (b) ^{133}Xe
   (c) ^{81m}Kr
   (d) ^{99m}Tc-technegas
12. Regarding ventilation/perfusion scan, the defect in ventilation scan is worse than that of perfusion. Which of the following diseases should be considered?
   (a) COPD
   (b) Cardiomegaly
   (c) Lobar pneumonia
   (d) All of the above
13. On a V/Q scan, an incomplete match indicates:
   (a) Asthma
   (b) Infarct
   (c) Pleural effusion
   (d) Sickle cell disease
14. Which statement regarding ventilation scan is NOT correct?
   (a) The down-scatter effect of high-energy Kr on Tc gate is important.
   (b) ^{99m}Tc-colloid scan can be utilized as aerosol.
   (c) ^{99m}Tc-technegas precipitation is less observed in the central airway than ^{99m}Tc-DTPA.
   (d) Aerosol scan can be performed before or after perfusion scan.

15. Regarding pulmonary perfusion scan, the reduction of particle number is NOT required in:
    (a) Pregnancy.
    (b) Pulmonary hypertension.
    (c) Right-to-left shunt.
    (d) Reduction of particle number is required for all items.
16. What is the most common source of non-acute emboli-mediated V/Q mismatch?
    (a) Previous unresolved pulmonary emboli
    (b) Pulmonary vasculitis
    (c) Fibrosing mediastinitis
    (d) Hilar carcinoma
17. Reversed mismatch is NOT a common finding in:
    (a) Lobar pneumonia
    (b) Pleural effusion
    (c) Cardiomegaly
    (d) Pulmonary vasculitis
18. The probability of pulmonary emboli is … when triple-match defects are observed on a pulmonary V/Q scan.
    (a) Low
    (b) High
    (c) Intermediate
    (d) Negative study
19. When PIOPED II criteria are applied, which finding is indicative of a low probability for pulmonary emboli?
    (a) Single-matched defect
    (b) Non-segmental defects
    (c) Subsegmental defects
    (d) Non-high/Non-low defects
20. Which of the following diseases represents ventilation defects in addition to perfusion defects?
    (a) Pleural effusion
    (b) Cardiac arrhythmia
    (c) Pulmonary infarction
    (d) Pulmonary hypertension
21. According to PIOPED II criteria, what is the likelihood of pulmonary emboli when perfusion defects are smaller than radiographic defects?
    (a) Very low
    (b) Low
    (c) Moderate
    (d) High

22. Pulmonary perfusion scan is requested for a patient with hemoptysis, dyspnea, and pleurisy. What is the possibility of pulmonary emboli before scintigraphy?
    (a) 29%
    (b) 31%
    (c) 74%
    (d) 87%
23. What is the reason for the hepatosplenic uptake on a pulmonary perfusion scan?
    (a) Right-to-left cardiac shunt
    (b) Free technetium in the radiotracer
    (c) Reduced technetium in the ^{99m}Tc- MAA complex
    (d) High level of aluminum in the kit
24. Which of the following statements about the recommendations for Tc-MAA application on a pulmonary perfusion scan is NOT correct?
    (a) Storing of the kit in a refrigerator before and after preparation.
    (b) Shaking of the prepared tracer in all stages.
    (c) The minimum number of administered particles for a uniform picture is one million.
    (d) Injection of the drug with larger needles.
25. Which of the following radiotracers does NOT need advanced equipment for radioprotection on a pulmonary ventilation scan?
    (a) ^{99m}Tc-technegas
    (b) ^{81m}Kr
    (c) ^{133}Xe
    (d) a and b
26. What is the reason behind the high activity of the head and kidneys on a pulmonary perfusion scan?
    (a) Inappropriate particle size
    (b) Possibility of metastasis
    (c) Existence of free technetium
    (d) Right-to-left shunt
27. What is the reason for a hot spot on a pulmonary perfusion scan?
    (a) Administration of radiotracer in the prone position
    (b) Obstruction of airways
    (c) Perfusion defect
    (d) Entrance of blood to the syringe
28. Activity is observed in the trachea and stomach during a pulmonary ventilation scan:
    (a) Left-to-right shunt.
    (b) The exam is performed by ^{99m}Tc-DTPA.
    (c) The exam is performed by ^{133}Xe.
    (d) The aerosol production system is contaminated.

29. In which patients is the reduction of particle count required?
    (a) Elderly patients
    (b) Patients with a high risk of emboli
    (c) Patients with asthma
    (d) Patients with pulmonary hypertension
30. On a perfusion–ventilation scan:
    (a) ^{133}Xe ventilation scan after a perfusion scan is the most appropriate scan because of the high quality of wash-out images.
    (b) A perfusion scan should be performed before a ventilation scan because if it is normal, there would be no need for a ventilation scan.
    (c) An aerosol scan is usually performed before a perfusion scan in the upright position.
    (d) A ventilation scan with carbon-labeled particles has a notable advantage over an aerosol scan.
31. Which of the following statements on V/Q SPECT is true?
    (a) V/Q SPECT has higher sensitivity and specificity than V/Q planar in the detection of PE.
    (b) The detection rates of the subsegmental defects are the same.
    (c) The V/Q SPECT should be conducted in a sitting position.
    (d) The ventilation SPECT is undertaken immediately after the perfusion SPECT without patient movement.
32. What is the radiotracer of choice for the evaluation of infants, children, or patients with low compliance?
    (a) ^{99m}Tc aerosols
    (b) ^{81}-Kr
    (c) ^{133}Xe
    (d) ^{81}-Rb
33. Regarding the pulmonary perfusion scan for pregnant women:
    (a) A pulmonary perfusion scan is recommended before ventilation scan.
    (b) A pulmonary ventilation scan is recommended before perfusion scan.
    (c) The sequence of the ventilation and perfusion scans is NOT important.
    (d) Ventilation and perfusion scans are contraindicated in pregnancy.
34. A middle-aged patient with acute dyspnea is evaluated. Chest X-ray is normal. V/Q scan finds a single segmental perfusion defect with a medium-size and normal ventilation. No risk factor for emboli and no evidence for DVT are found. What is the next step?
    (a) Pulmonary artery angiography
    (b) Pulmonary angiography with computerized tomography
    (c) Intravenous heparin and anticoagulant
    (d) Repeat of V/Q scan after 1 week

35. Two regions with large segmental perfusion defects are observed on the pulmonary perfusion scan of a patient suspected of having pulmonary emboli. Ventilation scan on the same day is required to interpret the study. Which of the following radiopharmaceuticals requires the computerized subtraction of ventilation and perfusion images for a precise interpretation?
    (a) ^{127}Xe
    (b) ^{81m}Kr
    (c) ^{99m}Tc-DTPA aerosol
    (d) ^{133}Xe
36. What is the advantage of ^{133}Xe on a pulmonary ventilation scan?
    (a) The possibility of imaging in different projections
    (b) Low energy of gamma ray
    (c) The possibility of a dynamic imaging of ventilation
    (d) High image resolution
37. What is the cigar sign?
    (a) Enlargement of a tight pulmonary artery on pulmonary radiography.
    (b) It is equivalent to the fissure sign on a pulmonary perfusion scan.
    (c) It is observed on a pulmonary ventilation scan.
    (d) It is observed on both pulmonary perfusion and ventilation scans.
38. The focal retention of xenon is reported on a pulmonary ventilation scan. What is the most probable diagnosis?
    (a) Pneumonia
    (b) Chronic bronchitis
    (c) Pulmonary emboli
    (d) Congestive heart failure
39. What is the maximum acceptable interval between chest X-ray and pulmonary perfusion if the goal is to compare the two tests?
    (a) 48 h
    (b) 5 days
    (c) 12 h
    (d) 4 h
40. What is the best injection technique if the goal is the homogenous diffusion of ^{99m}Tc-MAA in the entire field of both lungs?
    (a) Sitting position, slow and deep breathing, bolus injection of the radiopharmaceutical
    (b) Sitting position, breath-holding, bolus injection of the radiopharmaceutical
    (c) Supine position, breath-holding, radiopharmaceutical injection for 10 s
    (d) Supine position, slow breathing, radiopharmaceutical injection for 10 s
41. Ventilation and CXR are normal. However, an intermediate defect in the posterior inferior segment of the left lower lobe is observed on the perfusion scan. What is the possibility of pulmonary emboli according to the modified PIOPED criteria?
    (a) Very low
    (b) Low
    (c) Intermediate
    (d) High

42. What is the probability of pulmonary emboli according to the modified PIOPED criteria and to the following V/Q scan and CXR results? "Large perfusion defects that involve all lateral inferior and posterior inferior segments as well as the upper segment of the right lower lobe. Minor infiltration in the upper segment of the right lower lobe in CXR. Ventilation scan is normal."
    (a) Very low
    (b) Low
    (c) Intermediate
    (d) High
43. What is the probability of pulmonary emboli according to the modified PIOPED criteria and to the following V/Q scan and routine imaging methods? "Intermediate perfusion and ventilation defect in the lateral inferior segment of the right lower lobe, with a corresponding consolidation in the CXR."
    (a) Very low
    (b) Low
    (c) Intermediate
    (d) High
44. What is the probability of pulmonary emboli according to the modified PIOPED criteria and to the following V/Q scan and CXR results? "Two defects on the perfusion scan: one involves 75% of the lateral segment of the right middle lobe, and the other involves 90% of the upper segment of the right lower lobe. Ventilation scan is normal, whereas CXR shows Westermark's sign in the right lower lobe."
    (a) Very low
    (b) Low
    (c) Intermediate
    (d) High
45. For the diagnosis of pulmonary emboli with PET scan:
    (a) On-site cyclotron is NOT required.
    (b) Ventilation scan is performed with $^{15}O\text{-}CO_2$.
    (c) A rapid washout of CO_2 is observed in the embolic region.
    (d) A perfusion scan is performed.
46. The pulmonary perfusion scan shows a large perfusion defect corresponding to the CXR finding. What is the possibility of pulmonary emboli according to the Biello criteria?
    (a) High
    (b) Intermediate
    (c) Low
    (d) Very low
47. CT angiography demonstrates pulmonary emboli in a 69-year-old patient with dyspnea. Which abnormality is the least possible on chest X-ray?
    (a) Hampton's hump
    (b) Patchy opacities
    (c) Pleural effusion
    (d) Atelectasis

48. A ventilation–perfusion scan is performed for a patient with dyspnea. Multiple large matched defects are observed, and some regions have normal perfusion. Conversely, CXR is normal. What is the probability of pulmonary emboli?
    (a) Low
    (b) Intermediate
    (c) High
    (d) Very low
49. An 87-year-old woman with a history of COPD suddenly experiences dyspnea. V/Q scan shows a dominant hypoventilation and hypoperfusion region that completely occupies a lobe. What is the next recommended step?
    (a) Pulmonary arteriography
    (b) Bronchoscopy
    (c) Repeat after 48 h
    (d) MRI
50. About 5 cc of a solution containing 20 mCi of pertechnetate is added to a kit containing 150,000 particles of MAA. How much (cc) of this radiopharmaceutical must be injected for a perfusion scan of a patient with pulmonary hypertension?
    (a) 0.5
    (b) 0.7
    (c) 0.9
    (d) 1.5
51. Which item is NOT correct about ventilation scan?
    (a) The half-life of ^{127}Xe is greater than that of ^{133}Xe.
    (b) Ventilation scintigraphy with ^{127}Xe produces better-quality images than that with ^{133}Xe.
    (c) A medium-energy collimator must be applied for the scan with ^{127}Xe.
    (d) A ventilation scan with ^{127}Xe after a perfusion scan decreases the quality of images.
52. A defect is found on the perfusion scan of a patient with a history of dyspnea. The size of this defect in the CXR is greater than that on a perfusion scan. What is the risk of pulmonary emboli based on the PIOPED II criteria?
    (a) Very low
    (b) Low
    (c) Intermediate
    (d) High
53. Multiple hot spots are found in both lung fields on a pulmonary perfusion scan of a patient with suspected pulmonary emboli. What is the next suitable intervention?
    (a) Anticoagulants
    (b) Follow-up without treatment
    (c) Pulmonary ventilation scan
    (d) Repeat of the perfusion scan

54. In which view of the pulmonary perfusion scan is the observation of the stripe sign NOT reliable?
   (a) Anterior
   (b) Posterior
   (c) Posterior oblique
   (d) Lateral
55. Which statement about the radiation exposure of a patient on a pulmonary perfusion scan is correct?
   (a) It is less than the exposure on a chest X-ray.
   (b) It is equivalent to the exposure on a chest X-ray.
   (c) It is much less than the exposure on a lung CT.
   (d) It is equivalent to the exposure on a lung CT.
56. Pulmonary perfusion and ventilation scan is requested for a patient suffering from COPD. Which radiopharmaceutical is the most appropriate for a pulmonary ventilation scan?
   (a) ^{133}Xe-gas
   (b) ^{81m}Kr-gas
   (c) ^{99m}Tc-technegas
   (d) ^{99m}Tc-DTPA aerosol
57. A pulmonary perfusion scan is requested for a patient. The rapid termination of the scan is considered because of agitation and poor general condition. Which of the following scan views can be omitted?
   (a) Anterior
   (b) Posterior oblique
   (c) Anterior oblique
   (d) Lateral
58. A 39-year-old breastfeeding woman with dyspnea and hemoptysis is referred for a pulmonary perfusion scan. Which of the following statement about the discontinuation of breastfeeding after the ^{99m}Tc-MAA scan is correct?
   (a) Breastfeeding can be continued.
   (b) Breastfeeding must be discontinued for 24 h.
   (c) Breastfeeding must be discontinued at a time interval of 24–48 h after injection.
   (d) Breastfeeding must be discontinued at a time interval of 6–24 h after injection.
59. A patient is referred for a pulmonary perfusion scan. Which statement about the labeling of the MAA kit and its storage is correct?
   (a) It must be used in 3 h after labeling.
   (b) The labeled kit must be stored in a refrigerator.
   (c) The kit must be stored at room temperature before labeling.
   (d) The pH of the kit must be 8–9.

60. A patient is referred with a history of trauma and dyspnea from last week. A reverse mismatched defect is observed on the V/Q scan. What is the most probable cause of this pattern?
    (a) Acute pulmonary thromboemboli
    (b) Fat emboli
    (c) Functional intrapulmonary right-to-left shunt
    (d) Pulmonary vasculitis
61. A patient with an endobronchial obstruction due to a mucous plug is referred for a V/Q scan. What is the expected scan pattern?
    (a) A region with hypoperfusion and hypoventilation occupying a complete lobe
    (b) Segmental mismatched defect
    (c) Non-segmental mismatched defect
    (d) Normal scan
62. A patient with severe respiratory problems is referred for a pulmonary perfusion/ventilation scan. Which of the following radiopharmaceuticals can be used if a negative pressure room is NOT available?
    (a) ^{133}Xe gas
    (b) ^{127}Xe gas
    (c) ^{81m}Kr gas
    (d) ^{99m}Tc-technegas
63. In which of the following conditions should the minimum particle count be injected for a pulmonary perfusion scan?
    (a) Heart failure
    (b) COPD
    (c) Pulmonary hypertension
    (d) Systemic hypertension
64. Which of the following diseases has a similar pattern to that of emboli on a pulmonary perfusion/ventilation scan?
    (a) Bacterial pneumonia
    (b) Heart failure
    (c) COPD
    (d) Pulmonary vasculitis
65. What is the most common clinical symptom of pulmonary emboli?
    (a) Pleuritic pain
    (b) Tachypnea
    (c) Tachycardia
    (d) Cough
66. If the goal is to conduct a ventilation scan, which of the following radiotracers must be used before a perfusion scan?
    (a) ^{127}Xe
    (b) ^{81}Kr
    (c) DTPA aerosol
    (d) ^{133}Xe

67. A 56-year-old man is referred with dyspnea and chest pain. Multiple match defects in both lungs are observed on the perfusion and ventilation scans. What is the most probable diagnosis?
    (a) Pulmonary emboli
    (b) Pulmonary artery hypoplasia
    (c) Vasculitis
    (d) Asthma
68. New defects are found in the repeat of a pulmonary perfusion scan 1 week after the first scan of a patient with pulmonary emboli. Which of the following statements is NOT correct?
    (a) They can be due to the resolution of large defects and obstruction of other capillaries.
    (b) Changes in the regional pulmonary blood pressure can convert partial obstruction to complete obstruction.
    (c) They can be due to increased pleural effusion or pulmonary edema.
    (d) They are definitely due to the repeat of emboli.
69. Which of the following situations can cause a multifocal increase in uptake on a pulmonary perfusion scan with ^{99m}Tc-MAA?
    (a) Clotting in radiotracer syringe
    (b) Multiple pulmonary emboli
    (c) Presence of free ^{99m} technetium
    (d) Pulmonary parenchymal disease
70. What is the most common differential diagnosis of acute emboli on a pulmonary perfusion scan?
    (a) Fat emboli
    (b) Bronchogenic carcinoma
    (c) Vasculitis
    (d) Incomplete resolution of previous thromboemboli
71. Which of the following groups of patients with suspected emboli does NOT have the required criteria for the indication of venography of the lower extremities?
    (a) Normal V/Q scan, strong clinical suspicion
    (b) Low probability on the V/Q scan, intermediate clinical suspicion
    (c) Intermediate probability on the V/Q scan, low clinical suspicion
    (d) High probability on the V/Q scan, strong clinical suspicion
72. A patient is suspected of having pulmonary emboli. In which of the following conditions is pulmonary angiography with contrast contraindicated?
    (a) Peptic ulcer
    (b) Left bundle branch block
    (c) History of thrombocytopenia due to heparin
    (d) Intracranial neoplasm
73. Which of the following items is NOT necessary for a pulmonary perfusion scan?
    (a) Radiotracer injection in the supine position
    (b) Avoidance of clotting in the syringe
    (c) Imaging in the supine position
    (d) Shaking of the syringe before injection

74. All statements about pulmonary emboli are correct *except*:
    (a) Resolution begins 2 weeks after thrombosis.
    (b) One-third of patients are asymptomatic.
    (c) Dyspnea and tachypnea are the most critical clinical findings.
    (d) Radiologic findings are NOT specific.
75. On a perfusion scan with MAA:
    (a) The minimum count of administered particles is 500,000.
    (b) The minimum count of administered particles is 60,000–100,000.
    (c) The number of administered particles is equal between children and adults.
    (d) The number of administered particles is NOT important or harmful.
76. What is the first diagnostic step in diagnosing pulmonary emboli?
    (a) CXR and ECG
    (b) Measurement of the D-dimer
    (c) Pulmonary perfusion scan
    (d) Spiral CT scan
77. The stripe sign is observed on a pulmonary scan. What is the most probable diagnosis?
    (a) Pulmonary emboli
    (b) Pulmonary obstructive disease
    (c) Bronchogenic carcinoma
    (d) Pulmonary hypertension
78. Which of the following pulmonary ventilation radiotracers is produced by cyclotron?
    (a) ^{133}Xe
    (b) ^{81m}Kr
    (c) ^{99m}Tc-DTPA aerosol
    (d) ^{127}Xe
79. Which of the following pulmonary ventilation radiotracers is NOT appropriate for the measurement of regional ventilation?
    (a) ^{99m}Tc-DTPA aerosol
    (b) ^{133}Xe
    (c) ^{81m}Kr
    (d) ^{127}Xe
80. If … is used for a pulmonary perfusion scan, then the subsequent ventilation scan is NOT reliable.
    (a) ^{133}Xe
    (b) ^{81m}Kr
    (c) ^{99m}Tc-DTPA aerosol
    (d) ^{127}Xe
81. Which of the following interventions is rational if the goal is to prevent a false-positive interpretation in future scans of patients with acute pulmonary emboli and susceptibility for frequent embolism?
    (a) Radiography of lungs 3 months after acute emboli
    (b) Baseline CT scan 3 months after acute emboli
    (c) Baseline V/Q scan 3 months after acute emboli
    (d) Baseline MRI 3 months after acute emboli

82. Which of the following statements about chest X-ray for the evaluation of pulmonary emboli is NOT correct?
    (a) Radiographic findings are non-specific but suggestive.
    (b) Diaphragmatic rising and consolidation is a common finding.
    (c) Improvement of parenchymal defects takes about 1–4 weeks.
    (d) Cavitation is common in pulmonary infarction despite the absence of a secondary infection.
83. All of the following situations are considered contraindications for pulmonary artery arteriography *except*:
    (a) High risk for anticoagulant therapy
    (b) High right ventricular and pulmonary artery pressures
    (c) Renal failure
    (d) Left bundle branch block
84. About the pulmonary artery arteriography of patients with confirmed pulmonary emboli:
    (a) DVT is positive in more than 50% of these patients.
    (b) DVT is positive in less than 20% of these patients.
    (c) NO evident relationship exists between DVT and pulmonary emboli.
    (d) All patients have a history of DVT.
85. Which of the following parameters is indirectly represented by the total count of ^{81m}Kr in pulmonary static images?
    (a) Tidal volume
    (b) End-expiration volume
    (c) End-inspiration volume
    (d) Proximal respiratory zone volume
86. In the laboratory analysis of the D-dimer:
    (a) High incidence of false-negative results.
    (b) Rule out pulmonary emboli in patients with a low probability of pulmonary emboli.
    (c) It is NOT indicated as a screening method.
    (d) It is a completely specific test.
87. A segmental mismatched defect with an intermediate size is observed on a V/Q scan. What is the most probable diagnosis?
    (a) Pulmonary emboli with high probability
    (b) Pulmonary emboli with intermediate probability
    (c) Pulmonary emboli with low probability
    (d) Bronchogenic carcinoma
88. If two or more mismatched large perfusion defects are observed on a V/Q scan, what is the probability of pulmonary emboli according to the modified PIOPED criteria?
    (a) Low
    (b) High
    (c) Intermediate
    (d) Negative

89. On the perfusion/ventilation scan, the patterns of all of the following situations are similar to that of emboli *except*:
    (a) Atelectasis
    (b) Chronic perfusion insufficiency due to previous emboli
    (c) Intravenous addicts
    (d) Hilar or mediastinal diseases (usually bronchogenic carcinoma)
90. A 54-year-old patient with dyspnea is presented. Chest X-ray is normal. Perfusion of the left lung is normal, but the absence of the perfusion of the right lung is observed. What is the probability of pulmonary emboli according to the PIOPED II criteria?
    (a) High
    (b) Intermediate
    (c) Low
    (d) Very low
91. A woman on her nineth month of pregnancy is referred to the emergency room with sudden dyspnea and cough. Swelling of the superficial veins of the leg and tenderness of the leg are observed upon physical examination. What is the recommended method for diagnosis?
    (a) Thoracic CT
    (b) Lung perfusion scan
    (c) Pulmonary CT angiography
    (d) Treatment according to the primary diagnosis without nuclear imaging
92. What is the most common nonfatal complication of contrast pulmonary angiography?
    (a) Hemoptysis
    (b) Renal failure
    (c) Arrhythmia
    (d) Pneumonia
93. Which of the following methods provides the most diagnostic information aside from that on the ruling out of pulmonary emboli?
    (a) Perfusion/ventilation scan
    (b) Pulmonary angiography with contrast
    (c) Doppler sonography
    (d) CT angiography
94. If the pulmonary perfusion scan is normal for a patient with suspected pulmonary emboli, then a ventilation scan:
    (a) Is NOT required
    (b) Is required
    (c) Must be delayed
    (d) b and c
95. Which of the following diseases is associated with the Westermark's sign?
    (a) Localized pleural effusion
    (b) Pulmonary infarction
    (c) Regional oligemia
    (d) Pulmonary vascular dilatation

96. Which of the following diseases is associated Hampton's hump sign?
    (a) Localized pleural effusion
    (b) Pulmonary infarction
    (c) Weakened pulmonary vessels
    (d) Pulmonary vascular dilatation
97. Which of the following diseases is associated with the Fleischner sign?
    (a) Localized pleural effusion
    (b) Pulmonary infarction
    (c) Weakened pulmonary vessels
    (d) Prominent central pulmonary artery
98. A 44-year-old woman with a history of immobility for 3 months due to femoral neck fracture is presented with cough, chest pain, and dyspnea. She is taking OCP and antihypertensive drugs. She has tachycardia, tachypnea, and fever upon clinical examination. In addition, CXR shows a pleural-based infiltration and plural effusion. Her perfusion lung scan is unremarkable. What is the best next diagnostic test?
    (a) Ventilation scan
    (b) Pulmonary angiography
    (c) Spiral CT scan
    (d) Sputum smear
99. All the following statements regarding the assessment of pulmonary emboli on chest X-ray are true *except*:
    (a) Localized peripheral oligemia is the most common finding on chest X-ray.
    (b) Dilatation of the central pulmonary artery is commonly due to huge emboli.
    (c) Wedge-shaped opacity commonly occurs in the posterior and lateral costophrenic regions.
    (d) Opacity following emboli is resolved in 7–10 days.
100. Which of the following properly describes fat pulmonary embolism?
    (a) It occurs in the first 24 h post-trauma.
    (b) It develops hemorrhagic pulmonary edema with an air space pattern.
    (c) It is usually accompanied with pleural effusion.
    (d) CT angiography is the diagnostic modality of choice.
101. The lung perfusion scan shows a 2 cm defect without activity, whereas the ventilation scan and chest X-ray are normal. What is the probability of a pulmonary embolism occurring?
    (a) Less than 5%
    (b) 5–20%
    (c) 20–80%
    (d) More than 80%
102. Which of the following findings on central pulmonary emboli without infarction is the least likely to be found?
    (a) Localized peripheral oligemia
    (b) Volume loss
    (c) Distended proximal vessels
    (d) Air space opacification

103. A 58-year-old male smoker with suspected pulmonary embolism (PE) is presented. Based on clinical indicators, the probability for PE is high. Basal haziness and chronic obstructive pulmonary disease (COPD) changes on the chest X-ray are seen. What is the next best step?
   (a) CT angiography
   (b) D-dimer assay if it is abnormal and then CT angiography
   (c) V/P scan if the probability is high and then commencement of therapy
   (d) V/P scan if the probability is high and then CT angiography
104. A 39-year-old lady is presented to a university clinic with recent dyspnea and chest pain. CXR shows a density in the lower left lobe. In addition, a severe perfusion defect on the perfusion scan in the left lower lung with normal ventilation is reported. What is the most appropriate diagnosis?
   (a) Left lung emboli
   (b) Left lung infarction
   (c) Left lung emboli accompanied with infarction
   (d) Left lung pneumonia
105. The following is reported on a lung perfusion/ventilation scintigraphy: severe perfusion defect with a moderate ventilation defect in the left lower lung. What is the most appropriate diagnosis?
   (a) Left lung emboli
   (b) Left lung infarction
   (c) Left lung emboli accompanied with infarction
   (d) Left lung pneumonia
106. Which is the most accurate modality for the diagnosis of pulmonary emboli?
   (a) HRCT
   (b) Lung perfusion/ventilation scintigraphy
   (c) Angiography
   (d) MRI
107. To diagnose pulmonary emboli (PE), a V/Q scan should be performed rather than CT in all of the following conditions *except*:
   (a) Normal chest X-ray
   (b) Pregnancy
   (c) Low probability of PE
   (d) Patient in intensive care
108. Which ventilation scan produces the lowest radiation to a patient?
   (a) Xe.
   (b) Kr.
   (c) Tc-DTPA aerosol.
   (d) Radiation exposure is equal in all three tests.
109. In which of the following situations is a pulmonary perfusion scan NOT indicated for the diagnosis of pulmonary emboli?
   (a) Renal failure.
   (b) Anaphylactic reaction to contrast media.
   (c) Pregnancy.
   (d) Pulmonary perfusion scan is the method of choice in all patients with suspected pulmonary emboli.

110. Which of the following items is the advantage of CT pulmonary angiography (CTPA) over V/Q SPECT?
   (a) Radiation dose
   (b) Technical failure rate
   (c) Role and accuracy in follow-up
   (d) Specificity
111. Which of the following items is the advantage of V/Q SPECT/CT over V/Q SPECT?
   (a) Sensitivity
   (b) Specificity
   (c) Possible allergic reaction
   (d) Technical failure rate

5.3.1 Answer

	A	B	C	D		A	B	C	D
1			*		56	*			
2				*	57			*	
3			*		58		*		
4			*		59		*		
5		*			60			*	
6			*		61	*			
7				*	62				*
8		*			63			*	
9				*	64				*
10		*			65		*		
11			*		66				*
12				*	67				*
13		*			68				*
14				*	69	*			
15	*				70				*
16	*				71				*
17				*	72		*		
18			*		73			*	
19		*			74	*			
20			*		75		*		
21	*				76	*			
22			*		77		*		
23			*		78				*
24			*		79	*			
25		*			80	*			
26				*	81			*	
27				*	82				*
28		*			83	*			
29				*	84	*			

30		*			85	*			
31	*				86		*		
32		*			87		*		
33	*				88		*		
34		*			89	*			
35			*		90			*	
36			*		91		*		
37	*				92			*	
38		*			93	*			
39			*		94	*			
40				*	95			*	
41			*		96		*		
42				*	97				*
43			*		98				*
44				*	99		*		
45		*			100	*			
46		*			101			*	
47	*				102				*
48	*				103	*			
49		*			104	*			
50	*				105		*		
51				*	106			*	
52	*				107				*
53				*	108			*	
54				*	109				*
55				*	110				*
					111		*		

5.4 Non-embolic Disease of the Lungs

1. What is the best ventilation agent for the assessment of parenchymal lung diseases?
   (a) ^{133}Xe
   (b) ^{99m}Tc-DTPA aerosol
   (c) ^{81m}Kr
   (d) Technegas
2. Which radioaerosol is NOT used for the assessment of mucociliary clearance (MCC)?
   (a) ^{99m}Tc-sulfur colloid
   (b) ^{99m}Tc-HAS
   (c) ^{99m}Tc-iron oxide
   (d) ^{99m}Tc-DTPA
3. Mucociliary clearance (MCC) is normal in:
   (a) Chronic bronchitis
   (b) Acute asthma
   (c) Emphysema
   (d) Cystic fibrosis
4. Which radiopharmaceutical is NOT used in lung clearance studies?
   (a) 51Cr-EDTA
   (b) ^{99m}Tc-DTPA
   (c) ^{99m}Tc-HMPAO
   (d) ^{99m}Tc-HAS
5. The Marquardt–Levenberg method is used in:
   (a) Pulmonary endothelial study
   (b) Lung clearance study
   (c) Mucociliary clearance (MCC) study
   (d) V/Q study
6. Which test is recommended to diagnose COPD at the earliest time?
   (a) Pulmonary endothelial study
   (b) Mucociliary clearance (MCC) study
   (c) Lung clearance study
   (d) V/Q study
7. Which radiopharmaceutical is used on a pulmonary endothelial study?
   (a) ^{113m}In-transferrin
   (b) ^{99m}Tc-sulfur colloid
   (c) 51Cr-EDTA
   (d) ^{99m}Tc-HMPAO
8. Which of the following conditions result in the rapid clearance of mucociliary?
   (a) Smoking
   (b) Cystic fibrosis
   (c) Glucocorticoid administration
   (d) Oxygen therapy

9. Which statement corresponds to the pulmonary perfusion scan in a patient with primary pulmonary hypertension after a unilateral lung transplant?
   (a) Approximately symmetric perfusion on both sides.
   (b) Transient reduction in the perfusion of the transplanted lung.
   (c) Perfusion is mostly shifted to the transplanted lung.
   (d) Increased perfusion to the native lung that is reversed after a few weeks.
10. Which radiotracer is recommended for the differentiation of pulmonary Kaposi's sarcoma from lymphoma?
   (a) Thallium
   (b) Gallium
   (c) In-111-labeled liposome
   (d) FDG-PET
11. Perihilar pulmonary absorption is observed on the gallium scan of a patient with AIDS. Which one is the most probable?
   (a) Pneumocystis carinii
   (b) Infection with mycobacterium avium-intracellulare
   (c) Lymphocytic interstitial pneumonia
   (d) Diffuse infiltrative lymphocytosis syndrome
12. Which of the following better defines "curve a" in the expiration phase of pulmonary flow–volume graphs?
   (a) Normal inspiration
   (b) Obstructive lung disease
   (c) Restrictive lung disease
   (d) Normal expiration

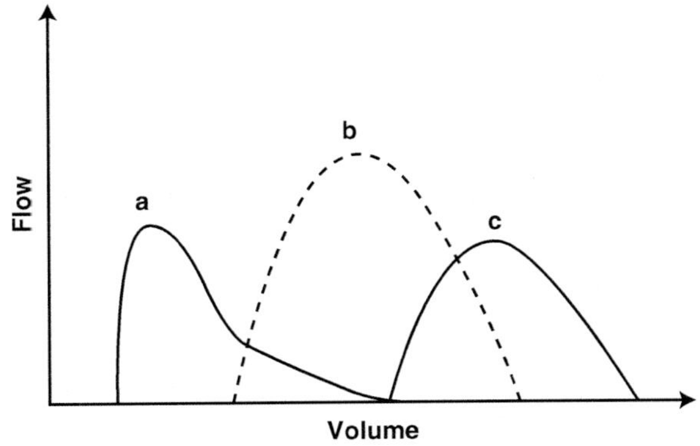

13. A pulmonary perfusion/ventilation scan is performed on a 38-year-old woman with sudden dyspnea and chest pain. The right lung does NOT appear on the perfusion scan and is smaller than the left lung on the ventilation scan. Radiography outcome is normal. What is the most probable diagnosis?
   (a) Previous surgery of the right lung
   (b) Extensive emboli
   (c) Extensive atelectasis
   (d) Takayasu disease

14. A homogenous view is reported in the washing phase of a ^{133}Xe ventilation scan. However, the wash-out phase shows a slow, nonhomogenous activity with retention of radioactivity in some spots. What is the most probable diagnosis?
    (a) Obstructive airway disease
    (b) Pulmonary emboli
    (c) Multiple tumoral lesions
    (d) Restrictive lung disease
15. Which of the following diseases is represented by an abnormal pulmonary ventilation scan?
    (a) Neoplasm-induced vascular pressure
    (b) Pulmonary vasculitis
    (c) Pulmonary infarction
    (d) Pulmonary emboli
16. Which radiopharmaceutical is NOT used for the evaluation of the activity of sarcoidosis?
    (a) Ga-67
    (b) F-18-FDG
    (c) Tc-99m-octreotide
    (d) All of the above
17. In the evaluation of a shunt in a child with Fallot's tetralogy:
    (a) Particle count must be less than 10,000.
    (b) Freshly prepared kits should be used.
    (c) Both.
    (d) None.
18. What is the minimum volume of a detectable hemoptysis with a labeled RBC scan?
    (a) 30 ml/24 h
    (b) 40 ml/24 h
    (c) 50 ml/24 h
    (d) 60 ml/24 h
19. Which of the following indices is used for the evaluation of intrathoracic shunts on a pulmonary perfusion scan?
    (a) Activity of the brain/lung
    (b) Activity of the right kidney/administered dose
    (c) Activity of the lung/right kidney
    (d) Activity of the brain/administered dose
20. In which of the following diseases is an alveolar clearance scan with radioaerosol indicated?
    (a) Chronic obstructive pulmonary disease (COPD)
    (b) Bronchiectasis and cystic fibrosis
    (c) Dysfunction of the pulmonary vascular endothelium such as acute respiratory distress syndrome (ARDS)
    (d) Interstitial lung disease (ILD)

21. What are the corresponding changes in alveolar compliance (AC) and airway resistance (AR) in a 55-year-old woman with idiopathic pulmonary fibrosis?
    (a) Decrease in AC, increase in AR
    (b) Decrease in AC, decrease in AR
    (c) Increase in AC, increase in AR
    (d) Increase in AC, decrease in AR
22. What are the corresponding changes in alveolar compliance (AC) and airway resistance (AR) in a 69-year-old man with chronic bronchitis?
    (a) Decrease in AC, increase in AR
    (b) Decrease in AC, decrease in AR
    (c) Increase in AC, increase in AR
    (d) Increase in AC, decrease in AR
23. Which item is NOT an indication for a quantitative pulmonary scan?
    (a) Evaluation and follow-up of patients with a congenital complicated heart disease
    (b) Before surgery or radiotherapy in patients with lung cancer
    (c) Infarction due to pulmonary emboli
    (d) Follow-up of patients with a lung transplant
24. Pneumonectomy of the right lung is indicated because of a right-to-left functional shunt for a 67-year-old patient with dyspnea. FVE1 is 1300 ml before surgery, and the proportion of the right lung in the conjugated image is 40% of the total. Which statement about the possibility of pneumonectomy is correct?
    (a) Dorsal image must be used for this evaluation; therefore, the calculated percentage of perfusion is not reliable.
    (b) Complete pneumonectomy of the right lung is possible.
    (c) Only partial pneumonectomy of the right lung is possible.
    (d) Pneumonectomy is NOT possible.
25. ^{99m}Tc-MAA injection is performed on the foot of a child with a Glenn shunt (SVC anastomosis of the right pulmonary artery) because of Fallot's tetralogy. What is the scan appearance?
    (a) All of the tracer accumulates in the right lung.
    (b) All of the tracer accumulates in the left lung.
    (c) Some of the radiopharmaceutical accumulates in the left lung and some in the systemic organs.
    (d) Some of the radiopharmaceutical accumulates in the right lung and some in the systemic organs.
26. A 75-year-old man underwent one-lung transplantation. V/Q scan is performed on the following day. A substantial shift of perfusion occurs toward the transplanted lung with a small shift of ventilation. What is the primary cause of the disease?
    (a) Pulmonary fibrosis
    (b) Chronic pulmonary emboli
    (c) Primary pulmonary hypertension
    (d) Emphysema

27. A patient is referred to the nuclear medicine center to evaluate the opening of a peritoneovenous shunt. The intraperitoneal administration of ^{99m}Tc-MAA is used for the scan. There is NO activity in the shunt or lungs until 1 h after injection. What is the best intervention for this patient?
    (a) Delayed imaging until 6 h
    (b) Reinjection of activity and imaging for 1 more hour
    (c) Immediate performance of thorax SPECT
    (d) Termination of the study and report of complete obstruction of the shunt
28. The focal retention of xenon is reported on a pulmonary ventilation scan. What is the most probable diagnosis?
    (a) Pneumonia
    (b) Chronic bronchitis
    (c) Pulmonary emboli
    (d) Congestive heart failure
29. Pulmonary perfusion scan is conducted on a patient with a history of dyspnea and cor pulmonale evidence. Which of the following patterns is indicative of a primary idiopathic pulmonary hypertension?
    (a) Non-segmental patchy defects
    (b) Segmental defects
    (c) Large defects
    (d) Solitary lobar defect
30. A patient with a history of severe primary pulmonary hypertension underwent surgery with no complication. A quantitative pulmonary perfusion scan is conducted. What is the perfusion of the transplanted lung immediately after and 1 month after surgery, respectively?
    (a) Approximately 90% and gradually decreases
    (b) Approximately 70% and gradually increases
    (c) Approximately 65% with no change over time
    (d) Approximately 20% and gradually increases
31. Which of the following methods is the most sensitive for the evaluation of obstructive airway diseases?
    (a) CXR
    (b) ^{133}X-single breath image
    (c) ^{133}X-equilibrium wash-in image
    (d) ^{133}X-wash-out phase
32. Pulmonary perfusion scan is performed for the detection of emboli, and activity is observed in the systemic organs. Which of the following views is recommended for the differentiation of a right-to-left shunt from the presence of free technetium–pertechnetate?
    (a) Kidneys
    (b) Thyroid
    (c) Stomach
    (d) Brain

33. Pulmonary clearance:
    (a) Clearance of the upper segments is faster than that of the lower segments because of the chronic administration of crack.
    (b) Rate of clearance decreases in alveolitis.
    (c) The normal rate of clearance is 20–30% per min.
    (d) It is NOT valuable for the early diagnosis of interstitial pneumonitis in AIDS.
34. Which of the following drugs does NOT inhibit mucociliary clearance in a breathing system?
    (a) Benzodiazepines
    (b) Glucocorticoids
    (c) Opiates
    (d) Barbiturates
35. What is the pattern of a ^{67}Ga pulmonary scan in patients with progressed systemic multiple sclerosis with pulmonary involvement?
    (a) Diffuse uptake mainly in the lower zones matched with chest X-ray.
    (b) Diffuse uptake mainly in the lower zones mismatched with chest X-ray.
    (c) Diffuse uptake mainly in the upper zones matched with chest X-ray.
    (d) Global multifocal pulmonary uptake mismatched with chest X-ray.
36. What is the formula for calculating the penetrating index in a mucociliary clearance study?
    (a) Peripheral activity of the right lung/central activity of the right lung
    (b) Central activity of the right lung/peripheral activity of the right lung
    (c) Peripheral activity of the left lung/central activity of the left lung
    (d) Central activity of the left lung/peripheral activity of the left lung
37. In which of the following conditions is right lung perfusion greater than that of the left lung?
    (a) Interventricular septal defect
    (b) Pulmonary artery stenosis
    (c) Pulmonary artery valve stenosis
    (d) Pulmonary artery stenosis and left-to-right shunt
38. What is the recommended method for bronchoscopy selection after the aspiration of a small material in children?
    (a) ^{133}Xe ventilation scan
    (b) Radiography
    (c) Fluoroscopy
    (d) MRI
39. What is the recommended radiotracer for the evaluation of pulmonary hemorrhage?
    (a) ^{99m}Tc-DTPA aerosol
    (b) ^{99m}Tc-SC
    (c) ^{99m}Tc-MAA
    (d) ^{99m}Tc-DTPA

40. Mucociliary (MCC) clearance:
    (a) MCC is normal in stable asthma patients.
    (b) ^{99m}Tc-MAA is the most common radioaerosol for the evaluation of MCC.
    (c) Oxygen therapy can cause mucociliary dysfunction.
    (d) The initial rapid phase represents the non-mucociliary clearance from the tracheobronchial tree.
41. Which of the following cells does NOT express transferrin receptors?
    (a) Lung cancer cells
    (b) Alveolar macrophages in pulmonary idiopathic fibrosis
    (c) Epithelioid cells of granuloma in sarcoidosis
    (d) Alveolar cells in interstitial pneumonia
42. Regarding the clearance of ^{99m}Tc-DTPA aerosol:
    (a) Clearance is slow in patients with adult respiratory distress syndrome.
    (b) Clearance is fast in smokers.
    (c) Clearance decreases in alveolitis.
    (d) Clearance decreases in children with hyaline membrane disease.
43. A 29-year-old woman comes to your clinic with acute dyspnea. Chest X-ray shows a decreased volume with attenuated vessels in the right lung. Ventilation/perfusion scintigraphy reveals a markedly diminished ventilation, delay in washout, vascular flow, and unilateral perfusion in the right lung. What is the most likely diagnosis?
    (a) Swyer–James syndrome
    (b) Primary central pulmonary artery occlusion
    (c) Hyponastic lung
    (d) Follicular bronchiolitis
44. All statements regarding pulmonary scintigraphy in children are correct *except*:
    (a) The number of alveoli increases fast in neonates and during the first and reaches the level of adults at the age of 8 years.
    (b) The injected particle count should not exceed 50,000 in neonates and 165,000 at the age of 1 year.
    (c) The recommended particle count is less than 10,000 for cases with severe neonatal lung disease.
    (d) The recommended particle count is about 100,000 for the quantitative evaluation of the right-to-left shunt
45. Which of the following radiotracers can be used for the measurement of mucociliary clearance?
    (a) ^{99m}Tc-MAA
    (b) ^{99m}Tc-SC
    (c) Tc-DTPA aerosol
    (d) a and b

5.4.1 Answer

	A	B	C	D
1				*
2				*
3			*	
4				*
5			*	
6		*		
7	*			
8			*	
9			*	
10		*		
11		*		
12		*		
13				*
14	*			
15			*	
16				*
17			*	
18			*	
19	*			
20			*	
21	*			
22			*	
23			*	
24		*		
25			*	
26			*	
27				*
28		*		
29	*			
30	*			
31				*
32				*
33	*			
34	*			
35		*		
36	*			
37	*			
38	*			
39		*		
40		*		
41				*
42		*		
43	*			
44				*
45				*

5.5 Gastrointestinal Bleeding

1. Which of the following agents is NOT used in Meckel's diverticulum scintigraphy?
   (a) Pentagastrin
   (b) Barium sulfate
   (c) Cimetidine
   (d) Glucagon
2. What pathological condition is associated with false-positive Meckel's diverticulum scintigraphy?
   (a) Duplication cyst
   (b) Intussusception
   (c) AVM
   (d) All of the above
3. Which item is NOT recommended to find the source of occult gastrointestinal bleeding on a ^{99m}Tc-labelad RBC scan?
   (a) Utilization of cinematic images
   (b) Shielding of the liver and spleen
   (c) Utilization of a large-field camera
   (d) In vitro labeling of RBC
4. In Meckel's diverticulum scan:
   (a) A positive Tc scan is still possible when parietal cells are absent in Meckel's diverticulum.
   (b) Similar to cimetidine, glucagon administration before scan reduces the Tc secretion and is beneficial.
   (c) Images are taken in two phases, namely, angiographic and static, for 30 min.
   (d) Fasting before scintigraphy is NOT necessary, especially for children.
5. If the goal is to localize the GI bleeding with labeled RBC scintigraphy, then:
   (a) Hemorrhagic gastritis is specifically detectable.
   (b) If bleeding appears in late views, the error of localization increases.
   (c) Vasopressin should be administered after a positive scan.
   (d) Cinematic images are not recommended.
6. Which item about the criteria for the diagnosis of GI bleeding with RBC is NOT correct?
   (a) Dynamic or serial static imaging should be applied.
   (b) Abnormal activity increases over time.
   (c) A focal region with an accumulated uptake that does not move along the intestine is the most specific finding.
   (d) Abnormal activity can move opposite of intestinal motility.

7. Meckel's scan is requested for a 16-month-old girl with melena. The patient underwent barium study 1 day ago, and she has taken cimetidine for 2 days. Which statement is correct?
   (a) The scan is negative regarding the existence of ectopic gastric mucosa.
   (b) The scan must be repeated.
   (c) Cimetidine administration is not sufficient.
   (d) The results are indicative of intestinal duplication.
8. ^{99m}Tc RBC scan is requested for the evaluation of GI bleeding. A high uptake in the stomach is observed at 1 h images without focal abdominal or pelvis activity. Which statement regarding the mentioned view is NOT correct?
   (a) It is associated with the time of generator elution.
   (b) It is associated with the RBC labeling technique.
   (c) Neck scintigraphy can help in the diagnosis.
   (d) Repeat of scan with ^{99m}Tc-SC is useful.
9. ^{99m}Tc-sulfur colloid scan is performed on a 34-year-old patient with melena for the localization of bleeding. Which of the following should be observed?
   (a) Fasting for at least 2 h.
   (b) The radiotracer must be changed if hepatic cirrhosis is predicted.
   (c) Imaging begins with 30 frames, with each frame for 60 s (a total of 30 min imaging).
   (d) 10 mCi of the radiotracer is administered through IV.
10. A 67-year-old woman with abdominal pain and a history of gastric cancer is evaluated. Liver hemangioma scintigraphy is requested because of the suspicious findings on CT scan from the previous day. The patient takes antihypertensive and antidiabetic medications. Which of the following agents or drugs does NOT affect the labeling of RBC?
    (a) Metformin
    (b) Recent contrast media
    (c) Amlodipine
    (d) Propranolol
11. In which of the following scintigraphy evaluations is fasting NOT required?
    (a) Gastric emptying scintigraphy for the diagnosis of gastric delay
    (b) Esophagus transit scintigraphy for the diagnosis of esophageal functional disorders
    (c) Bile duct scintigraphy for the diagnosis of acute cholecystitis
    (d) RBC scan for the diagnosis of GI bleeding
12. On the scintigraphic study of GI bleeding:
    (a) Some experts consider ^{111}In-RBC suitable for the detection of chronic intermittent GI bleeding.
    (b) If the hepatic function is normal, the serum half-life of Tc-sulfur colloid should be about 12.5–13.5 min.
    (c) ^{111}In is preferred over labeled Tc-pertechnetate for the diagnosis of active bleeding.
    (d) ^{99m}Tc-sulfur colloid is recommended for the diagnosis of upper GI bleeding.

13. In the scintigraphic detection of GI bleeding:
    (a) In vivo labeling of RBC increases the labeling efficiency in comparison with the in vitro method.
    (b) The required time for detecting the minimum volume of bleeding is longer for ^{99m}Tc-RBC than for sulfur colloid.
    (c) The sensitivity of the RBC scan for the diagnosis of intermittent bleeding is lesser than that of sulfur colloid scan.
    (d) Scintigraphy is more important than endoscopy if the goal is to detect upper GI bleeding.
14. In GI bleeding:
    (a) Scintigraphy after the once or twice passing of a substantial amount of blood with stool is NOT effective in the localization of bleeding.
    (b) Abdominal scan with RBC or sulfur colloid as a screening test is not helpful for the diagnosis of bleeding.
    (c) Radioisotope screening is NOT beneficial in the determination of time and region of invasive interventions.
    (d) If localization is not successful after the IV administration of a radiopharmaceutical, Tc-sulfur colloid enema may be used.
15. In Meckel's diverticulum scan:
    (a) Time has NO effect on the better observation of stomach mucosa after injection.
    (b) Fasting is NOT required for the scan.
    (c) Cimetidine does NOT inhibit the tracer uptake.
    (d) Gastric suction is always necessary.
16. Meckel's diverticulum scan is requested for a 4-year-old boy with mild diarrhea. What is the drug of choice for reducing intestinal peristalsis and the prolongation of washout?
    (a) Glucagon
    (b) Cimetidine
    (c) Pentagastrin
    (d) Diphenoxilate
17. Which item does NOT induce false-positive results in the ^{99m}Tc-RBC scan for GI bleeding?
    (a) Hemangioma
    (b) Alternative spleen
    (c) Esophageal varices
    (d) Necrotic tumor
18. Which item is the cause of both false-positive and false-negative findings on Meckel's diverticulum scan?
    (a) Bowel inflammation
    (b) Vascular aneurysm
    (c) Volvulus
    (d) Intussusceptions

19. For the preparation of a patient before Meckel's diverticulum scan:
    (a) Fasting is NOT required.
    (b) Bladder emptying is NOT required.
    (c) Laxative administration increases the diagnostic accuracy.
    (d) A recent study with oral barium brings false-negative results.
20. In which of Meckel's diverticulum imaging methods can stenosis of the diverticulum opening cause false-negative results?
    (a) Small intestine enterolysis
    (b) Small intestine transit
    (c) ^{99m}Tc- pertechnetate scan
    (d) Contrast angiography
21. Labeled RBC scintigraphy is performed for the evaluation of GI bleeding. A focal increase in uptake is observed in the RUQ persisting for 24 h. Which item corresponds to this finding?
    (a) The bleeding source is in the hepatic flexure.
    (b) The bleeding source is in the contact site of the jejunum with an ascending colon.
    (c) Retention in the renal pelvis is possible.
    (d) Liver hemangioma canNOT be excluded.
22. Total blood volume is measured on nuclear medicine based on:
    (a) Reverse transition
    (b) Isotope dilution
    (c) Reverse isotope dilution
    (d) Plasma dilution
23. Evaluation of GI bleeding in nuclear medicine:
    (a) Delayed imaging with labeled RBC provides prognostic value.
    (b) Confirmation of the bleeding is the main objective of the study.
    (c) Movement of activity in the intestine does NOT disturb accurate localization.
    (d) If sulfur colloid is used, serial imaging with reinjection of the radiopharmaceutical is NOT possible.
24. An area of increased red cell activity that does not move or progress within the bowel is usually NOT due to the site of
    (a) Ectatic aorta
    (b) Collateral vessels
    (c) Active bleeding
    (d) Aneurysm
25. False-positive findings as a result of urinary excretion of free pertechnetate can be eliminated when the images are acquired in the
    (a) Lateral view
    (b) Cinematic mode
    (c) Oblique view
    (d) SPECT

26. What percentage of patients with GI bleeding is positive only in delayed images?
    (a) Less than 30%
    (b) 30–50%
    (c) More than 70%
    (d) 27%
27. In Meckel's diverticulum scan:
    (a) Time passing after the radiotracer injection does NOT affect the appearance of gastric mucus.
    (b) Fasting is NOT required for the scan.
    (c) Cimetidine does NOT inhibit the uptake of the radiotracer.
    (d) Gastric suction is always necessary.
28. Which of the following situations does NOT induce false-positive findings in ^{99m}Tc-sulfur colloid scan for GI bleeding?
    (a) Paget's disease
    (b) Uptake in the transplanted kidney
    (c) Hemangioma
    (d) Ectopic spleen
29. A patient with a history of GI bleeding is presented. A focal region of uptake in the abdomen without a change of location during uptake is observed in ^{99m}Tc-sulfur colloid scan. What is the most probable diagnosis?
    (a) Paget's disease
    (b) Transplanted kidney
    (c) Extramedullary hematopoiesis
    (d) Accessory or ectopic spleen
30. If the goal is to enhance the sensitivity of Meckel's diverticulum scan with pertechnetate, which of the following drugs is NOT recommended?
    (a) Cimetidine
    (b) Phenobarbital
    (c) Glucagon
    (d) Pentagastrin
31. For the detection of acute GI bleeding:
    (a) ^{99m}Tc-SC scan cannot detect venous bleedings.
    (b) Angiography can detect a small amount of bleeding.
    (c) Varices and vascular disorders can be mistaken for bleeding in the initial views of the scan.
    (d) A constant focal activity in an abnormal region is primarily suggestive of bleeding.
32. A 3-year-old child is referred because of rectorrhage. What are the most probable diagnosis and radiotracer of choice, respectively?
    (a) Arteriovenous malformation, labeled RBC
    (b) Meckel's diverticulum, technetium–pertechnetate
    (c) Intestinal polyp, labeled RBC
    (d) Peptic ulcer, ^{99m}Tc-sulfur colloid

33. If the goal is to evaluate GI bleeding, what is the advantage of ^{99m}Tc-sulfur colloid over labeled RBC?
    (a) Ability to detect intermittent bleeding
    (b) Higher efficiency in detecting upper GI bleeding
    (c) Ability to detect a very low amount of bleeding
    (d) Possibility of the longer monitoring of a patient
34. Which of the following situations can cause false-negative findings in Meckel's diverticulum?
    (a) Ectopic kidney
    (b) Arteriovenous malformation
    (c) Necrotic mucosa
    (d) Inflammatory bowel disease
35. In the evaluation of gastrointestinal bleeding with labeled RBC:
    (a) Regional accumulation and bilateral spreading in delayed images indicate hemorrhage.
    (b) In vivo labeling of RBC is more efficient than in vitro.
    (c) Presence of free technetium in the kit does NOT affect the incidence of false-positive findings or the interpretation of the scan.
    (d) ^{99m}Tc-SC scan is more valuable than this method for evaluating intermittent bleeding.
36. Which of the following items increases the sensitivity of Meckel's diverticulum scan?
    (a) Bladder filling
    (b) Administration of glucagon
    (c) Administration of potassium perchlorate before scan
    (d) Feeding of the patient
37. What is the recommended radioisotope for the measurement of blood volume?
    (a) 57-Co
    (b) ^{111}-In
    (c) 51-Cr
    (d) 125-I
38. Which of the following items significantly decreases the labeling efficiency of Tc-labeled RBC?
    (a) Heparin
    (b) Fluoxetine
    (c) Anti-RBC antibody
    (d) Tetracycline
39. Which phrase regarding RBC labeling is NOT correct?
    (a) Technetium binds to globulin after cell entry.
    (b) Inadequate stannous ion increases free technetium and causes a higher background.
    (c) Higher stannous ion causes the reduction of technetium before cell entry and decreases the background.
    (d) Heparin induces the oxidation of stannous ion.

40. Which of the following factors can cause false-negative results on ^{99m}Tc scan for the diagnosis of Meckel's diverticulum?
    (a) Intussusception
    (b) Intestinal obstruction
    (c) Enteroliths in Meckel's diverticulum
    (d) Appendicitis
41. What is the best radiopharmaceutical for gastrointestinal (GI) bleeding?
    (a) ^{111}In-DTPA
    (b) ^{99m}Tc-sulfur colloid
    (c) ^{99m}Tc-DTPA
    (d) ^{99m}Tc-RBC
42. In RBC labeling with a modified in vivo method:
    (a) Incubation temperature decreases and hematocrit less than 20% inhibits labeling.
    (b) Incubation temperature increases and hematocrit less than 20% inhibits labeling.
    (c) Incubation temperature decreases and hematocrit more than 20% inhibits labeling.
    (d) Incubation temperature increases and hematocrit more than 20% inhibits labeling.
43. About the scintigraphic evaluation of gastrointestinal bleeding:
    (a) ^{111}Indium scintigraphy is more effective than ^{99m}Tc scan in detecting active bleeding.
    (b) The anatomic cause of bleeding can be discovered by scintigraphy, thus making it a suitable alternative for angiography or endoscopy.
    (c) If angiography is negative, scintigraphy alone canNOT be used for surgery.
    (d) A differential diagnosis of small intestinal bleeding from large intestinal bleeding can be performed according to the scan pattern.
44. Which of the following diseases is the least associated with ileum bleeding?
    (a) Crohn's disease
    (b) Intestinal infections
    (c) Neoplasm
    (d) Angiodysplasia
45. Which of the following statements regarding the study of gastrointestinal bleeding with ^{99m}Tc-sulfur colloid is NOT correct?
    (a) If the scan is negative, touché rectal method is recommended.
    (b) Constant activity is indicative of ectopic or accessory spleen.
    (c) Paget's disease and extramedullary hematopoiesis can cause false-positive results.
    (d) RAO view is recommended to attenuate the effect of liver activity.
46. In which region is gastrointestinal bleeding best localized?
    (a) Stomach
    (b) Duodenum
    (c) Small intestine
    (d) Colon

47. What is the minimum amount of detectable bleeding by scan?
    (a) 0.01 ml/min
    (b) 0.1 ml/min
    (c) 1 ml/min
    (d) 10 ml/min
48. A 38-year-old man is presented to the hospital with repeated rectal bleeding. His barium enema is unremarkable. What should be the next step for management?
    (a) Abdominal CT scan
    (b) RBC scintigraphy
    (c) Arteriography
    (d) Colonoscopy
49. What is the most sensitive modality for the evaluation of traumatic pancreas?
    (a) CT scan
    (b) MRI
    (c) Radionuclide scintigraphy
    (d) Ultrasonography
50. Which of the following statements about Meckel's diverticulum is NOT correct?
    (a) Meckel's diverticulum is a remnant of the vitelline duct, which is normally obliterated by 5–9 weeks of intrauterine life but persists in 1.5–3% of the population.
    (b) Complications occur in 10–20% of patients.
    (c) About 80% of symptomatic patients are under the age of 15 years.
    (d) Obstruction is the most common complication of Meckel's diverticulum in children.

5.5.1 Answer

	A	B	C	D
1		*		
2				*
3		*		
4	*			
5		*		
6			*	
7		*		
8				*
9				*
10	*			
11				*
12	*			
13		*		
14				*
15			*	

16	*			
17				*
18				*
19				*
20		*		
21				*
22		*		
23	*			
24			*	
25		*		
26			*	
27			*	
28			*	
29				*
30		*		
31			*	
32		*		
33			*	
34			*	
35	*			
36		*		
37			*	
38	*			
39			*	
40			*	
41				*
42	*			
43				*
44				*
45				*
46				*
47	*			
48				*
49	*			
50				*

5.6 Cholescintigraphy

1. What is the preferred cholescintigraphic tracer for patients with serum bilirubin higher than 10 mg/dl?
   (a) Disofenin
   (b) Mebrofenin
   (c) HIDA
   (d) DISIDA
2. In which case can morphine be administrated with confidence on cholescintigraphy?
   (a) Hyperamylasemia
   (b) Dilated cystic duct
   (c) During the first 60 min of examination in critically ill patients
   (d) Complete hepatic elimination of radioactivity
3. What is the most common source of false-positive findings in the diagnosis of acute cholecystitis?
   (a) Chronic cholecystitis
   (b) Prolonged fasting
   (c) Acalculous cholecystitis
   (d) Hepatitis
4. The rim sign on the HIDA scan:
   (a) It appears because of gallbladder perforation.
   (b) It appears because of a high radioactive entry to hepatic parenchyma due to overeating and inflammation.
   (c) Initial views are the best time for its observation.
   (d) When observed, it does not exclude morphine administration.
5. A rim sign is observed on the HIDA scan of a patient with pain in the RUQ. What is the most probable diagnosis?
   (a) Gallbladder dyskinesia
   (b) Gangrenous cholecystitis
   (c) Chronic cholecystitis
   (d) Biliary leakage
6. HIDA scan is performed on a 45-year-old woman with abdominal pain. About 0.5 h after beginning the scan and with the onset of clearance from hepatic parenchyma, an active margin of the gallbladder fossa is detected without the appearance of the gallbladder. Which item is the most appropriate decision to make?
   (a) Morphine injection
   (b) Cholecystokinin injection
   (c) Termination of scan
   (d) Continuation of scan for at least 4 h to observe the gallbladder

7. Cholecystography:
   (a) It is less sensitive for acalculous cholecystitis than for cholecystolithiasis.
   (b) The acceptable contraction of the gallbladder after CCK injection does NOT exclude cholecystitis.
   (c) Neither sonography nor CT scan can help in the diagnosis of pericholecystic abscess in patients with toxic acute cholecystitis.
   (d) Calcium blockers has NO effect on the CCK function.
8. About patients with cholecystectomy and Sphincter of Oddi dysfunction (SOD):
   (a) Biliary scintigraphy is NOT indicated for the follow-up of patients after the endoscopic opening of the Sphincter of Oddi.
   (b) Abnormal scintigraphy in patients with symptoms of relapse after treatment is NOT effective for diagnosis or therapy.
   (c) Abnormal scintigraphy before manometery increases the possibility of SOD.
   (d) Normal scintigraphy is NOT effective in diagnosing the obstruction of the Sphincter of Oddi.
9. Which finding in cholecystography is associated with the acute obstruction of the common bile duct?
   (a) Gallbladder appears 1 h after radiopharmaceutical injection.
   (b) Gallbladder does NOT appear even after morphine injection or delayed scan.
   (c) Gallbladder does NOT appear 30 min after morphine injection or delayed scan (after 4 h).
   (d) Bile ducts do NOT appear 1 h after radiopharmaceutical injection despite the notable liver uptake.
10. In patients with suspected acute cholecystitis examined by cholescintigraphy, which of the following basic imaging patterns is seen with the LEAST frequency?
    (a) Normal
    (b) Persistent GB non-visualization
    (c) Delayed GB visualization
    (d) Obstructive
11. A 58-year-old woman is referred to the emergency room with abdominal pain. Mirizzi syndrome is suggested by abdominal CT scan and ERCP. Which of the following findings is expected in cholecystography?
    (a) Gallbladder absence in delayed images up to 4 h after intestinal observation of activity
    (b) Intestinal observation of activity before 1 h and appearance of the gallbladder after another 1 h
    (c) Appearance of the gallbladder in 1–4 h with EF of less than 40%
    (d) Appearance of the gallbladder before 1 h with EF of more than 40%

12. Hepatobiliary scintigraphy is performed on a 63-year-old man with abdominal pain. Pericholecystic hot rim and a defect in the gallbladder are observed in 4 h. What is the most probable diagnosis?
    (a) Biloma due to a perforated gallbladder
    (b) Hydropic gallbladder
    (c) Gangrenous acute cholecystitis
    (d) Simultaneous chronic and acute cholecystitis
13. A scan is requested to rule out acute cholecystitis in a 46-year-old man with serum bilirubin of 12 mg/100 ml. What is the recommended dose of the technetium-labeled IDA agent?
    (a) 4 mCi
    (b) 6 mCi
    (c) 8 mCi
    (d) 10 mCi
14. What percentage of patients with symptomatic or asymptomatic chronic cholecystitis demonstrates a normal pattern?
    (a) Less than 30%
    (b) 30–50%
    (c) 55–85%
    (d) More than 86%
15. What is the diagnostic procedure of choice for the high clinical suspicion of a significant biliary tract complication following surgery?
    (a) ERCP
    (b) Cholescintigraphy
    (c) PTC
    (d) Sonography
16. Which statement about cholescintigraphy is NOT correct?
    (a) The rim sign on the scan is specific and sufficient for the diagnosis of acute cholecystitis, and morphine or delayed scan is NOT required for confirmation.
    (b) Scan findings are normal at least in 86–99% of cases with or without symptoms of chronic cholecystitis.
    (c) The absence of the appearance of the gallbladder and the rim sign after radiotracer injection in some patients is due to chronic cholecystitis confirmed by pathology.
    (d) The diagnostic accuracy of a morphine injection to confirm the opening of the cystic duct is similar to that of delayed scan (after 3 h or 4 h).
17. Hepatobiliary scintigraphy is performed on a patient with pain in the RUQ. Which of the following findings is indicative of acute cholecystitis?
    (a) Absence of the appearance of the gallbladder up to 2 h after radiotracer injection
    (b) Absence of the appearance of the gallbladder in the first 0.5 h if morphine is injected at the beginning of the scan
    (c) Absence of the appearance of the gallbladder up to 3 h after radiotracer injection
    (d) Absence of the appearance of the gallbladder at 0.5 h after morphine injection if morphine is injected in the 60th min of the scan

18. Hepatobiliary scintigraphy is performed on a patient with suspected acute cholecystitis. The gallbladder does NOT appear 1 h after radiotracer injection, although activity is detected in the intestines. Therefore, morphine is injected. Which statement is correct?
    (a) Acute cholecystitis is confirmed if the gallbladder does NOT appear in 30 min after morphine injection.
    (b) Chronic cholecystitis is confirmed if the gallbladder does NOT appear in 30 min after morphine injection.
    (c) Acute cholecystitis is most probably confirmed if the gallbladder appears in 30 min after morphine injection.
    (d) Imaging must be continued until 3 h after morphine injection to rule out chronic cholecystitis.
19. ^{99m}Tc-HIDA scan is performed on a patient with suspected acute acalculous cholecystitis. The gallbladder appears in the 45th min of the scan. Which of the following interventions is recommended if the goal is to increase the accuracy for the diagnosis of acute cholecystitis?
    (a) Morphine administration in the 60th min
    (b) Repeat of scan after intravenous CCK injection
    (c) Acquisition of 4 h delayed images
    (d) In-WBC scan
20. What is the preferred method for shortening the scan procedure in the diagnosis of acute cholecystitis?
    (a) Recommendation for 12 h fasting before the test
    (b) Termination of scan after 1 h
    (c) CCK injection 30 min before radiotracer injection
    (d) Injection of morphine if the gallbladder does NOT appear in 60 min
21. On hepatobiliary scintigraphy:
    (a) A patient with a marked reduction of gallbladder ejection fraction benefits from cholecystectomy.
    (b) The scan is abnormal in all cases with acute cholecystitis.
    (c) CCK is more commonly used than morphine for shortening the scan procedure.
    (d) Morphine decreases the incidence of false-negative findings of acute cholecystitis.
22. Which of the following conditions can cause false-negative results in the diagnosis of acute cholecystitis with gallbladder scintigraphy?
    (a) Acute acalculous cholecystitis
    (b) Prolonged fasting
    (c) Total parenteral nutrition
    (d) Non-fasting
23. Gallbladder ejection fraction is evaluated for a patient with chronic acalculous cholecystitis. Which of the following items is NOT considered an advantage of the slow infusion of CCK (30–60 min) over rapid infusion (1–2 min)?
    (a) More physiologic
    (b) No side effect
    (c) Lesser incidences of false-negative results
    (d) Better emptying

24. Which of the following situations is indicated in preferential gallbladder filling?
    (a) Decreased intra-CBD pressure
    (b) Increased gallbladder pressure
    (c) Biliary hypokinesia due to opium
    (d) Functional obstruction of the CBD
25. Which of the following conditions is associated with postcholecystectomy syndrome?
    (a) Common bile duct stimulation
    (b) Stimulation of the operated gallbladder
    (c) Sphincter of Oddi dysfunction
    (d) Choleductal stimulation
26. Which of the following statements about the rim sign is NOT correct?
    (a) The rim sign can be observed in biliary stasis.
    (b) The rim sign can be observed in hyperemia-induced radiotracer accumulation.
    (c) The sensitivity of the rim sign for acute gangrenous cholecystitis is high.
    (d) The rim sign is NOT sufficiently specific for acute cholecystitis to dismiss the requirement of a delayed scan or morphine injection.
27. On cholecystography for the diagnosis of acute cholecystitis:
    (a) A low dose of morphine (0.1 mg/kg) 60 min after radiotracer injection is the best method for the diagnosis of acute cholecystitis in patients with severe intermittent illness.
    (b) Morphine infusion is allowed in patients with symptoms of obstruction.
    (c) Morphine can help to evaluate suspected acute calculous/acalculous cholecystitis in patients with signs of a cystic duct.
    (d) The indication of morphine for patients with hyperamylasemia is agreed upon.
28. A patient with a history of cholecystectomy complains about pain in the RUQ after a fatty meal. Liver tests are abnormal, but the dilatation of the common bile duct is reported. What is the recommended method for a more accurate evaluation?
    (a) MRCP
    (b) ERCP
    (c) Cholescintigraphy
    (d) Sphincter of Oddi manometry
29. Which of the following statements about cholescintigraphy is NOT correct?
    (a) If the goal is to evaluate the Sphincter of Oddi dysfunction, then cholecystokinin is injected before the radiotracer.
    (b) Multiple injections of sincalide are possible in one study.
    (c) The delayed appearance of the intestines is NOT a specific finding for chronic cholecystitis.
    (d) If the rim sign is observed in the 1 h images, delayed imaging will NOT be required.

30. In the evaluation of gallbladder ejection fraction (GBEF) with fatty meal stimulation:
    (a) 5 g of fatty meal is required.
    (b) Calculation of GBEF should be performed 60 min after the fatty meal.
    (c) Maximum GBEF is 30 min after the fatty meal.
    (d) Fasting for 4 h before the scan is NOT required.
31. What is the best diagnostic method for chronic cholecystitis?
    (a) Hepatobiliary scan
    (b) Sonography
    (c) Oral cholecystography
    (d) Intravenous cholangiography
32. In which of the following studies is the Sostre score used?
    (a) Gastric emptying test
    (b) Evaluation of esophageal kinesis
    (c) Gastrointestinal bleeding
    (d) Hepatobiliary scan
33. A 49-year-old woman with severe abdominal pain is presented to the emergency department. On her physical examination, tenderness in the RUQ is observed. The probability of having gallstones is high. What should be the next modality in this patient's management?
    (a) Ultrasonography
    (b) Cholescintigraphy
    (c) OCG
    (d) ERCP
34. What is the most sensitive modality in the assessment of a cystic duct?
    (a) CT scan
    (b) MRI
    (c) Doppler ultrasonography
    (d) Cholescintigraphy
35. Which of the following findings properly describes Mirizzi syndrome?
    (a) Irregular mucous with an asymmetric increase in thickening of the gallbladder
    (b) Biliary obstruction, cholelithiasis, and cystic duct stone
    (c) Gallbladder dilatation and thickening without stone
    (d) Presence of echogenic foci in the dilated gallbladder wall
36. If the goal is to differentiate a choledochal cyst from other abdominal cysts, what is the most appropriate method for identifying the connection of the choledochal cyst with the bile ducts?
    (a) Transabdominal ultrasonography
    (b) MR cholangiopancreatography
    (c) Hepatobiliary scintigraphy
    (d) Endosonography

37. If the goal is to diagnose acute cholecystitis, when should morphine be injected on HIDA scintigraphy?
    (a) Concurrent with the HIDA injection for a quick procedure
    (b) When the gallbladder does NOT appear in 1 h despite the appearance of the intestines
    (c) Evident hepatic uptake without detectable secretion after 0.5 h
    (d) All of the above

5.6.1 Answer

	A	B	C	D
1		*		
2				*
3	*			
4				*
5		*		
6			*	
7	*			
8			*	
9				*
10				*
11	*			
12			*	
13		*		
14				*
15	*			
16	*			
17				*
18	*			
19				*
20				*
21	*			
22	*			
23			*	
24				*
25			*	
26			*	
27	*			
28		*		
29	*			
30		*		
31		*		
32				*
33	*			
34				*
35		*		
36			*	
37		*		

5.7 Neonatal Hyperbilirubinemia

1. Neonatal hyperbilirubinemia:
   (a) Estimated to occur in 1 out of 500,000 live births.
   (b) Males are more commonly affected than females.
   (c) There appears to be a genetic predilection.
   (d) There does not appear to be a genetic predilection.
2. In the diagnosis of neonatal hyperbilirubinemia:
   (a) The giant-cell transformation in histology can be present only in extrahepatic biliary atresia (EHBA).
   (b) The absent gallbladder is seen only in extrahepatic biliary atresia (EHBA).
   (c) The ultrasound is the diagnostic method for extrahepatic biliary atresia (EHBA).
   (d) A gallbladder larger than 1.5 cm is considered to indicate neonatal hepatitis.
3. The biliary tract is not seen even in the delayed views of the ^{99m}Tc-HIDA scan of a 3-month-old infant with hyperbilirubinemia. Otherwise, the infant is healthy. Which diagnosis is the least probable?
   (a) Cystic fibrosis
   (b) Alpha-1 antitrypsin deficiency
   (c) Alagille syndrome
   (d) Severe hepatitis
4. Biliary scintigraphy is performed on a 1-month-old infant with cholestatic icterus. The biliary tree is absent in the images. Which item is NOT probable?
   (a) Cystic fibrosis
   (b) Biliary atresia
   (c) Alagille syndrome
   (d) Alpha-1 antitrypsin deficiency
5. On a neonatal hepatobiliary scan:
   (a) No relationship exists between the amount of injected radiopharmaceutical and serum bilirubin.
   (b) The lateral view of the scan is NOT required for the observation of activity in the rectum.
   (c) Phenobarbital increases the specificity of ^{99m}Tc-IDA on biliary scintigraphy.
   (d) For infants younger than 2 months with biliary atresia, the liver–heart ratio 5 min after injection is similar to that of patients with neonatal hepatitis syndrome.
6. Which of the following findings is the most indicative of biliary atresia on hepatobiliary scintigraphy?
   (a) Decreased hepatic uptake, decreased serum clearance of the radiotracer, increased activity in the heart
   (b) Absence of the gallbladder and the common bile duct
   (c) Lack of activity in intestines up to 24 h after the administration of the radiotracer
   (d) Decreased hepatic uptake and increased renal clearance of the radiotracer

7. What is the first imaging step for a neonate with an increased level of serum bilirubin?
   (a) Hepatobiliary scintigraphy
   (b) Liver sonography
   (c) Abdominal CT scan
   (d) Hepatic scintigraphy with sulfur colloid
8. HIDA scan is indicated for neonates with suspected biliary atresia. Which statement is correct?
   (a) Intra- and extrahepatic bile ducts must be observed on a normal scan.
   (b) The administration of phenobarbital 2 days before scan increases the sensitivity of the test.
   (c) Diagnosis and treatment of the disease must be performed in the first 4 weeks after birth.
   (d) Biliary atresia and cystic fibrosis are always differentiable.
9. Which of the following statements about neonatal hepatobiliary scan and hyperbilirubinemia is NOT correct?
   (a) Retroviruses are the possible cause of biliary atresia and neonatal hepatitis.
   (b) The liver biopsy patterns of biliary atresia and neonatal hepatitis are similar.
   (c) Sonography is the first diagnostic method for neonatal conjugated hyperbilirubinemia.
   (d) Bile ducts usually appear on the scan, but the gallbladder is hardly observed.

5.7.1 Answer

	A	B	C	D
1				*
2				*
3				*
4				*
5			*	
6			*	
7		*		
8			*	
9				*

5.8 Nuclear Medicine in the Acute Care of Neurological Patients

1. The brain regions with rCBF of 12–22 ml/100 g/min are considered:
   (a) Misery perfusion
   (b) Penumbra regions
   (c) Luxury perfusion
   (d) Infarcted regions
2. Which MRI technique has become the method of choice for differentiating between irreversible damage and hypoperfused tissue?
   (a) Diffusion MRI
   (b) T2 MRI
   (c) T1 MRI
   (d) FLAIR MRI
3. What is the method of choice for the diagnosis of herpes simplex encephalitis (HSE)?
   (a) CT
   (b) PET/CT
   (c) MRI
   (d) ^{99m}Tc-HMPAO scintigraphy
4. Which scintigraphic agent is not recommended for the diagnosis of herpes simplex encephalitis (HSE)?
   (a) ^{99m}Tc-ECD
   (b) ^{99m}Tc-HMPAO
   (c) ^{99m}Tc-glucoheptonate
   (d) ^{99m}Tc-IMP
5. Which of the following findings does NOT appear on the brain scan of a patient with cerebrovascular accident?
   (a) Increased uptake in the same cerebellar hemisphere
   (b) Increased perfusion around the infarcted zone
   (c) Delayed parenchymal uptake and clearance of the involved hemisphere in the angiography phase
   (d) Shift of blood flow to the external carotid system
6. Evaluation of rCBF with SPECT is performed a few hours after stroke. In which of the following conditions is thrombolytic therapy indicated?
   (a) Acute complete absence of rCBF
   (b) No change in rCBF
   (c) Acute decrease in rCBF
   (d) Increase in rCBF
7. Brain MRI shows a focal lesion for an AIDS patient. Radiotracer accumulation in the same region is also reported on the ^{201}Tl SPECT scan. What is the most probable diagnosis?
   (a) Toxoplasmosis
   (b) Lymphoma
   (c) Tuberculosis
   (d) Fungal granuloma

8. Stroke penumbra after stroke:
   (a) It is observed before ischemic penumbra.
   (b) It is due to differentiation or disconnection.
   (c) It may be observed in subacute or chronic stroke.
   (d) This stage is before cell death and is reversible after reperfusion.
9. Oligemic zone after stroke:
   (a) It is observed before ischemic penumbra.
   (b) It is due to differentiation or disconnection.
   (c) It may be observed in subacute or chronic stroke.
   (d) This stage is before cell death and is reversible after reperfusion.
10. Diaschisis after stroke:
    (a) It is observed before ischemic penumbra.
    (b) It is due to differentiation or disconnection.
    (c) It may be observed in subacute or chronic stroke.
    (d) This stage is before cell death and is reversible after reperfusion.
11. Extended stroke penumbra after stroke:
    (a) It is observed before ischemic penumbra.
    (b) It is due to differentiation or disconnection.
    (c) It may be observed in subacute or chronic stroke.
    (d) This stage is before cell death and is reversible after reperfusion.
12. If the goal is to diagnose acute cerebral perfusion defects, how long after the event is the sensitivity of SPECT becomes higher than that of anatomical methods (CT and MRI)?
    (a) 72 h
    (b) 24 h
    (c) 48 h
    (d) 96 h
13. In which of the following conditions does FDG-PET overestimate the size of defect in brain trauma?
    (a) Cortical contusion
    (b) Intracerebral hematoma
    (c) Encephalomalacia due to trauma
    (d) Epidural hematoma
14. Which of the following statements regarding the application of PET in neurologic and psychiatric diseases is NOT correct?
    (a) Focal cerebral hypometabolism is observed in most subdural and epidural hematomas.
    (b) A relationship exists between the severity of hypometabolism and the Glasgow Coma Scale (GCS).
    (c) Hypometabolism and hypoperfusion of the thalamus on the dominant side are reported in patients with chronic refractory pain.
    (d) PET canNOT discriminate structural and functional defects in the brain.

15. Which of the following items about herpes simplex virus 1 (HSV-1) and 2 (HSV-2) is NOT correct?
    (a) HSV1 is common in adult and older children.
    (b) HSV1 causes a focal uptake in the temporal lobe.
    (c) The blood–brain barrier scan is commonly abnormal in viral infections of the brain.
    (d) HSV2 typically involves the frontal lobe.
16. What is the pattern of FDG and Tl uptake in AIDS-associated lymphoma and toxoplasmosis?
    (a) In contrast to toxoplasmosis, FDG and Tl uptake are NOT observed in lymphoma.
    (b) Both lymphoma and toxoplasmosis do NOT show FDG and Tl uptake.
    (c) Both lymphoma and toxoplasmosis show FDG and Tl uptake.
    (d) In contrast to toxoplasmosis, FDG and Tl uptake is observed in lymphoma.
17. Which scan is valuable for the evaluation of brain abscess?
    (a) Gallium scan
    (b) BBB imaging
    (c) CT scan
    (d) rCBF scan
18. In which of the following phases of cerebral infraction does the temporary loss of visibility of an infarct occur on the CT scan (fogging phenomenon)?
    (a) Acute (after hours)
    (b) Early subacute (after 1 week)
    (c) Late subacute (after 2 weeks)
    (d) Chronic (after 1 month)
19. Lesions causing acute stroke that are overlooked on a brain perfusion scan are commonly reported in:
    (a) Brain stem
    (b) Cerebellum
    (c) Cortex
    (d) Subcortical
20. A 48-year-old man is suspected to have brain death based on clinical symptoms and apnea test. Which of the following modalities has the highest diagnostic sensitivity and specificity?
    (a) ^{99m}Tc-HMPAO brain SPECT
    (b) ^{99m}Tc-pertechnetate cerebral perfusion
    (c) Electroencephalogram
    (d) ^{99m}Tc-DTPA cerebral perfusion

21. A patient with suspected herpes encephalitis is subjected to the ^{99m}Tc-HMPAO scan. What are the scan findings 1 day and 40 days after onset of the disease, respectively?
    (a) Mild increase in uptake, normal uptake
    (b) Severe increase in uptake, decrease in uptake
    (c) Severe increase in uptake on both scans
    (d) Decrease in uptake, increase in uptake
22. Which statement is NOT correct regarding the diagnosis of herpes simplex encephalitis with the ^{99m}Tc-HMPAO brain perfusion scan?
    (a) Increased uptake in the involved brain regions in the acute phase of the disease.
    (b) Increased uptake mainly in the temporal lobe.
    (c) The ^{99m}Tc-HMPAO scan is effective when the MRI is unremarkable.
    (d) Uptake in the involved brain regions increases over time.
23. What is the pattern of brain death in SPECT?
    (a) Diffuse cerebral distribution of Tc-HMPAO
    (b) Diffuse cerebral distribution of Tc-ECD
    (c) Empty skull
    (d) Observation of the sagittal sinus
24. In brain death:
    (a) Brain scintigraphy has NO role in the identification of brain death.
    (b) Hot nose sign is indicative of brain death.
    (c) Delayed cerebral activity after Tc-HMPAO injection is suggestive of brain death.
    (d) Barbiturates do NOT affect the scan pattern in brain death.
25. What is the preferred radiopharmaceutical for the confirmation of brain death in a patient in deep coma?
    (a) ^{99m}Tc-DTAP
    (b) ^{99m}Tc-ECD
    (c) ^{99m}TcO4−
    (d) ^{133}Xe
26. In acute viral encephalitis, the findings of which scan is NOT an increased uptake?
    (a) ^{99m}Tc-DTPA
    (b) ^{99m}Tc-HMPAO
    (c) ^{99m}Tc-IMP
    (d) ^{99m}Tc-ECD
27. About the evaluation of brain death in nuclear medicine:
    (a) An important sign in brain death is the lack of tracer activity in the superior sagittal sinus during the venous phase of the flow study.
    (b) In brain death, blood flow superior to the circle of Willis circulation may exist.
    (c) SPECT is necessary in all cases with suspected brain death.
    (d) Reduced flow in the scalp is also observed in brain death aside from reduced flow of ACA and MCA.

5.8.1 Answer

	A	B	C	D
1		*		
2	*			
3			*	
4	*			
5	*			
6			*	
7		*		
8				*
9	*			
10		*		
11			*	
12	*			
13				*
14	*			
15				*
16				*
17			*	
18			*	
19				*
20	*			
21		*		
22				*
23			*	
24				*
25		*		
26				*
27	*			

5.9 Radiolabeled Agents for the Localization of Infection and Inflammation

1. What is the gold standard scintigraphic technique for determining infection and inflammation?
   (a) ^{99m}Tc-MDP
   (b) ^{67}Ga
   (c) ^{99m}Tc-colloid
   (d) Radiolabeled leukocytes
2. What is the best scintigraphic technique for the diagnosis of spondylodiscitis?
   (a) ^{67}Ga
   (b) ^{99m}-Tc leukocytes
   (c) ^{111}In-leukocytes
   (d) ^{99m}Tc-colloid
3. ^{111}-In-WBC is performed on a 57-year-old man with fever of unknown origin (FUO). In the primary images, both lungs show radiotracer uptake. In the delayed images, lung activity is reduced, but hepatic uptake is increased. What is the best diagnosis?
   (a) Diffuse pulmonary vasculitis probably due to Wegener's granulomatosis
   (b) WBC damage during preparation
   (c) Drug-induced cholangitis
   (d) Normal view
4. In which of the following radiotracers does vascular permeability play the least important role in its accumulation in the infection site?
   (a) ^{67}Ga-citrate
   (b) ^{99m}Tc-HMPAO-WBC
   (c) Radiolabeled monoclonal antigranulocyte antibody
   (d) ^{111}In-IgG
5. Which method is the most effective in evaluating cerebral abscess?
   (a) ^{99m}Tc-MIBI scan
   (b) Thallium scan
   (c) MRT
   (d) CT scan
6. Which of the following regions does NOT show a radiotracer uptake on normal In-leucocyte scintigraphy?
   (a) Liver
   (b) Spleen
   (c) Breast
   (d) Bone scan
7. Radiotracer accumulation is found along the lateral and the diaphragmatic side of the liver and paracolic region on the gallium scan. Liver shows a marked decrease in uptake. What is the most probable diagnosis?
   (a) Hepatic failure
   (b) Peritonitis
   (c) Diffuse ascites
   (d) Infection of the supramesanteric space

8. If the goal is to evaluate infections, which one is NOT considered an advantage of In-leucocyte scan over gallium scan?
   (a) Higher specificity
   (b) Simple interpretation of the scan
   (c) High sensitivity for the detection of chronic infections
   (d) Better differentiation of abscess from tumor
9. In which of the following conditions is ^{99m}Tc- HMPAO-WBC preferred over ^{111}In-WBC?
   (a) A patient suspected to have an inflammatory bowel disease and quantitative calculation.
   (b) A patient with chronic fever but with no confirmed diagnosis.
   (c) A patient suspected to have urinary tract infection.
   (d) Precise localization of infection in a patient suspected to have abdominal abscess.
10. What is the mechanism of radiotracer accumulation at the infection site after ^{67}Ga-citrate injection?
    (a) Binding to lactoferrin, extravasal leakage, and binding to bacterial receptors and WBC at the infection site
    (b) Binding to leucocytes in blood circulation and accumulation at the infection site
    (c) Binding to transferrin, extravasal leakage, and binding to lactoferrin and siderophore at the infection site
    (d) Antigen–antibody bound between gallium and lactoferrin and binding to WBC receptors at the infection site
11. The In-WBC scan shows an increased uptake around the right shoulder joint, but the sulfur colloid scan is normal. What is the most probable diagnosis?
    (a) Loose prosthesis
    (b) Decreased bone marrow activity
    (c) Infection around the prosthesis
    (d) Tumoral infiltrations
12. Which organ is highly exposed to radiation after ^{111}In-WBC administration?
    (a) Spleen
    (b) Bone marrow
    (c) Gonads
    (d) Lungs
13. Which item is NOT the mechanism of ^{67}Ga uptake at the infection site?
    (a) Lymphocyte cell surface binding
    (b) Increase in vascular permeability
    (c) Bacterial siderophore binding
    (d) Macrophage uptake through iron binding
14. In which of the following conditions is gallium scan is preferred over ^{111}In-WBC?
    (a) Tissue encapsulation
    (b) Abdominal abscess
    (c) Inflammatory bowel disease (IBD)
    (d) Orthopedic infections

15. Which of the following complexes is used for WBC labeling in plasma and increases its viability and function?
    (a) ^{111}In complex with transferrin
    (b) ^{111}In complex with mercaptopyridine N-oxide and tropolone
    (c) ^{111}In-tropolone
    (d) ^{111}In-acetylacetone and tropolone
16. Which of the following patterns on the gallium scan is indicative of peritonitis in a child?
    (a) Haziness of the abdomen and pelvis, reduced uptake in the liver
    (b) Sporadic focal increase in activity in the abdomen and pelvis, increased activity in the liver
    (c) Accumulation of activity on the lateral and diaphragmatic sides of the liver, diffuse activity in the pelvis and abdomen, decreased liver uptake
    (d) Observation of a region without activity in the abdomen and pelvis, increased uptake in the liver
17. Gallium scan is performed on a patient. Diffuse abdominal uptake particularly in the liver and progression of liver uptake from the lateral border to the right subdiaphragmatic space are reported. What is the most probable diagnosis?
    (a) Hepatitis
    (b) Subdiaphragmatic abscess
    (c) Cellulitis
    (d) Peritonitis
18. For the labeling of leucocytes with technetium or indium:
    (a) In-labeled and ^{99m}Tc-labeled leucocytes have different normal distributions of activity.
    (b) The physiologic activity of ^{111}In-leukocyte in the kidneys and bladder sometimes interferes with the detection of renal defect.
    (c) High purity of the radionuclide is one of the advantages of ^{99m}Tc-labeling over indium.
    (d) No intestinal activity is observed 3 h after the intravenous administration of ^{99m}Tc-leucocyte.
19. A patient with severe and sudden spinal pain is presented. Laboratory tests show WBC of 18,000 and ESR of 56. What should be the first diagnostic procedure to be conducted?
    (a) X-ray and bone scan
    (b) X-ray and gallium scan
    (c) Gallium scan and bone scan
    (d) X-ray and sulfur colloid scan
20. A 45-year-old woman with history of L4–L5 disk surgery 20 months ago is referred with pain and intermittent fever. Bone scan shows an increased uptake in L4–L5, but the ^{111}In-WBC scan demonstrates a decreased activity. What is the most probable cause of this finding?
    (a) Acute infection
    (b) Metastasis in the region
    (c) Antibiotic administration for chronic infection
    (d) Low resolution of ^{111}In-WBC images

21. The ^{111}In-WBC scan is performed on a patient with suspected abdominal abscess. The appearance of which organ on the scan is considered normal?
    (a) Lung
    (b) Kidney
    (c) Small intestine
    (d) Colon
22. A 67-year-old woman with discopathy underwent surgical therapy 6 weeks ago. She is currently complaining about back pain. Blood test is normal, destructive changes are found on the radiography of the vertebral column, and an increased activity is detected in the delayed phase of the three-phase bone scan. Therefore, osteomyelitis is suspected. Which of the following diagnostic methods has the highest sensitivity and specificity?
    (a) ^{67}Ga SPECT
    (b) MRI
    (c) ^{111}In-labeled leukocyte scan
    (d) CT scan
23. A 32-year-old man is subjected to antibiotic therapy because of chronic osteomyelitis in the right medial tibia. What is the method of choice for therapeutic monitoring?
    (a) ^{67}Ga scan
    (b) ^{111}In-WBC scan
    (c) ^{99m}Tc-HMPAO-WBC scan
    (d) ^{201}Tl scan
24. A neonate with edema of the right ankle is referred for ^{111}In-WBC scan. What is the required blood volume for labeling?
    (a) 10 cc
    (b) 30 cc
    (c) 50 cc
    (d) 80 cc
25. Which item is the rarest cause of a false-positive result on the ^{99m}Tc-HMPAO-WBC scan?
    (a) Malignant bone tumors
    (b) Pulmonary emboli
    (c) Accessory spleen
    (d) Intermittent colon enema
26. Which of the following radiopharmaceuticals for a bone marrow scan demonstrates the least uptake in the liver and spleen?
    (a) ^{99m}Tc-nanocolloid
    (b) ^{99m}Tc-sulfur colloid
    (c) ^{99m}Tc-NS-Ab
    (d) ^{111}In-chloride

27. A 7-year-old child diagnosed with non-Hodgkin's lymphoma is subjected to chemotherapy. He suffers from granulocytopenia and is currently experiencing fever of unknown origin. A focal increase in uptake in the RLQ region is observed on the gallium scan and is present in the 24, 48, and 72 h images. What is the most probable diagnosis?
    (a) Infected appendicitis.
    (b) Typhlitis.
    (c) Delayed scan is also required for diagnosis.
    (d) Necrotizing proctitis.
28. In which of the following conditions is the discrepancy of reticuloendothelial and erythroblastic activity in the bone marrow the most common?
    (a) Metastatic lesions
    (b) Bone marrow infarction
    (c) Aplastic anemia due to chemotherapy
    (d) Radiation
29. About the application of bone marrow scan:
    (a) Radiography is more sensitive than bone marrow scan if the goal is the early detection of bone metastasis.
    (b) An increased activity in the involved region is observed in the primary stages of acute bone marrow infarction.
    (c) Bone marrow returns to its normal condition a few weeks after bone radiation.
    (d) Long bones are completely observed on the bone marrow scan of patients with sickle cell anemia.
30. What is the advantage of ^{99m}Tc-HMPAO over ^{111}-In for the labeling of WBC?
    (a) The scan can be completed in 2 h.
    (b) WBC must be separated.
    (c) It is more appropriate for the detection of chronic infection.
    (d) It is more appropriate for the detection of gastrointestinal and urinary infections.
31. In which of the following conditions is the In-leukocyte scan more effective than the gallium scan?
    (a) Evaluation of patients with fever of unknown origin without a history of surgery
    (b) Identification of the cause of fever in neutropenic patients
    (c) Diagnosis of chronic pulmonary granulomatosis defects
    (d) Evaluation of bone infection lesions
32. The uptake of ^{111}In-WBC is observed in all of the following conditions *except*:
    (a) Bacterial endocarditis
    (b) Active inflammatory bowel disease
    (c) Acute myocardial infarction
    (d) Transplanted kidney

33. In which of the following condition is the ^{111}In-labeled WBC scan has the least sensitivity?
    (a) A patient with fever and abdominal pain after hip surgery
    (b) A patient with ulcerative colitis and poor general condition for whom colonoscopy is NOT possible
    (c) A diabetic patient with suspected osteomyelitis of the metatarsal
    (d) A young man with fever and back pain after disk surgery
34. In the comparison between the gallium and ^{111}In-WBC scans:
    (a) The accumulation of ^{111}In-WBC in abscesses is greater than that of gallium.
    (b) Interpretation of the gallium scan is easier.
    (c) Gallium scan is more specific than ^{111}In-WBC scan in detecting infection.
    (d) ^{111}In-WBC shows a better uptake in chronic infections.
35. For the diagnosis of osteomyelitis with ^{111}In-leukocyte scan:
    (a) False-negative findings are observed in traumas and diabetes.
    (b) If this scan is conducted, bone scan with ^{99m}Tc-MDP is NOT required.
    (c) This scan is NOT useful for the diagnosis of vertebral osteomyelitis.
    (d) ^{111}In is more appropriate than ^{99m}Tc-HMPAO in children.
36. ^{111}In-IgG is the least valuable for the diagnosis of which type of infection?
    (a) Intrahepatic infections
    (b) Articular prosthesis infections
    (c) Pneumocystis carinii pneumonia
    (d) Early diagnosis of infection in patients with a compromised immune system
37. Bone marrow scan:
    (a) This scan is capable of differentiating between infarction and infection.
    (b) A radionuclide peripheral expansion is observed in most cases of multiple myeloma.
    (c) The scan is abnormal in the primary stages of polycythemia vera in most cases.
    (d) If the goal is to diagnose avascular necrosis of the femoral head in adults, accuracy of the radionuclide bone marrow scan is similar to that of bone scan.
38. Gallium scan:
    (a) CT scan and sonography are conducted prior to gallium scan for the diagnosis of phlegmon.
    (b) Gallium scan is NOT conducted prior to CT scan and sonography for the diagnosis of peritonitis.
    (c) Labeled-WBC scan is conducted prior to gallium scan for the detection of abdominal infection.
    (d) Gallium scan is currently NOT indicated for abdominal infections.

39. All of the following statements about the evaluation of infection with labeled leukocytes are correct *except*:
    (a) Imaging must be performed at least 4 h after injection if ^{99m}Tc-HMPAO is used for abdominal evaluation.
    (b) ^{111}In-WBC must be used for the evaluation of infection in the urinary tract.
    (c) ^{111}In-WBC is preferred for the quantitative evaluation of gastrointestinal inflammatory lesions.
    (d) ^{111}In-WBC is preferred for the concurrent evaluation of peripheral osteomyelitis with bone scan.
40. What is the recommended method for the therapeutic monitoring of a patient with malignant otitis externa?
    (a) Bone scintigraphy
    (b) Gallium scan
    (c) Nanocolloid scan
    (d) CT scan
41. Which of the following statements about WBC labeling with ^{111}In and ^{99m}Tc-HMPAO is NOT correct?
    (a) The labeling efficiency of ^{111}In-tropolon is less than that of ^{99m}Tc-HMPAO.
    (b) Complete plasma separation is required for ^{111}In-oxine.
    (c) ^{99m}Tc-HMPAO has greater affinity in the labeling of granulocytes.
    (d) ^{99m}Tc-HMPAO labeling is possible with a small amount of plasma.
42. Which of the following statements is correct?
    (a) CT scan can be used to detect phlegmon because it is a focal inflammatory defect.
    (b) When the clinical origin of sepsis is NOT clear, the labeled leukocyte scan can be used as the first diagnostic method.
    (c) Liver abscess can be diagnosed with gallium scan only.
    (d) Gallium scan can be used for differentiating between focal pancreatic abscess and pancreatitis.
43. Colloidal bone marrow scan:
    (a) The hepatosplenic uptake of nanocolloid is greater than that of sulfur colloid.
    (b) Sulfur colloid is recommended for the evaluation of bone marrow distant from the liver and spleen areas.
    (c) The background of sulfur colloid images are greater than that of nanocolloid.
    (d) The covering of the hepatosplenic region and dynamic imaging on a bone marrow scan are NOT beneficial.
44. In which of the following organs is the radiotracer uptake unremarkable 18–24 h after the injection of ^{111}In-leukocyte?
    (a) Bone marrow
    (b) Lungs
    (c) Spleen
    (d) Liver

45. Which of the following characteristics is considered an advantage of ^{67}Ga over ^{111}In-leukocyte?
    (a) Easier interpretation
    (b) More specific
    (c) Lack of accumulation in the colon and sterile wounds
    (d) Greater efficacy in chronic infections
46. In abdominal wall cellulitis:
    (a) Sonography is an efficient method for diagnosis.
    (b) CT scan is a suitable method for diagnosis.
    (c) The accuracy of the ^{67}Ga scan for diagnosis is high.
    (d) The anatomical features of cellulitis are clear.
47. In differentiating between subdiaphragmatic abscess and empyema, which modality is recommended?
    (a) CT scan
    (b) Ultrasonography
    (c) Radionuclide scintigraphy
    (d) All of the above
48. Which of the following statements about radioactive iron is NOT correct?
    (a) The quantitative evaluation of erythropoiesis can be performed by ^{52}Fe.
    (b) ^{52}Fe is more valuable than ^{99m}Tc-SC for the evaluation of bone marrow disorders in the thoracic and lumbar regions.
    (c) ^{52}Fe is indicated for the evaluation of suspected extramedullary hematopoiesis.
    (d) ^{57}Fe is a suitable alternative to ^{52}Fe because of its excellent photopeak.
49. Which of the following statements about In-chloride scan is NOT correct?
    (a) It binds to serum transferrin immediately after intravenous administration, and its half-life in plasma is 5 h.
    (b) Compared with ^{52}Fe scintigraphy, the higher dose of In-chloride is required for bone marrow evaluation.
    (c) The hepatosplenic uptake of In-chloride indicates erythropoiesis in these organs.
    (d) Five hundred rad of bone marrow radiation causes the absence of ^{52}Fe uptake but NOT In-chloride uptake.
50. Which type of cell is the least probable to react with NCA-95?
    (a) Promyelocytes
    (b) Myelocytes
    (c) Metamyelocytes
    (d) a and b
51. For the labeling of white blood cells:
    (a) Evaluation of sterility and apyrogenicity is critical after labeling.
    (b) Evaluation of leucocyte function is critical after labeling.
    (c) Imaging is performed 18–24 h after the injection of In-oxine WBC.
    (d) The presence of plasma does not interfere with the In-oxine labeling of blood cells.

52. Which of the following imaging methods earlier shows the positive findings of acute infection (e.g., osteomyelitis)?
    (a) ^{99m}Tc-MDP scan
    (b) ^{111}In-WBC scan
    (c) ^{68}Gallium scan
    (d) CT scan
53. The ^{111}In-labeled leukocyte scan is conducted prior to the ^{99m}Tc-labeled leukocyte scan in all of the following situations *except*:
    (a) Chronic infections (e.g., fever of unknown origin)
    (b) Suspected infection of the urinary tract
    (c) Quantification of the GI inflammatory process
    (d) Exact localization of the GI process
54. A 4-year-old boy is referred to the emergency ward with fever, lymphadenopathy, erythema, and edema of the cervical lymph nodes that began 5–6 days ago. Oral cephalexin was prescribed 3 days ago, but fever and edema have NOT yet diminished. The child is hospitalized and subjected to intravenous antibiotic therapy, but fever and edema continue for more than 48 h. Which of the following studies is recommended?
    (a) Gallium scan
    (b) Neck sonography
    (c) Thoracic CT scan
    (d) Neck and thorax MRI

5.9.1 Answer

	A	B	C	D
1				*
2	*			
3		*		
4		*		
5				*
6			*	
7		*		
8			*	
9				*
10			*	
11			*	
12	*			
13				*
14	*			
15		*		
16			*	
17				*
18	*			
19	*			

20			*	
21	*			
22	*			
23	*			
24	*			
25	*			
26			*	
27		*		
28				*
29				*
30	*			
31				*
32	*			
33				*
34	*			
35			*	
36	*			
37		*		
38			*	
39	*			
40		*		
41	*			
42		*		
43		*		
44		*		
45				*
46			*	
47				*
48				*
49			*	
50		*		
51			*	
52		*		
53				*
54			*	

5.10 Undiagnosed Fever

1. What is the most common tumor causing pyrexia of unknown origin (PUO)?
   (a) Colorectal cancer
   (b) Hodgkin's lymphoma
   (c) Non-Hodgkin's lymphoma
   (d) Hepatoma
2. Occult infection and pyrexia of unknown origin (PUO):
   (a) PUO is more likely to be associated with a neutrophilic infiltration.
   (b) Differentiating between PUO and occult infection is useful.
   (c) Patients categorized to have occult infection should be investigated with ^{67}Ga.
   (d) Patients categorized to have PUO should be investigated with labeled leukocytes
3. Infection is the name of
   (a) ^{99m}Tc-sulesomab
   (b) ^{99m}Tc-ciprofloxacin
   (c) ^{99m}Tc-anti-E-selectin
   (d) ^{99m}Tc-liposomes
4. Undiagnosed fever in pediatrics:
   (a) The interpretation of leukocyte scintigraphy in children is similar to that in adults.
   (b) ^{111}In-labeled cells are preferred over ^{99m}Tc-HMPAO for children.
   (c) ^{99m}Tc-HMPAO is preferred over ^{111}In-labeled cells for chronic sepsis in children.
   (d) The performance of leukocyte scintigraphy in children is different from that in adults.
5. A normal ^{67}Ga scan in the presence of obvious respiratory deterioration in an HIV patient indicates:
   (a) Very good prognosis.
   (b) Very poor prognosis.
   (c) It cannot determine the prognosis and needs further tests.
   (d) Good prognosis.
6. Fever of unknown origin (FUO) is observed in a patient after surgery. Abdominal graphy, sonography, and CT scan results are negative. What is the next step?
   (a) Scan with labeled leucocyte
   (b) Scan with labeled antibody
   (c) Gallium scan
   (d) Scan with ciprofloxacin
7. For the evaluation of a patient with fever of unknown origin:
   (a) Gallium scan is the first step.
   (b) ^{111}In-WBC scan is the first step.
   (c) Gallium scan should be considered as an imaging method for evaluating the patient.
   (d) ^{18}F-FDG is indicated when other methods canNOT provide a specific finding.

8. In the comparison between gallium and In-WBC scans for the evaluation of infectious and inflammatory processes:
   (a) In-WBC scan is more sensitive for the evaluation of sarcoidosis.
   (b) Gallium scan is preferred for the evaluation of abdominal abscess.
   (c) Gallium scan in the peripheral bones is more successful in detecting bone infection.
   (d) In-WBC scan is less sensitive for the detection of chronic osteomyelitis than that of the acute form.
9. A 64-year-old man with a history of fever for 4 weeks is evaluated. Laboratory tests are unremarkable. What is the recommended radiopharmaceutical for the diagnosis?
   (a) ^{67}Ga citrate
   (b) ^{99m}Tc-HMPAO-WBC
   (c) ^{111}In-WBC
   (d) NeutroSpec
10. What is the best radiopharmaceutical for the diagnosis of fever of unknown origin (FUO)?
   (a) Tc-HMPAO
   (b) ^{111}In-leukocyte
   (c) ^{67}Ga
   (d) ^{99m}Tc-IgG

5.10.1 Answer

	A	B	C	D
1		*		
2		*		
3		*		
4	*			
5		*		
6	*			
7			*	
8				*
9	*			
10			*	

5.11 Inflammatory Bowel Disease

1. All of the following are the principal indications for leukocyte imaging in inflammatory bowel disease (IBD) *except*:
   (a) Diagnosis of IBD especially ulcerative colitis (UC)
   (b) Ruling out of IBD in a patient with symptoms suggestive of IBD but without a diagnosis
   (c) Determination of disease distribution
   (d) Confirmation of disease relapse
2. ^{99m}Tc-HMPAO-labeled leucocyte scintigraphy reveals accumulated radioactivity in the rectum and descending colon. Which of the following items can cause such an accumulation?
   (a) Constipation
   (b) Ulcerative colitis
   (c) Pancolitis
   (d) Irritable bowel syndrome
3. A 44-year-old man with a history of IBD is experiencing fever. He has recently used antibiotics especially clindamycin. ^{111}In-WBC scan is performed to investigate the reason for the fever, and it shows generalized activity throughout the large bowel. What is the most probable diagnosis?
   (a) Scan is normal.
   (b) Pseudomembranous colitis should be considered.
   (c) Delayed scan is required for diagnosis.
   (d) b and c.
4. In-WBC scan is routinely performed 16–24 h after radiotracer injection. In which of the following conditions is a scan 2–4 h after injection also required?
   (a) Bone prosthesis
   (b) Diabetic foot
   (c) Vascular graft
   (d) Inflammatory bowel disease
5. Which of the following statements about imaging of patients with ulcerative colitis or Crohn's disease is NOT correct?
   (a) If the goal is to evaluate the whole colon in severe ulcerative colitis, scintigraphy with labeled leucocyte is preferred over colonoscopy.
   (b) If the goal is to evaluate patients with Crohn's disease suspected to have obstruction, CT scan and barium evaluation are more effective than scintigraphy.
   (c) ^{111}In-lukocyte scintigraphy is the gold standard for the diagnosis of ulcerative colitis.
   (d) Scintigraphy with labeled leukocyte is sometimes indicated for the differentiation between ulcerative colitis and Crohn's disease.
6. Which scan provides the best diagnostic findings in a patient with suspected inflammatory bowel disease?
   (a) ^{111}In-WBC
   (b) ^{99m}Tc polyclonal antibodies
   (c) ^{99m}Tc-HAMPAO WBC
   (d) ^{111}In-interleukin

7. A 47-year-old patient with a history of Crohn's is presented with diarrhea and bloody mucus that began in the previous week. What is the recommended method of evaluation?
   (a) Colonography with CT
   (b) ^{99m}Tc-HMPAO-WBC
   (c) ^{111}In-WBC
   (d) Small intestine transit with barium
8. Which of the following findings in the ^{99m}Tc-HMPAO-WBC scan of intestines has a positive predictive value of more than 90% for the diagnosis of inflammatory bowel disease?
   (a) No uptake in the 1 h scan, increased uptake in the 12 h scan
   (b) Increased uptake in the 1 h scan, decreased uptake in the 12 h scan
   (c) Increased uptake in the 1 h scan, increased intensity of initial uptake in the 3 h scan
   (d) No uptake in the 1 h scan, increased uptake in the 3 h scan
9. About ^{111}In-WBC scan:
   (a) The sensitivity of scan is NOT influenced by antibiotic therapy in chronic infections.
   (b) It is more sensitive for the detection of acute osteomyelitis than that of the chronic form.
   (c) The spleen receives most of the radiation during scan.
   (d) All of the above.
10. ^{111}In-labeled granulocyte is NOT indicated for the diagnosis of:
   (a) Ulcerative colitis
   (b) Paracolic abscess
   (c) Crohn's disease
   (d) Gastritis

5.11.1 Answer

	A	B	C	D
1	*			
2		*		
3		*		
4				*
5			*	
6			*	
7	*			
8			*	
9				*
10				*

5.12 Nuclear Imaging in Cardiovascular Infection and Cardiac Transplant Rejection

1. What is the frontline imaging method used for the diagnosis of prosthetic vascular graft infection during the late postoperative period?
   (a) MRI
   (b) CT
   (c) ^{67}Ga scintigraphy
   (d) ^{111}In-labeld leukocyte
2. What are the best modalities for the diagnosis of subacute endocarditis?
   (a) PET, MRI
   (b) Radionuclide angiogram, MRI
   (c) Echocardiography, Doppler ultrasonography
   (d) Echocardiography, MRI

5.12.1 Answer

	A	B	C	D
1		*		
2				*

5.13 The Immunocompromised Patient

1. ^{67}Ga scanning in immunocompromised patients is NOT recommended in:
   (a) Intra-abdominal infections
   (b) Lymphocytic interstitial pneumonitis
   (c) Mycobacterial lung involvement
   (d) Cytomegalovirus pneumonitis
2. A mild uptake around the hilum of the lung and an increased uptake in both orbits and adrenal glands are found on the gallium scan of a patient with AIDS. What is the most probable diagnosis?
   (a) Lymphocytic interstitial pneumonitis
   (b) Diffuse infiltrative lymphocytosis syndrome
   (c) Cytomegalovirus infection
   (d) Lymphoma with associated reaction
3. In which of the following conditions does ^{111}In-WBC have higher sensitivity than gallium scan?
   (a) Adult respiratory distress
   (b) Active pulmonary sarcoidosis
   (c) Pneumocystis carinii
   (d) None
4. What is the radiotracer of choice for the diagnosis of pneumocystis carinii in a patient with AIDS?
   (a) ^{111}In-IgG
   (b) ^{67}Ga-citrate
   (c) ^{111}In-WBC
   (d) ^{99m}Tc-anti-CD15
5. Diffused uptake of ^{67}Ga is observed in the lungs of a child with HIV. Swelling of the salivary glands, clubbing of fingers, and generalized lymphadenopathy are observed upon clinical examination. What is the most probable diagnosis?
   (a) Pneumocystis carinii pneumonia
   (b) Lymphocytic interstitial pneumonitis
   (c) Cytomegalovirus infection
   (d) Tuberculosis
6. Which of the following items is indicated by a normal gallium scan in a symptomatic patient with advanced AIDS?
   (a) Poor prognosis
   (b) Response to treatment
   (c) Saturated iron band capacity
   (d) Good prognosis
7. In which of the following conditions does ^{111}In-WBC have higher sensitivity than gallium scan?
   (a) Pulmonary active sarcoidosis
   (b) Adult respiratory distress syndrome
   (c) Pneumocystis carinii
   (d) Pneumonia in patients with AIDS

8. Gallium scan is performed on an HIV-positive patient with pulmonary symptoms. A radiopharmaceutical uptake is observed only in the lymph nodes. What is the most probable diagnosis?
   (a) Cytomegalovirus infection
   (b) Lymphoma
   (c) Bacterial pneumonia
   (d) Pneumocystis carinii
9. Which of the following diagnostic methods is the least valuable for a patient with herpes encephalitis?
   (a) Blood–brain barrier scan
   (b) ^{99m}Tc-HMPAO scan
   (c) ^{18}F-FDG-PET
   (d) CT scan
10. In cerebral HIV infection:
   (a) Multifocal reduced activity in brain ^{18}F-FDG-PET.
   (b) Multifocal increased activity in brain SPECT.
   (c) Thallium scan is NOT effective in differentiating between lymphoma and toxoplasmosis.
   (d) Increased uptake in ^{18}F-FDG-PET of patients with toxoplasmosis.
11. Which of the following methods provides high specificity and sensitivity for the diagnosis of problematic cases of brain abscess?
   (a) Blood–brain barrier scan
   (b) Labeled WBC scan
   (c) CT scan
   (d) MRI
12. In patients with brain lesions due to AIDS:
   (a) Ring sign in brain MRI is very specific for the diagnosis of the type of lesion.
   (b) Margin of the ring sign shows weak or no uptake on ^{201}Tl-SPECT in tuberculous lesions.
   (c) Margin of the ring sign shows a similar uptake in the scalp on ^{201}Tl-SPECT in toxoplasmosis.
   (d) The shape of the tuberculous lesions in MRI is completely different from that of toxoplasmosis.
13. Some ring lesions are observed in the brain MRI of a patient with AIDS. What is the method of choice for differentiating between toxoplasmosis and lymphoma?
   (a) Brain SPECT with ^{99}mTc-HMPAO
   (b) Brain SPECT with ^{201}Tl
   (c) Brain SPECT with ^{99}mTc-ECD
   (d) Brain SPECT with ^{68}Ga

14. Gallium scan is requested for an HIV+ patient with a history of PCP. An increased uptake is detected only in the upper segments of the lung. Which item is indicated by this finding?
    (a) Superimposed cytomegalovirus infection with necrosis in the medial segments
    (b) TB granuloma
    (c) Antimicrobial treatment
    (d) Superimposed Kaposi's sarcoma in the inferior segments
15. CT scan is performed on an HIV+ patient with focal neurologic symptoms. A large lesion is found in the frontal lobe. What is the recommended scan for differentiating between metastasis (lymphoma) and infection (toxoplasmosis)?
    (a) ^{67}Ga SPECT
    (b) ^{201}Tl SPECT
    (c) ^{18}F-FDG-PET
    (d) ^{99m}Tc-ECD SPECT
16. An increased uptake in the salivary glands is reported on the gallium scan of an AIDS patient. What is the most probable diagnosis?
    (a) Salivary gland malignancy
    (b) A normal finding for AIDS patients
    (c) Diffuse infiltrative lymphocytosis syndrome (DILS)
    (d) Opportunistic infection
17. A patient with chronic coronary artery disease and left ventricular dysfunction underwent heart transplantation. After surgery, he experiences fever, and multiple pulmonary nodules are found on radiography. What is the most probable diagnosis?
    (a) Nocardiosis
    (b) Pneumocystis carinii
    (c) Pneumococcus pneumonia
    (d) Aspergillus
18. What is the main finding of the pulmonary gallium scan for pneumocystis carinii pneumonia in a patient suffering from AIDS?
    (a) Negative gallium scan + abnormal radiography
    (b) Abnormal diffuse pulmonary uptake + normal radiography
    (c) Multifocal gallium uptake
    (d) Focal or regional gallium uptake
19. What is the main finding of the pulmonary gallium scan for actinomycosis in a patient suffering from AIDS?
    (a) Negative gallium scan + abnormal radiography
    (b) Abnormal diffuse pulmonary uptake + normal radiography
    (c) Multifocal gallium uptake
    (d) Focal or regional gallium uptake

20. What is the main finding of the pulmonary gallium scan for Kaposi's sarcoma in a patient suffering from AIDS?
    (a) Negative gallium scan + abnormal radiography
    (b) Abnormal diffuse pulmonary uptake + normal radiography
    (c) Multifocal gallium uptake
    (d) Focal or regional gallium uptake

5.13.1 Answer

	A	B	C	D
1	*			
2			*	
3	*			
4	*			
5		*		
6	*			
7		*		
8		*		
9				*
10	*			
11		*		
12		*		
13		*		
14			*	
15		*		
16			*	
17				*
18		*		
19			*	
20	*			

Suggested Readings

1. Ahmadzadehfar H, Biersack HJ, Freeman LM, Zuckier L. Clinical nuclear medicine. 2nd ed. Berlin: Springer; 2018.
2. Ell PJ, Gambhir SS. Nuclear medicine in clinical diagnosis and treatment. 3rd ed. Edinburgh, NY: Churchill Livingstone; 2004.
3. Sandler MP, Coleman RE, Patton JA, Wackers FJT, Gottschalk A. Diagnostic nuclear medicine. 4th ed. Philadelphia: Lippincott & Williams Wilkins; 2003.
4. Henkin RE. Nuclear medicine. 2nd ed. Philadelphia: Mosby Elsevier; 2006.

Nuclear Cardiology

6

6.1 Radiopharmaceuticals for the Study of the Heart

1. The critical organ for ^{201}Tl is:
   (a) Gallbladder
   (b) Kidneys
   (c) Ovaries
   (d) Large intestines
2. The shelf lives of ^{99m}Tc-MIBI and ^{99m}Tc-tetrofosmin are:
   (a) 15 h, 12 h
   (b) 12 h, 15 h
   (c) 15 h, 10 h
   (d) 10 h, 8 h
3. On a myocardial perfusion scan, which of the following factors can be considered an advantage of ^{99m}Tc-tetrofosmin over ^{99m} Tc-sestamibi?
   (a) Higher myocardial uptake
   (b) Rapid hepatic clearance
   (c) Lower pulmonary uptake
   (d) Lower price
4. The myocardial uptake pattern of which technetium agent is similar to that of ^{201}Tl?
   (a) ^{99m}Tc-sestamibi
   (b) ^{99m}Tc-tetrofosmin
   (c) ^{99m}Tc-furifosmin
   (d) ^{99m}Tc-NOET
5. A similar cardiac uptake pattern is usually observed between thallium and ^{99m}Tc-MIBG *except*:
   (a) Extensive ischemia in all three territories
   (b) Acute MI
   (c) Ventricular tachycardia and old MI
   (d) Arrhythmia

M. Assadi et al., *Principles of Nuclear Medicine*,
https://doi.org/10.1007/978-3-319-91701-6_6

6. In myocardial perfusion SPECT with ^{99m}Tc-teboroxime:
   (a) Imaging must be performed at least 1 h after injection.
   (b) Stress and rest images can be obtained with an interval of 2 h.
   (c) Hepatic and intestinal interfering activity is absent because of the renal elimination of the tracer.
   (d) It has lesser uptake than tetrofosmin on the cardiac first-pass study.
7. Which statement about the application of ^{82}Rb on cardiac scan is NOT correct?
   (a) It is directly injected from the generator to the patient.
   (b) Compared with thallium, a lower percentage of the administered dose is uptaken by myocardium.
   (c) Compared with ^{99m}Tc-MIBI, a higher percentage of the administered dose is uptaken by myocardium.
   (d) It behaves like a calcium analogue.
8. What happens to the ^{99m}Tc- teboroxime washout in the region of the heart with coronary stenosis?
   (a) Decrease
   (b) Increase
   (c) Similar to healthy myocardium
   (d) Without change
9. What percentage of the administered ^{201}Tl is uptaken by the heart?
   (a) 1–2%
   (b) 4–5%
   (c) 15–20%
   (d) 25–30%
10. Which of the following radiopharmaceuticals binds to phosphatidylserine on the surface of myocardial cells?
    (a) ^{99m}Tc-N-NOET
    (b) ^{99m}Tc-annexin V
    (c) ^{18}F-FDG
    (d) ^{99m}Tc-Teberoxime
11. Which radiopharmaceutical is used for the evaluation of the left ventricular function in both first-pass and gated SPECT studies?
    (a) ^{201}Tl
    (b) ^{99m}Tc-teboroxime
    (c) ^{99m}Tc-tetrofosmin
    (d) ^{82}Rubidium
12. Which method is NOT indicated for the evaluation of myocardial viability 1 month after myocardial infarction?
    (a) Echocardiography with low-dose dobutamine
    (b) Myocardial SPECT with sestamibi and nitrate administration in the rest phase
    (c) Myocardial SPECT with ^{123}I-MIBG in the rest phase
    (d) Myocardial SPECT with ^{201}Tl in the rest and redistribution phases

13. What is the relative advantage of ^{99m}Tc-tetrofosmin over ^{99m}Tc-sestamibi in the myocardial perfusion scan?
    (a) Better evaluation of myocardial viability
    (b) Rapid hepatic clearance
    (c) More accurate evaluation of myocardial function
    (d) The possibility of imaging in the rest phase in the first 5 min
14. In which of the following conditions is the linear increase in thallium uptake accompanied with the increase in myocardial perfusion?
    (a) In the physiologic range
    (b) Tissue acidosis
    (c) After physical exercise
    (d) Administration of vasodilators
15. Which radiotracer best shows the cardiac apex on the myocardial perfusion scan?
    (a) ^{99m}Tc-tetrofosmin
    (b) ^{99m}Tc-MIBI
    (c) ^{201}Tl
    (d) ^{99m}Tc-teboroxime
16. What is the critical organ for ^{99m}Tc-tetrofosmin?
    (a) Kidney
    (b) Gallbladder
    (c) Spleen
    (d) Liver
17. Which of the following radiotracers is NOT redistributed on the myocardial perfusion scan?
    (a) ^{201}Tl
    (b) Tc-NOET
    (c) Tc-teboroxime
    (d) Tc-furifosmin
18. Which of the following reagents is used on the hot spot scan for the detection of hypoxia?
    (a) Pyrophosphate
    (b) Antimyosin
    (c) Glucarate
    (d) Nitroimidazole
19. Which of the following radiotracers has the highest myocardial uptake?
    (a) ^{201}Tl
    (b) ^{99m}Tc-tetrofosmin
    (c) ^{99m}Tc-sestamibi
    (d) ^{99m}Tc-pyrophosphate

20. Anterior wall MI occurs in a 79-year-old patient with a history of drug treatment for hypertension and diabetes. Ejection fraction is about 45%, and blood sugar is NOT controlled in 2 weeks of hospitalization. If the evaluation of coronary arteries is desired, the postponing of which of the following tests is recommended?
    (a) Myocardial perfusion imaging
    (b) Coronary angiography
    (c) CT angiography
    (d) MR angiography

6.1.1 Answer

	A	B	C	D
1			*	
2				*
3		*		
4				*
5			*	
6		*		
7				*
8	*			
9		*		
10		*		
11			*	
12			*	
13		*		
14	*			
15	*			
16		*		
17				*
18				*
19	*			
20		*		

6.2 Radionuclide Ventriculography and the Assessment of Impaired Ventricular Function

1. Paradoxical septal motion is commonly seen in:
   (a) LBBB, aneurysm
   (b) LBBB, after CABG
   (c) Aneurysm, dilated cardiomyopathy
   (d) Dilated cardiomyopathy, after CABG
2. What is the effect of a high background activity on the calculated LVEF in radionuclide angiocardiography?
   (a) False decrease
   (b) False increase
   (c) Negative EF
   (d) No effect
3. What is the best criterion for the determination of cardiac shunt severity in first-pass studies?
   (a) Pulmonary to cardiac perfusion ratio (Qp/Qs)
   (b) Variance of perfusion of the shunt region in the unit of time
   (c) Average of the pulmonary perfusion in the left and right lungs
   (d) Variance of LVEF on both sides of the shunt
4. What is the assay of choice for the periodic evaluation of a patient receiving Adriamycin?
   (a) Stress echocardiography with dobutamine
   (b) Ergotamine angiography
   (c) Color Doppler
   (d) Radionuclide angiography (RNA)
5. In equilibrium radionuclide angiography (ERNA):
   (a) In vivo RBC labeling is preferred.
   (b) Anterior view (ANT) is the primary view of the scan.
   (c) Data acquisition is usually performed with the list mode.
   (d) Forward gating is the standard procedure.
6. Which of the following procedures can be applied for RV assessment?
   (a) Phase analysis of perfusion images
   (b) Gated myocardial perfusion SPECT
   (c) First pass
   (d) Gated blood pool SPECT
7. If the ventricular chamber is small, which of the following diagnostic errors is probable in the quantitative cardiac assessment with gated SPECT?
   (a) Lung–heart ratio overestimation
   (b) LVEF overestimation
   (c) EDV overestimation
   (d) RVEF overestimation

8. Which type of motion dysfunction demonstrates an extensive anteroseptal infarction and minimal viability in a gated myocardial SPECT study?
   (a) Hypokinesia
   (b) Akinesia
   (c) Dyskinesia
   (d) Paradoxical ventricular movement
9. Which type of motion dysfunction demonstrates a small region of inferolateral hibernation in a gated myocardial SPECT study?
   (a) Hypokinesia
   (b) Akinesia
   (c) Dyskinesia
   (d) Paradoxical ventricular movement
10. Which type of motion dysfunction demonstrates a left bundle branch block (LBBB) in a gated myocardial SPECT study?
   (a) Hypokinesia
   (b) Akinesia
   (c) Dyskinesia
   (d) Paradoxical ventricular movement
11. Which type of motion dysfunction demonstrates anteroapical aneurysm in a gated myocardial SPECT study?
   (a) Hypokinesia
   (b) Akinesia
   (c) Dyskinesia
   (d) Paradoxical ventricular movement
12. What is the most appropriate gamma camera system for the ERNA scan?
   (a) Multi-crystal LFOV
   (b) Single-crystal LFOV
   (c) Single-crystal SFOV
   (d) Multi-crystal SFOV
13. What is the method of choice for the determination of RVEF?
   (a) ECG-gated MPI
   (b) First pass
   (c) Rest study
   (d) ERNA
14. What is the abnormal finding of a cardiac test in the following time–activity curve?
   (a) Decreased TPFR and 1/3 FR
   (b) Increased PFR
   (c) Increased AFR
   (d) Decreased AFR

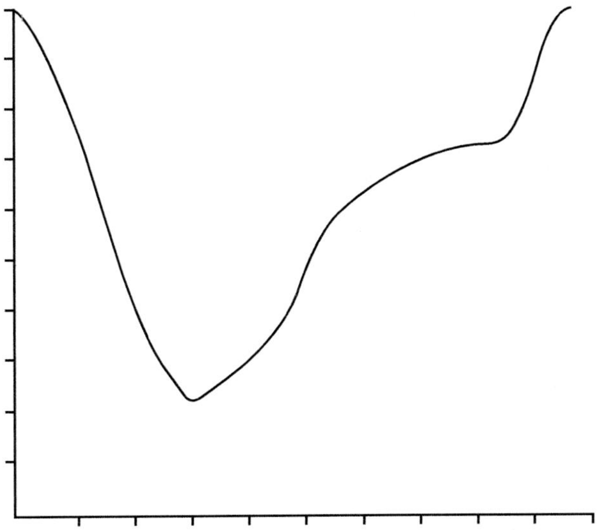

15. Which of the following disorders is specifically diagnosed by observing the local abnormal motion of myocardium in both stress and rest phases of ventriculography?
    (a) CAD
    (b) Cardiomyopathy
    (c) Valvular disease
    (d) Hypertension
16. Which method is recommended for the evaluation of circumflex territory in the stress condition?
    (a) ERNA
    (b) FPRNA
    (c) ERNA combined with FPRNA
    (d) Non-imaging probe
17. In normal condition, a significant increase in ventricular volume is observed following a small increase in diastolic pressure. This phenomenon happens to compensate for the:
    (a) Increase in afterload
    (b) Maintenance of lower compliance
    (c) Maintenance of constant preload
    (d) Decrease in performance
18. What is the best method for evaluating the left ventricular diastolic function?
    (a) First-pass angiography
    (b) Gated blood pool scintigraphy
    (c) Gated blood pool SPECT
    (d) Gated perfusion SPECT

19. What is the number of appropriate frames in each cardiac cycle for the evaluation of the left ventricular diastolic function with the MUGA procedure?
    (a) 8
    (b) 16
    (c) 32
    (d) 64
20. Which item about doxorubicin-induced cardiotoxicity is NOT correct?
    (a) Dose dependency.
    (b) It is reversible at 25%.
    (c) The side effects of doxorubicin are notable when a 5% reduction in LVEF occurs.
    (d) The drug must be discontinued when LVEF is below 45%.
21. Which statement about the evaluation of cardiac function with nuclear medicine modalities is NOT correct?
    (a) All Tc radiotracers can be used in the first-pass technique.
    (b) In gated blood pool, the method of RBC labeling significantly affects the final outcome.
    (c) The bolus administration of the radiotracer is critical in the first-pass technique.
    (d) The selection of an appropriate technique is critical in a patient with arrhythmia.
22. In the measurement of LVEF in radionuclide ventriculography:
    (a) If the spleen is included in the background ROI, LVEF is underestimated.
    (b) LAO view at 30° is the best view for imaging.
    (c) In the semiautomatic method, the left ventricle ROI must be extended at the end of systole.
    (d) The RBC labeling method has NO effect on LVEF measurement.
23. Which of the following variables is calculated by (EDV−ESV)/EDV?
    (a) Left ventricular diastolic function
    (b) Left ventricular systolic function
    (c) Left ventricular ejection fraction
    (d) Right ventricular diastolic function
24. Which of the following criterion is indicative of preload in a healthy heart?
    (a) End-systolic volume
    (b) End-diastolic volume
    (c) Systolic blood pressure
    (d) Myocardial contractility
25. What is the best septal view for the quantitative evaluation in a gated blood pool study?
    (a) Anterior
    (b) 40°–50° LAO
    (c) LL
    (d) 70° LL

26. The evaluation of ventricular function with stress is requested for a patient with a favorable physical condition. What is the preferred type of stress?
    (a) Stress with bicycle
    (b) Stress with treadmill
    (c) Atrial pacing
    (d) Infusion of dobutamine
27. Which finding in the evaluation of ventricular function is indicative of a left bundle branch block?
    (a) Septum movement toward the left ventricle chamber
    (b) Delayed contraction of the left atrium
    (c) Delayed contraction of the left ventricle
    (d) Paradoxical movement of the septum toward the right ventricle
28. What changes are observed on the first-pass scan because of the left-to-right shunt?
    (a) Simultaneous appearance of both ventricles
    (b) Simultaneous appearance of both atria
    (c) Appearance of the brain and kidneys
    (d) No dissociation between two atria
29. Which statement about first-pass radionuclide angiocardiography is NOT correct?
    (a) ^{99m}Tc-pertechnetate is the most common radiopharmaceutical used in this method.
    (b) Serial imaging is possible when ^{195}Au and ^{191m}Ir are used.
    (c) ^{99m}Tc-MAA is commonly used for the evaluation of left-to-right shunts.
    (d) The normal ratio of pulmonary perfusion to systemic perfusion (Qp/Qs) is 1.
30. What is the collimator of choice for a cardiac first-pass study?
    (a) LEGP
    (b) MEGP
    (c) LEUH
    (d) Pinhole
31. What is the choice technique of nuclear medicine for the evaluation of RV function?
    (a) Gated first-pass study
    (b) Gated equilibrium radionuclide angiography
    (c) First-pass study
    (d) Equilibrium radionuclide angiography
32. After cardiac surgery, a significant reduction of LVEF is observed for more than 24 h. What is the most common reason for this occurrence?
    (a) MI during surgery.
    (b) Sensitivity of myocardium to anesthetic drugs.
    (c) This phenomenon is transient, and no additional evaluation is required.
    (d) Multiple pulmonary microemboli.

33. Describe the sensitivity and specificity of dobutamine stress echocardiography in predicting cardiac events in diabetic patients.
    (a) More than that of nondiabetic patients
    (b) Less than that of nondiabetic patients
    (c) Similar to that of nondiabetic patients
    (d) Less than that of overweight nondiabetic patients
34. What is the most common application of resting MUGA cardiac study?
    (a) Cardiac injury after catheterization
    (b) Diagnosis of CAD
    (c) Diagnosis of heart valve disease
    (d) Adriamycin toxicity
35. Which view on the MUGA scan is the best for observing the right ventricle?
    (a) Posterior
    (b) Anterior
    (c) LPO
    (d) LAO
36. In which rhythmic disorders is the time of imaging in gated myocardial perfusion SPECT prolonged?
    (a) Sinus tachycardia
    (b) Sinus bradycardia
    (c) QT prolongation
    (d) Sinus arrhythmia
37. Which of the following items is necessary for the gated first-pass study before myocardial perfusion SPECT?
    (a) High-resolution collimator
    (b) Multi-crystal gamma camera
    (c) Bolus administration of the radiopharmaceutical in a low volume
    (d) Radiopharmaceutical administration with a double dose
38. Radionuclide ventriculography is NOT indicated for:
    (a) Comparing ejection fraction between the stress and rest phases
    (b) Evaluating myocardial systolic thickening
    (c) Diagnosing ventricular aneurysm after myocardial infarction
    (d) Detecting myocardial conduction disorders
39. Alternative R wave gating is recommended for the diagnosis of:
    (a) Adriamycin cardiotoxicity
    (b) Restrictive cardiomyopathy
    (c) Aortic insufficiency
    (d) Congenital heart disease
40. A 17-year-old girl with severe tricuspid failure is referred for PDA evaluation. QP/QS is 1.6 in the presented first-pass study, and the left ventricle is clearly observed in the serial images. What is the final interpretation of the left-to-right shunt?
    (a) No shunt
    (b) Minor shunt
    (c) Intermediate shunt
    (d) Interpretation is NOT possible

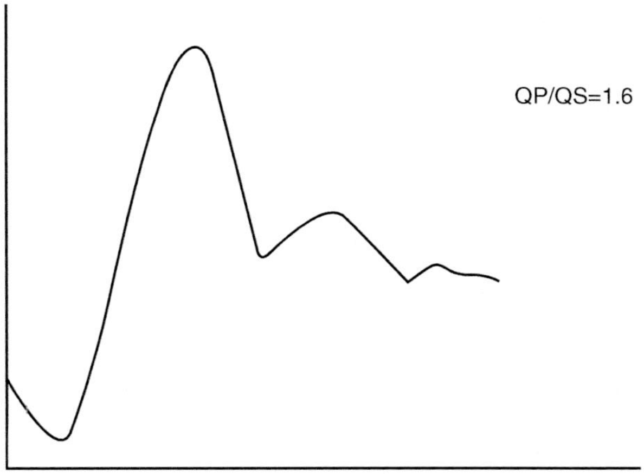

41. Which of the following items increases the accuracy of measuring the LVEF in a gated study?
    (a) Increase in administered dose
    (b) 256 × 256 matrix
    (c) High-sensitivity collimator
    (d) LFOV camera
42. The application of which of the following parameters provides the best resolution in myocardial gated SPECT?
    (a) End-diastolic volume
    (b) Summed frames
    (c) Frozen motion
    (d) End-systolic frames
43. The bolus administration of the radiopharmaceutical is performed in the right upper limb for the first-pass study. The right and left ventricles appear concurrently. What is the most probable diagnosis?
    (a) Pulmonary valve insufficiency
    (b) Tricuspid valve insufficiency
    (c) Constrictive pericarditis
    (d) Fallot tetralogy
44. In a cardiac index study on a resting MUGA scan after acute MI:
    (a) Global EF is the strongest prognostic factor for long-term morbidity.
    (b) EF is NOT a valuable prognostic factor for short-term morbidity.
    (c) Increased morbidity due to the low EF depends on the anatomic region of the myocardial defect.
    (d) The highest morbidity rate is about 40% when EF decreases.
45. What is the common normal range for EF in radionuclide and other techniques?
    (a) 45–55%
    (b) 50–65%
    (c) 55–75%
    (d) 65–85%

46. The dilatation of … is considered normal after heart transplantation.
    (a) Pulmonary artery trunk
    (b) Right atrium
    (c) Left atrium
    (d) Right ventricle
47. A gamma camera is used for a 16-frame gated myocardial perfusion SPECT without bad-beat rejection. Which of the following parameters is considered a stable parameter for the evaluation of left ventricular diastolic function?
    (a) Peak filling rate (PFR)
    (b) Time to peak filling (TTPF)
    (c) Mean filling fraction (1/2 FF)
    (d) Mean filling rate (MFR)
48. Doxorubicin-induced cardiomyopathy:
    (a) Acute toxicity occurs 48–72 h after injection.
    (b) Acute toxicity improves in 1 week after injection.
    (c) Chronic toxicity is NOT dose dependent.
    (d) Improvement of ejection fraction, which is observed in chronic administration, is due to cardiac hypertrophy.
49. Which view best shows the size of the left atrium in a myocardial blood pool study?
    (a) Anterior.
    (b) LAO.
    (c) LL and LPO.
    (d) Evaluation of the size of the left atrium is NOT possible with this method.
50. In myocardial perfusion and gated blood pool studies:
    (a) Reduced ejection fraction is less common than dyskinesia in patients with a coronary artery disease after exercise.
    (b) The left ventricle demonstrates hyperkinesia in idiopathic hypertrophic subaortic stenosis (IHSS).
    (c) A correlation does NOT exist between reversible defects and dyskinesia in coronary artery disease.
    (d) If dyskinesia is observed, the probability of ischemic heart disease (IHD) is NOT high.
51. A patient with dyspnea and chest pain is presented. Asymmetric septal hypertrophy, small size of the left ventricular chamber, diastolic disorder in ventricle filling, and increase in ejection fraction are found on radionuclide ventriculography. What is the most probable diagnosis?
    (a) Hypertrophic cardiomyopathy
    (b) Anteroseptal wall ischemia
    (c) Anteroseptal wall aneurysm
    (d) Right ventricular dilatation due to emphysema
52. Which of the following items best describes tardokinesis?
    (a) Decreased wall motility
    (b) Absence of wall motility
    (c) Delay in wall motility relative to the nearby regions
    (d) Extension of wall in systole

53. Which of the following items best describes dyskinesia?
    (a) Decreased wall motility
    (b) Absence of wall motility
    (c) Delay in wall motility relative to the nearby regions
    (d) Extension of wall in systole
54. Which of the following items best describes hypokinesia?
    (a) Decreased wall motility
    (b) Absence of wall motility
    (c) Delay in wall motility relative to the nearby regions
    (d) Extension of wall in systole
55. Which of the following items best describes akinesia?
    (a) Decreased wall motility
    (b) Absence of wall motility
    (c) Delay in wall motility relative to the nearby regions
    (d) Extension of wall in systole
56. Tracer reflux into the inferior vena cava and the subclavian vein is observed in the first-pass study. What is the most probable diagnosis?
    (a) Tricuspid regurgitation
    (b) Aortic stenosis
    (c) Pulmonary artery stenosis
    (d) Mitral regurgitation
57. What is the most appropriate radiopharmaceutical for the multi-gated acquisition scan (MUGA)?
    (a) ^{99m}Tc-HAS
    (b) ^{99m}Tc-MAA
    (c) ^{99m}Tc-SC
    (d) ^{99m}Tc-RBC
58. Which of the following modalities is the most appropriate for equilibrium radionuclide angiography?
    (a) Gamma camera with a small field of view (SFOV) equipped with LEAP collimator
    (b) Gamma camera with a large field of view (LFOV) equipped with LEAP collimator
    (c) Gamma camera with a small field of view (SFOV) equipped with slant hole collimator
    (d) Gamma camera with a small field of view (SFOV) equipped with high-sensitivity collimator
59. In hypertrophic cardiomyopathy:
    (a) Decreased ejection fraction.
    (b) The symmetric form is more common than the asymmetric.
    (c) Diastolic dysfunction is observed in most of patients.
    (d) Valve regurgitation is the most common cause of the disease.

60. What is the most valuable finding of a gated myocardial scan in pericardial effusion?
    (a) Increase in the distance between the liver and the right heart in the anterior view
    (b) Distance between the liver and the right heart as well as the enlargement of the silhouette of the left pericardium in the LAO view
    (c) Intense pericardium
    (d) Absence of the radiotracer in myocardium
61. Gated SPECT after exercise test:
    (a) It evaluates the stress myocardial function.
    (b) It is NOT different from routine SPECT for the detection of artifacts.
    (c) It is less applied because of its longer procedure.
    (d) It is more effective than the resting study for the diagnosis of myocardial dysfunctions.
62. On gated myocardial perfusion SPECT scan:
    (a) Contrast of images with 360° of rotation is better than those with 180° of rotation.
    (b) Changes in the wall count in the images obtained at the end of systole and diastole represent their thickness during ventricular contraction.
    (c) It has NO advantage over routine procedure for the differentiation of artifacts from perfusion defects.
    (d) MRI is the best method for the evaluation of wall motility with a marked decrease in perfusion.
63. What is the functional representative of harmony and intensity of ventricular contraction in different regions in ventriculography?
    (a) Phase and amplitude image
    (b) Ejection fraction image
    (c) Paradox image
    (d) Stroke volume image
64. What is the functional representative of stroke volume image relative to end-diastolic image in ventriculography?
    (a) Ejection fraction image
    (b) Paradox image
    (c) Stroke volume image
    (d) Phase and amplitude image
65. What is the functional representative of the subtraction of end-diastolic volume image from the end systolic volume in ventriculography?
    (a) Stroke volume image
    (b) Paradox image
    (c) Ejection fraction image
    (d) Phase and amplitude image
66. What is the functional representative of the subtraction of end-systolic image from the end diastolic image in ventriculography?
    (a) Stroke volume image
    (b) Paradox image
    (c) Ejection fraction image
    (d) Phase and amplitude image

67. Which of the following methods is the most suitable for equilibrium studies in radionuclide ventriculography?
    (a) ECG trigger with frame mode
    (b) Frame mode
    (c) List mode
    (d) List mode with exercise test
68. The phase images of radionuclide ventriculography are useful for the diagnosis of:
    (a) Conductive disorders
    (b) Systolic dysfunctions
    (c) Diastolic dysfunctions
    (d) Atrial contractibility disorders
69. What is the advantage of a myocardial gated blood pool scan over a first-pass study?
    (a) Quick procedure
    (b) Evaluation of left ventricular function during exercise
    (c) Better resolution for regional wall motion
    (d) Measurement of right ventricular ejection fraction
70. Which of the following factors underestimates the ejection fraction in a gated SPECT study?
    (a) Small size of the left ventricle
    (b) Zooming during imaging
    (c) Division of the cardiac cycle into eight frames
    (d) Zooming during the reconstruction of images
71. Which radionuclide has the most appropriate half-life for a pediatric radionuclide first-pass study?
    (a) ^{99m}Tc
    (b) ^{195m}Au
    (c) ^{178m}Ta
    (d) ^{191m}Ir
72. Which statement regarding the phase study in ventriculography is NOT correct?
    (a) The contraction times are calculated relative to the P wave in electrocardiography.
    (b) The contraction time can be determined for each pixel.
    (c) Iso-coloring represents the iso-phase.
    (d) It is useful for the detection of regions of ectopic arrhythmia.
73. Which of the following statements regarding the imaging angle in the radionuclide first-pass study is NOT correct?
    (a) If the goal is the study of shunts, some regions of the lungs especially the right lung must be present in imaging field even if it causes the exclusion of some regions of left ventricle.
    (b) If right ventricle is the main chamber of study, 30° RAO is the most suitable angle.
    (c) Left ventricular ejection fraction may be underestimated in LAO view.
    (d) Shallow LAO view is the best view for the exercise first-pass study.

74. In which of the following situations does a decrease in preload occur?
    (a) Aortic stenosis
    (b) Mitral stenosis
    (c) Aortic regurgitation
    (d) Mitral regurgitation
75. What is the best time to evaluate the LVEF in anthracycline chemotherapy with doses higher than 60 mg/m^2?
    (a) First week after the completion of chemotherapy
    (b) Second week after the completion of chemotherapy
    (c) Third week after the completion of chemotherapy
    (d) First week after the initiation of another chemotherapy cycle
76. A ventricular preload is:
    (a) End-diastolic myocardial tension
    (b) Resistance against the contraction of myocardial fibers
    (c) The quality of myocardial contraction
    (d) The relationship between diastolic pressure and left ventricular volume
77. What is the most common application of gated SPECT with consensus clinical approval?
    (a) Study of LVEF and ventricular volume
    (b) Study of breast artifact
    (c) Study of diaphragmatic artifact
    (d) Decrease in the effect of extra-cardiac activity
78. Which of the following statements about the exercise RNV study of the LVEF is NOT correct?
    (a) LVEF may NOT change in patients with coronary insufficiency.
    (b) LVEF may significantly decrease in patients with coronary insufficiency.
    (c) LVEF may increase in healthy subjects.
    (d) RVEF increases in patients with proximal RCA disease.
79. In which of the following studies does ERNA have the most important clinical role?
    (a) Regional and global systolic function study
    (b) RBBB study
    (c) LBBB study
    (d) Pacemaker rhythm study
80. All of the following statements about the study of left ventricular function in patients with cardiomyopathy are correct *except*:
    (a) In nonischemic cardiomyopathy, primary systolic dysfunction and ventriculomegaly are observed.
    (b) In ischemic cardiomyopathy, most of the abnormal regional changes are observed in the left ventricle.
    (c) In ischemic cardiomyopathy, left ventriculomegaly is severe without the enlargement of the right ventricle.
    (d) In nonischemic cardiomyopathy, right ventriculomegaly is observed without the enlargement of the left ventricle.

81. Which of the following statements is NOT considered a clinical indication for radionuclide angiography?
    (a) Evaluation of the global left ventricular function and prognosis in patients with ischemic heart disease
    (b) Evaluation before and after heart transplantation
    (c) Evaluation of left myocardial perfusion
    (d) Regional evaluation of cardiac wall dyskinesia in patients with ischemic heart disease
82. In which of the following situations is FPRA study conducted prior to ERNA?
    (a) Exercise left ventricular function study
    (b) Resting left ventricular function study
    (c) Bigeminal rhythm study
    (d) Evaluation of ischemia in the LCX artery territory
83. In which of the following conditions is the R-R interval tolerance of 30 ± 40 in ECG gated recommended?
    (a) Occasional extrasystoles
    (b) Intermittent extrasystoles
    (c) Atrial fibrillation
    (d) Absence of upright R wave
84. Which of the following statements regarding gated SPECT is NOT correct?
    (a) The size of the cardiac chamber may be underestimated in patients with a small ventricle.
    (b) LVEF may be overestimated in patients with a small ventricle.
    (c) LVEF may be overestimated in eight-frame gating imaging.
    (d) If the rejected beat is high, an extra frame can provide useful information for gate study.
85. All of the following parameters in ERNA are normal for a healthy subject at rest *except*:
    (a) PFR = 2.7 EDV/s
    (b) TPFR = 195 s
    (c) AFR = 1.5 EDV/s
    (d) PFR/AFR = 2.6
86. What is the best position for observing the left atrium in the MUGA study?
    (a) Anterior
    (b) LAO
    (c) RAO
    (d) LPO
87. Phase images of a scan shows that systolic contraction initiates from the apex and progresses toward the cardiac base. What is the most probable diagnosis?
    (a) Ventricular pacemaker
    (b) Left bundle branch block
    (c) Atrial pacemaker
    (d) Septal infarction

88. A symmetric halo surrounding the heart (separation of the heart from the lungs and liver) in pericardial imaging with blood pool agents is seen in:
    (a) Cholesterol pericarditis
    (b) Lipoma within pericardium
    (c) Fat surrounding the heart
    (d) All of the above
89. The end-systolic pressure–volume (PV) relation and the diastolic PV relation can be defined in a patient by constructing PV loops in different loading conditions. Which loop in the presented figure is acquired at a high preload and afterload?
    (a) Loop A
    (b) Loop B
    (c) Loop C
    (d) Loop C–loop A

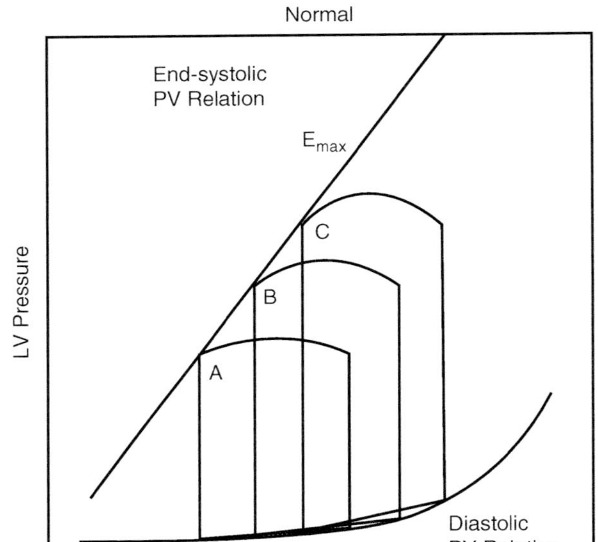

90. Which are the most appropriate studies for evaluating the following heart parameters, respectively?

    Ejection fraction measurement, diagnosis of ischemic and infarcted regions, assessment of congenital heart malformation, diagnosis of intracardiac tumors, diagnosis of aortic dissection, evaluation of left-to-right shunt, assessment of left ventricle dimension during systole and diastole

    (a) Radionuclide angiogram, radionuclide angiogram, MRI and Doppler echocardiography, MRI and transesophageal echocardiography, MRI and transesophageal echocardiography, Doppler echocardiography, M-mode echocardiography
    (b) Radionuclide angiogram, radionuclide angiogram, MRI and transesophageal echocardiography, MRI and transesophageal echocardiography, MRI and transesophageal echocardiography, Doppler echocardiography, transesophageal echocardiography
    (c) Radionuclide angiogram, transesophageal echocardiography, MRI and Doppler echocardiography, MRI and transesophageal echocardiography, MRI and transesophageal echocardiography, Doppler echocardiography, M-mode echocardiography
    (d) Radionuclide angiogram, Doppler echocardiography, MRI and Doppler echocardiography, MRI and transesophageal echocardiography, MRI and transesophageal echocardiography, Doppler echocardiography, M-mode echocardiography
91. Which of following techniques can assess ventricular wall motion?
    (a) Real-time echocardiography
    (b) Radionuclide angiogram
    (c) Cin-MRI
    (d) All of the above
92. What happens to the ejection fraction in gated myocardial blood pool imaging if the descending aorta is selected as the ROI for the background activity?
    (a) Underestimation of EF.
    (b) Overestimation of EF.
    (c) No change in the value of EF.
    (d) Both overestimation and underestimation of EF are possible.
93. What is the most appropriate time for valvuloplasty in aortic insufficiency (AI)?
    (a) When dysfunction of the left ventricle occurs at exercise on radionuclide ventriculography
    (b) When dysfunction of the left ventricle occurs at rest on radionuclide ventriculography
    (c) When the severity of the left ventricular dysfunction is moderate to severe
    (d) Observation of the first episode of hemoptysis
94. Which of the following aortic pathologies canNOT be studied by EqNA?
    (a) Moderate dilatation
    (b) Tortuosity
    (c) Dissection of the aorta
    (d) Aneurysm

95. What is the typical kinetic pattern of aneurysm?
    (a) Akinesia
    (b) Dyskinesia
    (c) Paradoxical motion
    (d) Tardokinesia
96. Which of the following radiotracers is NOT indicated for first-pass imaging?
    (a) ^{178}Ta
    (b) ^{191}Tr
    (c) ^{195}Au
    (d) ^{99m}Tc-MAA
97. Which of the following is NOT an advantage of the quantitative myocardial perfusion SPECT study?
    (a) Higher confidence in interpretation
    (b) Enhanced intra-observer and interobserver interpretation reproducibility
    (c) Measures the degree of abnormality
    (d) Provides entirely new information
98. What is the gold standard method for the evaluation of systolic myocardial function?
    (a) Radionuclide scan
    (b) Echocardiography
    (c) CT scan
    (d) MRI

6.2.1 Answer

	A	B	C	D		A	B	C	D
1		*			50		*		
2		*			51	*			
3	*				52			*	
4				*	53				*
5				*	54	*			
6				*	55		*		
7		*			56	*			
8		*			57				*
9	*				58	*			
10				*	59			*	
11			*		60	*			
12			*		61				*
13		*			62		*		
14			*		63	*			
15	*				64	*			
16	*				65		*		
17		*			66	*			
18			*		67	*			
19			*		68	*			

20			*		**69**			*	
21		*			**70**			*	
22				*	**71**				*
23			*		**72**	*			
24		*			**73**				*
25		*			**74**		*		
26	*				**75**			*	
27				*	**76**	*			
28	*				**77**	*			
29			*		**78**				*
30			*		**79**	*			
31	*				**80**				*
32	*				**81**			*	
33			*		**82**	*			
34				*	**83**			*	
35		*			**84**			*	
36				*	**85**		*		
37			*		**86**				*
38		*			**87**	*			
39		*			**88**				*
40				*	**89**			*	
41	*				**90**	*			
42			*		**91**				*
43				*	**92**		*		
44	*				**93**		*		
45			*		**94**			*	
46		*			**95**		*		
47		*			**96**				*
48				*	**97**				*
49			*		**98**				*

6.3 Infarct Avid Imaging and Myocardial Perfusion Scintigraphy Techniques Using Single-Photon Radiotracers

1. The critical organ of ^{111}In-antimyosin is:
   (a) Gallbladder
   (b) Kidneys
   (c) Large intestine
   (d) Liver
2. The presence of some ^{201}Tl uptake in an area of antimyosin uptake in a jeopardized myocardium indicates:
   (a) Ischemia
   (b) Prior infarction
   (c) Transmural infarction
   (d) Non-transmural infarction
3. In which of the following conditions can the reverse redistribution of thallium be observed?
   (a) Cardiomyopathy
   (b) Recent PTCA
   (c) Mitral valve prolapse
   (d) Hypertension
4. Which of the following indices is not usually measured in gated myocardial perfusion SPECT?
   (a) ESV
   (b) Diastolic function
   (c) EDV
   (d) EF
5. Tc-pyrophosphate scintigraphy is performed for a patient with myocardial infarction, and a doughnut-shaped image is detected on the anterior wall. What is the best interpretation of this finding?
   (a) Perfusion is normal in the central part.
   (b) Perfusion is reduced to 50–70% in the peripheral regions.
   (c) The patient experienced infarction more than a month ago.
   (d) The infarcted size is equal to the region with enhanced uptake.
6. If the goal is to diagnose MI, cardiac pyrophosphate scan has the highest sensitivity in:
   (a) Lateral infarction
   (b) Subendocardial infarction
   (c) Inferior infarction
   (d) Anterior infarction
7. Which of the following disorders demonstrates ^{111}In-antimyosin uptake?
   (a) Calcification
   (b) Amyloidosis
   (c) Doxorubicin toxicity
   (d) Pericarditis

8. A 180°-diametrical artifact defect in short-axis cardiac imaging is related to:
   (a) 180°-circular image acquisition
   (b) 360°-image acquisition
   (c) Image acquisition with a body contour circuit
   (d) Image acquisition with a dual-head camera
9. Which of the following conditions results in a reverse defect during a myocardial perfusion scan with ^{99m}Tc- MIBI?
   (a) Cardiomegaly
   (b) Percutaneous transluminal coronary angioplasty (PTCA)
   (c) Cardiomyopathy
   (d) Myocarditis
10. Which item is most likely to cause an inferior attenuation on a myocardial perfusion scan?
    (a) Abdominal wall fat
    (b) Further distance of the inferior wall from the detector
    (c) Thinner inferior wall
    (d) Lower count rate
11. Regarding the quantitative interpretation of myocardial perfusion, if the sum stress score (SSS) is 20 in a 20-segment model, what is the equivalent value in a 17-segment model?
    (a) 8.5
    (b) 17
    (c) 34
    (d) 68
12. Which of the following reduces the motion artifact in a myocardial SPECT evaluation?
    (a) 180° single-head systems, prone position of the patient
    (b) 180° single-head systems, circular movement of the head
    (c) 180° single-head systems, elliptical pattern of movement
    (d) Multi-detector systems with a 360° acquisition
13. A gated blood pool scan (forward at the initial two-thirds and reverse at the final one-third of the cardiac cycle) is performed on a patient. This procedure improves the precision of the measurement of:
    (a) Systole
    (b) Diastole
    (c) Early systole
    (d) End diastole
14. A 49-year-old man is referred to the emergency ward 12 h after the onset of chest pain; suspected changes in ST are found on the ECG. Which scan is more appropriate for the confirmation of acute infarction?
    (a) Technetium glutarate
    (b) Technetium pyrophosphate
    (c) Indium antimyosin
    (d) ^{201}Tl

15. Which view is used for detecting motion artifact on a myocardial perfusion scan?
    (a) Vertical long axis (VLA)
    (b) Cinematic view of the planar images
    (c) Horizontal long axis (HLA)
    (d) Short axis
16. Which artifact is associated with the hurricane sign, and which view is recommended for the best observation of this sign?
    (a) Field uniformity, horizontal long axis (HLA) view
    (b) Center of rotation (COR), horizontal long axis (HLA) view
    (c) Field uniformity, vertical long axis (VLA) view
    (d) Center of rotation (COR), vertical long axis (VLA) view
17. Which of the following mechanisms is involved in the concentration of Tc-99m phosphates?
    (a) Radiopharmaceutical influx
    (b) Macromolecular binding
    (c) Selective adsorption to tissue calcium sites
    (d) All of the above
18. What is the dual-radionuclide imaging protocol in the evaluation of myocardial perfusion?
    (a) Two phases of rest and stress scan in two subsequent days with 25–30 mCi of ^{99m}Tc-MIBI for each experiment
    (b) Administration of 3 mCi of thallium in the exercise phase followed by 2 mCi of thallium in the rest phase on the same day
    (c) Rest scan with 3–5 mCi of thallium followed by stress scan with 25–30 mCi of ^{99m}Tc-MIBI
    (d) Separate rest and stress scans with 25–30 mCi of ^{99m}Tc-MIBI followed by ERNA with labeled RBC
19. Which complex is recommended for the diagnosis of stunned myocardium?
    (a) MIBI (Cardiolite)
    (b) Misonidazole
    (c) Tetrofosmin (Myoview)
    (d) Teboroxime (Cardiotec)
20. Which of the following indices is used for the determination of LV pathologic remodeling on a myocardial perfusion scan?
    (a) Cedars–Sinai scoring
    (b) Sphericity index
    (c) LVEF
    (d) Center of rotation (COR) index
21. How long after acute MI does the ^{99m}Tc-PYP scan provide the highest sensitivity?
    (a) 6–12 h
    (b) 12–24 h
    (c) 72–96 h
    (d) 24–72 h

22. Which scan has the highest specificity for the diagnosis of acute MI?
    (a) ^{99m}Tc-PYP
    (b) ^{111}In-antimyosin
    (c) ^{99m}Tc-MIBI
    (d) ^{201}Tl-chloride
23. What is the correct rotation angle for cardiac SPECT with a 180° rotation?
    (a) From 45° RPO to 45° LAO
    (b) From 45° LPO to 45° RPO
    (c) From 45° RAO to 45° LPO
    (d) From 45° LAO to 45° RPO
24. Thallium is injected after the exercise test, and imaging is performed subsequently. A perfusion defect is found on the inferior wall on the stress scan, and it disappears in the resting phase. Which item is the most probable?
    (a) Diaphragmatic attenuation
    (b) Upward creep defect
    (c) MI of the inferior wall
    (d) Myocardial hibernation
25. A diaphragmatic attenuation artifact on a myocardial perfusion scan causes:
    (a) Decreased sensitivity
    (b) Decreased specificity
    (c) Increased sensitivity
    (d) Increased specificity
26. Which normal variant is attributed to the MPI scan with 180° cardiac tomography (instead of 360°)?
    (a) RV insertion defect
    (b) Septal shortening
    (c) Septal to lateral ratio less than 1
    (d) Apical thinning
27. A patient with severe chest pain is presented to the emergency room with suspected non-ST elevation MI. What is the recommended scan for the evaluation of myocardial necrosis in the early hours of referring?
    (a) ^{99m}Tc-PYP
    (b) ^{99m}Tc-glucaric acid imaging
    (c) Antimyosin antibody imaging
    (d) Rest thallium scan
28. Which item is replaced by the normalcy rate in the MPI statistical study?
    (a) Sensitivity
    (b) Specificity
    (c) Negative predictive value
    (d) Positive predictive value
29. Which filter is used for inhibiting the star artifact due to liver activity in the processing of MPI images with the FBP method?
    (a) Butterworth
    (b) OSEM
    (c) METZ
    (d) Ramp

30. What is the mechanism of Cu–ATSM accumulation in the myocardium?
    (a) Apoptosis
    (b) Necrosis
    (c) Receptor expression
    (d) Hypoxia
31. Which item is NOT considered a normal variant for myocardial perfusion SPECT scan?
    (a) Lower uptake in the midventricular short-axis slices of the septum
    (b) Coffee bean sign in the apical short-axis slices
    (c) Lower uptake on the inferoseptal wall of basal slices in women
    (d) Defect in the septal basal segment
32. Which of the following parameters can be evaluated by a gated SPECT myocardial perfusion scan with an eight frames/beat protocol?
    (a) Right ventricular ESV
    (b) Left ventricular EDV
    (c) Peak filling rate
    (d) Atrial filling rate
33. The myocardial chambers are absent on ^{99m}Tc-RBC ventriculography, and the background activity is high. Which item canNOT cause such a phenomenon?
    (a) Heparin in RBC labeling
    (b) Dextrose in radiotracer injection
    (c) Mannitol in radiotracer injection
    (d) Saline in radiotracer injection
34. Myocardial perfusion SPECT with exercise is performed on a patient weighing 85 kg. A defect with a reduced uptake on the inferior wall is observed. Which of the following items can cause a false-positive finding?
    (a) Center of rotation offset
    (b) Orbit-related artifact
    (c) Upward creep
    (d) Lateral chest wall attenuation
35. A patient with acute chest pain is referred to the emergency room. Which of the following statements about a myocardial perfusion scan in first 6 h is correct?
    (a) ^{201}Tl is the choice radiotracer.
    (b) Sensitivity of the scan after 4 h and cessation of chest pain is low.
    (c) The sensitivity of troponin I in this time interval is less than that of the scan.
    (d) A normal scan excludes the possibility of coronary artery disease.
36. In lung transplantation:
    (a) The right ventricular ejection fraction is improved.
    (b) The right ventricular ejection fraction does not change.
    (c) The left ventricular ejection fraction is improved.
    (d) The right ventricular ejection fraction is improved more in a unilateral transplantation than in a bilateral transplantation.

37. For a 49-year-old man with a 5-year history of diabetes and no clinical symptom of CAD:
    (a) A stress myocardial scan is indicated.
    (b) A stress myocardial scan is indicated if there is one other risk factor.
    (c) A stress myocardial scan is indicated if there are two other risk factors.
    (d) A stress myocardial scan is NOT required.
38. A 63-year-old man with no symptoms of heart disease is evaluated for coronary artery calcium scoring. In which of the following conditions is a myocardial scan with stress indicated?
    (a) Calcium score > 200 Agat score
    (b) Calcium score > 400 Agat score
    (c) Calcium score > 600 Agat score
    (d) Calcium score > 1000 Agat score
39. What is the recommended view on a planar myocardial perfusion scan if only one view is possible?
    (a) Anterior
    (b) Right anterior oblique
    (c) Left anterior oblique
    (d) Left lateral
40. What is the recommended position of the patient on a planar myocardial perfusion scan to decrease the attenuation effect of the diaphragm?
    (a) Left lateral decubitus
    (b) Right lateral decubitus
    (c) Supine
    (d) Prone
41. What is the best method to prevent upward creep in myocardial perfusion SPECT imaging?
    (a) Background subtraction
    (b) Fatty milk ingestion
    (c) Attenuation correction
    (d) Delaying of imaging for only a few minutes
42. A patient is presented with acute chest pain that started 4 days ago. A ^{99m}Tc-PYP scan is performed because of suspected myocardial infarction. Which of the following findings is indicative of a poor prognosis?
    (a) No myocardial uptake
    (b) Diffuse myocardial uptake
    (c) Focal uptake in the right ventricle
    (d) Doughnut sign
43. Which of the following corrections is critical if the goal is to prevent isotope cross talk on a myocardial perfusion scan with ^{99m}Tc-stress/^{201}Tl-rest?
    (a) Temporal list mode
    (b) Motion correction
    (c) Energy list mode
    (d) Variable temporal resolution method

44. Reverse redistribution is reported on a myocardial perfusion scan. Which of the following items is the least possible?
    (a) The patient has received thrombolytic treatment.
    (b) History of myocardial infarction.
    (c) Left ventricular dysfunction.
    (d) Previous coronary angioplasty.
45. About the diagnosis of acute myocardial infarction with In-antimyosin scan:
    (a) The negative report of this test is more valuable than that of ^{99m}Tc-PYP to rule out acute infarction.
    (b) The diagnosis of right ventricular infarction with an antimyosin planar scan is easier than with ^{99m}Tc-PYP.
    (c) Lateral infarction can cause false-negative results.
    (d) The relative activity of the heart to the sternum 10–12 h after radiotracer injection is used for imaging.
46. What is the best view for observing a membranous septum artifact in a myocardial SPECT scan?
    (a) Vertical long axis
    (b) Short-axis basal portion
    (c) Short-axis apical portion
    (d) Horizontal long axis
47. What is the best view for observing a diaphragmatic suppression artifact on a myocardial SPECT scan?
    (a) Short-axis basal portion
    (b) Horizontal long axis
    (c) Vertical long axis
    (d) Short-axis apical portion
48. What is the best view for observing a body contour artifact on a myocardial SPECT scan?
    (a) Short-axis basal portion
    (b) Horizontal long axis
    (c) Short-axis apical portion
    (d) Vertical long axis
49. In which coronary artery is the sensitivity and accuracy of myocardial scan minimal for the diagnosis of coronary artery disease?
    (a) LAD
    (b) LMCA
    (c) RCA
    (d) LCX
50. In the first-pass radionuclide angiography in children:
    (a) ^{99m}Tc-MAA is the most commonly used radiotracer.
    (b) Imaging in the upright position is preferred over the supine position.
    (c) Persistence of activity in the lungs and QP/QS > 2 is indicative of a left-to-right shunt.
    (d) High resolution parallel to the hole collimator is used for the test.

51. What happens to the sensitivity and specificity if a low cutoff and high-order Butterworth filter is used for myocardial reconstruction?
    (a) Decreased sensitivity and specificity
    (b) Increased sensitivity and specificity
    (c) Increased sensitivity and decreased specificity
    (d) Decreased sensitivity and increased specificity
52. In which of the following radiotracers is high radiochemical purity important to avoid interference by a high liver uptake?
    (a) ^{99m}Tc-MIBI
    (b) ^{99m}Tc-tetrofosmin
    (c) ^{99m}Tc-furifosmin (Q12)
    (d) ^{99m}Tc-teboroxime
53. What is the main purpose of acquiring long-axis images despite the fact that all walls can be evaluated in short-axis images?
    (a) Better evaluation of artifacts
    (b) Evaluation of the apex and basal segments of the heart
    (c) Evaluation of the relative shortness of the septum to the lateral wall
    (d) Better evaluation of the anterior and inferior walls
54. What is the most suitable filter for noise reduction in myocardial SPECT images?
    (a) Butterworth
    (b) Wiener
    (c) Hanning
    (d) Mets
55. Which statement regarding the ^{99m}Tc-PYP scan in myocardial infarction is NOT correct?
    (a) The doughnut sign is indicative of a poor prognosis.
    (b) A relationship exists between lesion size and prognosis.
    (c) Lesion size is underestimated after revascularization.
    (d) Radiotracer accumulation is higher in the margins than in the central regions of the lesion.
56. Which of the following factors is NOT considered an advantage of ^{111}In-antimyosin over ^{99m}Tc-PYP in evaluating acute MI?
    (a) Better evaluation of the inferior wall because of its negligible hepatic uptake.
    (b) Stable high sensitivity during 2 weeks after acute MI.
    (c) It becomes positive earlier than ^{99m}Tc-PYP.
    (d) Higher specificity.
57. Zoom factor (ZF) on a myocardial scan:
    (a) Higher zoom factors improve the uniformity of an image and its interpretation.
    (b) In an optimal planar image, the heart occupies one-third to one-fourth of the imaging field.
    (c) If zooming is NOT used, higher count density is required.
    (d) If a camera with a large field of view is used, a higher ZF produces a better outcome.

58. Which of the following statements regarding the black hole sign is NOT correct?
    (a) It represents aneurysm.
    (b) It is observed both in SPECT and planar methods.
    (c) It appears because of wall dyskinesia and the partial volume effect.
    (d) Perfusion can be normal in this condition.
59. What is the common pattern of a thallium differential uptake?
    (a) An exercise defect that improves or becomes normal in redistribution imaging but reappears after reinjection
    (b) A normal exercise region that appears as a defect in redistribution images and becomes normal after reinjection
    (c) An exercise defect that becomes larger in redistribution imaging but improves or becomes normal after reinjection
    (d) A normal exercise region that appears as a defect in redistribution imaging and after reinjection
60. What is the purpose of the 180° rotation in a myocardial SPECT study?
    (a) Decrease the attenuation effect
    (b) Decrease the attenuation effect and resolution changes due to depth
    (c) Increase the attenuation effect and resolution
    (d) Increase the attenuation effect but decrease the resolution
61. Regarding the polar map or bull's-eye:
    (a) The intensity of each pixel in the slice is indicative of the activity.
    (b) The intensity of each pixel in the slice is indicative of the radial position of the slice.
    (c) The position of each pixel is indicative of the radial activity in each slice.
    (d) The distribution of activity in a material represents the exterior to interior opening.
62. The partial volume effect can cause problems in nuclear medicine studies. Which of the following statements about this effect is correct?
    (a) If a hot spot in a cold background is smaller than twofold of the spatial resolution, it will appear larger and have less activity than that of the background.
    (b) If a hot spot in a cold background is smaller than twofold of the spatial resolution, it will appear smaller and have more activity than that of the background.
    (c) If a cold spot in a hot background is smaller than twofold of the spatial resolution, it will appear larger and have less activity than that of the background.
    (d) If a cold spot in a hot background is smaller than twofold of the spatial resolution, it will appear smaller and have less activity than that of the background.
63. Which of the following findings can be observed in the myocardial perfusion study of patients with hypertension?
    (a) Increased relative uptake in the inferior wall to the anterior wall
    (b) Increased relative uptake in the inferior wall to the septum
    (c) Increased relative uptake in the septum to the lateral wall
    (d) Increased relative uptake in the lateral wall to the anterior wall

64. Which of the following scans is recommended the least if the goal is to reduce the diaphragmatic effect on a myocardial perfusion scan?
    (a) Left lateral imaging in the supine position
    (b) Left lateral imaging in the right recumbent position
    (c) Left lateral imaging in the prone position
    (d) Study of wall motility on gated SPECT
65. The following statements about upward creep are correct *except*:
    (a) Cardiac rotation from vertical to horizontal.
    (b) It is due to deep breathing in the exercise phase and superficial breathing in the rest phase.
    (c) It is commonly observed on a ^{99m}Tc-MIBI scan.
    (d) It causes a false defect on the inferior wall.
66. Which item can cause a ring artifact in SPECT images?
    (a) Center of rotation error
    (b) Nonuniformity
    (c) Misalignment
    (d) Elliptical orbit instead of circular orbit
67. Which errors on myocardial SPECT can cause the hurricane sign and a smear in the apex, respectively?
    (a) Center of rotation error, center of rotation error
    (b) Nonuniformity, center of rotation error
    (c) Misalignment, nonuniformity
    (d) Center of rotation error, rotation axis error
68. The coffee bean appearance on myocardial SPECT is observed in which of the following situations and in which view, respectively?
    (a) Center of rotation error, short-axis view
    (b) Left bundle branch block, horizontal long axis
    (c) Hypertensive cardiomyopathy, horizontal long axis
    (d) Partial volume effect, short-axis view
69. Which of the following adjustments does NOT improve the orbit-related artifact?
    (a) Positioning of the heart at the center of rotation
    (b) Application of 360° imaging instead of 180° imaging
    (c) Application of a high-resolution collimator instead of LEGP
    (d) Selection of new axes in reconstructing the images
70. If the goal is to decrease the effect of a subdiaphragmatic abdominal activity on a ^{99m}Tc-MIBI cardiac scan, which of the following interventions is the least effective?
    (a) Imaging in the prone position instead of the supine position
    (b) Mild exercise during dipyridamole injection
    (c) Mild exercise with a high-fat regime
    (d) A lead shield on the liver
71. Which artifacts are produced by the offset of center of rotation and field non-uniformity on SPECT, respectively?
    (a) Coffee bean view and ring artifact
    (b) Hurricane sign and ring artifact
    (c) Coffee bean view and hurricane sign
    (d) Hurricane sign and coffee bean view

6.3.1 Answer

	A	B	C	D		A	B	C	D
1		*			37				*
2				*	38		*		
3		*			39			*	
4		*			40		*		
5		*			41				*
6				*	42				*
7			*		43			*	
8			*		44			*	
9		*			45	*			
10		*			46		*		
11		*			47			*	
12				*	48	*			
13		*			49				*
14			*		50			*	
15		*			51				*
16		*			52			*	
17				*	53		*		
18			*		54	*			
19		*			55			*	
20		*			56	*			
21				*	57		*		
22		*			58				*
23			*		59	*			
24		*			60		*		
25		*			61	*			
26	*				62	*			
27		*			63			*	
28		*			64			*	
29				*	65			*	
30				*	66		*		
31			*		67	*			
32		*			68				*
33				*	69				*
34			*		70				*
35			*		71		*		
36	*								

6.4 Positron Emission Tomography

1. In image reconstruction in PET using filtered back projection (FBP) and iterative reconstruction (IR) methods:
   (a) FBP has superior statistical quality than IR.
   (b) FBP has more flexibility than IR.
   (c) IR has better statistical quality and flexibility than FBP.
   (d) a and b.
2. Which of the following radiopharmaceuticals has a similar mechanism to that of ^{11}C-CO in myocardial imaging?
   (a) ^{99m}Tc-RBC
   (b) ^{82}Rb-chloride
   (c) ^{13}N-NH_3
   (d) ^{99m}Tc-sestamibi
3. Which of the following radiopharmaceuticals requires blood pool subtraction in a myocardial perfusion study?
   (a) ^{13}N-NH_3
   (b) Cu-PTSM
   (c) ^{15}O-H_2O
   (d) ^{11}C-acetate
4. Which PET radiotracer can be used for the simultaneous evaluation of myocardial perfusion and oxidative metabolism (MVO2)?
   (a) ^{15}O-H_2O
   (b) ^{11}C-acetate
   (c) ^{18}F-FDG
   (d) ^{15}O-oxygen
5. The myocardial uptake of which PET radiotracer does NOT depend on metabolism and is linearly related to perfusion?
   (a) ^{15}O-H_2O
   (b) ^{62}Cu-PTSM
   (c) ^{13}N-ammonia
   (d) ^{82}Rb
6. What happens to a subject with a healthy cardiac status after an intake of a high-carbohydrate meal?
   (a) Activation of lipolysis
   (b) Decreased glucose consumption in the oxidative metabolism of the heart
   (c) Decreased glucose transport into myocytes
   (d) Decreased plasma fatty acids
7. A 73-year-old man is referred for a cardiac PET scan. Which of the following radiopharmaceuticals can be administered both by injection and inhalation?
   (a) ^{15}O-H_2O
   (b) ^{11}C-acetate
   (c) ^{62}Cu-PTSM
   (d) ^{13}N-ammonia

8. What is the most appropriate radiopharmaceutical for myocardial perfusion with PET?
   (a) ^{18}F-FDG
   (b) ^{13}N-ammonia
   (c) ^{82}Rb
   (d) ^{11}C-palmitate
9. The preparation of nondiabetic patients for the evaluation of myocardial viability with FDG-PET includes all items *except*:
   (a) Having a light protein-rich breakfast
   (b) Glucose
   (c) Insulin infusion
   (d) Initiation of imaging 0.5 h after injection
10. What is the main reason for prioritizing PET scan over SPECT for myocardial study?
    (a) Measurement of regional blood flow
    (b) Evaluation of acute coronary artery syndrome
    (c) Determination of infarct size
    (d) Therapeutic monitoring in ischemia
11. Which of the following features distinguishes ^{18}F-FDG-PET from other imaging methods if the goal is the noninvasive imaging of atherosclerotic plaques?
    (a) Accumulation in plaque fibrous CAP
    (b) Accumulation in plaque endothelium
    (c) Accumulation in plaque macrophages
    (d) Accumulation in plaque cholesterol
12. What is the radiotracer of choice for the accurate evaluation of myocardial perfusion in ischemic regions in patients with CAD?
    (a) Radiolabeled microsphere
    (b) ^{82}Rubidium chloride
    (c) $^{15}O\text{-}H_2O$
    (d) ^{11}C-acetate
13. In which of the following situations is PET conducted prior to SPECT for the evaluation of ischemic heart disease?
    (a) Overweight patients
    (b) Underweight patients
    (c) Severe ischemia
    (d) Age > 77 years
14. In which of the following situations does myocardium use free fatty acids as energy source?
    (a) Fasting state
    (b) Glucose load (postprandial)
    (c) Hypoxia
    (d) Ischemia

15. Which of the following statements properly describes the value of a dual-PET study with metabolic and perfusion agents (e.g., 18 FDG vs. [13N]-NH_3) in cardiac sarcoidosis?
    (a) Normal perfusion, intense FDG uptake representing active acute inflammation
    (b) Reduced perfusion, intense FDG uptake representing the advanced stages of cardiac involvement
    (c) Reduced or absent perfusion, absent FDG uptake representing end-stage disease
    (d) All of the above
16. In the evaluation of which of the following parameters related to the imaging of atherosclerotic plaques is the strength of PET-MRI greater than that of PET-CT?
    (a) Stenosis
    (b) Microcalcification
    (c) Apoptosis
    (d) Fibrous cap

6.4.1 Answer

	A	B	C	D
1				*
2	*			
3			*	
4		*		
5	*			
6				*
7	*			
8		*		
9			*	
10	*			
11			*	
12			*	
13	*			
14	*			
15				*
16				*

6.5 Cardiac Stress

1. The ideal drug for stress myocardial perfusion imaging in patients with asthma is:
   (a) Dobutamine
   (b) Adenosine
   (c) Dipyridamole
   (d) Aminophylline
2. Slight exercise during dipyridamole administration on a myocardial perfusion scan will result in:
   (a) Enhanced clearannce of Tc
   (b) Higher vasodilatation
   (c) Lower drug side effects
   (d) Longer vasodilatation
3. What is the main advantage of adenosine over dipyridamole in a pharmacologic stress procedure?
   (a) Lower price and availability
   (b) No effect on heart rate
   (c) Lesser side effects
   (d) Shorter half-life and rapid vasodilatation
4. Which of the following drugs causes stress with vasoconstriction?
   (a) Ergonovine
   (b) Dopamine
   (c) Adenosine
   (d) Dipyridamole
5. Which item regarding the advantages of adenosine over dipyridamole is NOT correct?
   (a) Shorter half-life
   (b) More rapid vasodilatation
   (c) Lower dose of the administered radiotracer
   (d) Shorter protocol
6. According to the mechanism of dipyridamole-induced coronary vasodilatation, what happens if this drug is administered during chest pain?
   (a) Pain reduction
   (b) Pain exacerbation
   (c) No effect
   (d) Different effects depending on the patient's background
7. In which of the following conditions is dobutamine administration allowed?
   (a) Unstable angina
   (b) Patients with asthma
   (c) First week after MI
   (d) Severe stenosis of the aorta

8. Stress myocardial perfusion (by regadenoson, an adenosine derivative) is requested for a patient. On the examination day, the patient has taken labetalol (nonselective beta blocker and selective alpha-1 blocker), benazepril (angiotensin-converting enzyme inhibitor), hydrochlorothiazide, caffeine, and aspirin. What procedure would you recommend?
   (a) Postpone imaging until tomorrow and ask the patient not to take caffeine.
   (b) Use dipyridamole instead of regadenoson and perform imaging on the same day.
   (c) Use adenosine instead of regadenoson and perform imaging on the same day.
   (d) Use dobutamine instead of regadenoson and perform imaging on the same day.
9. Cardiac scan with exercise is requested for a patient. Basal blood pressure and heart rate are 140/80 mmHg and 67/min, respectively. Blood pressure and heart rate increase to 170/80 and 150, respectively, in the second step of the Bruce protocol. Which item indicates the discontinuation of the exercise test?
   (a) Decrease in systolic blood pressure to 160 mmHg
   (b) Decrease in diastolic blood pressure to 60 mmHg
   (c) 1.5 mm elevation of ST segment
   (d) Higher than 10 PVC per min
10. Myocardial perfusion with dipyridamole is requested for a 47-year-old woman with hypertension and atypical chest pain. She takes atenolol, Isordil, and enalapril. Which drug has NO effect on the sensitivity of the scan?
   (a) Atenolol
   (b) Isordil
   (c) Enalapril
   (d) a and b
11. Dipyridamole is used for stress induction on the myocardial perfusion scan. Which item is NOT correct?
   (a) Three to four times increase in coronary blood flow.
   (b) Maximum dilatation of the coronary flow is achieved 4 min after the completion of infusion.
   (c) Heart rate increases by 10 bpm.
   (d) Systolic blood pressure increases by 10 mmHg.
12. What is the maximum dosing rate of dobutamine for stress myocardial perfusion scan?
   (a) 20 μg/kg/min
   (b) 40 μg/kg/min
   (c) 70 μg/kg/min
   (d) 80 μg/kg/min
13. Which of the following findings in stress EKG is indicative of being high risk?
   (a) Increase in heart rate during exercise
   (b) ST changes of 1 mm that disappear at the end of the exercise
   (c) Non-sustained ventricular tachycardia that begins with exercise
   (d) Hypotension during exercise

14. Which item about cardiac stress with adenosine is NOT correct?
    (a) Adenosine increases cAMP content and induces the hyperpolarization of the membrane by binding to cellular receptors.
    (b) Adenosine increases the heart rate and decreases the blood pressure.
    (c) Heart block is the most dangerous side effect.
    (d) Concurrent benzodiazepine treatment is NOT contraindicated.
15. What is the drug of choice for the induction of cardiac stress?
    (a) Adenosine
    (b) Dipyridamole
    (c) Dobutamine
    (d) Arbutamine
16. In which of the following situations is the sensitivity of the exercise test low?
    (a) Multiple coronary stenosis
    (b) Single coronary stenosis
    (c) Females
    (d) Patients with an intermediate risk of CAD
17. Which drug is used to antagonize the effects of dobutamine?
    (a) Atropine
    (b) Theophylline
    (c) Aminophylline
    (d) Propranolol
18. Which of the following conditions is considered high risk for stress test?
    (a) Mitral stenosis
    (b) Unstable angina
    (c) Compensated left ventricle failure
    (d) Severe mitral valve regurgitation
19. Which drug is used with dobutamine to increase the heart rate on a myocardial perfusion scan?
    (a) Atropine
    (b) Epinephrine
    (c) Norepinephrine
    (d) Dipyridamole
20. In which of the following conditions is dobutamine-induced myocardial stress contraindicated?
    (a) Pulmonary bronchospastic disorders
    (b) AV block
    (c) Sensitivity to Na-bisulfate
    (d) Dipyridamole administration
21. A myocardial scan with stress is requested for a patient incapable of physical exercise. In which of the following conditions is dobutamine recommended for pharmacological stress?
    (a) Recent CVA
    (b) Sudden increase in blood pressure
    (c) AV block
    (d) Ventricular arrhythmia

22. Which statement about the pathophysiology of cardiac ischemia is NOT correct?
    (a) Two seconds of ischemia is enough to disturb myocardial contractility.
    (b) About 20–40 min of ischemia causes MI.
    (c) Abnormal findings is first observed on the perfusion scan, followed by echocardiography, and then EKG after ischemia.
    (d) A decrease in the demand/supply in myocardium is the WHO definition of heart ischemia.
23. The following all increase during dynamic exercise *except*:
    (a) Systolic blood pressure
    (b) Intramuscular forces
    (c) Oxygen consumption
    (d) Peripheral vascular resistance
24. Static exercise has the little effect on which of the following?
    (a) Systolic blood pressure
    (b) Intramuscular forces
    (c) Diastolic blood pressure
    (d) Cardiac parameters
25. A myocardial perfusion scan with physical stress is requested for a 65-year-old patient. Exercise test with Bruce protocol is performed. Blood pressure is 120/80 at the beginning. Blood pressure reaches to 160/90 and heart rate to 120 in the third part of the test. ST depression of 2 mm in precordial leads is observed in the EKG. What is the most appropriate decision?
    (a) Continuation of the exercise test
    (b) Radiotracer injection and immediate discontinuation of the exercise test
    (c) Radiotracer injection and continuation of the exercise test for 2 min
    (d) Discontinuation of the exercise test
26. The contraindications for the administration of adenosine in a myocardial stress test include all of the following *except*:
    (a) Chronic administration of dipyridamole
    (b) COPD
    (c) Wolff–Parkinson–White syndrome
    (d) Grade II block
27. Which of the following items is NOT an indication for the discontinuation of an exercise test?
    (a) Hypotension
    (b) ST depression of 2 mm
    (c) Fatigue
    (d) Ventricular arrhythmia
28. Dobutamine increases coronary blood flow through all of the following mechanisms *except*:
    (a) Increase in heart rate
    (b) Increase in myocardial contractility
    (c) Increase in blood pressure
    (d) Increase in vascular dilatation

29. Regarding the comparison between adenosine and dipyridamole:
    (a) Adenosine-induced vasodilatation is faster, stronger, and shorter than that induced by dipyridamole.
    (b) Dipyridamole decreases the serum concentration of adenosine.
    (c) In contrast to adenosine, dipyridamole increases cerebral and coronary blood flow and decreases renal blood flow.
    (d) Adenosine concentration decreases in ischemic tissues.
30. Regarding dobutamine pharmacological stress:
    (a) This drug increases blood flow comparable with dipyridamole.
    (b) This drug is contraindicated in patients who take xanthine derivatives.
    (c) This drug increases systolic blood pressure.
    (d) The sensitivity and specificity of this test are lesser than those of dipyridamole.
31. Dipyridamole in a myocardial perfusion scan:
    (a) Similar to nitroglycerin, it increases the coronary blood flow and the diameter of the epicardial vessels.
    (b) It increases the cellular uptake and metabolism of adenosine.
    (c) It changes neither the ejection fraction nor the ventricular afterload in healthy subjects.
    (d) In contrast to the exercise test, it induces little change in the heart rate, blood pressure, and myocardial oxygen demand.
32. Adenosine in indicated for stress induction in:
    (a) Patients with severe pulmonary obstructive diseases
    (b) Patients with unstable angina
    (c) Patients incapable of physical activity
    (d) Patients under treatment with oral dipyridamole
33. In which of the following conditions is an exercise test possible?
    (a) Significant aortic stenosis
    (b) Mitral valve prolapse
    (c) Treatment with beta blockers
    (d) Severe pulmonary diseases
34. What is the most appropriate intervention if the patient experiences chest pain during a myocardial perfusion scan with adenosine?
    (a) Intravenous injection of 25–50 mg aminophylline.
    (b) Sublingual TNG.
    (c) Intravenous morphine.
    (d) Discontinuation of adenosine infusion is usually sufficient.
35. Regarding a myocardial perfusion scan with adenosine:
    (a) Chest pain after injection is a good sign for the diagnosis of CAD.
    (b) The level of ST depression during infusion is related to the severity of CAD.
    (c) Adenosine is contraindicated in patients with first- and second-grade atrial blockade.
    (d) Persantine and benzodiazepines enhance adenosine effects.

36. A patient with severe pulmonary obstructive disease and treatment with theophylline and bronchodilators is referred for a myocardial perfusion scan because of atypical chest pains. What is the most appropriate method for stress induction?
    (a) Adenosine
    (b) Exercise
    (c) Dipyridamole
    (d) Dobutamine
37. About dobutamine:
    (a) The addition of atropine seems to enhance the sensitivity of the test in patients under treatment with beta blockers.
    (b) The inability to monitor dobutamine serum concentration is considered a problem because of its long-lasting effects.
    (c) Dobutamine must be used with caution in asthmatic patients because of the effects on bronchial B2 receptors.
    (d) Decrease in blood pressure during dobutamine infusion is predictive of a poor prognosis.
38. The discontinuation of all of the following drugs or reagents is recommended before myocardial perfusion with adenosine *except*:
    (a) Dipyridamole 12 h before the test
    (b) Methylene xanthines 24 h before the test
    (c) Coffee 12 h before the test
    (d) Calcium blockers 72 h before the test
39. What is the minimum required time interval after myocardial infarction for pharmacological stress by adenosine or dipyridamole?
    (a) 1–2 days
    (b) 2–3 days
    (c) 3–5 days
    (d) 6–7 days

6.5.1 Answer

	A	B	C	D
1	*			
2			*	
3				*
4	*			
5			*	
6		*		
7		*		
8	*			
9			*	
10			*	
11				*

12		*		
13				*
14				*
15	*			
16			*	
17				*
18		*		
19	*			
20			*	
21			*	
22				*
23				*
24				*
25	*			
26			*	
27		*		
28				*
29	*			
30			*	
31				*
32			*	
33		*		
34				*
35				*
36				*
37				*
38				*
39			*	

6.6 Detection of Coronary Artery Disease

1. The implementation of attenuation correction mainly leads to improve:
   (a) Specificity and sensitivity
   (b) Sensitivity and normalcy rate
   (c) Normalcy rate and specificity
   (d) Specificity, sensitivity, and normalcy rate
2. Which of the following factors is considered an advantage of electron beam tomography (EBT)?
   (a) Rapid scanning procedure
   (b) Higher radiation
   (c) Great specificity
   (d) The most accurate test for CAD
3. What is the greatest advantage of dual-isotope protocols over standard protocols in myocardial perfusion?
   (a) Quick scanning procedure
   (b) Higher specificity
   (c) Higher sensitivity
   (d) Lower radiation dose
4. What is the first change in cardiac ischemia?
   (a) Changes in metabolic pathways
   (b) Changes in ECG
   (c) Decreased contractility
   (d) Decreased range of ventricular wall motility
5. Regarding the calculated LVEF in stress gated SPECT during a myocardial perfusion scan:
   (a) It is always related to the stress period.
   (b) It is the average of EF in stress and rest.
   (c) It is always related to the rest period.
   (d) It depends on the apparatus settings and patient rhythm.
6. A normal myocardial perfusion scan is conducted on a patient with acute chest pain. What is the probability of CAD?
   (a) Low
   (b) Intermediate
   (c) High
   (d) Very unlikely
7. Myocardial perfusion SPECT appears to be normal. Which of the following findings is suggestive of three-vessel disease (3VD)?
   (a) TID of 1.1
   (b) ST depression of 1.5 mm
   (c) Reduced wash-out rate of thallium from myocardium
   (d) Increased diastolic blood pressure during exercise

8. An increased activity of the right to the left ventricle in the peak of exercise during a myocardial perfusion scan is suggestive of:
   (a) Severe disorder in the left circumflex artery
   (b) Hypertrophy of the left ventricle
   (c) Severe hypertension
   (d) Cardiomyopathy
9. LV dilatation, nonhomogenous uptake, and diffused hypokinesia are observed on a gated myocardial perfusion scan. What is the most probable diagnosis?
   (a) Ischemic cardiomyopathy
   (b) A three-vessel patient
   (c) Idiopathic cardiomyopathy
   (d) Diffuse subendocardial ischemia
10. What is the mechanism of nitrate enhancement on a myocardial perfusion scan with ^{99m}Tc-MIBI?
    (a) Increase in collateral artery blood flow
    (b) Decrease in heart rate
    (c) Increase in heart contractility
    (d) Steal phenomenon
11. A nonhomogenous activity of myocardium is found on a myocardial perfusion scan. An increase in the left ventricular size and a decrease in the ventricular wall motion and EF are observed. What is the most probable diagnosis?
    (a) 3VD
    (b) LBBB
    (c) Cardiomyopathy
    (d) Myocarditis
12. What is the minimum percentage of reversibility for the diagnosis of ischemia on a quantitative myocardial perfusion scan?
    (a) 5%
    (b) 10%
    (c) 25%
    (d) 40%
13. Which of the following pulmonary–cardiac uptake ratios is considered abnormal on a thallium scan?
    (a) Greater than 0.2
    (b) Greater than 0.3
    (c) Greater than 0.4
    (d) Greater than 0.5
14. Which of the following statements regarding the resting myocardial perfusion scan for a patient in the emergency room with suspected acute infarction is NOT correct?
    (a) Its negative predictive value is very high.
    (b) It has NO important role in the primary decision on therapeutic strategies.
    (c) It is a better diagnostic method than biomarkers.
    (d) If the scan findings are negative, early stress scintigraphy will be indicated.

15. Which statement about the transient dilatation of the left ventricle on a stress/rest myocardial perfusion scan is NOT correct?
    (a) It shows a left ventricular dysfunction due to stress.
    (b) It is indicative of a high risk for myocardium.
    (c) Global dilatation of the left ventricle is the reason for this finding.
    (d) Concomitant subendocardial ischemia is observed.
16. Cardiac scintigraphy reveals a marked dilatation of the left ventricle without the perfusion defect. Increased pulmonary uptake and right ventricular dilatation are also observed. What is the most probable diagnosis?
    (a) Extensive myocardial infarctus
    (b) Idiopathic cardiomyopathy
    (c) Ischemic cardiomyopathy
    (d) Heart valve disease
17. Myocardial scintigraphy with exercise is conducted on a patient with LBBB. A perfusion defect that extends to the apex is found on the anteroseptal wall. Which item is correct?
    (a) Myocardial ischemia.
    (b) The defect is not real and is due to LBBB.
    (c) Stress with dobutamine is preferred over exercise.
    (d) Resting scan is sufficient.
18. The resting myocardial perfusion scan of a patient with acute chest pain is normal. What is the risk of CAD?
    (a) Very low
    (b) Low
    (c) Moderate
    (d) High
19. Which statement about collateral vessels that are formed after coronary artery stenosis is NOT correct?
    (a) They are formed after an intermediate stenosis (about 50%).
    (b) They are formed 1–2 weeks after stenosis.
    (c) Their maximum activity is observed at 4 weeks after stenosis.
    (d) The resistance of these vessels is two to three times less than that of coronary arteries.
20. When is the appropriate time for sublingual TNG if the goal is to increase the reversibility of a defect on the ^{99m}Tc-MIBI cardiac scan?
    (a) Right before rest imaging
    (b) Right before injection of the radiopharmaceutical in rest imaging
    (c) Immediately after the termination of stress imaging
    (d) Concurrent with a fatty meal
21. All of the following items indicate left ventricle dysfunction after stress *except*:
    (a) Reverse defect in stress images
    (b) Lung uptake in stress images
    (c) Dilated left ventricle in stress images
    (d) A clear observation of the right ventricle in stress images

22. What is the recommended time for a myocardial perfusion scan after surgery or PTCA regardless of clinical symptoms?
    (a) 1 week
    (b) 4 weeks
    (c) 3 months
    (d) 8 months
23. What is the mechanism of sublingual TNG on a cardiac scan with ^{99m}Tc-MIBI?
    (a) Increase the redistribution
    (b) Increase the myocardial contractility
    (c) Increase the ventricular diastolic time
    (d) Increase the blood flow of collateral vessels
24. Cardiac demand is related to all of the following items *except*:
    (a) Heart rate
    (b) Contractility
    (c) Systolic wall stress
    (d) Oxygen-carrying capacity of blood
25. In which of the following conditions is the observation of a myocardial perfusion defect on a scan the most indicative of true ischemia?
    (a) Hypertrophic cardiomyopathy
    (b) LBBB
    (c) LVH
    (d) Dilated cardiomyopathy
26. What is the first recommended method for the evaluation of CAD in a diabetic patient?
    (a) Exercise test
    (b) CT angiography
    (c) Stress echo
    (d) Angiography
27. Which of the following items is indicated by the summed stress score in the grading of myocardial defects?
    (a) Extent of infarcted myocardium
    (b) Extent of ischemic myocardium
    (c) Extent of infarcted or hibernating myocardium
    (d) Extent of infarcted, ischemic, or jeopardized myocardium
28. The summed stress score of a patient is 8 on the quantitative myocardial perfusion scan with QPS software by the Cedars–Sinai Center. In which group is this patient categorized?
    (a) Near normal
    (b) Mild abnormal
    (c) Moderate abnormal
    (d) Severe abnormal

29. Which of the following items decreases the sensitivity of the myocardial perfusion scan for the detection of coronary artery disease in women?
    (a) Breast attenuation
    (b) Diaphragmatic attenuation
    (c) Sub-optimal stress
    (d) Orbit-related artifact
30. What is the cause of blinking in the dynamic image of gated SPECT?
    (a) Arrhythmia
    (b) Misalignment
    (c) Patient motion
    (d) Myocardial dysfunction
31. A myocardial perfusion scan with exercise is requested for a 7-year-old child with Kawasaki disease. The exercise MPI test is completed successfully, but a reversible perfusion defect is found on the inferior wall. Epicardial vessels are normal without stenosis in angiography. What is the therapeutic plan for this patient?
    (a) Limitation in sports
    (b) Full-dose administration of anti-ischemic drugs
    (c) Monitoring of myocardial perfusion defects until adolescence
    (d) RCA angioplasty
32. A 7% perfusion defect in the polar map image and an SSS of 8 are obtained from the MPI scan of a patient with a mild defect of the inferolateral wall. What is the best therapeutic plan?
    (a) Aggressive risk factor modification is recommended.
    (b) Angioplasty of the involved vessel is the choice treatment.
    (c) Arterioplasty of the involved vessel results is the best outcome.
    (d) Scan findings canNOT determine the therapeutic plan.
33. The myocardial perfusion scan shows a defect in the basal inferoseptal area. Which coronary artery is involved?
    (a) OM1
    (b) RCA
    (c) LAD
    (d) LCX
34. Which of the following findings indicates ischemic cardiomyopathy on the myocardial perfusion scan?
    (a) Fixed defect in the apex
    (b) Involvement of more than 40% of the pericardium on the scan
    (c) Fixed defect in the inferior area
    (d) Irregularity in the myocardial uptake of the radiotracer
35. A patient with a history of dyspnea and orthopnea is referred for a myocardial perfusion scan. Which of the following findings favors idiopathic dilated cardiomyopathy (the absence of coronary artery disease)?
    (a) Anterior wall akinesia
    (b) Dilatation of both ventricles and both atria
    (c) No increase in the LVEF during exercise test
    (d) Presence of stress-induced myocardial stunning

36. Regarding gated myocardial perfusion SPECT and the diagnosis of multivessel coronary disease (MCAD):
    (a) The sensitivity of the scan only for the diagnosis of CAD is higher than 90%.
    (b) The perfusion defect is observed in several territories in more than 80% of these patients.
    (c) The absence of TID excludes the possibility of MCAD.
    (d) The absence of a pulmonary uptake excludes the possibility of MCAD.
37. A 69-year-old man with a history of diabetes for 12 years and smoking for 32 years (one pack per day) underwent a cardiac scan with dipyridamole. The following parameters are obtained with the 20-segment method: SSS, 24, and SRS, 24. What percentage of the myocardium (left ventricle) is involved?
    (a) 12%
    (b) 21%
    (c) 30%
    (d) 36%
38. A patient with a history of atypical cardiac pains is suspected of having coronary artery disease. The thallium–persantine scan is normal, but the thallium–exercise scan shows a reversible anteroseptal defect. What is the most probable diagnosis?
    (a) LBBB
    (b) X syndrome
    (c) Mitral prolapse
    (d) Mild stenosis of LAD
39. Ischemia is detected on the anterior and lateral walls on the thallium myocardial perfusion scan. The involvement of which arteries is the most probable?
    (a) LCX and PDA
    (b) LAD
    (c) Left main artery
    (d) RCA, obtuse marginal
40. The right ventricle is observed on the resting thallium scan. What is the most probable cause of such a finding?
    (a) Decreased blood pressure
    (b) Decreased blood volume
    (c) A normal finding
    (d) Tachycardia
41. A dual-isotope study with ^{201}Tl and In-antimyosin Ab is performed on a patient with chest pain. A decrease in the thallium uptake in the anterior wall with a regional increase in antimyosin uptake in the same zone is observed. What is the most probable diagnosis?
    (a) Transmural anterior MI
    (b) Non-Q wave MI
    (c) Stunned myocardium
    (d) Subendocardial ischemia

42. Which of the following factors can cause false-negative findings on a planar myocardial perfusion scan?
    (a) Non-coronary heart disease
    (b) Sub-maximal exercise test
    (c) Activity of the pericardium
    (d) Diaphragm suppression of the inferior wall activity
43. Regarding the role of angiography for the diagnosis of coronary artery disease and myocardial ischemia:
    (a) The existence of coronary artery stenosis in angiography does NOT necessarily indicate myocardial ischemia.
    (b) Angiography identifies the collateral artery blood flow after stenosis.
    (c) The existence of coronary stenosis in angiography indicates an increase in the coronary reservoir capacity.
    (d) Angiography shows the extent of a small coronary artery involvement.
44. In which of the following situations is the ^{99m}Tc-MIBI scan the most efficient in the early hours after infarction if the goal is to determine the infarction size?
    (a) Extensive anterior infarction
    (b) Extensive posterolateral infarction
    (c) Extensive inferior infarction
    (d) Extensive anterolateral infarction
45. The maximum diagnostic value of the myocardial perfusion scan is in patients with a 40–70% possibility of having coronary artery disease. Which of the following patients is NOT included in this group?
    (a) A 62-year-old woman with atypical chest pain
    (b) A 52-year-old man with a positive exercise test
    (c) A 52-year-old diabetic woman
    (d) A 62-year-old man with typical angina pectoris
46. In a patient with myocardial infarction, ^{99m}Tc-sestamibi is administered before thrombolytic therapy. Which of the following items is indicated by the defect observed on the scan?
    (a) Myocardium at risk
    (b) Extent of infarcted myocardium
    (c) Extent of the viable myocardium around the infarcted region
    (d) Efficacy of thrombolytic therapy
47. What is the most appropriate radiotracer for the diagnosis and evaluation of cardiomyopathy?
    (a) Cardiolite
    (b) Myoview
    (c) Myoscint
    (d) ^{201}Tl
48. Which of the following diseases is represented by transient left ventricular dilatation during exercise or dipyridamole?
    (a) One-vessel coronary artery stenosis
    (b) RBBB
    (c) Primary cardiomyopathy
    (d) Multivessel severe coronary artery stenosis

49. A 79-year-old patient with LBBB is subjected to an exercise myocardial perfusion SPECT study. Which of the following artifacts are presented by this test?
    (a) Reversible lesion of the lateral wall
    (b) Fixed left ventricular dilatation
    (c) Transient left ventricular dilatation
    (d) Reversible septal lesion
50. Upward creep is the common cause of a false defect on the … myocardial wall.
    (a) Anterior
    (b) Septum
    (c) Inferior and inferolateral
    (d) Anteroseptal
51. Regarding unstable angina:
    (a) A myocardial perfusion defect is never observed during chest pain.
    (b) If a myocardial defect is observed during chest pain and disappears after the termination of chest pain, the sensitivity and specificity of this finding are high.
    (c) The shift in ST segment in ECG is relatively better than myocardial perfusion.
    (d) The specificity of myocardial perfusion is low.
52. What is the recommended method for a myocardial perfusion study in patients with LBBB?
    (a) Dobutamine perfusion scan
    (b) Exercise perfusion scan
    (c) MIBG perfusion scan
    (d) Dipyridamole perfusion scan
53. A normal uptake but a decrease in washout is observed from the normal ^{201}Tl activity curve of myocardium after exercise. What is the most probable diagnosis?
    (a) Normal
    (b) Mild ischemia
    (c) Severe ischemia
    (d) Recent thrombolysis
54. Which of the following situations can cause false-positive findings on an exercise myocardial perfusion scan?
    (a) Functionally nonsignificant, anatomically significant coronary stenosis
    (b) Functionally significant, anatomically nonsignificant coronary stenosis
    (c) Functionally and anatomically significant coronary stenosis
    (d) Functionally and anatomically nonsignificant coronary stenosis
55. Which of the following diseases is indicated by a pulmonary thallium uptake on a planar myocardial perfusion scan?
    (a) High left ventricular end-diastolic pressure (LVEDP)
    (b) Low right ventricular end-systolic volume (RVESV)
    (c) High right ventricular overload
    (d) Low cardiac index

56. Which of the following tests increases the diagnostic sensitivity of a gated SPECT MIBI study for the evaluation of CAD in patients with left ventricular hypertrophy (LVH)?
    (a) Transient ischemic dilatation study
    (b) Global wall motion study
    (c) Study of count density in end-diastole to end-systole interval
    (d) End-diastolic wall perfusion study
57. The recommended method for the diagnosis of CAD in a transplanted heart:
    (a) Coronary angiography
    (b) Clinical examination
    (c) Intravascular ultrasonography
    (d) Echo-dobutamine + thallium scan
58. Hypoperfusion of the inferior wall is reported on an exercise myocardial perfusion scan with technetium derivatives. Which of the following tests is effective in evaluating a true or false finding?
    (a) Repeat of scan with dobutamine
    (b) Scan in the supine–prone position
    (c) Repeat of scan with thallium
    (d) Administration of TNG
59. What is the optimal pretest probability for a myocardial perfusion scan?
    (a) 90–95%
    (b) 4–6%
    (c) 40–70%
    (d) 10–15%
60. Which of the following parameters is replaced by normalcy rate because of the inefficiency of angiography in confirming myocardial SPECT findings?
    (a) Accuracy
    (b) Sensitivity
    (c) Precision
    (d) Specificity
61. What is the reason for the difficult diagnosis of coronary artery disease in women?
    (a) The diverse clinical symptoms causes a delay in the exercise test.
    (b) The higher incidence of hypertension and left ventricular hypertrophy.
    (c) Requirement of prone imaging.
    (d) Equal risk for CAD at ages above 60 years in comparison with men.
62. Post-stress stunning is observed on the cardiac scan of a 65-year-old man. Which of the following statements is correct?
    (a) This finding is indicative of the lack of increase in ejection fraction during stress.
    (b) This finding is indicative of myocardial viability and low risk for CABG.
    (c) This finding is rare when the scan is performed immediately after stress.
    (d) This finding is commonly observed in multivessel coronary artery disease.

63. If the goal is to diagnose coronary artery disease, which of the following statements is correct about transient LV dilatation in the stress phase compared with the rest phase without evidence of myocardial ischemia in SPECT?
    (a) It is NOT valuable.
    (b) The sensitivity of this finding is high, but its specificity is low.
    (c) The specificity of this finding is high, but its sensitivity is low.
    (d) The sensitivity and specificity of this finding are high.
64. A 42-year-old man with chest pain is referred to the emergency ward. There is NO risk factor for atherosclerosis, but his ECG shows the possibility of ischemia. What is the probability of cardiac events occurring 72 h after hospitalization?
    (a) Very low risk (less than 1%)
    (b) Low risk (about 4%)
    (c) Intermediate risk (about 8%)
    (d) High risk (more than 16%)
65. A patient with chest pain is evaluated. Clinical examination shows a definite acute coronary syndrome, but there is NO specific finding in the ECG, and the cardiac markers are normal. A repeat of the ECG and cardiac markers after 6 h shows normal outcomes, and pain has NOT recurred. What is the recommended intervention?
    (a) No further evaluation is required, and the patient must be discharged.
    (b) The patient must be monitored in the CCU.
    (c) Drug treatment must be initiated, and the patient must be observed for 24 h in the emergency ward.
    (d) Echocardiography and exercise test are recommended.
66. How long is the warranty period after a normal myocardial perfusion scan?
    (a) 1 year
    (b) 2 years
    (c) 3 years
    (d) 4 years
67. Which coronary artery is the origin of the diagonal artery?
    (a) Left main coronary
    (b) Right coronary artery (RCA)
    (c) Left anterior descending (LAD)
    (d) Circumflex
68. A 51-year-old man with severe three-vessel atherosclerosis, severe left ventricular insufficiency, and ejection fraction of 15% in echocardiography is referred. What is the next intervention?
    (a) Myocardial perfusion scan at rest
    (b) Myocardial perfusion scan with dipyridamole
    (c) Myocardial perfusion scan with sub-maximal exercise
    (d) Cardiac transplantation

6.6.1 Answer

	A	B	C	D		A	B	C	D
1			*		35		*		
2	*				36	*			
3	*				37			*	
4	*				38	*			
5			*		39			*	
6				*	40				*
7			*		41		*		
8				*	42		*		
9			*		43	*			
10	*				44	*			
11			*		45				*
12			*		46	*			
13				*	47			*	
14		*			48				*
15			*		49				*
16		*			50			*	
17	*				51		*		
18		*			52				*
19	*				53		*		
20		*			54		*		
21	*				55	*			
22		*			56				*
23				*	57	*			
24				*	58		*		
25	*				59			*	
26	*				60				*
27				*	61	*			
28		*			62				*
29			*		63				*
30	*				64			*	
31			*		65				*
32	*				66		*		
33		*			67			*	
34		*			68	*			

6.7 Prognosis of Patients with Known or Suspected Coronary Artery Disease

1. All of the following statements regarding MPI indices is true *except*:
   (a) There is a good correlation between TID and lung uptake.
   (b) The C-M ratio is lineally correlated with LVEF.
   (c) TID is a strong predictor of future adverse cardiac events.
   (d) Lung uptake is closely related to LV dysfunction.
2. All of the following conditions indicate a high-risk exercise electrocardiographic stress test *except*:
   (a) ST depression of ≥2.0 mm
   (b) ST depression (≥1.0 mm) lasting >5 min in recovery
   (c) Exercise-induced non-sustained ventricular tachycardia
   (d) ST depression (≥0.5 mm) at a low workload
3. Which cardiac wall has the worst prognosis in MI?
   (a) Anterior extended to septum
   (b) Anterolateral
   (c) Lateral
   (d) Inferior
4. How long can a normal exercise myocardial scan in a patient without a history of CAD be credited?
   (a) 10 months
   (b) 1 year
   (c) 2 years
   (d) 5 years
5. What is the most common mechanism for the septal defect of LBBB on a myocardial perfusion scan?
   (a) Reduced perfusion of the lateral wall
   (b) Artifact (technical problems)
   (c) Stimulation of the parasympathetic system
   (d) Dilatation and dysfunction of the left ventricle
6. Which of the following situations can result in an overestimated EF?
   (a) Extensive aneurysm in the anterior left ventricle
   (b) Ischemic cardiomyopathy
   (c) LBBB
   (d) Inferior MI
7. Which of the following findings on a myocardial perfusion scan is considered high risk?
   (a) Transient dilatation of LV during exercise
   (b) Weak motion of the septum
   (c) Cardiomegaly
   (d) Dilatation of the right ventricle at rest

8. Which of the following findings on the gated scan of myocardial perfusion scintigraphy indicates a low-risk patient?
   (a) EF increase after stress
   (b) Increase in pulmonary uptake after stress
   (c) Transient dilatation of LV after stress
   (d) Appearance of RV after stress
9. A 45-year-old man without any risk factor is a candidate for inguinal hernia surgery:
   (a) Future events depend on the extent of perfusion defect.
   (b) The short-term prognosis depends on the presence of ischemia.
   (c) The long-term prognosis depends on the presence of a scar.
   (d) Risk assessment is not usually indicated for this patient.
10. About therapeutic monitoring with a myocardial perfusion scan of a patient with confirmed CAD:
    (a) Anti-ischemic drugs must be discontinued.
    (b) Cardiac stress is NOT necessary to be the same for comparison.
    (c) More than a 2% improvement of existing defects is considered significant.
    (d) A 4° change in SSS is indicative of the efficacy of treatment.
11. The right ventricle is observed on a cardiac perfusion scan with stress:
    (a) Sensitivity and specificity are high for the risk assessment of CAD.
    (b) The values of the exercise and dipyridamole tests are similar.
    (c) It can indicate left main disease.
    (d) All of the above.
12. What is the best method for estimating the prognosis of a patient with confirmed CAD?
    (a) ^{99m}Tc-MIBI
    (b) F-18-FDG
    (c) Rb-82
    (d) CT angiography
13. In which of the following patients is the risk of a heart event NOT high according to the ^{99m}Tc-MIBI scan?
    (a) A 54-year-old man with lung/heart ratio, 35% and EF, 45%
    (b) A 34-year-old woman with multiple defects on the anterior and inferior walls and EF: 55%
    (c) A 62-year-old man with a moderate scar on the anterior wall and EF: 30%
    (d) A 44-year-old woman with SSS of 15 and EF of 53%
14. What is the strongest predictor of the risk of death among both normal subjects and those with cardiovascular disease?
    (a) Inferolateral ischemia in myocardial perfusion imaging
    (b) Anterior ischemia in myocardial perfusion imaging
    (c) Poor functional capacity
    (d) Apex and septal ischemia in myocardial perfusion imaging

15. Which item does NOT indicate a high risk for a patient with CAD?
    (a) Pulmonary uptake of thallium
    (b) TID
    (c) Increase in the right ventricle uptake with exercise
    (d) Hypokinesia of the inferolateral septum
16. Regarding the right-to-left ventricular count ratio and the observation of the right ventricle during a myocardial perfusion scan:
    (a) If this ratio increases by 10% in the stress phase, it has a prognostic value.
    (b) If this ratio decreases by 10% in the stress phase, it has a prognostic value.
    (c) The abnormal increase in this ratio is specific for the diagnosis of a cardiac event with high risk.
    (d) The prognostic value of this finding is NOT reliable in pharmacologic stress.
17. What is the predicted order of prognosis (worse to best) in myocardial infarction according to the location of infarction?
    (a) Anterolateral, anteroseptal, inferior
    (b) Anteroseptal, inferior, anterior
    (c) Anteroseptal, anterior, inferior
    (d) Inferior, anterior, anteroseptal
18. Perfusion and metabolism by PET in myocardial stunning:
    (a) Both are normal.
    (b) Both show a defect.
    (c) Normal perfusion, abnormal metabolism.
    (d) Abnormal perfusion, normal metabolism.
19. Which of the following criteria is important in the estimation of the prognosis of CAD?
    (a) Rest LVEF
    (b) Age
    (c) Number of involved vessels
    (d) Arrhythmia at rest
20. The myocardial perfusion scan with stress is unremarkable. In which of the following groups is the probability of a cardiac event the soonest?
    (a) Diabetic male patients
    (b) Diabetic female patients
    (c) Patients with normal results after ETT
    (d) Patients younger than 40 years old
21. Which of the following statements about TID is the most appropriate?
    (a) It is observed because of subendocardial ischemia.
    (b) It is directly related to the observation of activity in the lungs.
    (c) The specificity of this phenomenon does NOT change with pharmacological or sports stress.
    (d) Quantitative methods are NOT required to interpret TID.

22. Patients who underwent a myocardial perfusion scan with single-isotope SPECT are selected. The ones with normal or nearly normal perfusion with SSS grade of 0–3 are divided into groups based on TID and stress type. Which group has the highest probability of fatal or nonfatal myocardial infarction in the coming 1 year?
    (a) The group that underwent a scan with dipyridamole and obtained TID of less than 1.2
    (b) The group that underwent exercise stress and obtained TID of more than 1.2
    (c) The group that underwent a scan with dipyridamole and obtained TID of more than 1.1
    (d) The group that underwent exercise stress and obtained TID of less than 1.1
23. What are the best predicting values for cardiac death and myocardial infarction on the MPI scan, respectively?
    (a) TID, SSS
    (b) TID, post-stress LVEF
    (c) Post-stress LVEF, SDS
    (d) SSS, post-stress LVEF
24. About direct and indirect quantitative studies of myocardial function with SPECT:
    (a) An inverse relationship exists between pulmonary uptake and capillary wedge pressure.
    (b) There is an absolute uptake of the radiopharmaceutical in myocardium.
    (c) A direct relationship exists between TID and LHR.
    (d) The sphericity index is the primary sign of CHF.
25. Which item best predicts the improvement of a region of the myocardium after revascularization?
    (a) Mild persistent defect in the rest–redistribution study with thallium
    (b) Mild persistent defect in the TNG–rest study with ^{99m}Tc-MIBI
    (c) Reversible defect in the stress–rest study with thallium
    (d) Severe persistent defect in the stress–rest study with thallium
26. Which item is NOT a high-risk marker on a myocardial perfusion scan?
    (a) Pulmonary uptake of ^{201}Tl
    (b) Persistent hepatic uptake of ^{99m}Tc-MIBI
    (c) Increase in the right ventricular uptake during stress
    (d) Transient LV ischemic dilatation
27. In which of the following patients is time to event the shortest after a normal myocardial perfusion?
    (a) A 53-year-old man without a history of CAD and with scan with physical stress
    (b) An 82-year-old man without a history of CAD and with scan with physical stress
    (c) A 52-year-old woman without a history of CAD and with scan with pharmacological stress
    (d) An 82-year-old woman without a history of CAD, with diabetes, and with scan with pharmacological stress

28. Which finding on the myocardial perfusion scan provides information about early events?
    (a) LVEF
    (b) Fixed defects
    (c) Reversible defects
    (d) RVEF
29. A myocardial perfusion SPECT scan is performed on a patient with a history of coronary artery disease. The sphericity index is 0.95. Which of the items describes the prognosis?
    (a) High probability of congestive heart failure
    (b) Low probability of cardiac events in the next 2 years
    (c) Presence of a high-risk tissue
    (d) Appropriate response to revascularization
30. Which of the following items indicates a poor prognosis on the myocardial scan of a patient with defects on the anterior walls in both scan phases?
    (a) EF < 50% with end-systolic volume >50 cc
    (b) EF < 45% with end-systolic volume >75 cc
    (c) EF < 50% with end-systolic volume >60 cc
    (d) EF < 45% with end-systolic volume >50 cc
31. The ejection fraction is 45% for a 59-year-old man with no history of recent MI or CAD. He underwent CABG 6 months ago. A stress-induced increase in EF of less than … after 1 year is indicative of restenosis.
    (a) 5%
    (b) 8%
    (c) 10%
    (d) 12%
32. Which of the following findings on the myocardial perfusion scan is indicative of a poor prognosis?
    (a) Infarcted region in the lower coronary artery zone
    (b) Fixed defect in the inferobasal area
    (c) Transient dilatation of the left ventricle in the stress phase
    (d) Septal ischemia in a patient with LBBB
33. Which of the following items is NOT indicative of a poor prognosis or coronary artery disease (CAD)?
    (a) Normal thallium scan with diffused slow washout
    (b) Transient dilatation of the left ventricle in ^{99m}Tc-MIBI images
    (c) Increase in pulmonary uptake in the 99mTc-MIBI scan
    (d) Mismatch in FDG-PET and ^{13}N-ammonia images
34. High-risk coronary artery disease in a myocardial perfusion study includes all items *except*:
    (a) X syndrome
    (b) Increase in thallium uptake after exercise
    (c) Significant ventricular dilatation immediately after exercise
    (d) Perfusion lesion in two or more coronary arteries

35. What is the annual mortality rate of patients with a mild myocardial perfusion defect and LVEF less than 45%?
    (a) More than 7%.
    (b) Less than 2%.
    (c) Less than 1%.
    (d) The annual mortality rate of these patients is NOT significantly different from that of patients with LVEF less than 45%.
36. What is the annual probability of a cardiac event in subjects with a normal myocardial perfusion scan?
    (a) 1% or less
    (b) More than 2%
    (c) 5%
    (d) 10%
37. Which of the following variables on a myocardial perfusion scan is critical in predicting cardiac death?
    (a) Summed stress score (SSS)
    (b) Summed difference score (SDS)
    (c) End-systolic volume (ESV)
    (d) End-diastolic volume (EDV)
38. In a medical center, all patients with suspected coronary artery disease (CAD) are directly subjected to angiography without previous assessment with noninvasive modalities, such as cardiac scan. How can the cost-effectiveness of this decision be described?
    (a) Higher cost but the method provides a better outcome.
    (b) More cases of unnecessary revascularization without a good outcome.
    (c) More cases of revascularization at a lower cost.
    (d) Lower cost and more efficient follow-up.
39. A 59-year-old man with an intermediate pretest likelihood of coronary disease is presented. The myocardial scan is positive, but angiography is unremarkable. What is the most appropriate interpretation?
    (a) CT angiography is required.
    (b) The patient's risk of cardiac events is four times greater than the normal population.
    (c) These findings are indicative of epicardial dysfunction.
    (d) Repeat of angiography is required.

6.7.1 Answer

	A	B	C	D		A	B	C	D
1	*				21	*			
2				*	22		*		
3	*				23			*	
4			*		24				*
5				*	25			*	

6				*	**26**			*	
7	*				**27**				*
8	*				**28**			*	
9				*	**29**	*			
10				*	**30**		*		
11			*		**31**	*			
12			*		**32**			*	
13	*				**33**			*	
14			*		**34**	*			
15				*	**35**	*			
16				*	**36**	*			
17			*		**37**	*			
18	*				**38**		*		
19	*				**39**		*		
20		*							

6.8 Assessment After Myocardial Revascularization

1. MPI post-CABG:
   (a) All symptomatic patients $\leq$5 years post-CABG may benefit from MPI.
   (b) All patients >5 years post-CABG may benefit from MPI.
   (c) All symptomatic and non-symptomatic patients $\leq$5 years post-CABG may benefit from MPI.
   (d) a and b.
2. When is the best time to undergo myocardial perfusion SPECT after balloon angioplasty (PCI)?
   (a) 1 week
   (b) 2 weeks
   (c) 4 weeks
   (d) 2 months
3. Cardiac metabolism and perfusion are evaluated using PET for a patient with myocardial infarction. Which of the following predicts an unsuccessful revascularization?
   (a) Matched
   (b) Mismatched
   (c) Reverse mismatched
   (d) Mild matched
4. Which of the following adverse effects is common in patients subjected to PCI?
   (a) MI
   (b) Cardiomyopathy
   (c) Silent ischemia
   (d) Cardiomegaly
5. Cardiac scintigraphy is requested for a 2-year-old child (weight: 10 kg) who underwent heart transplantation. What is the method of choice?
   (a) A 2-day protocol with 0.5 mCi of ^{201}Tl each day
   (b) A 1-day protocol with 1 mCi of ^{201}Tl and repeat with 0.5 mCi
   (c) A 2-day protocol with 2 mCi of ^{99m}Tc-MIBI each day
   (d) A 2-day protocol with 4 mCi of ^{99m}Tc-tetrofosmin each day
6. Which of the following ventriculography findings shows the least correlation with biopsy findings in a transplanted heart?
   (a) Ejection fraction
   (b) End-systolic volume
   (c) End-diastolic volume
   (d) Stroke volume
7. Which of the following items is indicated by a mismatch of FDG and ^{13}N-ammonia on a myocardial PET scan?
   (a) No change in the prognosis
   (b) No need for aggressive intervention
   (c) No risk of cardiovascular disease
   (d) High-risk patient

8. Regarding restenosis after PTCA:
   (a) The accuracy of exercise ECG is high for the diagnosis of restenosis in asymptomatic patients.
   (b) The accuracy of ^{201}Tl-SPECT is high for the detection of restenosis in asymptomatic patients.
   (c) Restenosis after PTCA is always accompanied by angina.
   (d) Rest–redistribution thallium imaging is the best method for diagnosis.
9. In the evaluation of myocardial viability, the improvement of LVEF after revascularization is:
   (a) Directly related to the extent of a dysfunctional viable tissue
   (b) Indirectly related to the extent of a dysfunctional viable tissue
   (c) Directly related to the extent of a functional viable tissue
   (d) Indirectly related to the extent of a functional viable tissue
10. Which of the following statements regarding the follow-up of patients who underwent coronary artery revascularization is NOT correct?
   (a) Exercise–electrocardiography is conducted prior to cardiac scan after CABG.
   (b) A routine myocardial perfusion scan is NOT required in asymptomatic patients after CABG.
   (c) The incidence of false-positive findings is high immediately after PTCA.
   (d) A cardiac scan 6 months after PTCA is beneficial in asymptomatic patients.
11. Which of the following statements about the evaluation of a patient after PTCA is NOT correct?
   (a) The diagnostic sensitivity of SPECT for restenosis in asymptomatic patients is less than that in symptomatic patients.
   (b) Electrocardiography is not reliable for the diagnosis of silent ischemia due to restenosis.
   (c) The extent of cardiac ischemia due to restenosis in symptomatic and asymptomatic patients is equal.
   (d) Restenosis does NOT change the risk of death.
12. PET scan shows an FDG–blood flow mismatch. The mortality rate in 1 year:
   (a) Is equal between drug treatment and revascularization
   (b) Is higher for drug treatment than for revascularization
   (c) Is higher for revascularization than for drug treatment
   (d) Depends on the type of revascularization (PTCA or CABG)
13. A patient complains about recurring chest pain after PTCA revascularization. What are the most common causes of pain 1 month after, 1–6 months after, and more than 6 months after PTCA, respectively?
   (a) Revascularization, restenosis, new defects
   (b) Revascularization, new defects, restenosis
   (c) New defects, restenosis, revascularization
   (d) New defects, revascularization, restenosis

6.8.1 Answer

	A	B	C	D
1				*
2			*	
3				*
4			*	
5				*
6	*			
7				*
8		*		
9	*			
10	*			
11	*			
12			*	
13	*			

6.9 Assessment of Myocardial Viability in Dysfunctional Myocardium

1. What percentage of irreversible defects on 3–4 h ^{201}Tl MPI shows a reversal in late imaging (24 h)?
   (a) 10–20%
   (b) 5–10%
   (c) 22–54%
   (d) 50–70%
2. What percentage of irreversible defects on 24 h ^{201}Tl MPI demonstrates metabolic activity and viability in PET?
   (a) 39%
   (b) 50%
   (c) 37%
   (d) 21%
3. Which of the following findings is indicative of hibernating tissue?
   (a) Reduced perfusion, reduced ^{18}F-FDG uptake
   (b) Reduced perfusion, normal ^{18}F-FDG uptake
   (c) Normal perfusion, normal ^{18}F-FDG uptake, ventricular hypokinesia
   (d) Normal perfusion, enhanced ^{18}F-FDG uptake
4. About congestive heart failure and cardiomyopathy:
   (a) Restrictive cardiomyopathy with diastolic dysfunction is presented with small heart chambers and normal EF.
   (b) Idiopathic cardiomegaly is presented with systolic dysfunction and decreased volume of both ventricles.
   (c) Ischemic cardiomegaly is presented with diastolic dysfunction, increased size of the right ventricle, and normal EF.
   (d) The primary goal of isotopic procedures is to determine EF.
5. What is the primary application of wall thickening on gated myocardial perfusion scintigraphy?
   (a) Differentiation of aneurysm from ventricular dilatation
   (b) Differentiation of MI from attenuation artifact
   (c) More specific detection of ischemia
   (d) More specific detection of reverse redistribution
6. Which of the following tracers is NOT indicated for the assessment of cardiac viability using PET?
   (a) ^{11}C-acetate
   (b) ^{15}O-H_2O
   (c) ^{8}F-fluoromethane
   (d) ^{82}Rb

7. In which of the following diseases is the evaluation of the viability of myocardium with nuclear medicine modalities useful?
   (a) A patient with non-Q wave MI with relapse of cardiac symptoms and temporary ST depression
   (b) A patient with hearth failure, three-vessel CAD, and LVEF <25%
   (c) A patient with a large stable defect on the lateral wall and LVEF = 50%
   (d) A patient with dilated cardiomyopathy
8. The basal EF is 55%, and it decreases to 40% after treatment with Adriamycin. What is the next step?
   (a) Continuation of drug treatment without dose adjustment, and follow-up scans should be conducted at shorter intervals
   (b) Continuation of treatment with reduction of Adriamycin dose
   (c) Confirmation of cardiac toxicity with transthoracic echocardiography
   (d) Discontinuation of Adriamycin
9. Which finding is indicative of tissue scar in a myocardial viability study?
   (a) Direct worsening in dobutamine stress echocardiography
   (b) Hyper-enhancement in MRI with contrast
   (c) Biphasic response in dobutamine stress echocardiography
   (d) End-diastolic wall thinness of 6 mm in MRI
10. All of the following items describe the advantages of PET in the evaluation of myocardial viability *except*:
   (a) Increased image resolution
   (b) Correction of photon attenuation
   (c) Correction of motion artifact
   (d) Evaluation of metabolic activity independent of perfusion
11. What is the gold standard for the assessment of myocardial viability?
   (a) Scan with ^{99m}Tc-MIBI and TNG
   (b) Thallium scan with rest–redistribution method
   (c) FDG-PET
   (d) Scan with tetrofosmin
12. The goal is to evaluate myocardial viability with Tc agents. What is the minimum level of uptake in the anterior and inferior walls for a better outcome, respectively?
   (a) 50% for both
   (b) 50% for both
   (c) 50% and 30%
   (d) 40% and 30%
13. ^{18}F-FDG and ^{13}N scan are performed to evaluate myocardial viability in a 75-year-old man. Which of the following findings on the anterior wall indicates non-viability?
   (a) Normal ^{13}N uptake, decreased ^{18}F-FDG uptake
   (b) Decreased ^{13}N uptake, normal ^{18}F-FDG uptake
   (c) Decreased ^{13}N uptake, decreased ^{18}F-FDG uptake
   (d) Normal ^{13}N uptake, normal ^{18}F-FDG uptake

14. Regions of decreased uptake are observed on the anteroseptal and inferolateral walls on the myocardial perfusion scan of a patient with a history of coronary artery disease. However, the FDG-PET scan shows only an increased uptake in the anteroseptal wall with absent uptake in the inferolateral wall. Which of the following is the best description of the viability of these walls?
    (a) Viable anteroseptal, viable inferolateral
    (b) Viable anteroseptal, nonviable inferolateral
    (c) Nonviable anteroseptal, viable inferolateral
    (d) Nonviable anteroseptal, nonviable inferolateral
15. Which group of patients with cardiovascular disease shows the least mortality rate?
    (a) Patients with a significant viable myocardial tissue subjected to drug treatment
    (b) Patients with a significant viable myocardial tissue subjected to revascularization
    (c) Patients with a significant scar in the myocardium subjected to revascularization
    (d) Patients with a significant scar in the myocardium subjected to drug treatment
16. A patient is referred for myocardial evaluation. No thallium uptake in the anteroseptal wall, akinesia of this wall in ventriculography, and FDG uptake in this region are observed in the tests. These findings indicate:
    (a) Hibernating myocardium
    (b) Stunned myocardium
    (c) Infarcted myocardium
    (d) Normal myocardium
17. About stunned and hibernating myocardium:
    (a) In hibernating myocardium, viability can be evaluated with thallium scan at rest.
    (b) Electrocardiography and functional changes in a stunned myocardium will be completely and simultaneously improved if blood flow is restored in 15–20 min.
    (c) Neither catecholamines nor calcium can change myocardial dysfunction.
    (d) Thallium scan findings on hibernating myocardium are similar to those of the PET scan.
18. A patient with a history of infarction and ventricular dysfunction is a candidate for bypass. Which of the following criteria is the most accurate for the assessment of viability?
    (a) Assessment of blood flow with SPECT
    (b) Assessment of wall motility with echocardiography
    (c) Assessment of systolic myocardial thickness with gated SPECT
    (d) Assessment of myocardial contractile reserve with dobutamine echocardiography

19. What is the most reliable method for identifying viable myocardium in a patient with a history of infarction and left ventricular dysfunction?
    (a) Quantitative study of sestamibi uptake
    (b) Evaluation of the redistribution of ^{201}Tl
    (c) FDG-PET scan
    (d) Sestamibi scan after the administration of TNG
20. All of the following statements about the reverse redistribution of thallium in infarction are correct *except*:
    (a) This phenomenon can be observed in the early days after infarction if the corresponding vessel is open.
    (b) The amount of this redistribution increases over time.
    (c) It represents myocardial salvaged.
    (d) It represents viability.
21. About the determination of myocardial viability:
    (a) Regional wall motion and wall thickening indices are accurate in differentiating hibernating myocardium from a scar.
    (b) Dobutamine echocardiography is accurate in predicting the efficacy of bypass surgery in viable unmasking dysfunctional myocardium.
    (c) The contractile reserve in hibernating myocardium is preserved and can be measured with low-dose dobutamine echocardiography.
    (d) The accuracy of a stress–redistribution ^{201}Tl cardiac scan is satisfactory for the differential diagnosis of hibernation and scan in coronary artery disease.
22. Regarding the determination of myocardial viability on a ^{99m}Tc-MIBI myocardial scan:
    (a) The efficacy of the ^{99m}Tc-MIBI scan is similar to that of thallium scan in severely ischemic myocardial regions.
    (b) ^{99m}Tc-MIBI underestimates viability in patients with chronic coronary artery disease and left ventricular dysfunction.
    (c) The probability of improving the myocardial regions with systolic dysfunction and reversible ischemia after revascularization is low.
    (d) The quantitative evaluation of resting ^{99m}Tc-MIBI perfusion defects does NOT have predictive value in functional improvement after revascularization.
23. Which of the following statements regarding the assessment of myocardial viability in late ^{201}Tl-redistribution scan is NOT correct?
    (a) The positive predictive value of this test is greater than 90%.
    (b) The negative predictive value of this method is better than that of rest–redistribution 3–4 h after stress.
    (c) About 37% of perfusion defects persisting 24 h after stress improve after bypass surgery.
    (d) About 39% of perfusion defects persisting 24 h after stress disappears after reinjection of thallium at rest.

24. About ^{201}Tl myocardial scan with reinjection method:
    (a) Data obtained from reinjection–redistribution are rarely similar to the previous three-image acquisition.
    (b) Reinjection immediately after stress scan and repeat of scan after 3–4 h produce favorable results.
    (c) A defect in stress reinjection that disappears in redistribution excludes viable myocardium.
    (d) When a fixed defect is found, the elimination of the redistribution phase from the stress reinjection scan decreases the reliability of the scan.
25. Regarding the assessment of myocardial viability on a rest–redistribution ^{201}Tl scan:
    (a) The results of the ^{201}Tl-redistribution scan with quantitative assessments are consistent with those produced by ^{201}Tl stress–reinjection imaging.
    (b) The specificity of rest–redistribution imaging is very high.
    (c) More than 90% of mild persistent defects on the rest–redistribution scan improve after revascularization.
    (d) The fixed defects in rest–redistribution with a relative redistribution on a stress scan do NOT indicate viability.
26. All items are correct about the evaluation of necrotic myocardium by gated perfusion study *except*:
    (a) The lack of increase in myocardial thickness in systole is an accurate criterion for the diagnosis of necrosis by itself.
    (b) The overestimation of necrosis is observed in this method.
    (c) The sensitivity of this method for detecting small necrosis is low.
    (d) The sensitivity of this method for detecting non-transmural necrosis is low.
27. Which of the following statements about the identification of myocardial viability with PET or SPECT in patients with coronary artery disease is NOT correct?
    (a) The improvement of symptoms and tolerance to exercise after revascularization is similar to that after drug treatment.
    (b) The survival rate of patients with/without infarction after revascularization is greater than that after medical treatment.
    (c) The results of PET and SPECT are consistent in terms of the high risk for medical therapy in patients with left ventricular dysfunction and viable myocardium.
    (d) The mortality rate before revascularization in patients without viability test is high.
28. Regarding PET scan for the identification of myocardial viability:
    (a) In blood flow mismatch, which is a sign of hibernating myocardium, the decrease in GLUT1 receptor density causes a metabolic shift from fatty acids to glucose.
    (b) The positive and negative predictive values of a blood flow mismatch for functional improvement after revascularization is greater than 95%.
    (c) The increase in ejection fraction after bypass graft is directly related to the level of blood flow mismatch.
    (d) The improvement of left ventricular function after bypass graft is NOT satisfactory when blood flow mismatch is accompanied by LVEF < 35%.

29. Myocardial viability:
    (a) Simultaneous histologic and scintigraphy studies show that hibernation accounts for 25% of all viable dysfunctional myocardia.
    (b) Intracellular disturbance and the production of nitric oxide without altering the intracellular components are reported in hibernating viable myocardium.
    (c) The improvement of resting myocardial function after revascularization is expected even if the density of healthy myocytes in a specific region of myocardium is less than 70%.
    (d) In stunning viable myocardium, intermittent stunning without a resting perfusion defect never results in chronic left ventricular failure.
30. Which of the following physiologic markers can best assess viability in nuclear cardiology?
    (a) Regional wall motion
    (b) Regional systolic wall thickening
    (c) Cell membrane integrity
    (d) Regional coronary blood flow
31. About the presence of viable or ischemic tissue on a stress perfusion scan in patients with acute myocardial infarction:
    (a) The presence or absence of ischemia does NOT influence future cardiac events.
    (b) The prognostic values of ischemia on a scan and stress EKG as well as the extent of coronary defects in angiography are similar.
    (c) The risk of cardiovascular events in patients with a large reversible perfusion defect is higher than that in patients with cardiac scar tissue.
    (d) The extent of ischemia and resting LVEF are NOT valuable in predicting long-term outcomes.
32. Which of the following statements about patients who are evaluated for myocardial viability is NOT correct?
    (a) The annual mortality rate of patients with viable myocardium and medical treatment is 16%.
    (b) The annual mortality rate of patients without viable myocardium who underwent bypass is 7.7%.
    (c) The annual mortality rate of patients without viable myocardium and medical treatment is 6.2%.
    (d) The minimum required extent of viable myocardium is 10% for 5% improvement of LVEF after revascularization.
33. Compare the radioisotopic methods, dobutamine echocardiography, and MRI for the evaluation of viability.
    (a) Only a small part of the viable regions in echocardiography shows normal or near-normal perfusion on a scan.
    (b) Dobutamine echocardiography is NOT indicated for patients with stunning.
    (c) Inotropic reserve in dobutamine echocardiography is NOT related to regional ^{201}Tl activity on a scan.
    (d) MRI canNOT differentiate between viable myocardium at risk from that without risk.

34. In which of the following situations is low-dose dobutamine effective?
    (a) Detection of mild myocardial defects
    (b) Detection of fixed myocardial defects
    (c) Better evaluation of viability of perfusion defects
    (d) Evaluation of myocardial uptake after the administration of TNG

6.9.1 Answer

	A	B	C	D
1			*	
2		*		
3		*		
4	*			
5		*		
6				*
7		*		
8				*
9		*		
10			*	
11			*	
12			*	
13			*	
14		*		
15		*		
16	*			
17	*			
18				*
19			*	
20		*		
21			*	
22		*		
23		*		
24				*
25	*			
26	*			
27	*			
28			*	
29		*		
30			*	
31			*	
32				*
33				*
34			*	

6.10 Myocardial Infarction: Assessment of Thrombosis

1. Following thrombolytic therapy for acute infarction, noninvasive imaging can best assess long-term patient risk based on:
   (a) LVEF
   (b) Myocardial ischemia
   (c) Myocardial motion and thickening
   (d) a and b

6.10.1 Answer

	A	B	C	D
1				*

6.11 Congenital Heart Disease

1. Which of the following congenital heart defects requires a shunt?
   (a) Aortic stenosis
   (b) Pulmonary stenosis
   (c) Coarctation of aorta
   (d) Truncus arteriosus
2. What is the most commonly used technique in cardiac shunt studies?
   (a) Gated SPECT
   (b) First-pass radionuclide angiography
   (c) Doppler echocardiography
   (d) b and c
3. What is the most useful technique for assessing right-to-left shunts?
   (a) MRI
   (b) First-pass radionuclide angiography
   (c) $^{15}C\text{-}O_2$ inhalation PET
   (d) Doppler echocardiography
4. What changes are induced by a left-to-right shunt in a pulmonary time–activity curve in first-pass studies?
   (a) Appearance of a third peak in the curve
   (b) Elongation of the first peak because of pulmonary redistribution of the radiotracer
   (c) Discontinuation of descending lines after the peak because of pulmonary redistribution of the radiotracer
   (d) Elongation of ascending lines and discontinuation of descending lines after the peak
5. Which of the following is indicated by the sphericity index of the heart?
   (a) Myocardial infarction
   (b) Myocardial ischemia
   (c) Pericarditis
   (d) Congestive heart failure
6. Which statement about patients with congenital heart disease is NOT correct?
   (a) A first-pass study is considered a precise method for evaluating a left-to-right shunt.
   (b) If the Qp/Qs ratio is higher than 3, the left-to-right shunt is considered large.
   (c) A continuous higher activity is observed in the left-to-right shunt.
   (d) Radiopharmaceutical administration to the left hand is recommended in a first-pass study.
7. PET scan with ^{13}N-ammonia (A) and ^{18}F-FDG (F) in the rest phase is performed after arterial switch operation (ASO) on a child with transposition of great arteries. Which PET finding indicates the requirement of coronary artery revascularization?
   (a) Normal A, decreased F.
   (b) Decreased A, normal F.
   (c) Decreased A, decreased F.
   (d) Imaging in the rest and stress phases is required for decision-making.

8. A neonate with congenital heart disease is referred for the evaluation of an endocardial shunt. The pulmonary time–activity curve in the first-pass study with pertechnetate is presented. The differential diagnosis includes:
   (a) Tricuspid atresia
   (b) Tetralogy of Fallot
   (c) Pulmonary atresia/intact septum
   (d) Truncus arteriosus

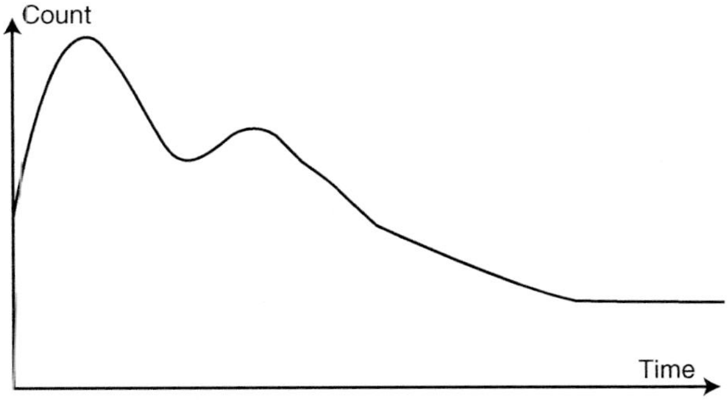

9. About the evaluation of left-to-right shunts:
   (a) This evaluation is NOT possible in patients with a poor general condition.
   (b) Myocardial dysfunction and valvular regurgitation underestimate the intensity of the shunt.
   (c) This evaluation is especially valuable in patients with VSD and PDA.
   (d) If the Qp/Qs > 3, the shunt is considered large.
10. The radiotracer is continuously observed in the lungs in first-pass angiocardiography. What is the most probable diagnosis?
    (a) Left-to-right shunt
    (b) Right-to-left shunt
    (c) Arteriovenous fistula
    (d) Bidirectional shunt
11. All of the following statements about pediatric cardiology are correct *except*:
    (a) The protocol of pharmacologic stress is identical to that in adults.
    (b) Radionuclide angiography is NOT a suitable method for the evaluation of ventricular function.
    (c) The right-to-left shunt can be estimated with first-pass angiography and the calculation of the area under the curve in radioactivity peaks.
    (d) Radionuclide ventriculography is conducted prior to echocardiography for the evaluation of cardiac function and ejection fraction in the transposition of the great arteries (TGA).

12. About thallium scan in Kawasaki disease:
    (a) A scan is required to diagnose aneurysm and coronary ectasia in the acute and subacute phases.
    (b) Thallium scan is normal in patients with normal coronary angiography.
    (c) If angiography is normal, restriction of daily activity is NOT required.
    (d) Thallium scan is always abnormal because of extensive microvascular involvement.
13. The left coronary artery originates from the pulmonary artery in a neonate. A myocardial perfusion scan is the least useful for the:
    (a) Primary diagnosis of disease
    (b) Determination of the severity of hypoperfusion
    (c) Determination of the improvement of perfusion and function after repair surgery
    (d) Determination of the indication of surgical revascularization

6.11.1 Answer

	A	B	C	D
1				*
2				*
3				*
4			*	
5				*
6				*
7		*		
8				*
9				*
10				*
11		*		
12			*	
13	*			

6.12 Single-Photon Imaging of Myocardial Metabolism: Role of Iodine-123 Fatty Acids and Fluorine-18 Deoxyglucose

1. All clinical applications of radioiodinated free fatty acids have been studied *except*:
   (a) Valvular heart disease
   (b) Congenital heart disease
   (c) CABG/PTCA
   (d) Hypertrophic cardiomyopathy

6.12.1 Answer

	A	B	C	D
1		*		

6.13 Clinical Applications of Positron Emission Tomography in Cardiology

1. A segment with impaired contractile function exhibits a maintained myocardial blood flow but decreased ^{18}F-deoxyglucose:
   (a) Perfusion–metabolism mismatch
   (b) Perfusion–metabolism match
   (c) Reverse mismatch
   (d) Mild match
2. Perfusion–metabolism mild match is seen in:
   (a) Transmural scar
   (b) Non-transmural scar
   (c) Mild ischemia
   (d) Severe ischemia
3. What is the main mechanism for hibernating myocardium?
   (a) Acute alterations in the cell membrane to protect the viability of myocytes
   (b) Defensive mechanism of the body to decrease oxygen demand
   (c) Increase in the number of mitochondria in the cytoplasm
   (d) Prevention of ischemia expansion to conductivity cells
4. Which of the following situations is indicated by an FDG–blood flow mismatch?
   (a) Myocardial metabolism shifts toward fatty acids.
   (b) Myocardial metabolism shifts toward glucose.
   (c) Myocardial metabolism shifts toward lactic acid.
   (d) The mentioned finding is not related to the source of energy for the myocardium.
5. The PET evaluation of myocardial viability is based on the:
   (a) Evaluation of oxidative metabolism with 11-C acetate
   (b) Evaluation of perfusable tissue with 15-O water
   (c) Evaluation of the uptake and washout of 82-rhobidium
   (d) Evaluation of glucose metabolism with 18-F FDG
6. Which of the following situations is indicated by an FDG–blood flow mismatch in the viable tissue of myocardium?
   (a) Higher consumption of glucose than of fatty acids and lactate
   (b) Higher consumption of fatty acids than of glucose
   (c) Higher consumption of lactate than of glucose
   (d) Higher consumption of fatty acids than of glucose

6.13.1 Answer

	A	B	C	D
1			*	
2		*		
3		*		
4		*		
5				*
6	*			

6.14 Myocardial Innervation: Imaging and Quantification

1. Regarding the in vivo evaluation of presynaptic neuronal function:
   (a) The accumulation and retention of the MIBG tracer increase in patients with idiopathic cardiomyopathy.
   (b) In patients with moderate heart failure, a significant decrease in cardiac ^{123}I-MIBG uptake is seen after a 6-month captopril treatment.
   (c) In patients with moderate heart failure, a significant decrease in cardiac ^{123}I-MIBG uptake is seen after a 6-month metoprolol treatment.
   (d) MIBG washout from the left ventricle could be a predictor of the response to beta-blockade in patients with heart failure.
2. About cardiac scintigraphy with MIBG:
   (a) Viable regions after infarction are a source of arrhythmia.
   (b) Cardiac uptake of MIBG increases in diabetic patients.
   (c) Cardiac uptake of MIBG and its washout decreases in patient with renal failure.
   (d) A low cardiac uptake of MIGB in heart failure indicates a good prognosis.
3. An increased uptake of technetium–annexin is reported in the whole myocardium of a 63-year-old man who underwent heart transplantation. What is the most probable diagnosis?
   (a) Myocarditis
   (b) Pericarditis
   (c) Rejection
   (d) Diffused infarctus
4. About cardiac receptors:
   (a) B2 is the dominant sympathetic receptor in myocardium.
   (b) M2 is the dominant parasympathetic receptor in the heart.
   (c) The number of muscarinic receptors in a transplanted heart is similar to that in a normal heart.
   (d) The density of beta receptors decreases in hypertrophic cardiomyopathy.
5. Which of the following situations demonstrates an increased uptake of ^{123}I-MIBG in the evaluation of myocardial innervations?
   (a) After treatment of heart failure by ACE I
   (b) After initiation of doxorubicin cardiotoxicity
   (c) In the primary stages of Parkinson's disease
   (d) In familial polyneuropathy disease
6. What is the radiopharmaceutical of choice for the evaluation of innervation in a transplanted heart?
   (a) ^{131}I-MIBG
   (b) ^{99m}Tc-MIBI
   (c) ^{201}Tl-chloride
   (d) ^{99m}Tc-tetrofosmin

7. About ^{123}I-MIBG scan and the pathophysiology of congestive heart failure in CHF:
   (a) Decrease in sympathetic activity in CHF
   (b) Increase in norepinephrine reservoir in the nerve terminals in CHF
   (c) Increase in the myocardial uptake of ^{123}I-MIBG
   (d) Increase in norepinephrine release from the nerve terminals in CHF
8. What is the main finding of a ^{123}I-MIBG scan after cardiac transplantation (denervation)?
   (a) Minimal cardiac uptake despite the satisfactory pulmonary uptake
   (b) Minimal uptake despite the satisfactory uptake
   (c) Very low pulmonary and cardiac uptake
   (d) Normal pulmonary and cardiac uptake
9. What is the scan of choice for the diagnosis of rejection of heart transplant?
   (a) FDG-PET scan
   (b) ^{99m}Tc-MIBI scan
   (c) Biopsy
   (d) ^{99m}Tc-PYP scan
10. Which of the following statements about cardiac scan with MIBG is NOT correct?
    (a) MIBG is uptaken and reserved in the sympathetic neurons.
    (b) MIBG uptake increases in a transplanted heart.
    (c) MIBG uptake decreases in myocardial infarctus.
    (d) MIBG uptake decreases in chemical or surgical sympathectomy.
11. An increase in circulating norepinephrine level can cause all of the following complications *except*:
    (a) Myocardial hypertrophy
    (b) Myocytes Ca^{++} overload
    (c) Arrhythmia
    (d) Hypersensitization of beta adrenoceptors
12. Which of the following statements about myocardial MIBG uptake and serum norepinephrine level in heart failure is NOT correct?
    (a) A decrease in MIBG uptake is associated with a decrease in norepinephrine in myocardium.
    (b) A decrease in MIBG uptake is associated with the normal serum norepinephrine level.
    (c) An increase in serum norepinephrine is the only known cause of a decreased MIBG uptake.
    (d) An increase in serum norepinephrine is a good prognostic marker.
13. In which of the following conditions is reinnervation observed as the initiation of ^{123}I-MIBG uptake in the left ventricular base?
    (a) CHF
    (b) Cardiomyopathy
    (c) Cardiac transplantation
    (d) Transmural infarction

14. Which of the following findings on an MIBG cardiac scan is expected in primary hypertrophic cardiomyopathy?
    (a) Increased uptake, decreased wash-out rate
    (b) Decreased uptake, decreased wash-out rate
    (c) Increased uptake, increased wash-out rate
    (d) Decreased uptake, increased wash-out rate
15. Decreased uptake and retention in myocardial imaging with ^{123}I-MIBG are NOT seen in:
    (a) Aortic insufficiency with heart failure
    (b) Aortic valvular stenosis with failure
    (c) Cardiac transplantation
    (d) Myocarditis
16. All of the following radiotracers are indicated for the evaluation of sympathetic and parasympathetic nerve terminals *except*:
    (a) ^{11}C-HED
    (b) ^{18}F-flourodopamine
    (c) ^{18}F-fluorometaraminol
    (d) ^{13}N-NH_3

6.14.1 Answer

	A	B	C	D
1				*
2	*			
3			*	
4				*
5	*			
6	*			
7				*
8	*			
9			*	
10		*		
11				*
12			*	
13			*	
14				*
15				*
16				*

6.15 Nuclear Medicine Techniques in the Assessment of Human Thrombosis and Atheroma

1. What is the method of choice for the imaging of thrombosis and atheroma?
   (a) ^{111}In-oxine-labeled platelets
   (b) FDG-PET
   (c) ^{111}In-oxine-WBC
   (d) LDL imaging
2. What is the preferred scanning procedure on scintigraphy of atheroma and thrombosis?
   (a) Antifebrin antibodies
   (b) Labeled RBC
   (c) Labeled fibrinogen
   (d) Labeled platelets
3. What is the mechanism of ^{111}In-platelet binding to the surface of active thrombosis?
   (a) Chemisorption
   (b) Compartmental localization
   (c) Cell sequestration
   (d) Capillary blockade
4. About the acute rejection of a heart transplant:
   (a) Changes in isotopic ventriculography are NOT consistent with the histologic findings of myocyte necrosis in endomyocardial biopsy.
   (b) The ratio of cardiac to pulmonary uptake 48 h after the injection of ^{111}In-antimyosin is consistent with the histologic criteria.
   (c) A decrease in gallium uptake is observed in ^{67}Ga.
   (d) An increase in perfusion is observed in ^{201}Tl scintigraphy.
5. What is the best method for the diagnosis of allograft vasculopathy in cardiac transplant?
   (a) Intracoronary ultrasonography
   (b) Coronary angiography
   (c) ^{13}N-ammonia PET scan
   (d) Doppler blood flow velocity measurement

6.15.1 Answer

	A	B	C	D
1	*			
2				*
3	*			
4		*		
5				*

Suggested Readings

1. Ahmadzadehfar H, Biersack HJ, Freeman LM, Zuckier L. Clinical nuclear medicine. 2nd ed. Berlin: Springer; 2018.
2. Ell PJ, Gambhir SS. Nuclear medicine in clinical diagnosis and treatment. 3rd ed. Edinburgh, NY: Churchill Livingstone; 2004.
3. Sandler MP, Coleman RE, Patton JA, Wackers FJT, Gottschalk A. Diagnostic nuclear medicine. 4th ed. Philadelphia: Lippincott & Williams Wilkins; 2003.
4. Henkin RE. Nuclear medicine. 2nd ed. Philadelphia: Mosby Elsevier; 2006.

Nuclear Medicine in Neurological and Psychiatric Diagnosis

7

7.1 Blood–Brain Barrier

1. In blood–brain barrier imaging:
   (a) Longitudinal sinuses reveal a higher tracer uptake than the brain.
   (b) Transverse sinuses reveal a higher tracer uptake than the brain.
   (c) Blood–brain barrier imaging is performed by ^{99m}-pertechnetate, ^{99m}Tc-DTPA, and ^{99m}Tc-glucoheptonate.
   (d) All of the above.
2. Which of the following is NOT a characteristic of the blood–brain barrier (BBB)?
   (a) High ionic permeability.
   (b) Existence of Na/K pump.
   (c) Low nonelectrolyte hydrophilic permeability.
   (d) It is a tight connection of endothelial cells.
3. Which of the following is a determinant of the transport of lipophilic agents from the blood–brain barrier (BBB)?
   (a) Na/K pump.
   (b) Calcium pump.
   (c) Glycoprotein pump.
   (d) The cerebral entry of lipophilic agents occurs without any intervention.
4. Which of the following factors is the least important in the permeability of the blood–brain barrier?
   (a) Lipophilicity.
   (b) Osmotic pressure.
   (c) Protein binding.
   (d) Hydrostatic pressure.

M. Assadi et al., *Principles of Nuclear Medicine*,
https://doi.org/10.1007/978-3-319-91701-6_7

5. Which of the following patterns of BBB imaging in neonates with asphyxia indicates high brain involvement?
   (a) Typical stroke pattern of uptake in one of the large cerebral arteries.
   (b) Abnormal uptake in the intermediary region of large cerebral arteries.
   (c) Skull cap-like increase in uptake.
   (d) Abnormal focal uptake in the basal ganglia.

7.1.1 Answer

	A	B	C	D
1				*
2	*			
3			*	
4				*
5			*	

7.2 Lipophilic Tracers: The Amines

1. Which of the following statements regarding lipophilic tracers is NOT true?
   (a) Penumbra region after CVA can be clearly demonstrated by iodine-123 IMP.
   (b) In a subacute stroke, the infarcted area shows a 40% perfusion decrease in iodine-123 IMP.
   (c) ^{99m}Tc-HMPAO and ^{99m}Tc-ECD display a nonlinear decreased uptake at high flow rates.
   (d) During luxury perfusion, an increased uptake is commonly observed with IMP.
2. What is the target organ of the ^{99m}Tc-ECD scan?
   (a) Gallbladder.
   (b) Kidney.
   (c) Intestine.
   (d) Bladder wall.
3. How long after the intravenous injection of labeled (A) ^{99m}Tc-ECD and (B) ^{99m}Tc-HMPAO can cerebral SPECT imaging be performed?
   (a) A, 30–90 min; B, 20–30 min.
   (b) A, 30–45 min; B, 45–90 min.
   (c) A, 15–20 min; B, 90–120 min.
   (d) A, 45–90 min; B, 30–45 min.
4. Which of the following radiopharmaceuticals is indicated for the evaluation of brain metabolism?
   (a) ^{99m}Tc-DTPA
   (b) ^{201}Tl
   (c) ^{127}Xe
   (d) ^{11}C-methionine.
5. Which characteristic is required for a technetium-containing radiopharmaceutical on a cerebral perfusion scan?
   (a) Colloidal
   (b) Electric charge
   (c) High molecular weight
   (d) Lipophilic and without electric charge
6. A patient with a history of chronic headache for 3 years is referred to evaluate the blood–brain barrier for brain tumor. Which of the following radiopharmaceuticals provides the best quality of images?
   (a) ^{99m}Tc-pertechnetate
   (b) ^{99m}Tc-DTPA
   (c) ^{99m}Tc-GHA
   (d) ^{111}In-granulocytes

7. What is the target organ of the ^{123}I-IMP scan?
   (a) Thyroid
   (b) Lung
   (c) Gallbladder
   (d) Lacrimal glands

7.2.1 Answer

	A	B	C	D
1				*
2				*
3		*		
4				*
5				*
6			*	
7		*		

7.3 Lipophilic Tracers for the Study of Regional Cerebral Blood Flow

1. The shelf lives of ^{99}Tc-exametazime and ^{99m}Tc-bicisate are:
   (a) 2 h, >4 h
   (b) 30 min, >6 h
   (c) 1 h, >8 h
   (d) 4 h, >4 h
2. ^{99}Tc-exametazime is more accumulated than ^{99m}Tc-bicisate in all of the following regions *except*:
   (a) Thalamus
   (b) Frontal lobe
   (c) Parietal lobe
   (d) Cerebellum
3. Which radiotracer is rapidly taken up in the brain in proportion to the regional blood flow and is retained there for a long period without a significant washout?
   (a) ^{99m}Tc-DMG-2MP
   (b) ^{99m}Tc-MRP20
   (c) ^{99m}Tc-T691
   (d) ^{201}Tl-DDC
4. Cerebral perfusion of a radiopharmaceutical:
   (a) The clearance of ^{99m}Tc-ECD is quicker than that of ^{99m}Tc-HAMPAO
   (b) Both radiopharmaceuticals are equally accumulated in the medial temporal lobe
   (c) The cerebellum picks up more ^{99m}Tc-ECD than ^{99m}Tc-HAMPAO
   (d) All of the above
5. Which one describes the most observed similarity between ^{99m}Tc-ECD and ^{99m}Tc-HAMPO on a cerebral perfusion scan?
   (a) The mechanism of absorption in the brain cells
   (b) Distribution of the radiodrug in the brain
   (c) PH of the lipophilic complex
   (d) Extent of cerebral uptake
6. Which of the following can be applied for the evaluation of brain tissue viability during cerebral scintigraphy?
   (a) ^{99m}Tc-HMPAO
   (b) ^{99m}Tc-ECD
   (c) ^{123}I-IMP
   (d) ^{133}Xe
7. Which item is NOT correct about the comparison between ^{99m}Tc-ECD and ^{99m}Tc-HMPAO?
   (a) ^{99m}Tc-ECD has a higher cerebral uptake.
   (b) Higher doses of ^{99m}Tc-ECD can be administered.
   (c) Imaging can be performed faster after the administration of ^{99m}Tc-HMPAO.
   (d) A luxury perfusion study can be performed with ^{99m}Tc-HMPAO.

8. In the evaluation of brain death:
   (a) ^{99m}TC-ECD is preferred over ^{99m}TC-DTPA.
   (b) SPECT should be used for a better diagnosis.
   (c) An uptake in the brain stem excludes the diagnosis of brain death.
   (d) Scintigraphy has no role in the diagnosis of brain death in children.
9. What is the standard radiopharmaceutical for the assessment of rCBF?
   (a) ^{133}Xe
   (b) ^{123}I-IMP
   (c) Tc-HMPAO
   (d) ^{18}F-FDG
10. About the brain scan of patients with brain death:
    (a) Radiopharmaceutical activity is observed in the carotid artery and in the anterior and medial cerebral arteries
    (b) The activity of the superior sagittal sinus and transverse is not due to background activity
    (c) First-pass images are not similar between ^{99m}Tc-HMPAO and ^{99m}Tc-pertechnetate
    (d) Cerebral perfusion can be preserved in children with cerebral injuries because of anoxia despite the clinical symptoms of brain death
11. A cerebral perfusion scan with ^{99m}Tc-ECD is requested for a patient. If the radiopharmaceutical is replaced with ^{99m}Tc-HMPAO, which lobes demonstrate the highest difference in uptake for these radiopharmaceuticals?
    (a) Occipital and parietal
    (b) Frontal and parietal
    (c) Occipital and temporal
    (d) Frontal and occipital
12. About brain perfusion and metabolism in children:
    (a) A remarkable uptake in the visual cortex and occipital lobe is reported in premature neonates
    (b) The uptake in the anterior bridge of the frontal lobes is equal to that in adults
    (c) Brain metabolism becomes similar to that of adults at the age of 9 years
    (d) Perfusion and metabolism of the cerebellum and brain stem are less than those of other organs at birth
13. Which of the following statements about brain SPECT is NOT correct?
    (a) The distribution of ^{99m}Tc-ECD in the brain indicates regional blood flow and enzymatic activity
    (b) In a patient with brain abscess under treatment with high-dose corticosteroids, ^{111}In- granulocytes accumulate in the abscess with high sensitivity
    (c) ^{201}Tl can be used for the evaluation of residual glioma tissue after radiation
    (d) The tumor avidities of ^{201}Tl and ^{99m}Tc-MIBI in the brain are identical
14. Which of the following factors decreases the efficacy of a radiotracer on a brain perfusion SPECT scan?
    (a) Low plasma protein binding
    (b) Molecular weight less than 400
    (c) Lipophilicity of more than 0.5
    (d) Rapid cerebral washout

15. What is the preferred radiopharmaceutical for the evaluation of cerebral mean transit time?
    (a) ^{99m}Tc-HAS
    (b) Xenon
    (c) ^{99m}Tc-HMPAO
    (d) 123I-IMP
16. Metas test is used for the therapeutic monitoring of:
    (a) Carotid artery ligation
    (b) Surgical treatment of epileptic attacks
    (c) Surgical treatment of Parkinson's disease
    (d) Drug treatment of schizophrenia
17. Brain perfusion scan is the least indicated for:
    (a) Acute cerebral ischemia
    (b) Cerebral infarction
    (c) Evaluation of ischemia after drug or surgical treatment
    (d) Diagnosis of migraine
18. Which statement regarding the comparison between the ^{99m}Tc-HMPAO and ^{99m}Tc-ECD radiotracers is NOT correct?
    (a) Brain extraction of ^{99m}Tc-HMPAO is higher.
    (b) The relative activity of brain to soft tissue is higher for ^{99m}Tc-ECD.
    (c) The serum clearance of ^{99m}Tc-HMPAO is faster.
    (d) The thalamus uptake of ^{99m}Tc-HMPAO is higher.
19. Compare 123I-IMP, ^{99m}Tc-HMPAO, and ^{99m}Tc-ECD.
    (a) 123I-IMP is the radiotracer of choice for measuring cerebral blood flow and is conducted prior to ^{99m}Tc-HMPAO and ^{99m}Tc-ECD.
    (b) A radiotracer with long shelf stability is required for the study of seizure attacks; therefore, NO difference can be found among ^{99m}Tc-ECD, 123I-IMP, and ^{99m}Tc-HMPAO.
    (c) Changes in the regional cerebral blood flow (rCBF) can be simply and accurately studied with a baseline brain scan and activation SPECT on 1 day.
    (d) Similar to 123I-IMP, ^{99m}Tc-ECD also overestimates the regions with higher blood flow.
20. Which of the following statements about the different radiotracers used on brain SPECT scan is NOT correct?
    (a) ^{99m}Tc-ECD is conducted prior to ^{99m}Tc-HMPAO for the evaluation of the ictal phase in epilepsy.
    (b) Benzodiazepine receptor imaging improves the identification of seizure focus.
    (c) Compared with 123I-IMP, ^{99m}Tc-ECD overestimates the regions of hyperperfusion.
    (d) Early imaging after the injection of 123I-IMP is indicated for the evaluation of the primary motor cortex.

7.3.1 Answer

	A	B	C	D
1		*		
2			*	
3		*		
4	*			
5			*	
6			*	
7			*	
8	*			
9	*			
10				*
11			*	
12		*		
13		*		
14				*
15	*			
16	*			
17				*
18			*	
19	*			
20			*	

7.4 Ligands for Neuroreceptor Imaging by Positron or Single-Photon Emission Computed Tomography

1. The imaging studies of muscarinic (M) receptors have been performed in:
   (a) Epilepsy
   (b) Depression
   (c) Schizophrenia
   (d) Alzheimer's disease (AD)
2. A patient with Alzheimer's is experiencing tremor and rigidity. Which radiotracer should be applied for the diagnosis of an associated Parkinson's disease?
   (a) ^{18}F-FDG
   (b) ^{18}F-flurodopa
   (c) ^{11}C-raclopride
   (d) ^{11}C-carfentanil
3. What is the receptor responsible for the accumulation of ^{123}I-IBZM in the brain?
   (a) Opiate
   (b) Benzodiazepine
   (c) Dopamine D2
   (d) Serotonin
4. The irreversible and severe reduction of the expression of cortical nicotine receptors:
   (a) Alzheimer's disease
   (b) Huntington's disease
   (c) Multiple sclerosis
   (d) Parkinson's disease
5. The radiotracer that shows the activity of dopamine receptors on a brain PET scan:
   (a) ^{11}C-scopolamine
   (b) ^{18}F-methylspiperone
   (c) ^{11}C-etorphine
   (d) ^{11}C-ephedrine
6. Muscarinic receptor imaging is NOT indicated for:
   (a) Schizophrenia
   (b) Alcoholism
   (c) Parkinson's disease
   (d) Alzheimer's disease
7. An increase in the density of dopamine receptors in the basal ganglia is reported on the dopamine receptor PET scan of:
   (a) Parkinson's disease
   (b) Schizophrenia
   (c) Huntington's disease
   (d) Idiopathic focal dystonia

8. Which neurotransmitter systems are imaged with SPECT in epileptic patients?
   (a) GABAergic and muscarinic cholinergic systems
   (b) GABAergic and dopaminergic D2R
   (c) Muscarinic cholinergic and dopaminergic D2R
   (d) Nicotinic and muscarinic cholinergic
9. Which of the following conditions shows a mild decrease in ^{123}I-iomazenil uptake?
   (a) Necrotic core (cerebral infarct)
   (b) Peri-infarct region
   (c) Misery perfusion
   (d) Remote differentiated areas
10. This SPECT imaging has also been suggested as a prognostic marker for aphasia in patients with cerebral infarction:
   (a) Serotonin transporter
   (b) Benzodiazepine receptor
   (c) Muscarinic cholinergic receptor
   (d) GABAergic transporter

7.4.1 Answer

	A	B	C	D
1			*	
2		*		
3			*	
4	*			
5		*		
6	*			
7		*		
8	*			
9		*		
10		*		

7.5 PET Tracers for Brain Scanning

1. About cholinergic neurotransmission:
   (a) A marked increase in muscarinic receptor binding in the basal ganglia in Huntington's disease.
   (b) A marked increase in nicotinic receptor density in AD.
   (c) Changes in cell number in the basalis of Meynert in AD.
   (d) It cannot differentiate AD from progressive nuclear palsy.
2. The gold standard PET tracer for D2 receptor:
   (a) N-^{11}C-methyl-spiperone.
   (b) N-^{18}F-methyl-spiperone.
   (c) ^{11}C-raclopride
   (d) N-^{18}F-fluoroethyl-spiperone.
3. All of the following PET radiotracers are used for the assessment of the β–amyloid deposit in AD *except*:
   (a) ^{11}C-BTA
   (b) ^{18}F-FDDNP
   (c) ^{18}F-FENE
   (d) ^{11}C-MADAM
4. In patients with rheumatoid arthritis (RA), substantial changes have been observed in the binding of:
   (a) ^{11}C-diprenorphine
   (b) ^{11}C-FLB457
   (c) ^{11}C-NNC
   (d) ^{11}C-SCH
5. PET is the method of choice for:
   (a) Migraine
   (b) Huntington's disease
   (c) Parkinson's disease
   (d) Chronic fatigue syndrome
6. Which of the following physiological parameters is best studied with ^{18}F-flurodeoxyuridine?
   (a) Increase in DNA synthesis
   (b) Increase in protein synthesis
   (c) Increase in glucose utilization
   (d) Hypoxia
7. Which of the following radiotracers is used in PET for the study of amino acid metabolism?
   (a) ^{18}F-FDG
   (b) ^{15}O-H_2O
   (c) ^{11}C-methionine
   (d) ^{11}C-scopolamine

8. Which of the following items does NOT properly describe the application of the corresponding radiotracer?
   (a) $^{15}O\text{-}H_2O$: blood flow
   (b) ^{18}F-FDG: glucose metabolism
   (c) ^{11}C-carfentanil: benzodiazepine receptor binding
   (d) ^{11}C-raclopride: dopamine receptor binding

7.5.1 Answer

	A	B	C	D
1			*	
2			*	
3				*
4	*			
5		*		
6	*			
7			*	
8			*	

7.6 Neuroactivation

1. Which brain SPECT imaging has the poorest resolution quality?
   (a) ^{99m}Tc-HMPAO
   (b) ^{99m}Tc-ECD
   (c) ^{123}I-IMP
   (d) ^{133}Xe

7.6.1 Answer

	A	B	C	D
1				*

7.7 Image Analysis Through Brain SPECT and PET

1. Which of the following statements regarding statistical parametric mapping (SPM) is NOT true?
   (a) It is a voxel-based statistical test.
   (b) It is the gold standard for the analysis of brain activity through PET and functional MRI.
   (c) It prevents inter-subject and inter-scan variability masking regional changes.
   (d) It can also be applied to cerebral blood perfusion.
2. Which of the following views is used for the efficient evaluation of cingulate gyrus?
   (a) 305° upward rotation of the head
   (b) Sagittal slices
   (c) Reconstructed 3D images
   (d) Transaxial midline view
3. Which region of the brain is the criterion for evaluating image resolution in the transaxial images of cerebral perfusion with SPECT?
   (a) Internal capsule
   (b) Cingulated gyrus
   (c) Basal ganglia
   (d) Hippocampus
4. … normally shows the minimum level of activity in a brain perfusion study with SPECT.
   (a) Basal ganglia
   (b) Visual cortex
   (c) White matter
   (d) Cerebellum
5. All of the following statements regarding the findings of PET in children are correct *except*:
   (a) The initiation of sensory and motor skills is associated with the increase in FDG uptake in the basal ganglia
   (b) The glucose metabolism of the frontal lobe in the first 4 months after birth is low, and it increases with the improvement of cognitive activity
   (c) The pattern and rate of brain metabolism become similar to those of adults at the ages of one and three years, respectively
   (d) The maximum rate of brain metabolism is at the age of 10–15 years
6. PET shows the hypoperfusion of … in hypoxemic–ischemic encephalopathy.
   (a) Cerebellum
   (b) Pons
   (c) Parasagittal
   (d) Basal ganglia
7. Exhibits the highest peak in the normal brain spectrum on MRS:
   (a) Choline
   (b) *N*-acetyl aspartate
   (c) Creatine
   (d) Lactate

8. Which of the following items is associated with the remarkable increase in the NAA level on MRS?
   (a) Brain infarction
   (b) Multiple sclerosis
   (c) Canavan disease
   (d) Mesial temporal sclerosis

7.7.1 Answer

	A	B	C	D
1	*			
2		*		
3	*			
4			*	
5				*
6			*	
7		*		
8		*		

7.8 SPECT Brain Imaging in Cerebrovascular Disease

1. The acetazolamide stress test is for assessing rCVR in patients with:
   (a) TIA
   (b) Epilepsy
   (c) Dementia
   (d) All of the above
2. AVM appears as:
   (a) High flow in ^{133}Xe, ^{99m}Tc-HMPAO, and ^{99m}Tc-ECD
   (b) Low flow in ^{133}Xe, ^{99m}Tc-HMPAO, and ^{99m}Tc-ECD
   (c) High flow in ^{133}Xe but low flow in ^{99m}Tc-HMPAO and ^{99m}Tc-ECD
   (d) Low flow in ^{133}Xe but high flow in ^{99m}Tc-HMPAO and ^{99m}Tc-ECD
3. In which cerebral disorder is the determination of the cerebral blood reservoir NOT indicated?
   (a) Carotid endarectomy
   (b) Subarachnoid hemorrhage
   (c) Arteriovenous malformation
   (d) Dementia
4. Luxury perfusion is NOT observed with:
   (a) ^{99m}Tc-HMPAO
   (b) ^{99m}Tc-ECD
   (c) ^{133}Xe
   (d) b and c
5. After acetazolamide administration, how long does it take for the cerebral blood flow to reach its maximum?
   (a) 10 min
   (b) 20 min
   (c) 60 min
   (d) 120 min
6. SPECT-rCBF has the least diagnostic sensitivity for:
   (a) Embolic CVA
   (b) Hemorrhagic CVA
   (c) Extensive CVA
   (d) Lacunar CVA
7. In which of the following conditions is evaluating the cerebrovascular reserve with acetazolamide NOT necessary?
   (a) Prediction of the surgical adverse effect in arteriovenous malformation
   (b) Determination of the type of dementia
   (c) Appropriate decision about the candidates for thrombolytic therapy
   (d) Prediction of the risk for infarction after subarachnoid hemorrhage

8. Cerebral perfusion is requested for evaluating the cerebrovascular reserve in a candidate for endarterectomy of the carotid artery. The patient is sensitive to cotrimoxazole and takes amlodipine. Which statement is correct?
   (a) The scan must be performed with 1 g of acetazolamide
   (b) The patient should be reminded of the possible experience of dizziness, hypotension, and tinnitus
   (c) Amlodipine must be discontinued
   (d) This scan is contraindicated for such a patient
9. About transient ischemic attach (TIA) and regional cerebral blood flow (rCBF) SPECT scan:
   (a) Sensitivity of the scan increases when it is performed a few days after an attack
   (b) Acetazolamide is not applied in this case
   (c) This scan is not valuable for identifying the severity of ischemia
   (d) This scan can be used for a follow-up study
10. What is the mechanism of misery perfusion in a cerebral stroke region?
    (a) Relative reduction of RCBF in comparison with rCMRglc.
    (b) Hypoperfusion or hypometabolism may be observed in the surrounding regions of infarction.
    (c) The existence of an ischemic and hyometabolic region in the margin of infarction.
    (d) Hypoperfusion and hypometabolism in the cortex of the opposite side.
11. Which of the following conditions indicates higher oxygen consumption in comparison with glucose in cerebral SPECT?
    (a) Crossed cerebellar diaschisis
    (b) Penumbral zone
    (c) Luxury perfusion
    (d) Infarct core
12. ^{99m}Tc-ECD perfusion SPECT before and after administering acetazolamide is performed on a 77-year-old man. Regions with a remarkable decrease in activity in the left hemisphere are observed on the acetazolamide images relative to the base scan. Which statement is correct?
    (a) Post-acetazolamide images must be repeated because normalizing the subcortical area is required.
    (b) This a normal response to acetazolamide.
    (c) The first therapeutic approach is endarterectomy of the left carotid artery.
    (d) A significant decrease in the cerebrovascular reserve is observed in the left carotid artery.
13. A cerebral perfusion scan is performed in the early hours after an acute brain stroke. Which finding predicts the best response to thrombolytic therapy?
    (a) No activity
    (b) Decrease of activity
    (c) Normal uptake
    (d) No activity in the center and an increased activity along the margins of the defect

14. About stroke:
    (a) Brain SPECT in the early hours of ictus has no advantage over CT or MRI in detecting cerebral ischemia
    (b) The size of the defect in the early hours after ictus is equal among brain SPECT, CT, and MRI
    (c) The difference in sensitivity among SPECT, CT, and MRI disappears after 72 h
    (d) The mechanisms of ^{99m}Tc-ECD and ^{99m}Tc-HMPAO cerebral uptake are identical
15. Which statement about TIA is NOT correct?
    (a) CT and MRI are NOT effective in the diagnosis
    (b) About 60% of TIA cases result in a complete stroke
    (c) The sensitivity of brain SPECT in TIA decreases over time
    (d) Acetazolamide in a cerebrovascular reserve study does NOT change the sensitivity of brain SPECT for an acute or a subacute attack
16. Which of the following diseases may exhibit normal acetazolamide response?
    (a) Alzheimer's disease
    (b) Stroke
    (c) TIA
    (d) AV malformation
17. About rCBF SPECT imaging in a patient with TIA:
    (a) Sensitivity of the test increases over time.
    (b) Sensitivity of the test is 40% during the first 24 h.
    (c) Acetazolamide does NOT change the sensitivity of test.
    (d) It is beneficial in therapeutic monitoring.
18. In which of the following zones is a decreased regional cerebral blood flow (rCBF) with increased oxygen extraction fraction (rOEF) observed on the PET scan of patients with brain stroke?
    (a) Luxury perfusion zone
    (b) Diaschisis zone
    (c) Penumbral zone
    (d) Infarcted zone
19. In which of the following brain regions is the reduced metabolism of glucose (CMR Glu) observed with the increase in age?
    (a) Frontal lobe and somatosensory cortex with a bilateral pattern
    (b) Basal ganglia
    (c) Occipital cortex, especially the visual cortex
    (d) Temporal and posteroparietal, with more involvement of the left side

20. Cerebral perfusion SPECT is performed on a patient with a history of TIA and shows more than 90% stenosis of the left carotid. A relative decrease in perfusion in the left hemisphere with crossed cerebellar intermediate diaschisis is also observed. Endarterectomy will be recommended if the acetazolamide scan shows:
    (a) Increased perfusion of the right hemisphere without reactivity of the left hemisphere
    (b) Decrease in crossed cerebellar diaschisis
    (c) Increased perfusion in the right hemisphere with a normalized activity of the left hemisphere
    (d) Increase in crossed cerebellar diaschisis
21. A cerebral perfusion SPECT scan with labeled ^{99m}Tc-ECD is performed 20 days after brain stroke because of an obstruction in the middle cerebral artery (MCA). A decreased perfusion in the left hemisphere and right cerebellum is observed. Which phenomenon is indicated for SPECT, and what is the outcome of the phenomenon?
    (a) Luxury perfusion, poor
    (b) Diaschisis, good
    (c) Luxury perfusion, good
    (d) Diaschisis, poor
22. Which of the following diagnostic methods is the effective for the diagnosis of TIA?
    (a) Conventional CT
    (b) Flow evaluation with SPECT at rest
    (c) ^{99m}Tc-HMPAO SPECT with acetazolamide
    (d) ^{99m}Tc-GHA SPECT
23. About the acetazolamide challenge in a brain perfusion study with ^{99m}Tc-HMPAO SPECT:
    (a) A slow intravenous injection of 1 g acetazolamide is first performed, and ^{99m}Tc-HMPAo is then administered after 20–25 min
    (b) A slow intravenous injection of ^{99m}Tc-HMPAO is first performed, and 1 mg acetazolamide is then administered intravenously after 5 min
    (c) Immediately after the intravenous injection of 1 g acetazolamide, ^{99m}Tc-HMPAO is administered intravenously
    (d) A slow intravenous injection of 1 g acetazolamide is first performed, and ^{99m}Tc-HMPAO is then administered after 5 min
24. A 69-year-old man with brain stroke is a candidate for thrombolytic therapy. What is the recommended diagnostic modality?
    (a) CT scan
    (b) Cerebral perfusion scan
    (c) Electroencephalography
    (d) FDG-PET scan

25. Which of the following modalities best shows the defects immediately after an acute stroke?
    (a) CT scan
    (b) MRI
    (c) Brain SPECT
    (d) Doppler ultrasonography
26. In which of the following diseases is the acetazolamide stress test performed for the differentiation between vascular and neural origins?
    (a) TIA
    (b) Stroke
    (c) Arteriovenous malformation
    (d) Dementia
27. Diaschisis in a patient with stroke is defined as:
    (a) Diaschisis is the relative reduction of rCBF in comparison with rCMR Glu
    (b) Diaschisis is the increase in rCBF in comparison with brain metabolism
    (c) Diaschisis is the reduction of metabolism and cortex perfusion of the opposite side of the infarct
    (d) Diaschisis is the reduction of metabolism on the infarct side
28. The ^{99m}Tc-HMPAO brain SPECT scan of a 79-year-old woman shows a decreased activity in the left brain hemisphere and right cerebellar hemisphere. What is the most probable diagnosis?
    (a) Metastasis to the left brain hemisphere and right cerebellar hemisphere
    (b) Cerebrovascular accident (CVA) of the left brain hemisphere and right cerebellar hemisphere
    (c) CVA of the left brain hemisphere
    (d) b and c
29. What is the recommended protocol for a ^{99m}Tc-HMPAO scan with acetazolamide in a patient with suspected TIA?
    (a) Bolus intravenous injection of acetazolamide 25 min after ^{99m}Tc-HMPAO
    (b) Acetazolamide infusion 10 min before the radiotracer and continued during the test
    (c) Slow intravenous injection of acetazolamide for 2 min and injection of ^{99m}Tc-HMPAO after 25 min
    (d) Acetazolamide infusion 10 min after ^{99m}Tc-HMPAO
30. A 19% increase in brain perfusion is observed after acetazolamide injection. What is the most probable diagnosis?
    (a) Transient ischemic attack
    (b) Normal
    (c) Multi-infarct dementia
    (d) Arteriovenous malformation
31. About diaschisis on a brain scan:
    (a) The possibility of its observation is high in a large infarction.
    (b) MRI usually shows abnormality in the corresponding region.
    (c) It is observed adjacent to the infarcted region.
    (d) It usually occurs 6 months after infarction.

32. Which item about the role of PET in a cerebrovascular attack is NOT correct?
    (a) PET detects the disorder and its extent earlier than other imaging modalities
    (b) An increase in oxygen extraction fraction is observed in the penumbral region
    (c) Luxury perfusion is observed along the margins of the infarct a few hours to few days after stroke
    (d) Crossed cerebellar diaschisis occurs because of the disconnection of the cerebro-ponto-cerebellar pathways
33. About brain infarction:
    (a) CT scan is positive in 50% of cases 8 h after brain infarction.
    (b) SPECT is positive in 90% of cases 8 h after brain infarction.
    (c) The prevalence of false-negative MRI results is around 50% in acute stroke.
    (d) The sensitivity of SPECT is high for the detection of lacunar infarction.
34. Regarding transient ischemic attack (TIA):
    (a) Acetazolamide does NOT affect the sensitivity of brain perfusion scan.
    (b) The sensitivity of brain perfusion scan decreases over time.
    (c) The diagnostic sensitivity of CT scan is higher than that of brain SPECT.
    (d) The sensitivity of CT scan increases over time.
35. Which of the following drugs or reagents is NOT indicated for the evaluation of cerebral blood flow reserve in patients with vascular obstructive disease?
    (a) Dipyridamole
    (b) Acetazolamide
    (c) Nitroglycerine
    (d) CO_2
36. Which of the following findings on a regional cerebral blood flow (rCBF) SPECT scan in the initial stages of a brain stroke predicts a poor prognosis?
    (a) Increase in regional uptake of the radiotracer
    (b) Normal radiotracer uptake
    (c) Decrease in the regional uptake of the radiotracer
    (d) Lack of regional uptake of the radiotracer
37. Which of the following statements regarding arteriovenous malformation (AVM) is NOT correct?
    (a) ^{133}Xe SPECT shows an increased blood flow in the AVM.
    (b) Patients with a reduced regional blood flow are at high risk for future ischemic events.
    (c) Patients with an increased regional blood flow around the AVM have a low risk for hemorrhagic events.
    (d) Hemorrhage, seizure, and relative cerebral ischemia are the main complications of AVM.
38. Which of the following methods is the most sensitive for the detection of vasospasm in patients with subarachnoid hemorrhage?
    (a) Transcranial Doppler
    (b) Contrast angiography
    (c) SPECT rCBF imaging
    (d) Brain CT scan

39. Which of the following statements about imaging of cerebrovascular diseases is NOT correct?
    (a) SPECT view may be normal 7 days after a brain stroke
    (b) SPECT shows a decreased cerebellar activity on the same side of the stroke
    (c) CT scan is NOT valuable for the diagnosis of TIA
    (d) SPECT is positive 24 h after TIA in more than 50% of cases
40. About cerebrovascular accident (CVA) in children:
    (a) Ischemic and hemorrhagic CVA account for 75% and 25% of CVA cases in children, respectively.
    (b) Children with CBF less than 10 ml/min/100 g shows abnormal brain development.
    (c) Stroke is surprisingly common in children, with new cases occurring as frequent as brain tumors.
    (d) Risk factors can be detected before CVA.
41. In the infarction of the bilateral thalamus and mesencephalon regions, which artery is the most likely to be occluded?
    (a) Recurrent artery of Huebner
    (b) Anterior choroidal artery
    (c) Posterior choroidal artery
    (d) Artery of Percheron

7.8.1 Answer

	A	B	C	D
1				*
2			*	
3		*		
4		*		
5		*		
6				*
7			*	
8				*
9				*
10	*			
11	*			
12				*
13		*		
14			*	
15				*
16	*			
17				*
18			*	
19	*			
20	*			
21				*

22			*	
23	*			
24	*			
25			*	
26				*
27			*	
28			*	
29			*	
30		*		
31	*			
32			*	
33		*		
34		*		
35			*	
36				*
37			*	
38		*		
39		*		
40			*	
41		*		

7.9 Nuclear Medicine in the Management of Patients with Epilepsy

1. In temporal lobe epilepsy (TLE):
   (a) ^{11}C-carfentanil shows an increased uptake, but ^{123}I-iodoexetimide shows a decreased uptake.
   (b) ^{11}C-carfentanil and ^{123}I-iodoexetimide show an increased uptake.
   (c) ^{11}C-carfentanil and ^{123}I-iodoexetimide show a decreased uptake.
   (d) ^{11}C-carfentanil shows a decreased uptake, but ^{123}I-iodoexetimide shows an increased uptake.
2. In frontal lobe epilepsy:
   (a) Ictal hyperperfusion is observed.
   (b) It is accompanied with ipsilateral basal ganglia hyperperfusion.
   (c) It is accompanied with contralateral cerebellar hyperperfusion.
   (d) All of the above.
3. What is the most sensitive method for the diagnosis of temporal lobe epilepsy (TLE)?
   (a) Interictal PET.
   (b) Ictal PET.
   (c) Interictal SPECT.
   (d) Ictal SPECT.
4. If seizure focus appears as an enhanced uptake on a cerebral perfusion scan, what is the maximum persistence time of the enhanced uptake region after the cessation of a temporal seizure?
   (a) 2 min
   (b) 5 min
   (c) 10 min
   (d) 20 min.
5. About brain scan of seizure disorders:
   (a) In the interictal phase, the sensitivity of brain SPECT with ^{99m}Tc–HMPAO is higher than that of cerebral PET.
   (b) In the ictal phase, a higher metabolic activity and a lower perfusion of neuroleptic site are observed.
   (c) In the ictal phase, the specificity of the scan depends on the time of injection.
   (d) In the interictal phase of extratemporal epilepsy, scan interpretation is problematic.
6. Which item about partial continuous epilepsy is NOT correct?
   (a) In the ictal scan, the radiopharmaceutical is injected at the beginning of a seizure attack, and the scan is performed after the attack.
   (b) Seizure focus is identified in 50–75% of patients subjected to a PET or SPECT scan in the interictal phase.
   (c) SPECT is preferred over PET in the ictal phase because of the short half-life of ^{18}F-FDG and its prolonged uptake.
   (d) The diagnostic sensitivity of ictal SPECT perfusion is similar to that of interictal PET.

7. What is the most sensitive method for the diagnosis of temporal lobe epilepsy?
   (a) MRI
   (b) Cerebral blood flow imaging
   (c) EEG
   (d) PET
8. Seizure focus perfusion in a patient with epilepsy:
   (a) Decreases in the ictal phase
   (b) Decreases in the early postictal phase
   (c) Increases in the interictal phase
   (d) Increases in the ictal and early postictal phase
9. About cerebral imaging for the evaluation of epilepsy:
   (a) The sensitivities of SPECT and PET are similar in the interictal phase.
   (b) Delayed imaging is recommended to prevent the observation of multiple regions of increased uptake caused by seizure propagation in ictal imaging.
   (c) A noticeable focal increase in activity on the SPECT scan in the ictal phase is also observed as an abnormal finding in MRI and CT.
   (d) Treatment-resistant epilepsy is usually extra temporal and shows no anatomical defect.
10. How is the seizure focus presented in the interictal phase on FDG-PET and cerebral perfusion SPECT, respectively?
   (a) Decrease, decrease
   (b) Increase, decrease
   (c) Increase, increase
   (d) Decrease, increase
11. A 27-year-old woman is referred because of a seizure attack. Medial temporal sclerosis is also detected by MRI and EEG. What is the recommended diagnostic method before surgery?
   (a) CT scan
   (b) Interictal FDG-PET
   (c) Interictal SPECT
   (d) Ictal FDG-PET
12. A 36-year-old woman with refractory seizure attacks is evaluated. The MRI and EEG results are ambiguous, and extratemporal epileptic foci are suspected. What is the preferred diagnostic modality?
   (a) Interictal PET
   (b) Ictal/interictal SPECT
   (c) Ictal PET
   (d) Interictal SPECT
13. Which item is preferred regarding the application of ^{18}F-FDG-PET and SPECT on a seizure patient candidate for surgery?
   (a) Ictal SPECT, ictal PET
   (b) Interictal SPECT, ictal PET
   (c) Interictal PET, ictal PET
   (d) Interictal PET, ictal SPECT

14. A patient is subjected to a brain perfusion study because of refractory seizure. When is the right time for an injection to observe the reduced perfusion defect with maximum sensitivity?
    (a) Ictal phase.
    (b) Postictal phase.
    (c) Interictal phase.
    (d) 5 min before seizure.
15. MRI and brain perfusion scan are performed on a 3-year-old child with refractory seizure. Which of the following findings is the most probable?
    (a) Decreased extratemporal perfusion + abnormal MRI in that region.
    (b) Decreased perfusion of the temporal lobe + abnormal MRI in that region.
    (c) Decreased perfusion of the temporal lobe + normal MRI in that region.
    (d) Decreased extratemporal perfusion + normal MRI in that region.
16. FDG-PET is performed before temporal lobectomy on an epileptic patient. In which of the following conditions is the probability of a seizure after surgery high?
    (a) High-grade hypometabolism in the temporal lobe.
    (b) Unilateral restriction of the seizure focus in the temporal lobe.
    (c) Thalamic hypometabolism.
    (d) Generalized increase in metabolism in the interictal phase.
17. The inferotemporal lobe is involved in a patient with partial epilepsy. Which section of the brain SPECT study is the most appropriate for the evaluation of this lobe?
    (a) Sagittal
    (b) Transaxial
    (c) Oblique
    (d) Coronal
18. About patients with temporal lobe epilepsy:
    (a) The diagnostic sensitivity of interictal SPECT is similar to that of MRI.
    (b) All patients show focal hypoperfusion in the interictal phase.
    (c) Interictal SPECT is important for a better interpretation of ictal studies.
    (d) SPECT can be used for the differentiation between unilateral and bilateral seizure foci.
19. About temporal lobe epilepsy:
    (a) Ictal encephalography with electrodes on head skin can localize the seizure focus in all patients.
    (b) The sensitivity of MRI for the detection of seizure focus is similar to that of PET scan.
    (c) Asymmetric metabolism on the brain PET scan is similar to the asymmetric perfusion on SPECT.
    (d) Ictal brain PET scan is easy and capable of detecting seizure focus similar to SPECT.

20. Long-term administration of sodium valproate in children with the absence of seizure causes:
    (a) Increased density of benzodiazepine receptors
    (b) Decreases density of benzodiazepine receptors
    (c) Increased density of dopamine D2 receptors
    (d) Decreased density of dopamine D2 receptors
21. What changes are observed in the metabolism and perfusion of a seizure focus in the interictal phase in comparison with brain normal tissue?
    (a) Hyperperfusion and hypometabolism
    (b) Hypoperfusion and hypometabolism
    (c) Hypoperfusion and hypermetabolism
    (d) Hyperperfusion and hypermetabolism
22. About the evaluation of seizure focus in the temporal lobe:
    (a) The patterns of a brain perfusion scan in the ictal and postictal phases are similar
    (b) The patterns of brain perfusion scan in the ictal, interictal, and postictal phases are similar
    (c) Brain perfusion scan has the maximum sensitivity in the interictal phase if the goal is to localize the seizure focus
    (d) The diagnostic value of a brain perfusion scan is similar between generalized and partial seizures
23. Epileptogenic regions on an FDG scan show … and … in the ictal and interictal phases, respectively.
    (a) Hypermetabolism, hypometabolism
    (b) Hypermetabolism, hypermetabolism
    (c) Hypometabolism, hypometabolism
    (d) Hypometabolism, hypermetabolism
24. Which brain regions are the most common epileptogenic zones in a partial seizure?
    (a) Frontal and parietal
    (b) Temporal and parietal
    (c) Frontal and occipital
    (d) Temporal and frontal
25. What is the sensitivity of PET if the goal is to localize the epileptogenic zone in temporal lobe epilepsy?
    (a) 80%
    (b) 60%
    (c) 70%
    (d) 90%
26. A patient with a multiple seizure type and low IQ is presented. EEG shows a repetitive 1–2.5 Hz spike wave pattern, and a Lennox–Gastaut syndrome is suspected. What is the expected pattern of a PET scan?
    (a) Unilateral focal hypometabolism
    (b) Unilateral diffuse hypometabolism
    (c) Bilateral diffuse hypometabolism
    (d) All of the above

27. When is the most appropriate time to administer sedatives in children for brain scan?
    (a) During IV catheterization at the beginning of the study
    (b) Concurrent with the injection of the radiotracer
    (c) Before radiotracer injection in the restroom
    (d) Before imaging
28. Which of the following statements regarding the findings of a brain scan and brain development of children is NOT correct?
    (a) Cisternography must be initiated earlier in children than in adults
    (b) The pattern of rCBF uptake and rCMRglc becomes similar to that of adults at the age of 2 years
    (c) rCMRglc increases until 9 years of age and decreases to the level of adults during late adolescence
    (d) Maximum rCBF uptake and rCMRglc at birth is observed in sites with high development
29. In a seizure:
    (a) Seizure foci show a high uptake of ^{11}C-flumazenil and ^{123}I-iomazenil
    (b) PET is the preferred method for ictal imaging
    (c) Ictal imaging increases the sensitivity of the localization of a seizure focus by 50–75%
    (d) Acquired epileptic aphasia (Landau–Kleffner syndrome) in the temporal lobe is commonly bilateral

7.9.1 Answer

	A	B	C	D
1	*			
2				*
3		*		
4		*		
5				*
6				*
7				*
8				*
9				*
10	*			
11		*		
12		*		
13				*
14		*		
15				*
16			*	
17				*
18			*	
19		*		

20		*		
21		*		
22	*			
23	*			
24				*
25			*	
26				*
27				*
28		*		
29				*

7.10 Nuclear Medicine and the Management of Patients with Parkinsonian Disorders

1. A dopamine transporter system (DaT) scan is abnormal in:
   (a) AD
   (b) Benign essential tremor
   (c) Dopa-responsive dystonia
   (d) Early-onset Parkinson's disease
2. Which of the following is the method of choice if the goal is to evaluate clinical progress and therapeutic effectiveness in Parkinson's disease?
   (a) F-18-FDG-PET
   (b) C-15-CO_2 PET
   (c) C-11-nomifensine PET
   (d) F-18-fluorodopa PET
3. Which of the following radiotracers is used for the diagnosis of Parkinson's in the early stages?
   (a) Tc-99m-DAT
   (b) F-18-FDG
   (c) C-11-carfentanil
   (d) I-123-raclopride
4. A patient with bradykinesia, tremor, and rigidity is referred for the differentiation of parkinsonism from essential tremor. What is the radiotracer of choice, and what is the pattern of uptake in the involved region?
   (a) ^{18}F-FDG, decreased uptake
   (b) ^{18}F-Dopa, increased uptake
   (c) ^{99m}Tc-DAT, decreased uptake
   (d) None
5. Which of the following SPECT or PET findings is associated with Parkinson's disease?
   (a) Decreased perfusion and metabolism in the temporoparietal region
   (b) Scattered focal decrease in uptake and metabolism in the cerebral cortex
   (c) Decreased ^{18}F-fluorodopa in the striatum
   (d) Severe decrease in metabolism in the lenticular nuclei
6. The reduced metabolism of the basal ganglia on a brain PET scan is associated with:
   (a) Alzheimer's disease
   (b) Dementia with Lewy bodies
   (c) Huntington's disease
   (d) Parkinson's disease
7. CNS disorders are associated with changes in perfusion/metabolism. What are the significant changes in the brain scan of patients with Binswanger's disease?
   (a) Decreased rCBF and rCMRO2 in white matter
   (b) Decreased metabolism and perfusion in the caudate and putamen nuclei
   (c) Increased glucose metabolism in the lenticular nucleus of the opposite side
   (d) Decreased whole brain metabolism, particularly in the temporal and parietal lobes

8. CNS disorders are associated with changes in perfusion/metabolism. What are the significant changes in the brain scan of patients with dystonia?
   (a) Decreased rCBF and rCMRO2 in white matter
   (b) Decreased metabolism and perfusion in the caudate and putamen nuclei
   (c) Increased glucose metabolism in the lenticular nucleus of the opposite side
   (d) Decreased whole brain metabolism, particularly in the temporal and parietal lobes
9. FDG-PET is performed on a subject with confirmed Parkinson's. The hypometabolism of the ... indicates the intensity of bradykinesia.
   (a) Basal ganglia
   (b) Cortex
   (c) Inferior thalamus
   (d) Striatum
10. What changes in FDG-PET are indicative of progressive supranuclear palsy?
   (a) Hypometabolism of the cerebellum and striatum
   (b) Hypermetabolism of the lenticular nuclei
   (c) Hypometabolism of the caudate and putamen
   (d) Hypometabolism of the basal ganglia and cortex
11. What changes in FDG-PET are indicative of Wilson's disease?
   (a) Hypometabolism of the cerebellum and striatum.
   (b) Hypermetabolism of the lenticular nuclei.
   (c) Hypometabolism of the caudate and putamen.
   (d) Hypometabolism of the basal ganglia and cortex.
12. What changes in FDG-PET are indicative of Huntington's disease?
   (a) Hypometabolism of the cerebellum and striatum
   (b) Hypermetabolism of the lenticular nuclei
   (c) Hypometabolism of the caudate and putamen
   (d) Hypometabolism of the basal ganglia and cortex
13. Bilateral hypometabolism in the parietotemporal regions is observed on FDG-PET. PET imaging with ^{18}F-flurodopa shows a decreased activity of the putamen for the same patient. What is the most probable diagnosis?
   (a) Parkinson's disease with dementia
   (b) Idiopathic torsional dystonia
   (c) Progressive supranuclear palsy
   (d) Alzheimer's disease
14. What is the diagnostic method of choice for the evaluation of genetically susceptible cases for Huntington's disease?
   (a) Brain SPECT
   (b) CT scan
   (c) FDG-PET scan
   (d) MRI

15. A patient with tremor, bradykinesia, and rigidity is referred. The ^{123}I-IBZM scan shows a decreased striatal uptake, and the ^{123}I-FP-CIT scan shows a decreased uptake in both putamens. Which item is the best interpretation?
    (a) Secondary parkinsonism
    (b) Parkinsonism
    (c) High-dose L-dopa is required
    (d) The scan results exclude the possibility of progressive supranuclear palsy
16. A decreased perfusion in the striatum is observed on the brain SPECT scan of a patient. What is the most probable diagnosis?
    (a) Alzheimer's disease
    (b) Multiple infarct dementia
    (c) Parkinson's disease
    (d) Grand mal epilepsy
17. A decrease in radiotracer uptake is observed in the caudate nucleus of a young adult patient on the ^{18}F-FDG brain scan. Which of the following diseases is predicted?
    (a) Petit mal
    (b) Adrenoleukodystrophy (ALD)
    (c) Parkinson's disease
    (d) Huntington's disease
18. A decrease in glucose metabolism and perfusion in the caudate and putamen is observed on the brain PET and SPECT scans. What is the most probable diagnosis?
    (a) Pick's disease
    (b) Wilson's disease
    (c) Dementia due to AIDS
    (d) Huntington's disease
19. A decrease in metabolism and perfusion in the lenticular nuclei is observed on the brain PET and SPECT scans. What is the most probable diagnosis?
    (a) Dementia due to AIDS
    (b) Wilson's disease
    (c) Pick's disease
    (d) Huntington's disease
20. What is the PET scan pattern for a patient with progressive supranuclear palsy?
    (a) Global decrease in brain glucose metabolism mainly in the superior frontal cortex
    (b) Decrease in glucose metabolism in the caudate and putamen
    (c) Scattered focal decrease in glucose metabolism in the parietal and temporal lobes
    (d) Diffuse ^{15}O (oxygen) hypometabolism in the posterior parietal and temporal lobes
21. Which of the following statements about Parkinson's disease is NOT correct?
    (a) PET scan usually shows a normal pattern of metabolism.
    (b) Dementia accompanied with Parkinson's does NOT change the FDG-PET scan pattern.
    (c) This disease has a presynaptic dopaminergic dysfunction.
    (d) The ^{18}F-DOPA scan shows a decreased uptake in the putamen.

22. On a brain scan:
    (a) Global brain perfusion increases in the aura phase of migraine.
    (b) Decreased rCBF in the caudate and increased rCBF in the putamen are observed in Huntington's disease.
    (c) A high thallium uptake in the cerebral lesion of AIDS patients rules out granulomatosis.
    (d) Thallium uptake in the glioma tumor site indicates recurrence or necrosis.
23. ^{123}I-β-CIT is indicated for:
    (a) Parkinson's disease
    (b) Minimal cognitive impairment
    (c) Prion disease
    (d) Lewy body dementia
24. What is the main advantage of a dopamine transporter (DAT) SPECT study in Parkinson's disease?
    (a) Evaluation of the disease progression
    (b) Definite diagnosis
    (c) Primary diagnosis
    (d) All of the above
25. Which type of the Parkinson's syndromes best responds to L-dopa treatment?
    (a) Parkinson's disease (PD)
    (b) Multiple system atrophy (MSA)
    (c) Essential tremor
    (d) Progressive supranuclear palsy (PSP)
26. All of the following statements regarding the findings of SPECT in parkinsonism are correct *except*:
    (a) Dopamine transporter (DAT) SPECT can discriminate between multiple system atrophy (MSA) and progressive supranuclear palsy (PSP).
    (b) Dopamine D2 receptor SPECT can discriminate among Parkinson's disease (PD), MSA, and PSP.
    (c) A patient with symptoms of Parkinson's must be primarily evaluated with DAT SPECT.
    (d) DAT SPECT is effective in diagnosing patients with clinically uncertain Parkinson's syndrome.
27. What is the pattern of rCMRglc uptake in a patient with choreoathetoid cerebral palsy?
    (a) Unilateral hypometabolism on the opposite side of neural symptoms without crossed cerebellar diaschisis
    (b) Hypometabolism in the thalamus and lenticular nucleus without a focal defect
    (c) Regions of hypometabolism matched with anatomical defects and clinical symptoms
    (d) Regions of hypometabolism mismatched with anatomical defects and clinical symptoms

28. A patient with tremor is referred for ^{18}F-Dopa PET scan. A diffuse and symmetrical decreased uptake is observed in the striatal regions. What is the most probable diagnosis?
    (a) Corticobasal degeneration
    (b) Parkinson's disease (PD)
    (c) Progressive supranuclear palsy
    (d) Essential tremor

7.10.1 Answer

	A	B	C	D
1				*
2				*
3	*			
4			*	
5			*	
6			*	
7	*			
8			*	
9		*		
10				*
11	*			
12			*	
13	*			
14			*	
15			*	
16			*	
17				*
18				*
19		*		
20	*			
21	*			
22			*	
23	*			
24				*
25	*			
26	*			
27		*		
28			*	

7.11 Anxiety Disorders and Effective Disorders

1. In obsessive compulsive disorder (OCD), abnormal metabolism is seen in the:
   (a) Temporal cortex
   (b) Orbitofrontal cortex
   (c) Parietal cortex
   (d) Hippocampus
2. In panic disorders, no abnormality is seen in the:
   (a) Posterior cingulate
   (b) Parietotemporal region
   (c) Hippocampus
   (d) Orbitofrontal cortex
3. A significant decrease in iomazenil uptake is observed on the brain SPECT of PTSD patients in the:
   (a) Temporal lobe
   (b) Frontal lobe
   (c) Parietal lobe
   (d) Occipital cortex
4. In depressed patients, a reduction is seen in the:
   (a) Orbitofrontal cortex
   (b) Subgenual cingulate
   (c) Amygdala
   (d) Dorsolateral prefrontal region
5. Which of the following findings is observed in chronic fatigue syndrome?
   (a) Decreased nonhomogeneous uptake in the cortex
   (b) Decreased diffuse uptake in the cortex
   (c) Transient reduction of the total cerebral blood flow
   (d) Decreased perfusion in the brain stem
6. PET is valuable for the evaluation of psychiatric disorders. What is the pattern of glucose metabolism in different psychiatric disorders?
   (a) Hypofrontalism is observed in schizophrenia, particularly in young patients.
   (b) Decreased glucose metabolism of the subcortical regions in comparison with the cortical regions is notable in patients with depression.
   (c) A bilateral increase in glucose metabolism in the caudate nucleus is notable in obsessive compulsive disorder.
   (d) Increased glucose metabolism of the frontal and temporal lobes is observed in alcoholism.
7. In mild cognitive impairment, brain SPECT shows reduced perfusion in the:
   (a) Temporal lobe
   (b) Parietal, frontal, visual cortex
   (c) Frontal lobe
   (d) Posterior cingulate gyrus

8. Cerebral perfusion with SPECT is performed on a patient with unipolar major depression. Normal perfusion is expected in the:
   (a) Right limbic region
   (b) Anterior frontal cortex
   (c) Caudate nucleus
   (d) Anterior cingulate gyrus
9. What changes in FDG-PET are indicative of anorexia nervosa?
   (a) Hypometabolism of the caudate nuclei
   (b) Global cortex hypometabolism
   (c) Parahippocampal gyrus hypermetabolism
   (d) Hypermetabolism of the frontal lobe and caudate nuclei
10. What changes in FDG-PET are indicative of obsessive-compulsive disease?
   (a) Hypometabolism of the caudate nuclei
   (b) Global cortex hypometabolism
   (c) Parahippocampal gyrus hypermetabolism
   (d) Hypermetabolism of the frontal lobe and caudate nuclei
11. What changes in FDG-PET are indicative of major depression?
   (a) Hypometabolism of the caudate nuclei
   (b) Global cortex hypometabolism
   (c) Parahippocampal gyrus hypermetabolism
   (d) Hypermetabolism of the frontal lobe and caudate nuclei
12. Decrease in frontal cortex flow and changes in the basal ganglia and perfusion of the temporal lobe are reported on the brain SPECT scan. What is the most probable diagnosis?
   (a) Primary generalized epilepsy
   (b) Schizophrenia
   (c) Anxiety disorder
   (d) Temporal lobe epilepsy
13. FDG-PET shows hypermetabolism in the orbitofrontal lobe and caudate nuclei. What is the most probable diagnosis?
   (a) Schizophrenia with negative symptoms
   (b) Obsessive-compulsive disorder
   (c) Anxiety disorders
   (d) Long-term cocaine addiction
14. Which of the following statements regarding the PET findings in psychiatric diseases is NOT correct?
   (a) Therapeutic effects can be monitored with receptor imaging.
   (b) PET is capable of differentiating patients with schizophrenia from malingering subjects.
   (c) PET shows a global dysfunction in patients with major depression.
   (d) Hypoperfusion on PET scan is NOT related to the severity of depression.
15. Regarding the findings of PET in bipolar disorders:
   (a) PET is capable of discriminating between bipolar and unipolar patients.
   (b) Brain metabolism is normal in unipolar patients.
   (c) Brain metabolism in mania is normal but shows a decrease in the depression phase of bipolar patients.
   (d) All of the above are correct.

16. What is the receptor involved in post-cerebrovascular attack (CVA) depression?
    (a) D2 dopamine receptors
    (b) Serotonin-s2 receptors
    (c) GABA receptors
    (d) 5HT1A receptors
17. Which brain region shows hypermetabolism in obsessive-compulsive disorder (OCD)?
    (a) Infrofrontal
    (b) Orbitofrontal
    (c) Superofrontal
    (d) Posterofrontal
18. Which brain regions show hyperperfusion in the rest phase and during panic attacks, respectively?
    (a) Right parahypocampal region at rest; temporal, clastrum, and lateral putamen during attack
    (b) Temporal, clastrum, and lateral putamen at rest; right parahypocampal region during attack
    (c) Left parahypocampal region at rest; temporal, clastrum, and medial putamen during attack
    (d) Temporal, clastrum, and lateral putamen at rest; left parahypocampal region during attack
19. Which brain regions show hypometabolism after the administration of benzodiazepine in patients with generalized anxiety disorder?
    (a) Occipital and left frontal
    (b) Parietal and left frontal
    (c) Occipital and right frontal
    (d) Parietal and right frontal
20. Which of the following statements about attention deficit disorder (ADD) is NOT correct?
    (a) Decreased rCMRglc in the premotor and superior prefrontal cortices.
    (b) Decreased rCMRglc in the left anterior frontal lobe in adolescent ADD.
    (c) rCMRglc abnormalities in PET changes are altered by acute stimulant therapy or clinically effective chronic stimulant therapy.
    (d) Dopamine SPECT imaging shows an increase in striatal uptake in adolescent ADD.

7.11.1 Answer

	A	B	C	D
1		*		
2	*			
3		*		
4				*
5				*

6			*	
7				*
8	*			
9	*			
10				*
11		*		
12		*		
13		*		
14				*
15				*
16		*		
17		*		
18	*			
19			*	
20			*	

7.12 Addictions

1. Which part of the brain is approximately involved in all types of addiction?
   (a) Temporal lobe
   (b) Frontal lobe
   (c) Parietal lobe
   (d) Occipital lobe
2. Cerebral perfusion scintigraphy is performed on a patient with alcohol withdrawal syndrome. Which part of the brain has the highest increase in blood perfusion?
   (a) Temporal lobe
   (b) Frontal lobe
   (c) Cerebellum
   (d) Brain stem
3. Which item properly describes the most expected PET finding in the corresponding diseases?
   (a) Global increase in brain metabolic activity in alcoholism
   (b) Cocaine administration in a cocaine-addicted subject increases the metabolism of the cortex
   (c) Temporal lobe shows the height abnormality in schizophrenia
   (d) Global decrease in brain perfusion and metabolism in depression
4. Which of the following disorders demonstrates reduced metabolism of the whole brain on a brain FDG scan?
   (a) Anxiety disorders
   (b) Acute ingestion of alcohol
   (c) Cocaine abuse
   (d) Obsessive-compulsive disorder
5. ^{11}C-N-methylspiperone is used for evaluating a patient. Which receptor is responsible for the cerebral uptake of this radiotracer?
   (a) Opioid
   (b) Dopamine
   (c) Serotonin
   (d) Acetylcholine
6. What are the SPECT or PET scan findings on alcoholic patients?
   (a) Hypoperfusion mainly in the frontal and parietal cortex as well as global brain hypometabolism
   (b) Hypoperfusion in the prefrontal, frontal, and basal ganglia as well as global brain hypometabolism
   (c) Cerebellar hypoperfusion and metabolism as well as hyperperfusion in the right temporal and prefrontal cortex
   (d) Hyperperfusion in the cerebellum, basal ganglia, orbitofrontal, and prefrontal cortex

7. What are the SPECT and PET scan findings on cocaine addict patients?
   (a) Hypoperfusion mainly in the frontal and parietal cortex as well as global brain hypometabolism
   (b) Hypoperfusion in the prefrontal, frontal, and basal ganglia as well as global brain hypometabolism
   (c) Cerebellar hypoperfusion and metabolism as well as hyperperfusion in the right temporal and prefrontal cortex
   (d) Hyperperfusion in the cerebellum, basal ganglia, orbitofrontal, and prefrontal cortex
8. Which of the following changes is observed on the ^{99m}Tc-HMPAO brain SPECT of heroin addicts after withdrawal?
   (a) Brain hypoperfusion after 3 days.
   (b) Improvement of global brain perfusion after 3 weeks.
   (c) Improvement of global brain perfusion after 2 days.
   (d) NO difference is found in brain perfusion before and after withdrawal.
9. About the SPECT or PET scan of alcoholic patients:
   (a) Alcohol does NOT change the cerebellum blood flow.
   (b) Acute alcohol withdrawal increases the cerebral flow or metabolism, especially in the frontal lobe.
   (c) Toxic levels of alcohol increases glucose metabolism in the cerebral and cerebellar cortex.
   (d) A positive relationship exists between the age and period of alcohol administration and the metabolic changes in the frontal, parietal, and temporal cortex.
10. What is the most expected pattern of brain SPECT and PET in patients abusing ecstasy?
    (a) Hyperperfusion in the visual cortex and caudate nucleus.
    (b) Glucose hypermetabolism, especially in the striatum.
    (c) Negative correlation between the dose of ecstasy and brain metabolism.
    (d) Increase in the serotonin transporter (5HTT) level in the brain cortex.
11. In cocaine addicts:
    (a) ^{15}O-H_2O PET scan shows a decreased cerebral blood flow, especially in the prefrontal cortex.
    (b) FDG-PET shows a global brain increase in glucose metabolism after the intravenous administration of euphorogenic doses of cocaine.
    (c) FDG-PET shows hypometabolism in the orbitofrontal cortex and basal ganglia in the first week after cocaine withdrawal in addicts with normal neurologic symptoms.
    (d) NO relationship exists between the dose and period of cocaine abuse and the metabolic changes on the PET scan.

12. About opioid addiction:
    (a) Brain SPECT shows hyperperfusion in the frontal and parietal cortex as well as decreased activity in the thalamus of opiate addicts.
    (b) ^{99m}Tc-HMPAO brain SPECT shows decreased activity in the anterior cingulate cortex, amygdala, and thalamus in hydromorphine addicts.
    (c) ^{99m}Tc-HMPAO brain SPECT shows NO perfusion change in the frontal and parietal lobes in heroin addicts.
    (d) FDG-PET shows brain glucose hypometabolism in morphine intoxication.
13. Which statement about the cerebral effects of alcohol is false?
    (a) Global brain hypometabolism is observed in alcoholism.
    (b) Alcohol-associated hypometabolism is dominant in the right temporal and frontal regions.
    (c) The acute administration of alcohol decreases metabolism in the occipital and prefrontal lobes and in the cerebellum.
    (d) The acute administration of alcohol decreases the metabolism of regions with a high density of benzodiazepine receptors.
14. Which of the following statements about the cerebral effects of cocaine is NOT correct?
    (a) Basal ganglia receive the maximum cocaine uptake.
    (b) The acute administration of cocaine induces cortical and subcortical hypometabolism, which is associated with euphoria.
    (c) Cocaine mainly affects the right hemisphere.
    (d) Craving induces hypometabolism of the frontal lobe and basal ganglia in cocaine addicts.

7.12.1 Answer

	A	B	C	D
1		*		
2		*		
3				*
4		*		
5		*		
6			*	
7		*		
8		*		
9		*		
10			*	
11	*			
12				*
13		*		
14			*	

7.13 Management of Patients with Schizophrenia

1. The antipsychotic drug risperidone causes a decrease in metabolism in the:
   (a) Hippocampus
   (b) Insula
   (c) Cerebellum
   (d) Frontal lobe
2. Which of the following diseases is associated with increased density of dopamine receptors in the basal ganglia when evaluated with the dopamine receptor PET scan?
   (a) Parkinson's disease
   (b) Schizophrenia
   (c) Huntington's disease
   (d) Idiopathic focal dystonia
3. Muscarinic receptor scintigraphy is NOT useful in the evaluation of:
   (a) Schizophrenia
   (b) Alcoholism
   (c) Parkinson's disease
   (d) Alzheimer's disease
4. The reduced uptake of ^{99m}Tc-ECD in the … is expected on the brain perfusion scan of a patient with schizophrenia
   (a) Frontal lobe
   (b) Parietal lobe
   (c) Temporal lobe
   (d) Occipital lobe
5. A patient with a long-term history of schizophrenia is referred for a brain perfusion PET scan. A decrease in perfusion in the dorsolateral prefrontal cortex is observed on the scan. Which of the following syndromes is expected?
   (a) Psychomotor poverty syndrome
   (b) Disorganization syndrome
   (c) Reality distortion syndrome
   (d) Patients with predominantly positive symptoms
6. Which statement about dopamine receptor imaging is NOT correct?
   (a) The density of dopamine receptors in the caudate and putamen increases in some cases of schizophrenia
   (b) The most intense and persistent uptake on the scan is reported in the thalamus
   (c) The density of dopamine D2 receptors decreases with age
   (d) The density and affinity of these receptors can be quantitatively evaluated
7. Which of the following findings about CT, PET, or SPECT scan of patients with schizophrenia is NOT correct?
   (a) Significant increase in activity in the left putamen
   (b) Defect in global brain perfusion and metabolism
   (c) Decrease in glucose metabolism in the frontal lobe
   (d) Decrease in perfusion and metabolism in the left basal ganglia

8. The main system involved in schizophrenia is:
   (a) Cholinergic
   (b) Adrenergic
   (c) Opioidergic
   (d) Dopaminergic
9. Which of the following statements about PET findings on schizophrenia is NOT correct?
   (a) An increase in the activity of the basal ganglia, especially the left globus pal, is observed.
   (b) Dysfunction of the frontal lobe, especially on the left side, is reported.
   (c) The intensity of hypometabolism is related to the positive symptoms of schizophrenia.
   (d) Patients with positive symptoms of schizophrenia are usually younger, and hypofrontality is absent in these patients.
10. What is the pattern of the regional cerebral blood flow (RCBF) in patients with schizophrenia and disorganization syndrome?
   (a) Increased RCBF in the right anterior cingulate gyrus
   (b) Increased RCBF in the medial temporal lobe
   (c) Decreased RCBF in the dorsolateral prefrontal cortex
   (d) Decreased RCBF in the lateral temporal lobe

7.13.1 Answer

	A	B	C	D
1	*			
2		*		
3	*			
4	*			
5	*			
6		*		
7				*
8				*
9		*		
10	*			

7.14 PET and SPECT Imaging in Evaluating Alzheimer's Disease and Related Dementias

1. Hypometabolism and hypoperfusion affecting the cortical, subcortical, and cerebellar areas:
   (a) AD
   (b) Huntington's disease
   (c) Parkinson's dementia
   (d) Vascular dementia
2. Similar to AD but less sparing of the occipital cortex and possibly the cerebellum:
   (a) Huntington's disease
   (b) Parkinson's dementia
   (c) Lewy body dementia
   (d) Frontotemporal dementia
3. Similar to AD but more sparing of the mesiotemporal area and less sparing of the visual cortex:
   (a) Parkinson's dementia
   (b) Huntington's disease
   (c) Frontotemporal dementia
   (d) Vascular dementia
4. Caudate and lentiform nuclei are affected early, with a gradual development of the diffuse cortical involvement:
   (a) Parkinson's dementia
   (b) Huntington's disease
   (c) Vascular dementia
   (d) AD
5. In which of the following dementias is the occipital lobe less likely to be compromised?
   (a) Lewy body
   (b) Parkinsonism
   (c) Pick's disease
   (d) a and b
6. A cerebral perfusion scan is performed on a patient suspected to have Alzheimer's. A decreased perfusion is observed in the inferior parts of both temporal and parietal lobes along the medial and inferior surface of the cortex. These findings indicate the... stage of Alzheimer's.
   (a) Early
   (b) Intermediate
   (c) Late
   (d) Advanced
7. Bilateral parietal hypometabolism on a cerebral PET scan is the hallmark of which disease?
   (a) Alzheimer's disease
   (b) Parkinson's disease
   (c) Bilateral parietal subdural hematoma
   (d) Bilateral parietal stroke

8. What type of dementia is due to neurodegeneration?
   (a) Alzheimer's disease
   (b) Vascular dementia
   (c) Frontal lobe dementia
   (d) Lewy body dementia
9. A decreased uptake of ^{99m}Tc-HMPAO in the posterior parietofrontal and occipital lobes is found on the cerebral perfusion scan. What is the most probable diagnosis?
   (a) Alzheimer's dementia
   (b) Pick's disease
   (c) Lewy body disease
   (d) Vascular dementia
10. Which of the following diseases is associated with the bilateral decrease in metabolism in the frontal and anterior temporal lobes?
    (a) Pick's disease
    (b) Parkinson's disease
    (c) Huntington's disease
    (d) Wilson's disease
11. Dementia:
    (a) Pick's disease is the most common type of dementia
    (b) In Alzheimer's disease, the incidence of involvement of the right lobe is greater than that of the left lobe
    (c) The involvement of the frontotemporal lobe is observed in Pick's disease
    (d) Alzheimer's disease is the second most common form of dementia
12. About the evaluation of Alzheimer's disease by PET:
    (a) The temporal lobe shows the highest change in metabolism.
    (b) The extent of involvement of the lobes is high in severe Alzheimer's disease but NOT the intensity of hypometabolism.
    (c) Therapeutic monitoring is the most important application of PET in Alzheimer's disease.
    (d) Metabolism is usually not affected in the left midfrontal lobe.
13. CNS disorders are associated with changes in perfusion/metabolism. What are the significant changes on the brain scan of patients with Alzheimer's disease?
    (a) Decreased rCBF and rCMRO2 in white matter
    (b) Decreased metabolism and perfusion in the caudate and putamen nuclei
    (c) Increased glucose metabolism in the lenticular nucleus of the opposite side
    (d) Decreased whole brain metabolism, particularly in the temporal and parietal lobes
14. Brain SPECT shows reduced perfusion of the … in patients with diffuse Lewy body disease.
    (a) Temporal lobe
    (b) Parietal, frontal, visual cortex
    (c) Frontal lobe
    (d) Posterior cingulate gyrus

15. An 85-year-old man with symptoms of dementia is evaluated. Bilateral coronal shrinkage of the hippocampus is found in the MRI. rCBF SPECT reveals a bilateral reduced perfusion of the inferotemporal lobe with dominancy of the left side. What is the most probable diagnosis?
    (a) Pick's disease
    (b) Diffuse Lewy body disorder
    (c) Early Alzheimer's disease
    (d) Multi-infarct dementia
16. The appearance of the adrenal on a scan with ... is considered normal.
    (a) ^{11}C-HED
    (b) ^{11}C-epinephrine
    (c) ^{18}F-FDG
    (d) ^{131}I-MIBG
17. A mild decrease in perfusion is found in the parietal, temporal, and visual cortex of a 75-year-old man with dementia. What is the most probable diagnosis?
    (a) Vascular dementia
    (b) Minor cognitive dysfunction
    (c) Lewy body dementia
    (d) Pick's disease
18. What is the percentage of demented patients who will have mixed dementia, usually vascular dementia (VD) and AD?
    (a) 20–40%
    (b) 5–10%
    (c) 15–20%
    (d) 40–50%
19. Which of the following neuronal metabolite levels measured by magnetic resonance spectroscopy imaging (MRSI) has been shown to be elevated in Alzheimer's disease (AD) and may represent the earliest marker of the AD process?
    (a) Myoinositol
    (b) N-acetyl aspartate (NAA)
    (c) Choline-containing metabolites (Cho)
    (d) Creatine-containing metabolites (Cr)
20. Which brain region rarely shows hypoperfusion in Alzheimer's dementia?
    (a) Parietal cortex
    (b) Posterior temporal cortex
    (c) Sensorimotor cortex
    (d) Posterior cingulate cortex
21. What is the most common finding on Alzheimer's disease on a brain perfusion SPECT scan with ^{133}Xe?
    (a) Multifocal decreased perfusion in the cerebral cortex
    (b) Bilateral defects in the parietal or posterotemporal regions
    (c) Multiple defects in the frontal cortex
    (d) Unilateral defects in the parietal and posterotemporal cortex

22. What is the best brain SPECT view for the early diagnosis of Alzheimer's disease?
    (a) Coronal.
    (b) Transaxial.
    (c) Sagittal.
    (d) All of the abovementioned views are equally valuable.
23. A generalized decrease in metabolism and perfusion in the prefrontal cortex is observed on the brain PET and SPECT scans. What is the most probable diagnosis?
    (a) Dementia due to AIDS
    (b) Pick's disease
    (c) Wilson's disease
    (d) Huntington's disease
24. Decreased metabolism in the subcortical area rather than in the gray matter cortex is reported on the brain PET and SPECT scans. What is the most probable diagnosis?
    (a) Pick's disease
    (b) Wilson's disease
    (c) Dementia due to AIDS
    (d) Huntington's disease
25. In Binswanger's dementia:
    (a) CT scan shows a symmetric bilateral increase in white matter in the periventricular area.
    (b) PET scan shows changes in the perfusion and oxygen metabolism in white matter such as the cortex.
    (c) PET scan shows lower oxygen consumption in white matter than in Alzheimer's disease or vascular dementia.
    (d) Brain SPECT provides more information about white matter than gray matter.
26. Which of the following statements about the PET scan of patients with Alzheimer's disease is NOT correct?
    (a) Patients with NO white matter defect in the MRI do NOT show a metabolic defect in the temporal and parietal lobes.
    (b) Some studies indicate prioritizing the PET scan over MRI and CT scan for the diagnosis of Alzheimer's disease.
    (c) SPECT is NOT indicated for the differential diagnosis of Alzheimer's and multi-infarct dementia, although a relative decrease in temporo–cerebellar perfusion is beneficial.
    (d) Decreased perfusion in the prefrontal cortex is more evident in depression than in Alzheimer's disease.
27. FDG-PET shows decreased metabolism in progressed primary aphasia and Pick's disease. In which brain regions is this finding noticeable in the mentioned diseases, respectively?
    (a) Left temporal and parietal, bilateral frontal and anterotemporal
    (b) Bilateral parietal and temporal, bilateral frontal and posterotemporal
    (c) Left temporal and parietal, bilateral temporal and parietal
    (d) Left anteroparietal and posterotemporal, left temporal and parietal

28. What is the most sensitive method for the differential diagnosis of vascular dementia from other cerebral disorders?
    (a) PET
    (b) SPECT
    (c) MRI
    (d) Spiral CT
29. Which of the following findings is NOT observed on the SPECT-rCBF scan of Alzheimer's disease?
    (a) Hypoperfusion in the inferotemporal lobes
    (b) Hypoperfusion in the superior occipital lobe
    (c) Severe hypoperfusion in the superior temporal lobes
    (d) Hypoperfusion in the medial and superior parietal cortex
30. What is the common sign of Alzheimer's disease in the early stages?
    (a) Hypoperfusion in the posterior cingulate cortex
    (b) Hypoperfusion in the occipital lobe
    (c) Hypoperfusion in the sensory/motor
    (d) Hypoperfusion in the striatum
31. A brain perfusion SPECT scan is requested for a 79-year-old patient with suspected dementia. In addition to the decreased uptake in the parietal lobe and posterior cingulate, a decreased uptake is also observed in the visual cortex and the frontal lobe. The sensorimotor cortex and basal ganglia are normal. Which type of dementia is the most probable?
    (a) Early Alzheimer's disease
    (b) Multi-infarct dementia
    (c) Frontotemporal dementia
    (d) Lewy body dementia
32. Bilateral frontal hypoperfusion is reported on the brain perfusion SPECT scan of a 69-year-old man, who is referred with symptoms of amnesia and diagnosis of dementia. What is the most probable diagnosis?
    (a) Alzheimer's disease
    (b) Pick's disease
    (c) Multi-infarct dementia
    (d) AIDS-associated dementia
33. MR spectroscopy shows a decreased global NAA and an increased myoinositol level. What is the most likely diagnosis?
    (a) Hypoxic–ischemic encephalopathy
    (b) Alzheimer's disease
    (c) Multiple sclerosis
    (d) Canavan's disease

7.14.1 Answer

	A	B	C	D
1				*
2			*	
3	*			
4		*		
5			*	
6		*		
7	*			
8			*	
9			*	
10	*			
11			*	
12			*	
13				*
14		*		
15			*	
16				*
17			*	
18			*	
19			*	
20			*	
21		*		
22				*
23		*		
24			*	
25			*	
26	*			
27	*			
28	*			
29		*		
30	*			
31				*
32		*		
33		*		

7.15 Nuclear Medicine and Drug Studies on the Brain

1. What is the most common subtype of the dopamine receptor in the brain?
   (a) D1
   (b) D2
   (c) D3
   (d) D5
2. Which of the following effects is NOT induced by neuroleptic drug treatment?
   (a) Significant increase in metabolism in the left temporal lobe
   (b) Increase in metabolism of other cortical regions
   (c) Alteration of the anteroposterior gradient
   (d) Increased metabolism in the basal ganglia

7.15.1 Answer

	A	B	C	D
1	*			
2			*	

7.16 Cerebrospinal Fluid Physiology, Clearance Flow Studies, and Cerebrospinal Fluid Shunt Studies

1. Dilated ventricles may be filled with the radiotracer from reflux. However, the tracer clears normally or shows only mild delay in passage over the hemispheres by 24 h. Large subarachnoid spaces are usually found:
   (a) Obstructive hydrocephalus
   (b) Communicating (nonobstructive) hydrocephalus
   (c) Communicating hydrocephalus (ex vacuo)
   (d) Normal pressure hydrocephalus (NPH)
2. Which of the following is a normal CSF shunt tracer pattern?
   (a) No flow
   (b) No ventricular reflux
   (c) No peritoneal activity
   (d) Transit time of 42 min
3. In the evaluation of cerebral shunts:
   (a) ^{99m}Tc-DTPA (5 mCi) is administered
   (b) Transit time up to 1 h is normal
   (c) The absence of a ventricular reflux indicates a closed shunt
   (d) Observation of the kidneys indicates an open shunt
4. Radiotracer is injected into one of the ventricles on a cisternography scan. Subsequently, it is detected in other ventricles and basal cisterns, but its transmittance across the hemispheres is weak and dissymmetric. The radiotracer uptake is also weak, and some activity remains in the ventricles after 24 h. What is the diagnosis?
   (a) Hydrocephalus with normal pressure
   (b) Nonobstructive communicating hydrocephalus
   (c) Ex vacuo communicating hydrocephalus
   (d) Obstructive hydrocephalus
5. Which statement regarding the evaluation of cerebral shunts is NOT correct?
   (a) This assessment is less valuable in children than in adults.
   (b) Sensitivity and specificity of the scan are high in localizing obstruction.
   (c) The scan view is different between children and adults.
   (d) The cerebrospinal fluid has different views depending on the type of shunt.
6. For the diagnosis of CSF leakage on CSF scintigraphy:
   (a) CSF scintigraphy can accurately detect the location of CSF leakage.
   (b) The combination of scintigraphy and quantitative methods (counting of the activity of intranasal cotton) can be applied to detect all (100%) CSF fistulas.
   (c) Scintigraphy in the prone position is preferred to improve the accuracy of the scan.
   (d) Anterior and posterior cranial views are the best views for the diagnosis of these defects.

7. About CSF leakage:
   (a) Pyrogenic meningitis is the most troubling complication.
   (b) The spontaneous form begins in 1 week and finishes in 1 month.
   (c) Rhinorrhea is the only symptom of traumatic form.
   (d) It is NOT an adverse effect of rhinoplasty.
8. Which item indicates the proper function of a shunt in radionuclide cisternography?
   (a) Accumulation of activity in the beginning of the peritoneal shunt
   (b) Reflux to the ventricular system
   (c) Persistence of activity in the ventricles after several hours
   (d) Lack of appearance of the parotid glands after 30 min
9. In radionuclide cisternography for the evaluation of hydrocephalus:
   (a) 2, 12, and 24 h images must be prepared for children.
   (b) CSF flow in adults is faster than that in children.
   (c) ^{99m}Tc-DTPA is the radiopharmaceutical of choice.
   (d) Reflux of activity to the lateral ventricles indicates a proper injection.
10. What is the advantage of ^{111}In-DTPA over ^{99m}Tc-DTPA for the evaluation of CSF leakage?
    (a) Availability.
    (b) Lower radiation.
    (c) Higher resolution.
    (d) Possibility of the diagnosis of minor intermittent leakages.
11. Cisternography with a bolus injection of low-volume labeled DTPA in the sitting position is performed on a 15-year-old boy. The distribution of the radiopharmaceutical is slow in imaging. Which item affects the rate of radiopharmaceutical distribution?
    (a) Rate of injection
    (b) Age
    (c) Volume of injection
    (d) Position of the patient
12. Intra-reservoir injection of the radiopharmaceutical is performed to evaluate the patency of a ventriculoperitoneal shunt. Twenty-five hours later, the focal accumulation of the radiopharmaceutical is observed in the RUQ. Which statement is correct?
    (a) Accumulation is seen in the hydronephrotic kidney; therefore, a complete obstruction of the shunt is diagnosed.
    (b) Obstruction is NOT present, and the pattern of accumulation is a natural variance.
    (c) Obstruction is NOT present, but a CSF pseudocyst exists.
    (d) Relative obstruction and CSF pseudocyst are diagnosed.
13. Which of the following regions naturally appears in normal radionuclide cisternography?
    (a) Internal auditory canal
    (b) Internal ventricles
    (c) Nasal cavity
    (d) Sylvian fissures

14. A 48-year-old man with a history of head trauma presents gait ataxia, urinary incontinence, and memory loss. Dilatation of the brain ventricles is found on the CT scan. Cisternography reveals early entrance of the tracer into the ventricles and its appearance in the cortex of the hemispheres after 72 h. What is the most probable diagnosis?
    (a) Normal pattern of the tracer flow
    (b) Indeterminate communicating hydrocephalus
    (c) Non-communicating obstructive hydrocephalus
    (d) Normal pressure hydrocephalus
15. What is the most accurate method to define the anatomy and pathology of leptomeningeal metastases?
    (a) MRI
    (b) CT
    (c) Radionuclide CSF flow study
    (d) MRI + radionuclide CSF flow study
16. Which of the following situations does NOT cause non-communicating obstructive hydrocephalus?
    (a) Subarachnoid hemorrhage
    (b) Dandy–Walker cyst
    (c) Arnold–Chiari malformation
    (d) Aqueductal stenosis
17. What is the pharmaceutical of choice for CSF scintigraphy?
    (a) ^{131}I-HAS
    (b) ^{99m}Tc-DTPA
    (c) 169Yb-DTPA
    (d) ^{111}In-DTPA
18. Which statement about the diagnosis of CSF leakage by CSF scan is NOT correct?
    (a) The patient is recommended to remain in the supine position until the beginning of the scan
    (b) The incidence of false-negative results decreases with the Valsalva maneuver and the compression of the internal jugular vein
    (c) ^{99m}Tc-DTPA is preferred over ^{111}In-DTPA for the diagnosis of minor intermittent leakage
    (d) The scan is best conducted 1–3 h after intrathecal injection
19. Cisternography is performed on a patient. The radiotracer immediately enters the lateral ventricles and remains for 24–48 h, but it is NOT observed around the hemispheres. What is the best interpretation of this occurrence?
    (a) This patient may benefit from a ventriculoperitoneal shunt.
    (b) This finding is normal.
    (c) A ventriculoperitoneal shunt is NOT beneficial.
    (d) This patient definitely has hydrocephalus with normal pressure.

20. Radionuclide cisternography is NOT indicated for:
    (a) Evaluation of shunts
    (b) Evaluation of cerebrospinal fluid (CSF) leakage
    (c) Diagnosis of hydrocephalus and its typing
    (d) Evaluation of brain infarction
21. A peritoneovenous shunt is used in a patient with ascites, and radionuclide cisternography is requested. The lungs are clearly observed in the delayed images after the intraperitoneal injection of the radioisotope. What is the diagnosis?
    (a) Obstruction along the shunt.
    (b) Shunt valve malfunction.
    (c) Technical error in the radiotracer preparation.
    (d) The shunt is open and functional.
22. Which statement about the role of cisternography in patients with normal pressure hydrocephalus (NPH) is NOT correct?
    (a) Treatability of dementia is the main importance of diagnosis of this disease.
    (b) The scan can be normal in this disease.
    (c) Patients with classic findings on the scan may show a better response to the CSF shunt.
    (d) Cerebral hemispheres appear earlier than normal in these patients.
23. How long after the intrathecal injection of radiotracer does activity appear around the convexity of cerebral hemispheres in a normal cisternogram?
    (a) 4 h
    (b) 6 h
    (c) 24 h
    (d) 48 h
24. If the goal is to investigate the reasons for hydrocephalus, in which of the following situations does cisternography have the least efficacy for diagnosis?
    (a) Increased secretion due to choroid plexus papilloma
    (b) Obstruction due to intraventricular hemorrhage
    (c) Aqueductal stenosis
    (d) Normal pressure hydrocephalus
25. Which of the following methods is the most valuable for the diagnosis of hydrocephalus?
    (a) ^{111}In-DTPA imaging
    (b) CT and MRI.
    (c) Pneumoencephalography
    (d) Intracarotid sonography
26. Regarding normal pressure hydrocephalus:
    (a) Brain hyperperfusion is found in the periventricular area.
    (b) MRI is NOT necessary for ruling out situations that present clinical symptoms of hydrocephalus.
    (c) Reflux in cerebral ventricles is NOT a reliable marker for the prediction of successful shunting.
    (d) The diagnostic value of the CT scan with metrizamide contrast media is less than that of isotopic cisternography.

27. About the radionuclide study of CSF leakage:
    (a) Activity of more than 1.5-fold of the plasma is suggestive of CSF leakage.
    (b) First imaging must be performed 6–12 h after intrathecal injection.
    (c) ^{99m}Tc-DTPA is the radiotracer of choice.
    (d) Imaging must be performed in the supine position.
28. If a radiotracer is injected intrathecally (in the subarachnoid space of lumbar vertebrae), where can it normally be detected after 12 h?
    (a) Basal cistern
    (b) Frontal poles and Sylvian fissure
    (c) Cerebral convexities
    (d) Arachnoid villi in the sagittal sinus
29. Which bone fracture is the most common cause of CSF leakage?
    (a) Ethmoid
    (b) Temporal
    (c) Frontal
    (d) Parietal
30. Which of the following conditions causes high pressure of CSF leakage?
    (a) Congenital anomalies
    (b) Bone atrophy
    (c) Osteomyelitis
    (d) Tumors
31. Which of the following statements regarding the interval between trauma and CSF leakage is NOT correct?
    (a) CSF leakage occurs immediately or 48 h after trauma
    (b) CSF leakage may occur years after trauma
    (c) Rhinorrhea due to spontaneous CSF leakage usually improves spontaneously
    (d) About 50–70% of cases of rhinorrhea due to traumatic CSF leakage improve spontaneously in one week
32. Which of the following statements regarding the diagnostic tests for CSF leakage is NOT correct?
    (a) The negative findings of the glucose oxidase strip test are more valuable than the positive results.
    (b) Radionuclide cisternography is the primary and routine method for the localization of CSF leakage.
    (c) Radionuclide cisternography is the method of choice for the evaluation of vertebral leakage.
    (d) Radionuclide cisternography is NOT capable of localizing leakage.
33. Which of the following findings is absent in normal pressure hydrocephalus (NPH)?
    (a) Ataxia.
    (b) Dementia.
    (c) Colloid cyst.
    (d) Ventricular dilatation.

34. Regarding the role of radionuclide cisternography for the evaluation of shunts:
    (a) Radionuclide cisternography can determine which patients with normal pressure hydrocephalus (NPH) can benefit from ventriculoperitoneal shunting.
    (b) Radionuclide cisternography is the best prognostic method for ventriculo-peritoneal shunting in patients with NPH.
    (c) An open patent shunt indicates the proper functioning of the shunt.
    (d) The absence of the appearance of the parotid glands in shuntography with ^{99m}Tc after 10 min indicates distal obstruction.
35. Which of the following statements regarding the radionuclide assessment of normal pressure hydrocephalus (NPH) is false?
    (a) There is no activity in the subarachnoid space above the hemisphere.
    (b) Clinical manifestation has an important role in the scan pattern.
    (c) In the early stages, radionuclide is localized in the lateral ventricles.
    (d) The activity is seen longer than 24 h in the ventricles.

7.16.1 Answer

	A	B	C	D
1			*	
2				*
3			*	
4		*		
5	*			
6		*		
7	*			
8		*		
9	*			
10				*
11			*	
12				*
13				*
14				*
15	*			
16	*			
17				*
18			*	
19	*			
20				*
21				*
22				*
23			*	
24	*			
25		*		
26			*	

27	*			
28			*	
29	*			
30				*
31			*	
32		*		
33			*	
34	*			
35				*

7.17 Clinical PET-MRI in Neuropsychiatric Disorders

1. The most common neurodegenerative disease is Alzheimer's disease (AD), which accounts for approximately ...% of all patients with dementia:
   (a) 70%
   (b) 80%
   (c) 60%
   (d) 50%
2. An MRI clinical dementia protocol includes all of the following items *except*:
   (a) 3D T1-weighted magnetization-prepared rapid acquisition gradient-echo (T1-MPRAGE) sequence
   (b) T2-weighted fluid attenuation inversion recovery (FLAIR) sequence and T2-weighted BLADE or turbo spin-echo (TSE) sequence
   (c) Susceptibility-weighted imaging (SWI) sequence or gradient-echo T2-weighted sequence
   (d) Diffusion-weighted imaging (DWI)
3. Which of the following tracers is NOT categorized as an amyloid tracer?
   (a) [18F] florbetapir
   (b) [18F] flutemetamol
   (c) [18F] florbetaben
   (d) [11C] raclopride
4. All of the following statements regarding PET with amyloid tracers are true *except*:
   (a) Increased amyloid binding constitutes a risk factor, which may appear decades before the symptom onset.
   (b) A negative amyloid PET scan does not exclude neurodegeneration by other causes.
   (c) If an AD typical parietotemporal metabolic deficit cannot be explained by structural lesions, then it needs further examination by amyloid tracers.
   (d) Amyloid imaging is largely used as a supplementary examination when FDG-PET results are ambiguous.
5. Which of the following metabolite patterns on proton magnetic resonance spectroscopy (1H-MRS) indicates brain malignancy?
   (a) Increased ratio of choline–*N*-acetylaspartate
   (b) Increased ratio of choline–creatine
   (c) Increased creatine–*N*-acetylaspartate
   (d) a and b.
6. Regarding functional MRI (fMRI) and diffusion-tensor imaging (DTI) tractography:
   (a) May be used to identify the eloquent cortex (specifically motor and speech).
   (b) May be applied to distinguish white matter tracts.
   (c) Can be used to assess the safe margins of tumor resection.
   (d) All of the above are correct.

7.17.1 Answer

	A	B	C	D
1				*
2				*
3				*
4			*	
5				*
6				*

Suggested Readings

1. Ahmadzadehfar H, Biersack HJ, Freeman LM, Zuckier L. Clinical nuclear medicine. 2nd ed. Berlin: Springer; 2018.
2. Ell PJ, Gambhir SS. Nuclear medicine in clinical diagnosis and treatment. 3th ed. Edinburgh, NY: Churchill Livingstone; 2004.
3. Sandler MP, Coleman RE, Patton JA, Wackers FJT, Gottschalk A. Diagnostic nuclear medicine. 4th ed. Philadelphia: Lippincott & Williams Wilkins; 2003.
4. Henkin RE. Nuclear medicine. 2nd ed. Philadelphia: Mosby Elsevier; 2006.
5. Henriksen OM, Marner L, Law I. Clinical PET/MR imaging in dementia and neuro-oncology. PET Clin. 2016;11(4):441–52.

Nuclear Medicine in Renal Disorders

8

8.1 Overview of Renal Nuclear Medicine

1. Which renal disorder can be studied by nuclear medicine techniques?
   (a) Impotence
   (b) Mass lesion
   (c) Residual urine
   (d) All of the above
2. Renal scintigraphy is performed with ^{99m}Tc-DTPA and ^{99m}Tc-DMSA. The ^{99m}Tc-DTPA scan is unremarkable, but a poor uptake in the kidneys is reported on the ^{99m}Tc-DMSA scan. What is the most probable diagnosis?
   (a) Diabetic nephropathy
   (b) Chronic renal failure
   (c) Tubulointerstitial disease
   (d) Acute renal failure

8.1.1 Answer

	A	B	C	D
1				*
2			*	

M. Assadi et al., *Principles of Nuclear Medicine*,
https://doi.org/10.1007/978-3-319-91701-6_8

8.2 Radiopharmaceuticals: Their Intrarenal Handling and Localization

1. The maximum kidney radiation dose is from:
   (a) 51Cr-EDTA
   (b) ^{67}Ga
   (c) ^{99m}Tc-DMSA
   (d) ^{99m}Tc-glucoheptonate
2. What happens when the interval between the preparation of the ^{99m}Tc-DMSA kit and its administration is prolonged and the solution is exposed to air?
   (a) Increased filtration and elimination
   (b) Increased hepatic and decreased renal uptake
   (c) Appearance of the stomach
   (d) Increased uptake by renal medullary parenchyma
3. What characteristic is essential for a radiopharmaceutical to be used in GFR determination?
   (a) Neutral charge
   (b) Rapid distribution in the intra- and extracellular fluid
   (c) Protein binding of at least 50%
   (d) Conversion to active metabolites after administration
4. Which one is NOT considered a disadvantage of ^{99m}Tc-MAG3 over iodine-131 OIH?
   (a) Increased hepatobiliary excretion
   (b) Different renographies
   (c) Lower renal clearance
   (d) Protein binding
5. Which of the following radiopharmaceuticals provides low-quality images in patients with reduced renal function?
   (a) ^{123}I-OIH
   (b) ^{99m}Tc-MAG3
   (c) ^{99m}Tc-DTPA
   (d) ^{99m}Tc-EC
6. If the goal is to measure the GFR, a radiopharmaceutical must have all the following characteristics *except*:
   (a) Active filtration from glomeruli
   (b) No protein binding
   (c) No breakdown during filtration
   (d) No reabsorption
7. Hepatobiliary uptake is observed with:
   (a) ^{99m}TC-MAG3
   (b) ^{99m}TC-DMSA
   (c) ^{131}I-OIH
   (d) ^{99m}TC-DTPA

8. What is the main segment for ^{131}I-OIH and ^{99m}Tc-MAG3 secretion?
   (a) Proximal segments of the distal tubules
   (b) Distal segments of the proximal tubules
   (c) Proximal segments of the proximal tubules
   (d) Distal segments of the distal tubules
9. What is the major disadvantage of ^{99m}Tc-DTPA?
   (a) Metabolic changes after filtration
   (b) Weak reproducibility of the calculated GFR
   (c) Underestimated GFR
   (d) Tubular uptake
10. What is the radiotracer of choice for the measurement of effective renal plasma flow (ERPF)?
   (a) ^{131}I-OIH
   (b) ^{99m}Tc-MAG3
   (c) ^{99m}Tc-EC
   (d) ^{99m}Tc-HAG3
11. Which radiopharmaceutical is recommended for a more accurate assessment of GFR?
   (a) ^{99m}Tc-DTPA
   (b) ^{99m}Tc-MAG3
   (c) 51Cr-EDTA
   (d) ^{131}I-OIH
12. After preparing the ^{99m}Tc-DMSA kit, it is injected into a patient without completing the incubation time. What is the expected view?
   (a) Decreased renal uptake, appearance of the liver
   (b) Decreased renal uptake, appearance of bones
   (c) Increased urinary secretion of ^{99m}Tc-DMSA, appearance of bones
   (d) Increased urinary secretion of ^{99m}Tc-DMSA, appearance of the liver
13. What is the reason for the reduced uptake of ^{99m}Tc-DMSA in acute pyelonephritis?
   (a) Tubular necrosis
   (b) Ischemia
   (c) Fibrotic changes
   (d) Urodynamic changes
14. Which of the following radiopharmaceuticals can be used for static imaging of the renal cortex?
   (a) ^{99m}Tc-glucoheptonate
   (b) ^{99m}Tc-MAG3
   (c) ^{99m}Tc-DTPA
   (d) ^{99m}Tc-EC
15. Which characteristic is critical for a radiopharmaceutical to be used in the assessment of renal plasma flow?
   (a) It must be excreted only by glomerular filtration.
   (b) It must be excreted only by tubular secretion.
   (c) It must NOT be reabsorbed in the tubules.
   (d) It must have the maximum extraction ratio in the renal first pass.

16. Which of the following radiopharmaceuticals produces the maximum radiation to the kidneys per 1 mCi of injection?
    (a) ^{99m}Tc-DMSA
    (b) ^{99m}Tc-MAG3
    (c) ^{99m}Tc-DTPA
    (d) ^{99m}Tc-GH
17. Which of the following radiopharmaceuticals is uptaken in the target organ with active transport?
    (a) ^{99m}Tc-MAA
    (b) ^{99m}Tc-MDP
    (c) ^{99m}Tc-sulfur colloid
    (d) ^{99m}Tc-MAG3
18. Which of the following radiopharmaceuticals produces the most radiation to the kidneys?
    (a) ^{99m}Tc-DTPA
    (b) ^{131}I-OIH
    (c) ^{99m}Tc-GHA
    (d) ^{99m}Tc-MAG3
19. What is the radiopharmaceutical of choice for the evaluation of chronic pyelonephritis?
    (a) ^{131}I-OIH
    (b) ^{99m}Tc-GHA
    (c) ^{99m}Tc-DTPA
    (d) ^{67}Ga
20. In which of the following conditions is renal scintigraphy with ^{99m}Tc-DMSA NOT valuable?
    (a) Diagnosis of acute pyelonephritis
    (b) Differential diagnosis of a cyst from a kidney tumor
    (c) Diagnosis of renal infarction
    (d) Differential diagnosis of pseudotumors from factual tumors
21. What is the radiopharmaceutical of choice for the evaluation of kidney trauma?
    (a) ^{99m}Tc-DTPA
    (b) ^{131}I-OIH
    (c) ^{99m}Tc-GHA
    (d) ^{99m}Tc-DMSA
22. Which of the following radiotracers has the highest renal extraction fraction?
    (a) ^{125}I-OIH
    (b) ^{99m}Tc-MAG3
    (c) ^{99m}Tc-DMSA
    (d) ^{131}I-OIH
23. Which of the following radiopharmaceuticals is characterized by tubular secretion, high resolution, and the minimum level of kidney radiation?
    (a) ^{99m}Tc-GHA
    (b) ^{99m}Tc-DMSA
    (c) ^{99m}Tc-DTPA
    (d) ^{99m}Tc-MAG3

24. Which of the following is NOT an advantage of ^{99m}Tc-MAG3?
    (a) It is a Tc-labeled radiotracer for renal tubules.
    (b) It has a low protein-binding capacity.
    (c) Its renogram curve is similar to that of ^{131}I-OIH.
    (d) The renal images of ^{99m}Tc-MAG3 are better than those of ^{131}I-OIH.
25. Which of the following radiotracers is reabsorbed in the renal tubules?
    (a) TcO4
    (b) ^{99m}Tc-MAG3
    (c) ^{99m}Tc-DMSA
    (d) ^{99m}Tc-EC
26. Which of the following drugs or situations is the least probable to interfere with the ^{99m}Tc-DMSA uptake?
    (a) Probenecid
    (b) Renal tubular acidosis
    (c) Cisplatin toxicity
    (d) Mercury toxicity
27. The renal excretion of which radiotracer highly depends on the tubular extraction rate (TER)?
    (a) ^{99m}Tc-MAG3
    (b) ^{131}I-OIH
    (c) ^{99m}Tc-DTPA
    (d) ^{99m}Tc-DMSA
28. Although the assessment of renal perfusion requires angiography (the Fick principle), it can be measured with:
    (a) ^{131}I-hippuran
    (b) ^{99m}Tc-MAG3
    (c) ^{99m}Tc-EC
    (d) ^{51}Cr-EDTA
29. What is the main determining factor of ultrafiltration?
    (a) Size
    (b) Electric charge
    (c) Filtration pressure
    (d) Hydrostatic pressure
30. What are the recommended radiotracers for the evaluation of tubular secretion and filtration, respectively?
    (a) ^{131}I-hippuran, ^{51}Cr-EDTA
    (b) MAG3, EC
    (c) DTPA, ^{51}Cr-EDTA
    (d) DMSA, ^{131}I-hippuran
31. The cine-mode images of … can be used to evaluate ureteral contraction.
    (a) ^{99m}Tc-MAG3
    (b) ^{99m}Tc-DMSA
    (c) ^{99m}Tc-EDTA
    (d) ^{99m}Tc-EC

32. What are the radiotracers of choice for the measurement of renal plasma flow (RPF) and effective renal plasma flow (ERPF), respectively?
    (a) Para-aminohippurate (PAH), ortho-iodohippurate (OIH)
    (b) ^{51}Cr-EDTA, ^{99m} Tc-MAG3
    (c) ^{99m} Tc-MAG3, ortho-iodohippurate (OIH)
    (d) ^{51}Cr-EDTA, ^{131}I-hippuran
33. What is the gold standard for the measurement of GFR?
    (a) ^{51}Cr-EDTA
    (b) Inulin
    (c) Polyfructosan
    (d) b and c
34. What are the recommended radiotracers for the evaluation of renal collecting systems?
    (a) ^{51}Cr-EDTA, ^{99m} Tc-MAG3
    (b) ^{51}Cr-EDTA, ^{131}I-Hippuran
    (c) ^{99m} Tc-MAG3, ortho-iodohippurate (OIH)
    (d) ^{99m} Tc-EC, ^{99m} Tc-DTPA
35. If the goal is to evaluate the renal function in tumors or infections, ^{99m} Tc-DMSA and glucoheptonate are indicated for the study of:
    (a) Renal tubular acidosis
    (b) Gentamicin toxicity
    (c) Cisplatin toxicity
    (d) Distal tubular dysfunction
36. Which technetium complex produces the minimum radiation to the kidneys and gonads, respectively?
    (a) ^{99m}Tc-DMSA, ^{99m}Tc-MAG3
    (b) ^{99m}Tc-MAG3, ^{99m}Tc-DMSA
    (c) ^{99m}Tc-DMSA, ^{99m}Tc-GH
    (d) ^{99m}Tc-DTPA, ^{99m} c-MAG3
37. Which technetium complex produces the minimum radiation to the whole body and bladder, respectively?
    (a) ^{99m}Tc-DMSA, ^{99m}Tc-MAG3
    (b) ^{99m}Tc-MAG3, ^{99m}Tc-DMSA
    (c) ^{99m}Tc-DMSA, ^{99m}Tc-GH
    (d) ^{99m}Tc-DTPA, ^{99m}Tc-MAG3
38. About diethylene triamine pentaacetic acid (DTPA):
    (a) It overestimates GFR in comparison with inulin.
    (b) Protein binding of the radiotracer is about 20%.
    (c) It is filtrated from the glomeruli without tubular secretion or reabsorption.
    (d) It produces low-quality images in comparison with ^{99m}Tc-EC and ^{99m}Tc-MAG3.
39. All of the following statements about ^{51}Cr-EDTA are true *except*:
    (a) The protein binding of this radiotracer is greater than that of ^{99m}Tc-DTPA.
    (b) Imaging is problematic because of low photon flux.
    (c) It is stable and relatively pure, and it produces low radiation exposure to the body.
    (d) It is an ideal radiotracer for measuring GFR in both children and adults.

40. All of the following statements about ^{125}I-iothalamate are true *except*:
    (a) It is a glomerular reagent but has minor tubular secretion.
    (b) The protein binding of this radiotracer is greater than that of ^{99m}Tc-DTPA.
    (c) The impurities of this radiotracer are high.
    (d) It can help to estimate clearance.
41. All of the following statements about ^{131}I- or ^{123}I-hippuran are true *except*:
    (a) It can be used to measure ERPF.
    (b) Free iodine is the main impurity.
    (c) Hippuran may underestimate the value of ERPF.
    (d) It has high protein binding.
42. What is the recommended radiotracer for the measurement of ERPF?
    (a) Para-aminohippurate (PAH) clearance
    (b) ^{99m}Tc-MAG3
    (c) ^{131}I-OIH
    (d) ^{99m}Tc-EDTA
43. ^{99m}Tc-mercaptoacetyltriglycine (MAG3):
    (a) The purity of this radiotracer is high (95%), and air exposure before heating increases its purity.
    (b) ^{99m}Tc-MAG3 also has hepatic excretion.
    (c) It has a higher renal extraction rate than ^{131}I-OIH and PAH.
    (d) The protein binding of this radiotracer is high.
44. All of the following statements about ^{99m}Tc-DMSA are true *except*:
    (a) The lack of ^{99m}Tc-DMSA uptake indicates the absence of renal function.
    (b) Air exposure of the kit decreases the purity of the radiotracer.
    (c) The lower the urine pH is, the lower the renal uptake of ^{99m}Tc-DMSA.
    (d) An absent ^{99m}Tc-DMSA uptake in an obstructive uropathy dose necessarily indicates severe loss of function.
45. All of the following statements about ^{99m}Tc-GH are true *except*:
    (a) The quality of images with ^{99m}Tc-GH is better than that with ^{99m}Tc-DMSA.
    (b) Imaging 1–3 min after injection can be used to evaluate the relative renal function.
    (c) An acid–base imbalance does NOT affect the uptake of ^{99m}Tc-GH.
    (d) The simultaneous evaluation of the urinary system and the renal cortex is possible.
46. Which of the following radiotracers is described by low protein binding, short renal retention time, and plasma clearance equal to GFR because it has NO extrarenal clearance and is an ideal radiotracer for measuring GFR in children and adults?
    (a) ^{99m}Tc-GH
    (b) ^{51}Cr-EDTA
    (c) Iothalamate
    (d) ^{99m}Tc-DTPA
47. What is the most appropriate radiotracer for the calculation of functional renal mass?
    (a) ^{51}Cr-EDTA
    (b) ^{99m}Tc-GH
    (c) ^{99m}Tc-MAG3
    (d) ^{99m}Tc-DMSA

48. Which of the following radiotracers is characterized by 10% of protein binding, excretion dominantly from the glomeruli, and lack of tubular reabsorption or secretion?
    (a) ^{99m}Tc-MAG3
    (b) Iothalamate
    (c) ^{123}I-OIH
    (d) ^{99m}Tc-DTPA
49. Which of the following radiotracers is a glomerular radiologic contrast media labeled with ^{125}I?
    (a) Iothalamate
    (b) OIH
    (c) DTPA
    (d) Inulin
50. Which renal isotope has a maximum percentage protein binding in blood?
    (a) ^{99m}Tc-DTPA
    (b) ^{99m}Tc-EDTA
    (c) ^{99m}Tc-MAG3
    (d) ^{99m}Tc-DMSA
51. Which of the following radiotracers has a minimum protein binding and glomerular excretion, respectively?
    (a) ^{99m}Tc-DMSA, ^{99m}Tc-MAG3
    (b) ^{99m}Tc-MAG3, ^{99m}Tc-DTPA
    (c) ^{99m}Tc-DTPA, ^{99m}Tc-MAG3
    (d) ^{99m}Tc-DMSA, ^{99m}Tc-DTPA
52. Differential renal function with … indicates the function of proximal collecting tubules and loop of Henle.
    (a) ^{99m}Tc-MAG3
    (b) ^{99m}Tc-DTPA
    (c) ^{99m}Tc-DMSA
    (d) ^{99m}Tc-EC
53. What is the radiotracer of choice for indirect radionuclide cystogram?
    (a) ^{99m}Tc-MAG3
    (b) ^{99m}Tc-DTPA
    (c) ^{99m}Tc-DMSA
    (d) ^{99m}Tc-EC

8.2.1 Answer

	A	B	C	D
1			*	
2		*		
3	*			
4		*		
5			*	
6	*			

7	*			
8		*		
9			*	
10	*			
11				*
12		*		
13		*		
14	*			
15				*
16	*			
17				*
18			*	
19		*		
20		*		
21			*	
22				*
23				*
24		*		
25	*			
26	*			
27	*			
28	*			
29			*	
30	*			
31	*			
32	*			
33				*
34			*	
35				*
36			*	
37				*
38				*
39	*			
40			*	
41				*
42	*			
43			*	
44	*			
45	*			
46		*		
47				*
48				*
49	*			
50			*	
51			*	
52			*	
53	*			

8.3 Dynamic and Static Renal Imaging

1. Which radiopharmaceutical in renography has the least effective radiation dose (mSv/MBq)?
   (a) ^{99m}T-DTPA
   (b) ^{99m}Tc-MAG3
   (c) ^{123}I-OIH
   (d) ^{99m}Tc-EC
2. The F-15 protocol on a diuretic renal scan will:
   (a) Reduce false-positive cases
   (b) Reduce equivocal cases
   (c) Reduce the need for urinary catheter
   (d) All of the above
3. Which item causes false-negative findings on a diuretic renal scan?
   (a) High-grade hydrourolithiasis
   (b) Not too large renal pelvis with good kidney function
   (c) Hydronephrosis in one of the kidneys with 15% of normal function and a healthy kidney on the other side
   (d) Unilateral hydronephrosis in a 2-week-old newborn with a urinary catheter
4. Which renal dysfunction is presented in the following DPTA renogram?

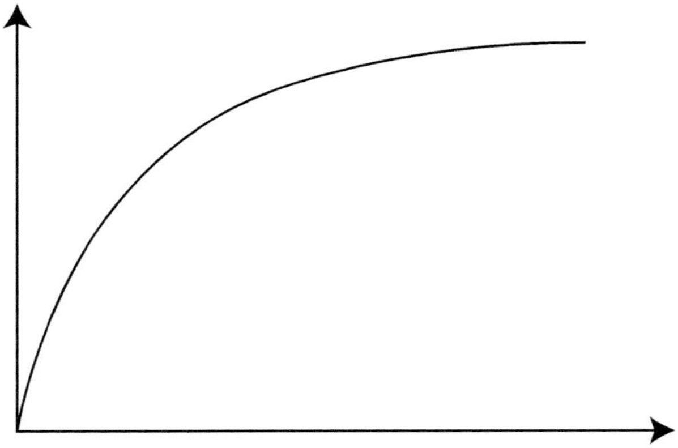

   (a) Glomerulopathy
   (b) Involvement of interstitial tissue
   (c) Decreased pressure gradient between the glomerulus and Bowman's capsule
   (d) All of the above
5. The ^{99m}Tc-DTPA scan shows the kidneys, primary blood pools, and gradual elimination. The OIH scan reveals a gradual accumulation of the radiotracer in the renal parenchyma. What is the best diagnosis?
   (a) Prolonged urinary obstruction
   (b) Aminoglycoside-induced nephrotoxicity
   (c) Tubular acidosis
   (d) Nephropathic diabetes

6. What is the primary process in radiation nephritis?
   (a) Nephrosclerosis
   (b) Nephritis
   (c) Necrosis
   (d) Vascular shunt
7. The early appearance of the inferior vena cava on a renal perfusion scan indicates all of the following conditions *except*:
   (a) Injection in the femoral vein
   (b) Intrarenal arteriovenous fistula
   (c) Extrarenal arteriovenous fistula
   (d) A rare but natural phenomenon
8. Which of the following statements about the effects of angiography and angioplasty with nonionic contrast media on renal scintigraphy is true?
   (a) This study alters the renal blood circulation.
   (b) Renal scintigraphy should be postponed for 2 months after such studies.
   (c) This contrast media agent has no effect on any type of renal scan.
   (d) Renal scintigraphy should be postponed for 1–2 weeks after such studies.
9. What is the primary effect of dehydration on the renogram?
   (a) Elongation of all three phases
   (b) Rapid phase one, elongation of phase two
   (c) Rapid phase three, elongation of phases one and two
   (d) Elongation of phases two and three
10. Which parameters are affected by the hydration of the patient on renal scintigraphy with ^{99m}Tc-MAG3?
   (a) Flow phase, initial cortical uptake, excretory phase
   (b) Flow phase, initial cortical uptake, relative renal function
   (c) Flow phase, excretory phase, relative renal function
   (d) Initial cortical uptake, excretory phase, relative renal function
11. Which parameter is critical for the assessment of the relative renal function with a dynamic renal scan?
   (a) Patient's distance from the apparatus
   (b) Labeling efficiency
   (c) Sensitivity
   (d) Uniformity of the detector
12. Only one kidney with a normal size, morphology, and cortex is reported in the sonography of a 30-year-old man. Therefore, he is referred for dynamic renal scintigraphy. What is the recommended position for the scan?
   (a) Imaging in the prone position
   (b) Simultaneous anterior and posterior imaging
   (c) Posterior imaging of the pelvis
   (d) Imaging in the sitting position

13. A 6-year-old child with viral gastroenteritis and diarrhea from yesterday is referred for a dynamic renal scan with ^{99m}Tc-MAG3. The urine tests on the same day of the scan before scintigraphy are as follows: WBC, 0–1; RBC, 1–2; and specific gravity, 1.028. Which of the following scan findings is the least reliable?
    (a) Renal perfusion phase
    (b) Renal exertion phase
    (c) Differential renal function
    (d) A dynamic renal scan is NOT possible because of the underlying disease
14. Kidney transplantation from a 32-year-old subject with brain death is performed on an 18-year-old patient with chronic renal failure. Twenty-four hours later, renal scintigraphy with ^{99m}Tc-MAG3 is requested because of low urinary excretion. The uptake is weak and slow, and it reaches its maximum at the end of the study (30th min). Nevertheless, the images show adequate perfusion of the transplanted kidney. What is the most probable diagnosis?
    (a) ATN
    (b) Cyclosporine toxicity
    (c) Acute rejection
    (d) Urinary tract obstruction
15. A 17-day-old neonate with suspected prenatal stenosis of the UPJ is referred for renal ^{99m}Tc-DTPA scan. Which statement according to the well-tempered renography and age is correct?
    (a) Age is NOT important.
    (b) The scan is best postponed for 2 weeks.
    (c) The scan is possible with adequate hydration.
    (d) The scan is possible with the administration of diuretic.
16. What is the best method for the differentiation of horseshoe from pseudo-horseshoe kidneys on ^{99m}Tc-DMSA renal scintigraphy?
    (a) Acquisition of anterior view after emptying of the bladder
    (b) Repeat of scan with ^{99m}Tc-DTPA
    (c) Acquisition of oblique view with magnification
    (d) Shielding of the bladder and repeat of scan in the posterior view
17. A 3 cm × 2 cm mass in the lateral margin of the left kidney is detected in the sonography of a 29-year-old man with pain in the left flank. Moreover, a regional increase in uptake is observed in this area on the ^{99m}Tc-DMSA scan. What is the most probable diagnosis?
    (a) Hamartoma
    (b) Acute pyelonephritis
    (c) Bertin's column hypertrophy
    (d) Pelvis cyst
18. If the F-15 protocol is used instead of the F-20 protocol in diuretic renogram, what happens to the initial uptake and differential renal function, respectively?
    (a) No change, decrease
    (b) Increase, no change
    (c) Increase, increase
    (d) Decrease, no change

19. What is the best imaging method for evaluating a patient with blunt trauma of the abdomen?
    (a) Abdominal sonography
    (b) Hepatobiliary scintigraphy
    (c) Abdominal CT scan
    (d) Renal scintigraphy with ^{99m}Tc-GHA
20. A renal lesion with absent perfusion and function indicates all of the following diseases *except*:
    (a) Lymphoma
    (b) Calyx diverticulum
    (c) Hamartoma
    (d) Hematoma
21. Which of the following diagnostic methods produces the most comprehensive data for renal evaluation?
    (a) IVP
    (b) Ultrasonography
    (c) CT scan
    (d) Radionuclide scintigraphy
22. All of the following statements about renogram are correct *except*:
    (a) The first phase in the first minute indicates perfusion and renal entrance of 10% of the administered radiotracer.
    (b) Nephrotoxic drugs that cause ATN can induce the retention of tubular radiotracers.
    (c) Delayed secretion in renogram is observed in patients under treatment with cyclosporine and aminoglycosides even in asymptomatic patients.
    (d) The difference in kidney depth is more dominant in the supine position than in the sitting position.
23. Which renogram index represents clearance and is associated with serum creatinine?
    (a) Time to maximum counts (Tmax)
    (b) Time to half-peak counts (T½)
    (c) Percentage fall at 20 min
    (d) 20 min to peak activity ratio
24. What percentages of ^{99m}Tc-DMSA and ^{99m}Tc-GH are fixed in the cortex after injection, respectively?
    (a) 20% and 10–15%
    (b) 40% and 10–15%
    (c) 10–15% and 20%
    (d) 10–15% and 40%
25. Which of the following findings on the ^{99m}Tc-DMSA scan of children below 2 years old is considered a normal one?
    (a) Nonhomogenous uptake in the internal kidney
    (b) Hypoactivity of kidney bridges
    (c) Nonhomogenous uptake in the lateral kidney
    (d) Abnormal borders

26. The size of the kidney reaches its maximum:
    (a) At age 1
    (b) At age 6
    (c) At age 10
    (d) At age 12
27. Which of the following methods overestimates the size of kidneys?
    (a) Renal scintigraphy
    (b) CT scan
    (c) Sonography
    (d) IVP
28. False-positive outcomes of ^{99m}Tc-DMSA SPECT include all of the following items *except*:
    (a) Bertin's column
    (b) Intrarenal septum
    (c) Hypoactivity of the upper bridge
    (d) Hypoactivity of the lower bridge
29. The ratio of d/c is related to which of the following parameters in a typical renogram curve?

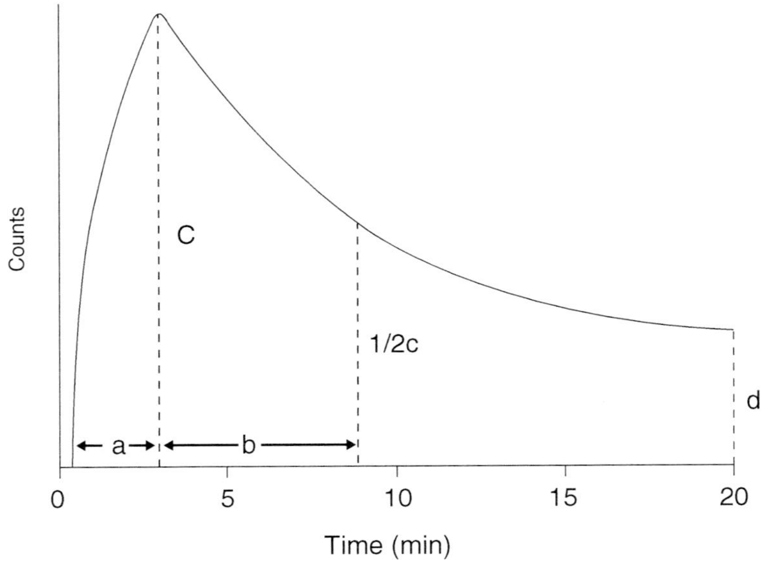

    (a) Time to peak
    (b) Residual cortical activity
    (c) Mean transit time
    (d) Time to half-peak

8.3.1 Answer

	A	B	C	D
1			*	
2		*		
3		*		
4			*	
5		*		
6	*			
7				*
8				*
9				*
10	*			
11				*
12		*		
13		*		
14	*			
15		*		
16			*	
17			*	
18		*		
19			*	
20			*	
21	*			
22				*
23		*		
24		*		
25	*			
26				*
27				*
28				*
29		*		

8.4 Quantitative Evaluation of Clearance

1. The standard deviation of the measurement of clearance by a gamma camera is approximately:
   (a) 10%
   (b) 20%
   (c) 30%
   (d) 5%
2. After correcting the physical decay of the radionuclide used, the clearance (Cl) can then be calculated as follows:
   where N is the average number of motor steps per minute (min^{-1}), D is the administered activity dose per motor step (cps), and c is the plasma concentration of the clearance agent (cps/ml).
   (a) (N × D)/c
   (b) (N × c)/D
   (c) (c × D)/N
   (d) (D − c)/N
3. The standard deviation of the gamma camera clearance measurement results is approximately:
   (a) 5%
   (b) 10%
   (c) 15%
   (d) 20%
4. Which of the following renal diseases presents a greater reduction of ERPF in comparison with GFR?
   (a) Rejection of transplanted kidney
   (b) ATN
   (c) Renal artery stenosis
   (d) Glomerulonephritis
5. Which of the following should be performed when the goal is to assess GFR with a gamma camera?
   (a) Fowler's position for better urinary drainage
   (b) Imaging up to 6 min
   (c) Administration of at least 10 mCi of ^{99m}Tc-DTPA
   (d) Administration of a low-dose diuretic before the injection of ^{99m}Tc-DTPA
6. Compare the extraction fraction (EF) between ^{99m}Tc-MAG3 and ^{99m}Tc-DTPA.
   (a) They are approximately equal.
   (b) The EF of ^{99m}Tc-DTPA is higher.
   (c) The EF of ^{99m}Tc-MAG3 is higher.
   (d) EF depends on the administered dose.
7. What is the radionuclide method of choice for the evaluation of chemotherapy-induced nephrotoxicity in children?
   (a) GFR
   (b) ERPF
   (c) First-pass evaluation and determination of T1/2
   (d) Evaluation of renal cortex and calculation of relative renal function

8. When is the appropriate time for measuring GFR on a ^{99m}Tc-DTPA dynamic renal scan?
   (a) Perfusion phase
   (b) Exactly before the excretion phase
   (c) Concurrent with the stabilization of the pyelocaliceal system
   (d) Rapid excretion phase after furosemide injection
9. A 58-year-old woman with chronic headache has taken NSAIDs (ibuprofen and aspirin) for several years. Inulin clearance is performed with a suspected decreased renal function. During the slow intravenous injection of inulin, the patient has urine excretion of 360 cc in 1 h. If the average inulin concentration in serum and urine is 1 mg/ml and 10 mg/ml, respectively, what is the inulin clearance (GFR)?
   (a) 45 ml/min
   (b) 90 ml/min
   (c) 60 ml/min
   (d) 30 ml/min
10. In which renal disease does the filtration fraction (GFR/ERFP ratio) increase despite the decreased GFR?
    (a) Renal artery stenosis
    (b) Acute renal transplant rejection
    (c) Contrast- induced nephropathy
    (d) Renal obstruction
11. Which item about the advantages and disadvantages of GFR calculation with Gate's method is true?
    (a) Possibility of measuring differentiated GFR
    (b) Longer imaging process
    (c) The requirement of blood sample
    (d) The requirement of urine sample
12. Which statement about GFR is NOT correct?
    (a) CT scan can be applied to measure GFR.
    (b) Measuring GFR with MRI is NOT possible.
    (c) Depth correction is performed through the gamma camera method.
    (d) About 1.5 mCi of ^{99m}Tc-DTPA is sufficient for the gamma camera method.
13. The obtained value of GFR with ^{99m}Tc-DTPA is 5% less than its actual value. What is the reason for this finding?
    (a) Binding of 5% of ^{99m}Tc-DTPA to tubular epithelial cells.
    (b) About 5% of the radiopharmaceutical remains at the injection site.
    (c) Binding of 5% of ^{99m}Tc-DTPA to plasma proteins.
    (d) About 5% of the radiopharmaceutical remains in the syringe.
14. Which property of ^{99m}Tc-DTPA is NOT appropriate for measuring GFR?
    (a) Tubular secretion
    (b) Tubular reabsorption
    (c) Plasma protein binding
    (d) Renal metabolism

15. Which formula is appropriate for renal filtration fraction?
    (a) ERPF/GFR
    (b) GFR/ERPF
    (c) (GFR + ERPF)/2
    (d) (ERPF − GFR)/2
16. All of the following available techniques for plasma and/or urinary clearance determination are based on the during slope principle *except*:
    (a) Feedback-controlled infusion
    (b) Multiple blood sampling
    (c) Single-sample method
    (d) External counting methods
17. Which of the following statements about the radiotracers used in measuring effective renal plasma flow is NOT correct?
    (a) Dissociation from plasma protein is required for renal transport
    (b) Renal metabolism is required
    (c) High renal extraction fraction is required
    (d) Urinary and plasma detection preferably with radioassay
18. A 57-year-old man is referred with increased BUN and creatinine as well as proteinuria 2 days after contrast myelography. Which radioisotopic quantitative parameter can help to evaluate accurately the suspected contrast-induced nephropathy?
    (a) GFR
    (b) ERPF
    (c) Filtration fraction
    (d) 20 min/peak activity ratio
19. What is the gold standard for the quantitative evaluation of renal clearance?
    (a) Multiple blood sampling
    (b) Single blood method
    (c) External counting method
    (d) Feedback-controlled infusion
20. Which of the following methods can be used for measuring GFR, ERPF, and renal clearance?
    (a) Two-compartment model
    (b) Stewart–Hamilton principle
    (c) Single-compartment model
    (d) Feedback-controlled infusion
21. If the goal is to assess the GFR and the tubular function or ERPF by the two-compartment model, at least …and … samples are required, respectively.
    (a) 3 h, 2 h
    (b) 2 h, 2 h
    (c) 3 h, 1 h
    (d) 2 h, 2 h

22. What samples are required to measure the GFR by the single-compartment (slope/intercept) model? Is this model suitable for research applications?
    (a) 2–3 h sample, yes
    (b) 3–4 h, yes
    (c) 2–3 h, no
    (d) 3–4 h, no
23. Which model is similar to the Steward–Hamilton principle (which uses the dilution technique) and when is the proper time for sampling if the goal is to measure the GFR?
    (a) Two-compartment model, 3–4 h for glomerular and 1–2 h for tubular agents
    (b) Two-compartment model, 1–2 h for glomerular and 3–4 h for tubular agents
    (c) One-compartment model, 3–4 h for glomerular and 1–2 h for tubular agents
    (d) One-compartment model, 3–4 h for glomerular and 1–2 h for tubular agents
24. Which of the following parameters can be measured with the single-sample method?
    (a) TER
    (b) ERPF
    (c) Clearance
    (d) All of the above
25. If the goal is to determine the GFR and tubular function by the single-sample method, … and … samples are required, respectively; and tubular function is … in patients with low plasma oncotic pressure and a large extracellular space.
    (a) 2–3 h, 20–50 min; overestimated
    (b) 2–3 h, 20–50 min; underestimated
    (c) 1–2 h, 2–4 h; overestimated
    (d) 1–2 h, 2–4 h; underestimated
26. The urinary tract (kidneys, bladder, and ureter) must be shielded in the external counting method. When is the proper time of sampling, and what is the correct formula for calculating the clearance?
    (a) 10–20 min, Stewart–Hamilton principle
    (b) 2–3 min, Stewart–Hamilton principle
    (c) 20–50 min, gate formula
    (d) 2–3 min, gate formula
27. What are the normal values for blood and renal transit times, respectively?
    (a) 5–10 s, 3–5 min
    (b) 5–10 s, 5–7 min
    (c) 10–15 s, 5–7 min
    (d) 1–15 s, 3–5 min
28. Which of the following radiotracers does NOT change the transit time on the renal scan of patients with renovascular hypertension (RVH)?
    (a) ^{99m}Tc-MAG3
    (b) ^{99m}Tc-DTPA
    (c) ^{123}I-OIH
    (d) ^{99m}Tc-DMSA

8.4.1 Answer

	A	B	C	D
1		*		
2	*			
3				*
4		*		
5		*		
6			*	
7	*			
8		*		
9			*	
10			*	
11	*			
12		*		
13			*	
14			*	
15		*		
16	*			
17		*		
18			*	
19				*
20				*
21			*	
22				*
23	*			
24				*
25	*			
26	*			
27	*			
28				*

8.5 Measurement and Interpretation of Renal Transit Times

1. All of the following deconvolution analysis methods are used for measuring the renal transit time *except*:
   (a) Iterative approach
   (b) Laplace transform
   (c) Fourier transform
   (d) Stewart–Hamilton principle
2. Which item has the least effect on the prolongation of renovascular transit time?
   (a) Primary stages of ATN
   (b) Decreased cardiac output
   (c) Age
   (d) Renal artery stenosis in the transplanted kidney
3. In which of the following conditions can creatinine clearance overestimate the GFR calculation?
   (a) Hypertension
   (b) Transplanted kidney
   (c) ATN
   (d) Chronic renal diseases
4. The goal is to assess the relative renal function in healthy kidneys. How long is the interval between the injection of the tracer and imaging for ROI selection?
   (a) ^{99m}Tc-GHA: 15–20 min
   (b) ^{99m} Tc-MAG3: 30–60 min
   (c) ^{99m} Tc-DTPA: 5–10 min
   (d) ^{99m} c-DMSA: 2–3 h
5. What is the sign of chronic glomerulonephritis on renal scintigraphy?
   (a) Symmetrical enlargement of the kidneys without photopenic defect and scar
   (b) Normal perfusion and ERPF
   (c) Elongation of the ^{123}I-OIH transit
   (d) Increased renal uptake of the labeled leucocyte despite the normal gallium uptake
6. Renal transit time is valuable in all of the following conditions *except*:
   (a) Renal artery stenosis
   (b) Ureter obstruction
   (c) Renal infection
   (d) Acute rejection of the renal graft

8.5.1 Answer

	A	B	C	D
1				*
2	*			
3				*
4				*
5			*	
6			*	

8.6 Role of PET in Renal Nuclear Medicine

1. PET is particularly useful in measuring:
   (a) GFR
   (b) Renal blood flow
   (c) Angiotensin–receptor imaging
   (d) Functional cortical mass
2. This radiotracer is used for measuring GFR with PET:
   (a) ^{64}Cu
   (b) ^{68}Ga
   (c) ^{15}C-RBC
   (d) ^{18}F-fluorocaptopril

8.6.1 Answer

	A	B	C	D
1		*		
2		*		

8.7 Renal Infection

1. Variance of results in subsequent cystograms is observed in up to:
   (a) 10%
   (b) 20%
   (c) 5%
   (d) 1%
2. Which of the following statements regarding reproducibility in reporting ^{99m}Tc-DMSA is NOT true?
   (a) Reproducibility in the reporting of ^{99m}Tc-DMSA is excellent.
   (b) The addition of SPECT imaging increases the risk of false-positive images.
   (c) The addition of SPECT imaging increases the risk of the interobserver variability.
   (d) The ^{99m} Tc-DMSA reporting of only the normality or abnormality of kidneys is more reproducible.
3. What is the primary cause of a decreased ^{99m}Tc-DMSA uptake by the renal cortex in acute pyelonephritis?
   (a) Bacterial toxin and increased regional pH
   (b) Superoxide production by neutrophils and tubular injury
   (c) Interstitial tissue edema
   (d) Localized edema and tubular dysfunction
4. The DSMA scan is performed on an 8-year-old girl with a history of fever and urinary infection. Reduced activity is observed in the upper pole of the kidney in the posterior view, but the cortical uptake is normal in the LPO view. What is the most probable diagnosis?
   (a) Hypertrophied column of Bertin
   (b) Improving pyelonephritis
   (c) Extension of the superior calyx of the left kidney
   (d) Suppressive effect of the spleen on the left kidney
5. Which of the following about renal scintigraphy with ^{99m}Tc-DMSA is NOT correct?
   (a) It has higher sensitivity than IVP for the detection of renal scar in children.
   (b) Radiation of patients with ^{99m}Tc- DMSA is lower than that with IVP.
   (c) If pyelonephritis remains untreated, renal failure is a possibility.
   (d) Proper and on-time diagnosis and treatment of pyelonephritis do NOT play a role in the prevention of a renal scar.
6. What is the main reason for the reduced cortical ^{99m}Tc-DMSA uptake in acute pyelonephritis?
   (a) Bacterial toxin and increased regional pH
   (b) Superoxide production in neutrophils and tubular destruction
   (c) Interstitial tissue edema
   (d) Regional ischemia and tubular dysfunction

7. About ^{99m}Tc-DMSA scan in patients with VU reflux and pyeloplastic surgery:
   (a) The scan is NOT indicated for this condition.
   (b) Patients with a normal scan benefit the most from surgery.
   (c) Patients with an abnormal scan benefit the most from surgery.
   (d) Both normal and abnormal scans benefit equally from surgery.
8. Which of the following findings on ^{99m}Tc-DMSA renal scintigraphy is indicative of chronic pyelonephritis?
   (a) Uptake defect in the upper and lower renal poles
   (b) Multiple regions of reduced uptake with different degrees in the whole kidney
   (c) Diffusely reduced uptake and enlargement
   (d) Reduced uptake and size
9. Which of the following findings is NOT observed on the ^{99m}Tc-DMSA scan of a patient with acute pyelonephritis?
   (a) A region with decreased activity
   (b) Multiple regions with decreased activity
   (c) Diffused reduction of activity
   (d) Decreased size of the kidney
10. Which of the following views on a ^{99m}Tc-DMSA scan indicates acute pyelonephritis with low probability?
    (a) Focal cortical defect
    (b) Irregular kidney borders
    (c) Multiple cortical defects
    (d) Unilateral diffused reduction of activity
11. If the goal is to follow up on acute pyelonephritis, what is the minimum interval for ^{99m}Tc-DMSA scintigraphy after the initiation of treatment?
    (a) 4 weeks
    (b) 6 weeks
    (c) 8 weeks
    (d) 12 weeks
12. Which of the following findings is indicative of acute pyelonephritis on ^{99m}Tc-DMSA scintigraphy?
    (a) Reduced uptake in the left upper pole in the posterior view with a flat shape in the LPO view
    (b) Indentation of the counter kidney between medullary pyramids
    (c) Reduced focal uptake on both sides of the transverse band of the increased uptake in a kidney with a duplex collecting system
    (d) Reduced focal uptake in the upper and lower poles without change in size or deformity
13. About acute renal infection:
    (a) Acute pyelonephritis is usually associated with cystoureteral reflux.
    (b) Scar formation after acute pyelonephritis is independent of reflux.
    (c) Evaluation of the kidney parenchyma with a ^{99m}Tc-DMSA scan is limited to cases with ureteral reflux.
    (d) Diffuse reduction of uptake in an enlarged kidney is the most common view of a ^{99m}Tc-DMSA scan in acute pyelonephritis.

14. A reduction in size of both kidneys is observed on ^{99m}Tc-DMSA scintigraphy in all of the following diseases *except*:
    (a) Glomerulonephritis
    (b) Diabetic nephropathy
    (c) Polycystic kidney
    (d) Polyarteritis nodosa (PAN)

8.7.1 Answer

	A	B	C	D
1		*		
2			*	
3				*
4				*
5				*
6				*
7			*	
8				*
9				*
10		*		
11				*
12				*
13		*		
14			*	

8.8 Pediatric Nephro-urology

1. What are the most appropriate dose and time of diuretic administration on the renal scintigraphy of children, respectively?
   (a) 0.5 mg/kg on the 5th min
   (b) 1 mg/kg on the 20th min
   (c) 2 mg/kg on the 30th min
   (d) 3 mg/kg on the 20th min
2. Which item is considered the key point of radionuclide study in children?
   (a) Selection of a radiotracer with low activity
   (b) Acquisition of high-quality images with the lowest radiation for the patients
   (c) Precise preparation of the radiotracer
   (d) Appropriate method for radiotracer administration
3. Which statement about pyelonephritis in infants is NOT correct?
   (a) Clinical and laboratory examinations are not reliable for the diagnosis of pyelonephritis and lower UTI.
   (b) Acute pyelonephritis usually occurs without VU reflux.
   (c) The formation of scar tissue in kidneys does NOT depend on reflux.
   (d) Evaluation of the renal cortex is only recommended when reflux exists.
4. What is the advantage of indirect radionuclide cystography?
   (a) It is preferred over the direct method for neuropathic bladder in children.
   (b) The radiation dose is less than that of the direct method.
   (c) The possibility of the simultaneous evaluation of renal morphology and function.
   (d) It is more sensitive than the direct method in neonates.
5. The following are the advantages of direct radionuclide cystography *except*:
   (a) Its average exposure of gonads to radiation is much less than that of VCUG radiology.
   (b) It is more sensitive than VCUG radiology for the diagnosis of intermittent refluxes.
   (c) It is more efficient than VCUG in evaluating the urethra.
   (d) The total sensitivity of this method is higher than that of VCUG.
6. Renal cortex scintigraphy with ^{99m}Tc-DMSA is requested for a 9-year-old child with a history of urinary infection. Serum creatinine and dynamic renal scan with ^{99m}Tc-EC are normal. ^{99m}Tc-DMSA cortical scan shows a significantly reduced uptake in both kidneys along with increased liver uptake. Therefore, a repeat of the scan is recommended to differentiate between proximal tubular dysfunction and technical errors. What factors should be noted in the repeat test?
   (a) Injection less than 2 h after the preparation of tracer
   (b) Utilization of ^{99m}Tc-DMSA kit for every two patients and immediate injection after the addition of ^{99m}Tc
   (c) Preparation of the tracer for each patient separately if the kit is used for several subjects
   (d) Administration of at least 10 mCi of ^{99m}Tc-DMSA for each patient

7. What is the minimum age limit for the ^{99m}Tc-DMSA scan in the diagnosis of renal scar?
   (a) 4 weeks
   (b) 8 weeks
   (c) 12 weeks
   (d) 16 weeks
8. Indirect radionuclide cystourethrography is requested for a 7-year-old child. What is the most suitable radiopharmaceutical for the detection of vesicoureteral reflux?
   (a) ^{99m}Tc-DTPA
   (b) ^{99m}Tc- MAG3
   (c) ^{99m}Tc-DMSA
   (d) ^{99m}Tc-sulfur colloid
9. Cortical defect is found on the renal scintigraphy with ^{99m}Tc-DMSA of a 2.4-year-old boy suspected of having kidney infection. What is the next diagnostic step?
   (a) Direct radionuclide cystography (DRC)
   (b) Micturating cystourethrography (MCU) with X-ray
   (c) Indirect radionuclide cystography (IRC)
   (d) Intravenous pyelography (IVP)
10. A 5-year-old girl with dysuria, pain in the lower abdomen, and fever of 39°°C is presented. WBC of 10–15, RBC of 3–4, and several bacteria are reported in the urine test. What is the recommended method for localizing the infection?
   (a) Direct radionuclide cystography
   (b) Indirect radionuclide cystography
   (c) Scan with ^{99m}Tc-MAG3
   (d) Scan with ^{99m}Tc-DMSA
11. In which of the following patients is indirect radionuclide cystography recommended?
   (a) A 7-month-old infant with first urinary infection
   (b) A 1.5-year-old child with second urinary infection
   (c) A 5-year-old child with urinary incontinence
   (d) A 7-year-old child with intermittent urinary infection
12. A 12-month-old girl with anorexia, agitation, fever (38.5 °C), and change in urine color underwent antibiotic therapy for urinary infection. You have been consulted about the method of choice for urinary reflux. Conduct a comparison between VCUG (voiding cystourethrography) and DRNC (direct radionuclide cystography).
   (a) The sensitivity of VCUG is higher than that of DRNC.
   (b) VCUG is preferred because of the possibility of the involvement of the posterior ureteral valve.
   (c) None of these methods has priority over the other for this patient.
   (d) The rate of radiation exposure in DRNC is less than that in VCUG.

13. A 3-year-old girl with a history of first urinary infection in the previous month underwent DRNC. After the complete emptying of the bladder and sonography, normal saline with ^{99m}Tc-pertechnatae is injected into the bladder in a sterile condition. Entrance rate significantly decreases after 100 ml of injection. What is the best answer if the technician asks about the necessity of completely filling the bladder?
    (a) Bladder filling must be continued for at least 120 ml.
    (b) The filling phase can be stopped, and the voiding phase can be initiated.
    (c) Bladder filling must be continued for at least 150 ml.
    (d) Bladder filling must be continued for at least 180 ml.
14. A 3-month-old girl with a breastfeeding problem, inappropriate weight gain, and minor fever is subjected to a ^{99m}Tc-DMSA scan for urinary infection. A small scar is obtained in the right upper pole. VCUG scan shows a grade IV reflux on the right side, no reflux on the left side, and normal bladder and urine volumes. The mother asks about the spontaneous improvement (without surgery) of the reflux. Which of the following variables indicates the least possibility of spontaneous improvement?
    (a) Reflux grade IV
    (b) Age (infant)
    (c) Sex (girl)
    (d) Normal bladder
15. Hydronephrosis is detected in prenatal ultrasonography in the right kidney of a 5-day-old premature neonate. What is the primary recommended imaging method?
    (a) IVU
    (b) US
    (c) ^{99m}Tc-MAG3 scan
    (d) ^{99m}Tc-DTPA scan
16. About multicystic dysplastic kidney:
    (a) It is bilateral in most cases.
    (b) It is more common in girls than in boys.
    (c) VCUG must be performed in all cases.
    (d) It is presented as a marked nonhomogenous uptake on a ^{99m}Tc-DMSA scan.
17. Which of the following interventions is recommended for a girl with grade V reflux?
    (a) Follow-up of the patient and radiologic VCUG every 6 months
    (b) Follow-up of the patient and radionuclide cystogram every 6 months
    (c) Referral for surgery
    (d) Follow-up of the patient and prophylactic antibiotic therapy for 5 years
18. Which modality is the most sensitive for the evaluation of pyelonephritis?
    (a) Sonography
    (b) ^{99m}Tc-DMSA scan
    (c) IVP
    (d) Dynamic renography

19. About kidneys with a doublex system:
    (a) Reflux is commonly observed in the upper pole.
    (b) Obstruction is commonly observed in the lower pole.
    (c) Ureterocele is commonly observed in the lower pole.
    (d) Urinary obstruction is usually accompanied by ureterocele.
20. Compare VCUG and radionuclide cystogram.
    (a) The absorbed radiation dose is higher in radionuclide cystography.
    (b) VCUG is more sensitive for the evaluation of urinary reflux.
    (c) VCUG must be used for the evaluation of the posterior urethral valve.
    (d) Grading is better performed with radionuclide cystography.
21. A 7-year-old child with a history of grade IV vesicoureteral reflux and fever is referred for ^{99m}Tc-DMSA scintigraphy. A defect is observed in the right upper pole. When is the most appropriate time for the repeat of scan after treatment?
    (a) 1 month
    (b) 2 months
    (c) 4 months
    (d) 1 year
22. ^{99m}Tc-DTPA scan is normal for an 8-year-old boy, but a lower renal uptake is observed on the ^{99m}Tc-DMSA scan. What is the most probable diagnosis?
    (a) Chronic renal failure
    (b) Tubulointerstitial renal disease
    (c) Vesicoureteral reflux
    (d) Dehydration
23. Describe the sensitivity and specificity of a renal scan, respectively, for the evaluation of renal vein thrombosis in neonates with a history of severe dehydration.
    (a) High sensitivity, high specificity
    (b) High sensitivity, low specificity
    (c) Low sensitivity, high specificity
    (d) No sensitivity and specificity
24. About direct radionuclide cisternography:
    (a) It is NOT more sensitive than radiography.
    (b) Reflux appears only during voiding.
    (c) Its radiation is higher than that of radiography.
    (d) It must be performed only with ^{99m}Tc-sulfur colloid.
25. Radiologic cystography is preferred over radionuclide cystography in:
    (a) Follow-up of children who underwent surgical or medical therapy for reflux
    (b) Evaluation of an 8-year-old boy for first urinary infection
    (c) Evaluation of the asymptomatic sister of a boy with reflux
    (d) Serial evaluation of a child with a neurogenic bladder

26. Which of the following statements regarding acute pediatric pyelonephritis is NOT correct?
    (a) It is NOT associated with reflux in most cases.
    (b) Imaging techniques are NOT required to differentiate it from lower urinary tract infections.
    (c) Lack of treatment can cause irreversible renal injuries.
    (d) Renal scar is independent of the presence or absence of reflux.
27. About children with vesicoureteral reflux:
    (a) Appearance of a reflux indicates pyelonephritis.
    (b) Clinical and laboratory examinations are useful and sufficient for differentiating acute pyelonephritis from lower urinary tract infections.
    (c) Early diagnosis and antibiotic therapy exclude a renal scan despite the presence of reflux.
    (d) The sensitivity of a ^{99m}Tc-DMSA scan for the diagnosis of pyelonephritis is similar to that of sonography.
28. About the first urinary tract infection of a 9-month-old girl:
    (a) ^{99m}Tc-DMSA scan and direct cystography are the first intervention.
    (b) ^{99m}Tc-DMSA scan and direct cystography are recommended if renal sonography is abnormal and hydronephrosis is absent.
    (c) ^{99m}Tc-DMSA scan is NOT required if renal sonography is normal.
    (d) Renal sonography and cystography are recommended if ^{99m}Tc-DMSA is normal.
29. What is the disadvantage of renal cortical imaging with ^{99m}Tc-DMSA in comparison with ^{99m}Tc-GHA?
    (a) Higher gonadal dose
    (b) Lower image contrast
    (c) Interference of gallbladder activity with the right kidney
    (d) Higher renal radiation per MBq
30. If the indicated dose of ^{99m}Tc-DMSA is 100 MBq for adults, what is the recommended dose for a 3-year-old child?
    (a) 25 MBq
    (b) 30 MBq
    (c) 50 MBq
    (d) 40 MBq
31. About radionuclide cystogram:
    (a) The sensitivity of indirect cystogram with ^{99m}Tc-DTPA and that with ^{99m}Tc-MAG3 are equal.
    (b) A normal direct cystogram excludes reflux.
    (c) The indirect method is preferred over the direct one in girls older than 1 year because of the lower radiation rate.
    (d) The results of two different evaluations may not be similar for an infant because of the intermittent characteristic of reflux.

32. A very agitated neonate is a candidate for cystography. What is the drug of choice for sedation and increased compliance?
    (a) Pentobarbital injection
    (b) Pentobarbital suppository
    (c) Diazepam injection
    (d) Chloral hydrate
33. Which of the following radiopharmaceuticals produces the best quality of images on the renal scintigraphy of a 26-day-old neonate?
    (a) ^{99m}Tc-DTPA
    (b) ^{99m} c-MAG3
    (c) ^{99m}Tc-DMSA
    (d) ^{99m}Tc-GHA
34. Which of the following findings on the ^{99m}Tc-DTPA renal scintigraphy of a healthy neonate is considered abnormal?
    (a) Poor appearance of the kidneys
    (b) Slow renal transit time
    (c) Flattening of the renogram curves
    (d) Higher background activity
35. A total of 1 mCi of the radiotracer is required for a child candidated for renal scintigraphy with ^{99m}Tc-DMSA. ^{99m}Tc-DMSA is replaced with 3 mCi of ^{99m}Tc-GHA because the kit was unavailable. Which item is expected?
    (a) Increased cortical exposure rate.
    (b) Cortical exposure rate is equal in both radiotracers.
    (c) Decreased cortical exposure rate.
    (d) Gonadal exposure rate is equal in both methods.
36. All of the following statements regarding a pseudo-horseshoe kidney in children are correct *except*:
    (a) It is usually associated with meningocele.
    (b) It is usually associated with vertebral column deformations.
    (c) Renal malposition exists.
    (d) An isotope scan canNOT differentiate this disease from a true horseshoe kidney.
37. What is the advantage of indirect radionuclide cystography?
    (a) Diagnosis of all cases of reflux in the filling phase
    (b) No need for catheterization
    (c) Low compliance of patient for urination
    (d) Lower radiation dose
38. What is the most common cause of a palpable mass in the flank of neonates?
    (a) Hydronephrosis due to UVJ obstruction and Wilms' tumor
    (b) Hydronephrosis due to reflux and neuroblastoma
    (c) Congenital megaureter and polycystic kidney
    (d) Hydronephrosis due to UPJ obstruction and multicystic dysplastic kidney

39. About the diagnosis of acute infantile pyelonephritis with ^{99m}Tc-DMSA:
    (a) SPECT is recommended.
    (b) Planar imaging with a pinhole collimator is considered sufficient.
    (c) The sensitivity and accuracy of SPECT increase significantly.
    (d) A lower dose of ^{99}mTc-DMSA is required in SPECT.
40. Which of the following statements about renal vein thrombosis is NOT correct?
    (a) In neonates, it is usually observed in the first month after birth.
    (b) Rim activity around the kidneys on the ^{99m}Tc-DTPA scan indicates collaterals in the renal capsule.
    (c) In neonates, it is usually bilateral.
    (d) Radionuclide methods are conducted prior to anatomical methods for diagnosis.
41. About imaging of suspected pyelonephritis:
    (a) Utilization of SPECT on the ^{99m}Tc-DMSA scan increases the incidence of false-positive results.
    (b) Repeat of the ^{99m}Tc-DMSA scan after 1 month is recommended if cortical defect is present in acute pyelonephritis.
    (c) Rapid tubular washout is the main mechanism of cortical defect on a ^{99m}Tc-DMSA scan.
    (d) In acute pyelonephritis, cortical defects are mainly observed in the middle segment, which is thicker than the other segments.
42. A 1-month-old neonate is referred with dehydration, symptoms of renal failure, and mild macroscopic hematuria. A bilateral palpable mass in the flank is observed upon physical examination, and the rim sign is seen on the ^{99m}Tc-DTPA renal scan. What is the most probable diagnosis?
    (a) RVT
    (b) RAS
    (c) RVH
    (d) Bilateral renal embolism
43. GFR at birth is about 20% of the corrected adult value, and it reaches only to 45% by 2 weeks of age. The adult levels are reached at:
    (a) 1–2 years of age
    (b) 12–18 months of age
    (c) 1–6 months of age
    (d) 6–12 months of age
44. Which of the following statements regarding urinary tract infection (UTI) in pediatrics is false?
    (a) Most cases of acute pyelonephritis occur in the absence of demonstrable vesicoureteral reflux (VUR).
    (b) Once acute pyelonephritis occurs, the subsequent development of renal scarring is independent of the presence or absence of reflux.
    (c) IVU has high sensitivity for the diagnosis of pyelonephritis.
    (d) ^{67}Ga and ^{111}In-WBS procedures may be reliable for the diagnosis of acute pyelonephritis and provide information about the morphology and function of the kidneys.

45. What is the least common scintigraphic pattern in acute pyelonephritis on a ^{99m}Tc-DMSA scan?
    (a) Decreased cortical uptake in the upper pole and midzone
    (b) Decreased cortical uptake in the lower pole and midzone
    (c) Decreased cortical uptake in the upper and lower poles
    (d) Diffusely decreased tracer uptake in an enlarged kidney
46. An 18-year-old girl presents with repeated urinary tract infections. Sonography shows severe hydronephrosis and an echogenic mass 20 mm × 9 mm in size in the right kidney. Moreover, a 15 mm stone is found near the mass. Urine also contains echogenic particles. The right kidney shows no function in the renogram. What is the most likely diagnosis?
    (a) Congenital UPJ stenosis accompanied with stone and secondary infection
    (b) Pyonephrosis in the background of UPJ stenosis and stone
    (c) Xanthogranulomatous pyelonephritis (XGPN)
    (d) Angiomyolipoma (AML) and stone
47. Which of the following statements properly describes the characteristics of a medullary sponge kidney?
    (a) Both kidneys are usually enlarged.
    (b) It is an autosomal dominant inherent disease.
    (c) Dilatation in the collecting system and papilla.
    (d) It is part of the differential diagnosis of renal tubular acidosis.
48. Which of the following items regarding a medullary sponge kidney is not true?
    (a) Susceptible to infection and stone.
    (b) May be focal or unilateral.
    (c) Striation in IVP is a characteristic.
    (d) Risk for renal failure.
49. If a suspected hypertrophied column of Bertin is found on the sonography of an adult patient, what will you choose as the confirmatory diagnostic test?
    (a) ^{99m}Tc-DMSA scan
    (b) Contrast CT scan
    (c) Percutaneous biopsy
    (d) Intravenous pyelography
50. What percentage of patients with renal scar will experience hypertension?
    (a) 10–18%
    (b) 20–30%
    (c) 30–40%
    (d) 5–10%
51. Reflux nephropathy is responsible for … of cases with ESRD.
    (a) 20–30%
    (b) 10–20%
    (c) 30–40%
    (d) 5–10%

52. What is the most accurate method for differentiating between upper and lower urinary tract infections?
    (a) Presentation of symptoms of sepsis
    (b) Erythrocyte sedimentation rate (ESR)
    (c) Separate catheterization of the ureter and bladder in a sterile condition
    (d) Urine β2-microglobulin
53. All of the following statements regarding the ^{99m}Tc-DMSA scan in urinary infections are correct *except*:
    (a) None of the cases of pyelonephritis will be overlooked with the combination of the ^{99m}Tc-DMSA scan and ultrasonography.
    (b) Radionuclide VCUG is the next step after an abnormal ^{99m}Tc-DMSA scan and sonography.
    (c) ^{99m}Tc-DMSA scan shows transient lesions in acute infection, but renal scar is possible if the lesions remain for more than 6 months.
    (d) About 40% of the administered dose of ^{99m}Tc-DMSA binds to the proximal collecting tubule (PCT).
54. Which of the following statements about the application of different radiotracers in urinary tract infection is NOT correct?
    (a) ^{99m}Tc-glucoheptonate is dominantly filtrated, although 10% of the administered dose binds to the distal collecting tubule (DCT).
    (b) Although gallium is specific for pyelonephritis, it is NOT commonly used.
    (c) The ^{111}In-WBC scan is more specific than gallium for the detection of infection and is commonly used for this purpose.
    (d) Lower radiation exposure and no need for blood sampling are considered the advantages of a NAC-95 (Tc-antigranulocyte) scan.
55. All of the following statements regarding the protocol for the ^{99m}Tc-DMSA scan are correct *except*:
    (a) ^{99m}Tc-DMSA scan is the radiotracer of choice for cortical imaging, especially in neonates and infants.
    (b) The pediatric dose of ^{99m}Tc-DMSA is calculated by [(age +1)/(age +7)] × adult dose.
    (c) A pinhole collimator is recommended for the ^{99m}Tc-DMSA scan.
    (d) The more accurate the imaging (application of a pinhole collimator) is, the higher the uniformity of the final image on a ^{99m}Tc-DMSA scan.
56. All of the following statements regarding ^{99m}Tc-DMSA scan are correct *except*:
    (a) Serial scans are required for evaluating acute and chronic lesions.
    (b) An uptake in the lesion with cortical thinning and decreased kidney size indicates chronic disease and scar.
    (c) The mechanism of the decreased uptake of ^{99m}Tc-DMSA in pyelonephritis is single factorial.
    (d) ^{99m}Tc-DMSA scan is the method of choice for differentiating between upper and lower urinary tract infections (UTI).

57. Which of the following statements regarding the application of sonography in urinary tract infections (UTI) is NOT correct?
    (a) Sonographic signs of pyelonephritis include the disappearance of the distinction between the cortex and the medulla, enlargement, hypoechoic regions or those with change in echo, and dilatation of the pelvis.
    (b) Sonography overestimates pyelonephritis.
    (c) Sonography can help to characterize a lesion on a ^{99m}Tc-DMSA scan.
    (d) Pyelonephritis without reflux is NOT common in children.
58. What is the recommended drug for the sedation of children?
    (a) Intranasal midazolam
    (b) Oral chloral hydrate
    (c) Diazepam
    (d) a and b
59. When do the pediatric values of GFR and tubular function reach the level of adults, respectively?
    (a) Adolescence, at age 3 years
    (b) At birth, at age 1 year
    (c) At age 1 year, at age 1 year
    (d) At age 3 years, at age 3 years
60. If the goal is to eliminate the problem of extravascular fluid on a pediatric renal scan, what is the recommended radiotracer with 90% of protein binding?
    (a) ^{99m}Tc-EC
    (b) ^{99m}Tc-MAG3
    (c) ^{99m}Tc-DTPA
    (d) ^{123}I-OIH
61. GFR at birth is about … and reaches to 80% of the level of adults at the age of ….
    (a) 20 ml/min, 3 years
    (b) 30 ml/min, 2 years
    (c) 20 ml/min, 2 years
    (d) 30 ml/min, 3 years
62. The fastest renal maturation occurs:
    (a) In the first 2 months after birth
    (b) At the age of 1–6 months
    (c) Before 1 year old
    (d) In adolescence
63. The lack of renal maturity decreases the ^{99m}Tc-DMSA uptake. Therefore, the ^{99m}Tc-DMSA scan is best performed at the age of:
    (a) 2 months
    (b) 6 months
    (c) 3 months
    (d) 1 year

64. Which of the following items about ^{99m}Tc-MAG3 is NOT correct?
    (a) Lower radiation and high-quality images.
    (b) Blood sampling in the 20th min is required for a quantitative study.
    (c) Differential renal function indicates tubular excretion.
    (d) It is recommended for infants below 2 years old.
65. The following are the advantages of direct radionuclide cystography *except*:
    (a) High sensitivity for the diagnosis of reflux.
    (b) A urodynamic study can be conducted simultaneously.
    (c) Radiation is relatively less than that of voiding cystourethrography (VCUG).
    (d) It provides a relatively good anatomical resolution.
66. What are the recommended methods for the diagnosis and follow-up of urinary reflux in girls and boys below 3 years old with urinary tract infection, respectively?
    (a) Direct radionuclide cystography (DRC) for both diagnosis and follow-up in girls; voiding cystourethrography (VCUG) for diagnosis and DRC for follow-up in boys
    (b) VCUG for diagnosis and DRC for follow-up in girls; DRC for both diagnosis and follow-up in boys
    (c) DRC for both diagnosis and follow-up in girls and boys
    (d) VCUG for both diagnosis and follow-up in girls and boys
67. The child must be toilet trained for indirect renal cystography (IRC). …. is used as the radiotracer in this method, and imaging is conducted … min after injection.
    (a) ^{99m}Tc-MAG3, 10–20
    (b) ^{99m}Tc-DTPA, 30–60
    (c) ^{99m}Tc-MAG3, 30–60
    (d) ^{99m}Tc-DTPA, 10–20
68. The evaluation of which phase of reflux is problematic with indirect radionuclide cystography (IRC)?
    (a) Filling phase
    (b) Voiding phase
    (c) Post-void phase
    (d) All phases
69. All of the following statements regarding reflux and urinary infection are correct *except*:
    (a) Reflux is an intermittent phenomenon and is independent of urine volume.
    (b) Pelvis dilatation secondary to ureteropelvic junction obstruction (UPJO) is the most common type of hydronephrosis.
    (c) Sonography is recommended on the day of hospitalization for a child with acute pyelonephritis.
    (d) A ^{99m}Tc-DMSA scan is recommended 2 weeks after hospitalization for a child with acute pyelonephritis.
70. Which of the following parameters is accurate for studying the diuretic effects in a renogram?
    (a) T1/2 (time of half-activity)
    (b) T75 (time of excretion of 75% of activity)
    (c) Pelvic excretion efficiency (PEE)
    (d) Tmax

71. The results of diuretic renography are reliable after the age of:
    (a) 4 months
    (b) 3 months
    (c) 2 months
    (d) 1 month
72. What is the minimum required level of GFR for a ^{99m}Tc-MAG3 scan?
    (a) 40 ml/min
    (b) 30 ml/min
    (c) 20 ml/min
    (d) 50 ml/min
73. If the goal is to evaluate an ectopic kidney, which scan and what additional view are necessary?
    (a) ^{99m}Tc-MAG3, anterior pelvis
    (b) ^{99m}Tc-DMSA, posterior pelvis
    (c) ^{99m}Tc-MAG3, posterior pelvis
    (d) ^{99m}Tc-DMSA, anterior pelvis
74. All of the following statements regarding renogram and blood pressure are correct *except*:
    (a) Renal problems are the most common cause of hypertension in children over 1 year old.
    (b) Captopril-enhanced scintigraphy can be used for the evaluation of renovascular hypertension.
    (c) If the goal is to evaluate RVH in pediatrics, Doppler sonography>^{99m}Tc-MAG3 scan>captopril renal scan>^{99m}Tc-DMSA scan is the right order of diagnostic interventions.
    (d) If the goal is to evaluate RVH in pediatrics, captopril renal scan>Doppler sonography>^{99m}Tc-MAG3 scan>^{99m}Tc-DMSA scan is the right order of diagnostic interventions.
75. Which of the following studies must be conducted earlier if the goal is to evaluate the complications of kidney transplantation?
    (a) Sonography.
    (b) Isotopic scan.
    (c) Both sonography and isotopic scan must be conducted in 1 day.
    (d) Sonography is conducted first, followed by isotopic scan after a few days.
76. The determination of which parameter is critical for each renal scan?
    (a) Blood flow
    (b) GFR (1–3 min)
    (c) Differential renal function
    (d) 20 min transit time
77. Which of the following items regarding the relationship between the findings of renal scan and the complications of kidney transplantation is NOT correct?
    (a) Good perfusion with retention: ATN, cyclosporine toxicity, and obstruction
    (b) Lack of perfusion: renal vein or artery thrombosis
    (c) Decrease in perfusion and function: acute or chronic rejection
    (d) Preserved perfusion with decreased function: ATN, hyperacute rejection, cyclosporine toxicity

78. How long after kidney transplantation is a base ^{99m}Tc-DMSA scan required for all children?
    (a) 2 months
    (b) 3 months
    (c) 1 month
    (d) 4 months
79. What are the radiotracer of choice and the dose for radionuclide retrograde cystography (RRC), respectively? Which organ receives the highest radiation?
    (a) ^{99m}Tc-SC, 1 mCi, gallbladder
    (b) ^{99m}Tc-DTPA, 2 mCi, gallbladder
    (c) ^{99m}Tc-DTPA, 2 mCi, bladder
    (d) ^{99m}Tc-SC, 1 mCi, bladder
80. Which formula is used for the calculation of the maximum capacity of the bladder for infants?
    (a) [age (year) +2] × 30 ml
    (b) [age (year) +30] × 2 ml
    (c) [age (month) +2] × 30 ml
    (d) [age (month) +30] × 2 ml
81. In addition to missed torsion, scrotal scintigraphy shows the bull's eye sign in:
    (a) Abscess
    (b) Hematoma
    (c) Neoplasm with necrosis
    (d) All of the above
82. The false-negative findings of testicular torsion in scrotal scintigraphy include:
    (a) Spontaneous detorsion
    (b) Incomplete torsion
    (c) Inguinal testis
    (d) All of the above
83. The ratios of epididymitis to torsion in patients younger and older than 20 years are … and …, respectively.
    (a) 1.5, 9
    (b) 2.5, 8
    (c) 9, 1.5
    (d) 8, 2.5
84. Which of the following diseases induces a unilateral kidney enlargement?
    (a) Acute tubular necrosis
    (b) Multiple myelomas
    (c) Diabetic glomerulosclerosis
    (d) Acute pyelonephritis

85. An 8-year-old girl is referred with urinary infection. Three months after treatment and a negative urine culture, cystogram shows grade III bilateral retrograde reflux. She has two older sisters and one brother with no symptoms or history of urinary infection. Which of the following diagnostic methods is recommended for the evaluation of her siblings?
    (a) ^{99m}Tc-DTPA scan to evaluate the existence of a renal scar
    (b) Renal sonography
    (c) Radionuclide retrograde cystography
    (d) Retrograde voiding cystourethrography
86. In which of the following situations is Foley catheterization NOT required to rule out upper tract obstruction on a diuretic scan?
    (a) Possibility of reflux
    (b) Possibility of neurogenic bladder
    (c) Pelvic kidney
    (d) Possibility of bilateral UPJO
87. Which of the following methods is the most accurate for the evaluation of renal anatomy, obstruction, and differential function?
    (a) Sonography
    (b) ^{99m}Tc-DTPA
    (c) MR urography
    (d) ^{99m}Tc-DMSA scan

8.8.1 Answer

	A	B	C	D		A	B	C	D
1		*			45				*
2		*			46			*	
3				*	47			*	
4			*		48				*
5			*		49	*			
6			*		50	*			
7			*		51		*		
8		*			52			*	
9		*			53				*
10				*	54			*	
11				*	55				*
12				*	56			*	
13	*				57				*
14	*				58				*

15			*		**59**	*			
16			*		**60**		*		
17			*		**61**				*
18		*			**62**		*		
19				*	**63**			*	
20			*		**64**		*		
21			*		**65**				*
22		*			**66**	*			
23				*	**67**			*	
24		*			**68**	*			
25		*			**69**				*
26		*			**70**			*	
27			*		**71**	*			
28		*			**72**			*	
29				*	**73**				*
30				*	**74**				*
31				*	**75**			*	
32				*	**76**			*	
33		*			**77**				*
34		*			**78**			*	
35		*			**79**				*
36				*	**80**	*			
37		*			**81**				*
38				*	**82**				*
39		*			**83**	*			
40				*	**84**				*
41	*				**85**		*		
42	*				**86**				*
43				*	**87**			*	
44				*	**88**				

8.9 Nuclear Medicine in the Clinical Diagnosis and Treatment of Obstructive Uropathy

1. What is the action of furosemide?
   (a) Acts in the ascending limb of the loop of Henle
   (b) Blocks the active reabsorption of chloride
   (c) Blocks the active reabsorption of sodium
   (d) All of the above
2. Which of the following conditions results in a sawtooth sign in a renogram?
   (a) Vesicoureteral reflux
   (b) Severe dilatation of the collecting system
   (c) Intra-bladder urine pressure
   (d) Relative stenosis in UPJ
3. What happens in a renal scan with a persistent and augmented renal obstruction?
   (a) Delayed and reduced perfusion, cortical retention, and delayed secretion
   (b) Cortical retention and delayed secretion, with no significant change in perfusion
   (c) Reduced cortical uptake
   (d) Renogram fall in the third stage
4. In which of the following disorders does filtration fraction (GFR/ERPF) NOT significantly change?
   (a) Renal artery thrombosis
   (b) Acute rejection
   (c) Post-captopril
   (d) Renal obstruction
5. About obstructive renal disorders:
   (a) Pathologic glomerular changes are persistent.
   (b) Glomerular dysfunction occurs earlier than tubular dysfunction.
   (c) No change is observed in the second stage of the renogram.
   (d) An increase is found in the slope of the third stage of the renogram.
6. If renal obstruction is NOT complete, in the renogram:
   (a) The parenchymal phase will NOT change.
   (b) The perfusion phase is elongated.
   (c) The excretion phase is delayed.
   (d) ERPF decreases.
7. The renogram of a child suspected to have unilateral hydronephrosis is evaluated. A fall in the curve is observed after furosemide injection, and then the curve ascends with a short interval. What is the most probable diagnosis?
   (a) Obstruction of UV
   (b) UV reflux
   (c) Flow-dependent obstruction
   (d) Improved obstruction

8. About renal obstruction:
   (a) Glomerular function is disturbed earlier than tubular function.
   (b) The first stage of a renogram is shortened, but the second stage remains unchanged.
   (c) Glomerular dysfunction is observed for a longer time on the scan.
   (d) The second stage of a renogram remains unchanged, and the third stage is elongated.
9. Renal scintigraphy is performed on a child suspected to have a flow-dependent obstruction. What is the pattern of the renogram after the injection of furosemide?
   (a) Ascending followed by descending
   (b) Decrementing (step by step descending of the curve)
   (c) Descending followed by ascending
   (d) Intermittent descending and ascending
10. About ureteropelvic junction obstruction (UPJO) in infants:
   (a) This type of obstruction is the rarest cause of hydronephrosis at birth.
   (b) It is common in girls.
   (c) Severe VU reflux can cause partial obstruction of the UPJ.
   (d) Stenosis due to the pressure of the inferior aberrant renal artery rarely causes UPJO.
11. In severe nephroptosis, what is the proper medical position to detect obstructive uropathy on a renal scan?
   (a) Supine.
   (b) Semi-erect.
   (c) Prone.
   (d) It is independent of patient position.
12. Which regions in a diuresis renogram are selected as the ROI for the evaluation of urinary tract drainage with hyperureteronephrosis?
   (a) Whole kidney, pelvis, and ureter
   (b) Whole kidney and pelvis without ureter
   (c) Renal cortex and pelvis without calices
   (d) Renal cortex without calices and pelvis
13. Which of the following disorders can cause the stepwise phenomenon in the third phase of a diuresis renogram of the right kidney?
   (a) VU reflux
   (b) Duplex system
   (c) Ureter stone and retrograde peristalsis of the ureter
   (d) Increase in peristalsis of the pyelocaliceal and ureter
14. In which of the following cases is a pseudo-horseshoe kidney observed?
   (a) Patients with sacrum atresia
   (b) Patients with meningomyelocele and severe deformities of the vertebra
   (c) Patients with fused crossed ectopic kidney
   (d) Patients with a single pelvic kidney

15. Diuretic renography is indicated for the evaluation and differentiation of renal obstruction from nonobstructive dilatation of the pyelocaliceal system. What is the recommended time for furosemide injection?
    (a) 15 min before injection of the radiopharmaceutical
    (b) 10 min after injection of the radiopharmaceutical
    (c) 20 min after injection of the radiopharmaceutical
    (d) Concurrent with the injection of the radiopharmaceutical
16. A patient with hydronephrosis is subjected to diuretic renography with the F+20 protocol. The GFR of the right hydronephrotic kidney is 10 ml/min, and the furosemide response is equivalent. What is the next step?
    (a) Diuretic renography with the F-15 protocol
    (b) Repeat of scan with the F+20 protocol after 3 or 6 months
    (c) CT scan
    (d) Perfusion–pressure flow test (Whitaker)
17. Which of the following factors can cause false-negative findings in the diagnosis of obstruction with diuretic renography?
    (a) Age < 1 month
    (b) Vesicoureteral reflux
    (c) Intrarenal pelvis
    (d) Differential renal function < 20%
18. In obstructive uropathy:
    (a) The presence of urinoma is indicative of a non-acute complete obstruction.
    (b) The cortical transit time remains normal in acute obstruction.
    (c) Dilatation of the collecting system occurs immediately after acute obstruction.
    (d) The glomerular function becomes abnormal earlier than the tubular function.
19. Which of the following changes is induced by the early injection of furosemide on the dynamic renal scan of a child with severe unilateral dilatation of the pelvis and calices?
    (a) Better observation of nonobstructive stasis
    (b) False delay in the radiotracer washout and increase in false-positive results in detecting the obstruction
    (c) Increased radiotracer washout and increase in false-negative results in detecting the obstruction
    (d) It changes neither the wash-out rate nor the final outcome
20. Which of the following signs can help to differentiate reflux nephropathy from obstruction?
    (a) Presence or absence of ureteral dilatation
    (b) Involvement of bilateral kidneys
    (c) Generalized decrease in cortical thickness
    (d) Marked dilatation of the upper pole calices

21. All of the following statements regarding the urinary system are correct *except*:
    (a) Pacemakers for ureteral pain are located in minor cycles.
    (b) About one bolus of urine volume is excreted every 2–6 min from the calices to the ureter and moves downward at a rate of 2–5 cm/s. The volume of boluses increases with the increase in flow, but their number remains constant.
    (c) The normal pressure of a renal calyx is 4–10 cmH_2O but increases to 60 cmH_2O in obstructions.
    (d) Increase in blood pressure secondarily increases the renal flow through PGF2, but renal flow decreases in the next 24 h and reaches 40–70% of its normal level. Finally, GFR decreases.
22. All of the following statements regarding urinary tract obstruction are correct *except*:
    (a) Obstruction is rarely complete.
    (b) Sonography can show parenchymal and lower urinary tract obstructions.
    (c) The sitting position is recommended for the evaluation of obstruction in diuretic renography.
    (d) CT scan is NOT commonly indicated for the evaluation of obstruction.
23. What is the most appropriate screening test for obstruction?
    (a) Sonography
    (b) CT
    (c) MRI
    (d) IVP
24. What is the radiotracer of choice for diuretic renography?
    (a) ^{99m}Tc-DTPA
    (b) ^{99m}Tc-EC
    (c) ^{99m}Tc-MAG3
    (d) ^{123}I-OIH
25. Regarding renogram:
    (a) The upper region of the kidney is preferred as the ROI of the background.
    (b) The peak of the renogram normally appears in 2–5 min.
    (c) Phase I of the renogram indicates perfusion and a less positive slope.
    (d) Phase III of the renogram indicates voiding, and the normal findings in this phase exclude obstruction.
26. What are the reasons for the stepwise and sawtooth patterns in the renogram, respectively?
    (a) Intense ureteral peristaltic movements, reflux, or a duplex renal system
    (b) Reflux or intense ureteral peristaltic movements, duplex renal system
    (c) Duplex renal system, intense ureteral peristaltic movements
    (d) Reflux, duplex renal system

27. Which of the following statements regarding the assessment of a relative or split function is NOT correct?
    (a) Phase II or uptake of the renogram is used to assess the relative or split function.
    (b) The 1st–2.5th min images of ^{99m}Tc-MAG3 and ^{123}I-OIH as well as the 2nd—3rd min images of ^{99m}Tc-DTPA are used to assess the relative or split function.
    (c) A split function with ^{99m}Tc-DTPA demonstrates the tubular function.
    (d) A split function with ^{123}I-OIH demonstrates ERPF.
28. All of the following situations can cause a false-positive obstruction in a renogram *except*:
    (a) Dehydration
    (b) Severely dilated pyelocaliceal system
    (c) Compression effect of a full bladder
    (d) Renal stones
29. Which of the following statements about furosemide is NOT correct?
    (a) Furosemide is the diuretic of choice for the evaluation of equivocal obstruction.
    (b) The ascending loop of Henle is the site of action of furosemide.
    (c) The maximum level of urine flow increased with furosemide is five times the normal value.
    (d) The therapeutic dose of furosemide for adults and children is 40 mg and 0.5 mg/kg, respectively, and the maximum response appears 15 min after injection.
30. Response to furosemide is NOT predictable at age below …, and the minimum GFR for its effectiveness is …
    (a) 2 months, 30 ml/min
    (b) 1.5 months, 16 ml/min
    (c) 3 months, 20 ml/min
    (d) 1.5 months, 25 ml/min
31. All of the following diseases or conditions interfere with the effect of furosemide *except*:
    (a) Acute tubular necrosis
    (b) Fanconi syndrome
    (c) Massive dilatation of the renal system
    (d) Pyelonephritis
32. Tandem obstruction is defined as:
    (a) Obstruction in multiple points of the urinary system, where the scan only detects the most severe one
    (b) Obstruction in the lower urinary tract, which is hardly detected by scan
    (c) Obstruction in the upper urinary tract, which is easily detected by scan
    (d) Obstruction in the intrarenal tubules, which are easily detected by scan

33. Identify the proper timing of the study in F+20 and F-15 diuretic renography.
    (a) F+20, until 15 min after the injection of furosemide; F-15, until 15 min after the injection of the radiotracer
    (b) F+20, until 15 min after the injection of the radiotracer; F-15, until 15 min after the injection of furosemide
    (c) F+20, until 15 min after the injection of furosemide; F-15, until 15 min after the injection of furosemide
    (d) F+20, until 15 min after the injection of the radiotracer; F-15, until 15 min after the injection of the radiotracer
34. In diuretic renography, urinary catheterization is required in all of the following situations *except*:
    (a) Voiding defect.
    (b) Lower tract obstructions.
    (c) High residual urine.
    (d) Catheterization is generally recommended for all patients.
35. Which of the following statements is NOT correct about urinary obstruction?
    (a) When hydration is good and GFR is more than 16 ml/min, an equivocal outcome indicates relative obstruction.
    (b) The F-15 protocol is recommended for relative obstruction, and it decreases equivocal results to 1/5; if equivocal outcomes are observed again (in 3% of cases), the study must be repeated after 3–6 months.
    (c) The F-15 protocol can be conducted on patients with GFR < 16 ml/min to evaluate urinary obstruction.
    (d) T1/2 clearance in a quantitative study is the time for a 50% decrease in renal activity.
36. What conditions are described by I, II, IIIa, and IIIb curves, respectively?
    (a) I, normal; II, obstructed; IIIa, dilated unobstructed; IIIb, equivocal
    (b) I, normal; II, obstructed; IIIa, equivocal; IIIb, dilated unobstructed
    (c) I, normal; II, delayed decompensate; IIIa, equivocal; IIIb, obstructed
    (d) I, normal; II, obstructed; IIIa, dilated unobstructed; IIIb, delayed decompensate

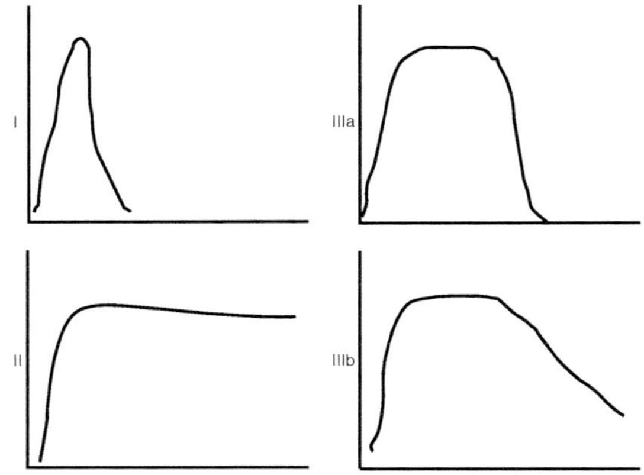

37. What is the most common cause of delayed decompression (delayed double peak), and in which protocol (F+20 or F-15) is it most commonly reported?
   (a) Presence of the radiotracer in the catheter, which enters into the system with an injection of furosemide, F-15
   (b) Reflux, F-15
   (c) Obstruction, F+20
   (d) Presence of the radiotracer in the catheter, which enters into the system with an injection of furosemide, F+20
38. All of the following statements about peak elimination rate (Emax) are correct *except*:
   (a) Emax less than 7% indicates obstruction.
   (b) Emax of 7–14% indicates an intermediate outcome of the scan.
   (c) Emax of greater than 14% indicates normal condition.
   (d) Emax is an accurate method and shows the percentage of the eliminated activity in unit of time.
39. Saline is administered at a rate of … in the Whitaker test (perfusion pressure flow study), and pressure of more than … indicates obstruction and less than… excludes obstruction.
   (a) 10 cc/min, 20 cmH_2O, 15 cmH_2O
   (b) 50 cc/min, 20 cmH_2O, 15 cmH_2O
   (c) 10 cc/min, 20 cmH_2O, 10 cmH_2O
   (d) 10 cc/min, 22 cmH_2O, 15 cmH_2O
40. What is the corresponding rate of perfusion pressure flow study (PPFS) and diuretic renography?
   (a) 40–50%
   (b) 53–85%
   (c) 80–90%
   (d) 90–100%
41. All of the following statements regarding renogram are correct *except*:
   (a) Alternative to diuretic renography; the selection of two different ROI around the renal parenchyma and around the kidneys can be used to assess parenchyma transit time.
   (b) Obstruction is indicated if transit time in both ROI is prolonged.
   (c) Stasis without obstruction is indicated if renal transit time is prolonged, but parenchyma transit time is normal.
   (d) In contrast to diuretic renography, ROI drawing in a renogram is independent of the dilatation of the system and is related to plasma concentration and protocol of injection of the radiotracer.
42. Four main questions must be considered for the management of a dilated system. A radionuclide scan canNOT answer which of the following questions?
   (a) What is the cause?
   (b) Is the intervention appropriate?
   (c) What intervention is appropriate?
   (d) What is the outcome?

43. All of the following statements regarding renal obstruction are correct *except*:
    (a) Measurement of a split function before and after compression is indicated for the selection between the removal of the stone or the kidney when a kidney stone with intermediate function exists.
    (b) The most common and malignant complication of urinary schistosomiasis is ureteral hypotonia.
    (c) Ureterocele is the cyst formation in the submucosal segment of the ureter that moves into the bladder and causes filling defects and obstruction.
    (d) In a doublex system, obstruction is commonly observed in the ureter connected to the upper bridge, and the ureter connected to the lower bridge is more susceptible to reflux and infection.
44. All statements regarding urinary diversion are correct *except*:
    (a) In a standard ileal loop diversion, posterior imaging is performed for 15 min, and then furosemide is injected for loop imaging and excretion.
    (b) The prevalence of obstruction in a standard ileal loop diversion is 18–18.4%.
    (c) A sawtooth pattern is dominantly observed in the drainage phase and indicates obstruction.
    (d) A regular isotopic scan for the determination of GFR is NOT required for these patients.
45. Which of the following statements about obstruction in pregnancy is NOT correct?
    (a) The cause of obstruction in pregnancy is hormonal or mechanical.
    (b) Dilatation of the urinary system is more dominant on the right side.
    (c) Ruling out of obstruction is required at the time of the clinical presentation of infection.
    (d) Sonography-guided decompression is a simple method for de-obstruction. When this method is NOT possible, IVP and diuretic renography are recommended.
46. What is the recommended method for the routine evaluation of asymptomatic patients after extracorporeal shock wave lithotripsy (ESWL)?
    (a) Abdominal radiography
    (b) Renal sonography
    (c) IVU
    (d) Abdominal radiography + renal sonography

8.9.1 Answer

	A	B	C	D
1				*
2	*			
3	*			
4				*
5		*		
6	*			

7			*	
8	*			
9			*	
10			*	
11		*		
12	*			
13			*	
14		*		
15	*			
16				*
17			*	
18				*
19		*		
20				*
21				*
22		*		
23				*
24			*	
25			*	
26	*			
27			*	
28			*	
29			*	
30		*		
31				*
32	*			
33	*			
34				*
35			*	
36	*			
37				*
38				*
39				*
40		*		
41				*
42	*			
43			*	
44				*
45				*
46				*

8.10 Vascular Disorders, with Emphasis on Hypertension

1. In patients with high clinical suspicion of renovascular hypertension and history of iodine allergy, it is preferred to recommend:
   (a) Computed tomography angiography (CTA)
   (b) Magnetic resonance angiography (MRA)
   (c) Captopril scintigraphy
   (d) Doppler sonography (DS)
2. In identifying renal artery stenosis with a captopril renal scan, which one is the least effective?
   (a) More than 2 min increase of peak time
   (b) More than 30% alteration of the cortical retention ratio
   (c) More than 20% decrease in the total renal flow
   (d) More than 10% increase in the differential function
3. Which of the following has the least effect on a positive renal scan with ACE inhibitors?
   (a) Cortical uptake ratio
   (b) Renogram pattern
   (c) Tmax
   (d) Flow curve
4. A renal perfusion scan is completed for a patient. A focal and transient increase in flow is found in the medial segments. A reduced uptake is also observed in the excretion phase. What is the most probable diagnosis?
   (a) Urinary leakage
   (b) Renal artery aneurysm
   (c) Renal hematoma
   (d) Arterial thrombosis
5. What is the effect of a reduced renal blood flow on prostaglandin E2 secretion?
   (a) No effect
   (b) Increase in PGE2 secretion
   (c) Decrease in PGE2 secretion
   (d) PGE2 secretion discontinues
6. Renal scintigraphy is performed on a patient suspected to have RVHT. Which of the following findings is the least valuable?
   (a) Unequal size of the kidneys
   (b) Delayed appearance of activity in the renal pelvis
   (c) A focal retention of activity in the parenchyma
   (d) Unequal perfusion of the kidneys
7. What is the positive pathologic finding of aspirin renography in unilateral RVH?
   (a) Quick Tmax with rapid perfusion
   (b) ^{123}I -OIH retention and elongation of Tmax in the renogram
   (c) Quick washout and early Tmax
   (d) Nonhomogenous cortical retention of ^{123}I -OIH

8. Small vessels are involved in all of the following renovascular hypertensive diseases *except*:
   (a) Systemic lupus erythematosus
   (b) Hemolytic uremic syndrome
   (c) Scleroderma
   (d) Renal vein thrombosis
9. About aspirin renography:
   (a) Aspirin increases the renal blood flow and GFR.
   (b) The total sensitivity of this procedure is lower than that of a captopril scan.
   (c) Discontinuation of ACEI drugs is NOT required before the test.
   (d) All NSAIDS must be discontinued 24 h before the test.
10. Renal artery stenosis is confirmed in a patient with hypertension. If renal function is good, what is the next step?
   (a) Drug treatment
   (b) Captopril scan
   (c) Revascularization
   (d) Follow-up with MR angiography
11. Which diuretics are contraindicated in the RVH study with captopril renal scintigraphy?
   (a) All diuretics
   (b) Ca-excreting diuretics
   (c) K-excreting diuretics
   (d) Na-excreting diuretics
12. What is the finding on exercise renography in patients with essential hypertension?
   (a) Unilateral increase in ERPF
   (b) Elongation of the parenchymal transit time in both kidneys
   (c) Bilateral decrease in GFR and ERPF
   (d) Reduced uptake of ^{99m}Tc-MAG3 in both kidneys
13. Which of the following findings is indicative of renal vascular hypertension (RVH)?
   (a) Relapse of hypertension
   (b) Grade 1 retinopathy
   (c) Abdominal bruit
   (d) Refractory hypertension
14. In which of the following conditions is extravasation and urinoma predicted?
   (a) Partial urinary tract obstruction
   (b) Nonobstructive urinary extension
   (c) Chronic mild urinary obstruction
   (d) Acute complete urinary obstruction
15. Renal scintigraphy is performed with ^{99m}Tc-DTPA. A transient focal increase in medullary uptake is found in the angiography phase. A decreased renal uptake is also observed in the excretion phase. What is the most probable diagnosis?
   (a) Renal artery aneurysm
   (b) Urinary leakage
   (c) Kidney hematoma
   (d) Arterial thrombosis

16. The renogram grade with captopril administration is 2B with no change in the base scan. What is the possibility of hypertension?
    (a) High
    (b) Low
    (c) Intermediate
    (d) Intermediate to high
17. The inferior vena cava appears on one frame after the aorta, concurrent with the kidney in the perfusion phase of a ^{99m}Tc-DTPA renal scan. What is the most probable diagnosis?
    (a) Renal failure
    (b) Arteriovenous fistula
    (c) Aneurysm of the aorta
    (d) Normal view of the scan
18. Which of the following findings is indicative of renovascular hypertension in captopril renography with ^{99m}Tc-MAG3?
    (a) 20 min to peak ratio: 36% in the captopril phase and 22% in the absence of captopril
    (b) 20 min to peak ratio: 49% in the captopril phase and 39% in the absence of captopril
    (c) Ratio of right-to-left kidney function: 46–54% in captopril phase and 49–51% in the absence of captopril
    (d) Time to peak: 360 s for captopril and 280 s in the absence of captopril
19. Aspirin induces …in renography.
    (a) Increased prostaglandin E2 production
    (b) Decreased renin production in the kidney
    (c) Increased angiotensin II production
    (d) Decreased cardiac output
20. A 67-year-old woman has been under treatment with furosemide, losartan, and nifedipine for 8 months for hypertension. Despite the treatment with three drugs, she still has uncontrolled hypertension. Therefore, captopril-enhanced renography is requested. Which of the following items properly describes the requirements for the preparation before the scan?
    (a) Discontinuation of losartan is NOT necessary.
    (b) Discontinuation of furosemide is NOT necessary.
    (c) Discontinuation of nifedipine is NOT necessary.
    (d) A low-salt regime is NOT necessary.
21. Captopril-enhanced renography is requested for a 57-year-old man who is taking atenolol for hypertension. Creatinine is normal, and the patient has drunk three glasses of water. He has NOT taken any diuretic for 3 days. One hour after oral administration of a 50 mg captopril tablet, systolic blood pressure is 90 mmHg, and diastolic blood pressure is NOT detectable. What is the best intervention?
    (a) Discontinuation of atenolol and repeat of scan after 2 days
    (b) Slow injection of enalaprilat instead of captopril and repeat of scan after 10 min
    (c) Supine position with elevated feet and re-measurement of blood pressure
    (d) Administration of losartan tablet instead of captopril and repeat of scan after 1 h

22. A 47-year-old man with recently diagnosed hypertension is evaluated. What is the most suitable diagnostic method to predict the benefits of surgical renal artery revascularization?
    (a) Selective angiography of renal artery
    (b) Renal scintigraphy before and after captopril
    (c) Doppler sonography of renal arteries
    (d) Measurement of renin in peripheral blood
23. Which statement about renovascular hypertension due to transplanted kidney artery stenosis is NOT correct?
    (a) Scan view of the kidney is NOT distinguishable from that of chronic rejection.
    (b) Renal retention is observed in captopril-enhanced ^{99m}Tc-DTPA renography.
    (c) Captopril-enhanced ^{99m}Tc-DMSA scan is indicated for diagnosis.
    (d) The view of a captopril-enhanced ^{99m}Tc-DMSA scan is similar to that of acute rejection.
24. Reduced primary uptake and bilateral symmetric parenchymal retention are observed in the renogram after ACEI administration. Which item is the least possible?
    (a) Bilateral renal artery stenosis
    (b) Injection site extravasation
    (c) Dehydration
    (d) Hypotension
25. The renogram baseline is grade 4 with no change after ACEI administration. What is the probability of RVHT?
    (a) High
    (b) Intermediate
    (c) Low
    (d) Very low
26. Renal function is NOT severely reduced, and the intermediate possibility of RVH is reported after ACEI administration. What is the next step?
    (a) Standard angiography
    (b) CTA or MRA
    (c) Doppler sonography
    (d) Follow-up
27. What is the gold standard for the diagnosis of RAS?
    (a) CT angiography
    (b) Arteriography
    (c) Captopril renography
    (d) Doppler ultrasonography
28. A captopril-enhanced renal scan is requested for a 69-year-old woman with a history of IHD, refractory hypertension, and suspected renal artery stenosis. The administration of which antihypertensive drug can postpone her scan?
    (a) TNG
    (b) Prazocine
    (c) Dipyridamole
    (d) Losartan

29. In which of the following group of patients is captopril-enhanced renography the most valuable to determine the evolution of renovascular hypertension?
    (a) Renal artery stenosis in a single kidney and agenesis of the opposite side
    (b) Bilateral renal artery stenosis
    (c) Renal artery stenosis in the presence of parenchymal kidney disease
    (d) Unilateral renal artery stenosis without the involvement of the opposite side
30. Which of the following radiopharmaceuticals is appropriate for the evaluation of renovascular hypertension if the intensity of the differential renal function in the involved kidney is less than 25%?
    (a) ^{99m}Tc-DTPA
    (b) ^{99m}Tc-MAG3
    (c) ^{131}I-OIH
    (d) ^{99m}Tc-DMSA
31. What is the pharmaceutical of choice for the detection of segmental stenosis of the renal artery?
    (a) ^{99m}Tc-MAG3
    (b) ^{99m}Tc-DTPA
    (c) ^{99m}Tc-GHA
    (d) d.^{123}I-OIH
32. Which statement about captopril renography is NOT correct?
    (a) Controlling blood pressure during the study is necessary.
    (b) ^{99m}Tc-MAG3 is the preferred radiotracer when renal function is reduced.
    (c) Captopril and enalapril must be discontinued 3 and 5 days before the test, respectively
    (d) A low-salt diet is recommended a few days before captopril administration.
33. Which of the following conditions can cause false-negative results in the diagnosis of renal artery stenosis?
    (a) Renal failure
    (b) Diabetic nephropathy
    (c) Lupus nephritis
    (d) Obstructive uropathy
34. Regarding renovascular hypertension (RVH):
    (a) Normal blood pressure excludes renal artery stenosis.
    (b) Fibromuscular disease is the most common cause of renal artery stenosis.
    (c) 25% of blood pressure cases are due to RVH.
    (d) Angioplasty is efficient in patients with a positive captopril scan.
35. Which of the following items is the least probable in renovascular hypertension due to renal artery stenosis?
    (a) Activation of the renin–angiotensin system
    (b) Decrease in afferent arteriole pressure
    (c) Decrease in efferent arteriole tonicity
    (d) Increase in angiotensin II

36. Which of the following diseases is considered one of the most common causes of hypertension due to renal artery stenosis?
    (a) Neurofibromatosis
    (b) Renal artery aneurysm
    (c) Atherosclerosis
    (d) Congenital renal artery stenosis
37. In aspirin renography:
    (a) Prostaglandin secretion increases.
    (b) Renin secretion increases.
    (c) The diagnostic sensitivity of this method is higher than that of captopril renography.
    (d) It is similar to ACE inhibitor renography.
38. The bilateral worsening of renal dysfunction after captopril is observed in the renogram. Differential diagnosis includes all of the following situations *except*:
    (a) Hypotension during test
    (b) Dehydration
    (c) Unilateral renal stenosis
    (d) Bladder fullness
39. Captopril renography is requested for a patient with refractory hypertension. The patient is under treatment with amlodipine, spironolactone, and metoprolol. What is the best recommendation for the preparation before the scan?
    (a) Discontinuation of amlodipine and spironolactone 96 h before the scan.
    (b) Discontinuation of amlodipine 48 h and metoprolol 72 h before the scan.
    (c) Discontinuation of spironolactone 48 h before the scan.
    (d) Discontinuation of drugs is NOT required, but discontinuation of a low-salt regimen a few days before the scan is required.
40. About renal artery stenosis (RAS):
    (a) RAS is the cause of 4–5% of all cases of hypertension.
    (b) RAS in children is unilateral in 35–70% of all cases.
    (c) RAS does NOT typically cause hypertension.
    (d) Stenosis of more than 50% is required for the induction of hypertension in patients with RAS.
41. Which of the following items describes the similarity of renal artery stenosis (RAS) caused by atherosclerosis to fibrous muscular dysplasia?
    (a) More common in men
    (b) More common in youth
    (c) More commonly bilateral
    (d) Bilateral in the medial or distal renal artery
42. When is captopril renography indicated for a patient with hypertension?
    (a) Hypertension for more than 3 years
    (b) Aged 25–55 years
    (c) Observation of two small kidneys on sonography
    (d) Refractory hypertension

43. What is the most reliable finding of renal artery stenosis (RAS), which is observed in 55% of cases?
    (a) Abdominal bruit
    (b) Grade II and III retinopathy
    (c) Malignant or accelerated hypertension
    (d) Septal hypertrophy in echocardiography
44. Which of the following findings is indicative of the definite diagnosis of renovascular hypertension (RVH)?
    (a) Positive captopril renal scan
    (b) Improvement of hypertension after revascularization
    (c) Stenosis of more than 80% in angiography
    (d) Severe stenosis on Doppler sonography
45. Which of the following statements about captopril renography is NOT correct?
    (a) Captopril must be discontinued 3 days before the test.
    (b) Enalapril must be discontinued 5 days before the test.
    (c) All antihypertensive drugs must be discontinued 10 h before the scan except alpha blockers.
    (d) When systolic blood pressure is less than 130 mmHg, the administration of captopril is NOT recommended.
46. All of the following statements about captopril renography are true *except*:
    (a) ACE inhibitors in renovascular hypertension decrease RPF and GFR and deteriorate renal function.
    (b) The sensitivity of the test is low if the 20 min/peak retention ratio is higher than 30%.
    (c) A 2-day protocol is preferred when the patient has discontinued antihypertensive medications.
    (d) The sensitivity of the test with tubular agents, such as ^{99m}Tc-MAG3, is greater than that with glomerular agents, such as ^{99m}Tc-DTPA.
47. What are the required doses of MAG3 and ^{131}I- or ^{123}I- OIH for the baseline and post-ACE inhibitor renography, respectively?
    (a) 7.5, 1.5 mCi; 0.3 and 2 mCi
    (b) 1.5, 7.5 mCi; 0.3 and 2 mCi
    (c) 0.3 and 2 mCi; 1.5, 7.5 mCi
    (d) 2 and 0.3 mCi; 1.5, 7.5 mCi
48. All of the following statements regarding the interpretation of captopril renography are true *except*:
    (a) Renal function below 42% on the base scan indicates the high probability of renal artery stenosis (RAS).
    (b) RAS is highly probable if the post-ACEI scan shows more than a 10% difference in renal function and when there is a 2-min delay in Tmax.
    (c) The post-ACEI scan may show minor lesions even in severe RAS.
    (d) Improvement of time to peak on the post-ACEI scan indicates the intermediate probability of RAS.

49. What is the least recommended radiotracer for captopril renography in a patient with high serum creatinine?
    (a) ^{99m}Tc-MAG3
    (b) ^{99m}Tc-DTPA
    (c) ^{123}I-OIH
    (d) ^{131}I-OIH
50. What is the administered dose of enalapril for injection 15 min before the radiotracer in ACEI renography?
    (a) 0.01–0.02 mg/kg to a maximum of 25 mg
    (b) 0.04–0.05 mg/kg to a maximum of 2.5 mg
    (c) 0.01–0.02 mg/kg to a maximum of 2.5 mg
    (d) 0.01–0.02 mg/kg to a maximum of 25 mg
51. Which of the following variables can be evaluated with renal perfusion imaging?
    (a) Renal vascularity
    (b) Arteriovenous malformation
    (c) Arteriovenous fistula
    (d) All of the above
52. What is the most common congenital renal vascular anomaly?
    (a) Renal vein duplication
    (b) Renal artery duplication
    (c) Arteriovenous malformation
    (d) Renal artery aneurysm
53. What is the most common cause of renal artery obstruction?
    (a) Invasive methods (e.g., catheterization of the umbilical artery)
    (b) Fat emboli
    (c) Dissecting the aneurysm of the abdominal aorta
    (d) Emboli of atherosclerotic plaques
54. All of the following statements regarding hypertension and kidneys are true *except*:
    (a) Exercise renography is indicated for the evaluation of essential hypertension.
    (b) Disease progression in renal artery stenosis (RAS) due to arteriosclerosis is greater than that due to fibromuscular dysplasia.
    (c) Renal artery stenosis necessarily indicates renovascular hypertension (RVH).
    (d) Renal reabsorption of salt and water increases in renal artery stenosis.
55. If the goal is to evaluate renovascular hypertension (RVH), what are the specificities of measurement of renin in the renal vein before and after captopril stimulation, respectively?
    (a) 50% and 90%
    (b) 80% and 95%
    (c) 90% and 80%
    (d) 70% and 90%

56. What percentage increase of the 20 min/peak ratio is considered positive on captopril scintigraphy?
    (a) 20%
    (b) 30%
    (c) 15%
    (d) 10%
57. What is (are) the main cause(s) of a false-negative outcome in captopril renography?
    (a) Chronic administration of angiotensin-converting enzyme inhibitors (ACEI)
    (b) Overhydration
    (c) Dehydration
    (d) a and b
58. Which of the following items does NOT properly describe the time of discontinuation of the corresponding drugs before captopril-enhanced renal scintigraphy?
    (a) Captopril, 3 days
    (b) Lysinopril, 1 week
    (c) Enalaprilate, 1 week
    (d) Enalapril, 1 week
59. All of the following statements regarding captopril scintigraphy are true *except*:
    (a) The sensitivity and specificity of the test are greater than 90%.
    (b) Bilateral involvement and renal failure do NOT decrease the sensitivity of the test.
    (c) Captopril scintigraphy enhances the renal scan pattern of patients with essential hypertension.
    (d) The pattern of obstruction on a captopril scan may be similar to that of renal artery stenosis.
60. Which of the following forms of renovascular hypertension (RNH) best responds to angioplasty, and which one shows the highest rate of recurrence?
    (a) Renal artery stenosis (RAS) due to atherosclerosis, RAS due to fibromuscular dysplasia (FMD)
    (b) RAS due to atherosclerosis, RAS due to atherosclerosis
    (c) RAS due to FMD, RAS due to FMD
    (d) RAS due to FMD, RAS due to atherosclerosis
61. If the goal is the differential diagnosis of atherosclerotic renovascular hypertension (RVH) from fibromuscular RVH, which of the following findings is suggestive of the atherosclerotic renovascular form?
    (a) Absence of carotid bruit
    (b) Progressive pattern to complete obstruction of renal artery
    (c) Absence of familial history of hypertension
    (d) Age below 50 years

8.10.1 Answer

	A	B	C	D
1		*		
2			*	
3				*
4		*		
5			*	
6				*
7		*		
8				*
9		*		
10	*			
11				*
12		*		
13			*	
14				*
15	*			
16			*	
17		*		
18		*		
19		*		
20				*
21			*	
22		*		
23		*		
24	*			
25		*		
26		*		
27		*		
28				*
29				*
30		*		
31	*			
32				*
33	*			
34				*
35			*	
36			*	
37				*
38			*	
39			*	
40			*	
41			*	
42				*
43	*			
44		*		

45			*	
46			*	
47		*		
48				*
49		*		
50		*		
51				*
52		*		
53			*	
54			*	
55	*			
56			*	
57				*
58			*	
59		*		
60			*	
61		*		

8.11 Renal Failure

1. What is the method of choice to exclude renal obstruction in the presence of multiple cysts?
   (a) High-dose urography
   (b) Helical CT
   (c) Sonography
   (d) ^{99m}Tc-MAG3 scintigraphy
2. A renal radionuclide study is performed twice on a patient. Primary blood pool and gradual disappearance of the kidneys are observed on the ^{99m}Tc-DTPA scan. The gradual accumulation of the radiotracer in renal parenchyma is found on the ^{123}-OIH scan. What is the best diagnosis?
   (a) Chronic urinary obstruction
   (b) Aminoglycoside-induced nephrotoxicity
   (c) Tubular acidosis
   (d) Diabetic nephropathy
3. In acute tubular necrosis:
   (a) Renal retention of the radiotracer is NOT observed.
   (b) Renal excretion to the bladder is functional.
   (c) The urinary collecting system is clearly observed.
   (d) The collecting system and bladder do NOT appear.
4. Which of the following statements about renal function is NOT correct?
   (a) Dialysis must be conducted in GFR below 5–10 ml/min.
   (b) Urine volume and creatinine level are NOT suitable criteria for the evaluation of renal function.
   (c) Renal scintigraphy is especially important in emergency cases of acute renal failure (ARF)
   (d) The ascending segment of the loop of Henle is the most sensitive part of the kidney to ischemia.
5. Which of the following causes of chronic renal failure does NOT induce anemia?
   (a) Diabetes
   (b) Hypertension
   (c) Polycystic kidney
   (d) Glumerulonephritis
6. What is the only method for ruling out obstruction in multicystic kidney disease?
   (a) High-dose urography
   (b) Low-dose urography
   (c) Diuretic renography with ^{99m}Tc-DTPA
   (d) Diuretic renography with ^{99m}Tc-MAG3
7. Which of the following items does NOT properly describe the pattern of acute tubular necrosis on a renal scan?
   (a) Very early peak with decreased uptake of ^{99m}Tc-DTPA.
   (b) Progressive uptake and retention of ^{123I}-OIH and ^{99m}Tc-MAG3.
   (c) Increased uptake of gallium.
   (d) ^{99m}Tc-DTPA provides a more specific scan pattern than tubular agents.

8. Which of the following statements regarding renal failure is NOT correct?
   (a) The lack of uptake of ^{99m}Tc-MAG3 and ^{123}I-OIH in acute tubular necrosis (ATN) does NOT necessarily indicate a poor prognosis.
   (b) ^{99m}Tc-DTPA scan is recommended for the diagnosis of rhabdomyolysis.
   (c) The pattern of a renal scan with all tubular agents in bilateral pyelonephritis is similar to that in ATN.
   (d) The evaluation of fever of unknown origin is critical in patients who undergo dialysis, and gallium scan is recommended for the detection of renal infection, which is common in these patients.
9. Which of the following scans shows a normal pattern in interstitial nephritis?
   (a) ^{68}Ga
   (b) ^{99m}Tc-DTPA
   (c) ^{99m}Tc-DMSA
   (d) ^{99m}Tc-MAG3
10. All of the following items regarding hemolytic uremic syndrome (UHS), a form of thrombotic microangiopathy, are correct *except*:
    (a) It is usually associated with hypotension and is common in children.
    (b) Prothrombin time (PT) is normal.
    (c) ^{99m}Tc-MAG3 uptake indicates a good prognosis.
    (d) The scan pattern shows hypoperfusion.
11. Which of the following items about renal scintigraphy in acute glomerulonephritis is NOT correct?
    (a) Enlargement of the kidneys.
    (b) Hypoperfusion.
    (c) The scan can help in the diagnosis.
    (d) Acute glomerulonephritis is usually accompanied with proteinuria

8.11.1 Answer

	A	B	C	D
1	*			
2		*		
3				*
4			*	
5			*	
6	*			
7			*	
8		*		
9		*		
10	*			
11			*	

8.12 Renal Space-Occupying Lesions and Trauma

1. Which radiotracer specifically accumulates in renal cell carcinoma?
   (a) ^{99m}Tc-glucoheptonate
   (b) ^{99m}Tc-DMSA
   (c) a and b
   (d) None
2. Which of the following renal problems is commonly observed after radiotherapy of the abdomen?
   (a) Hematuria
   (b) Proteinuria
   (c) Hematoma
   (d) Renal vein thrombosis
3. What is the minimum detectable size of a tumor on renal scintigraphy?
   (a) 3 cm
   (b) 1 cm
   (c) 4 cm
   (d) 2 cm
4. What are the least and most valuable methods for the evaluation of intrarenal mass, respectively?
   (a) Scintigraphy, MRI
   (b) IVP, sonography
   (c) IVP, CT
   (d) MRI, scintigraphy
5. Which space-occupying lesion exhibits an uptake of renal radiotracers?
   (a) Oncocytoma
   (b) Cyst
   (c) Mesoblastic nephroma
   (d) a and c
6. If the goal is to evaluate kidney trauma, which radiotracer is NOT indicated? In addition, renal scintigraphy is performed in … phases.
   (a) ^{99m}Tc-MAG3, double
   (b) ^{99m}Tc-DMSA, double
   (c) ^{99m}Tc-GH, triple
   (d) ^{99m}Tc-DMSA, triple

8.12.1 Answer

	A	B	C	D
1				*
2		*		
3				*
4			*	
5				*
6				*

8.13 Renal Transplant Evaluation

1. Short-segment stenosis following renal transplant is probably due to:
   (a) Rejection
   (b) Surgical intimal injury
   (c) Turbulent flow
   (d) Reaction to the suture material
2. A substantial decrease in perfusion and function of the transplanted kidney is observed on the renal scan of the day after surgery. Which one is the least probable?
   (a) Arterial thrombosis
   (b) Venous thrombosis
   (c) Acute tubular necrosis (ATN)
   (d) Acute rejection
3. In contrast-induced nephrotoxicity, which of the following radiotracers results in the blood-pool view with gradual vanishing?
   (a) ^{99m}Tc-DTPA
   (b) ^{99m}Tc-MAG3
   (c) ^{123}I-OIH
   (d) ^{99m}Tc-GHA
4. Which of the following statements regarding hyperacute rejection is true?
   (a) It usually occurs 5 days to years following transplant.
   (b) It is predominantly cell mediated (T cell).
   (c) It is irreversible and due to the close allogenic matching between donor and host.
   (d) Scintigraphy usually shows a reduced perfusion, while function is relatively maintained.
5. In kidney transplantation, normal parenchymal transit is observed in:
   (a) ATN
   (b) Acute rejection
   (c) Cyclosporine-induced severe toxicity
   (d) Stable chronic rejection

6. Angiography of a normal transplanted kidney is depicted below. Which radiopharmaceutical is used for such an evaluation?
   (a) ^{99m}TC-MAG3
   (b) ^{99m}TC-EC
   (c) ^{131}I-OIH
   (d) ^{99m}TC-DTPA

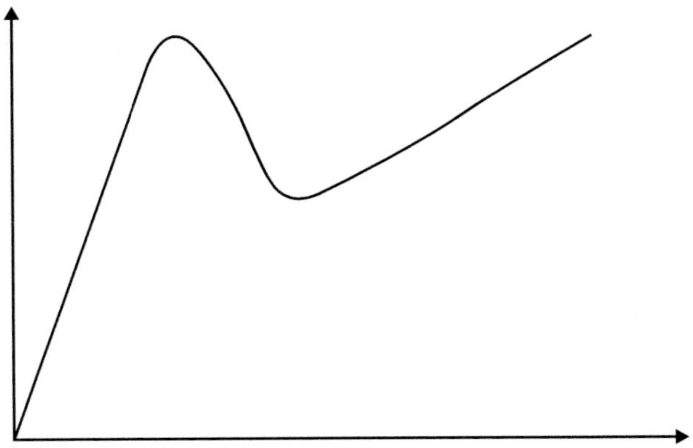

7. What are the ^{99m}Tc-DTPA scintigraphy findings on a patient with ATN?
   (a) Reduced perfusion, reduced cortical uptake
   (b) Reduced perfusion, normal cortical uptake
   (c) Normal perfusion, reduced cortical uptake
   (d) Reduced perfusion, retention in collecting system
8. Which of the following situations can cause false-negative findings in the diagnosis of rejection of transplanted kidney by a ^{99m}Tc-sulfur colloid scan?
   (a) Coexisting rejection and infection in the first week
   (b) Intense administration of corticosteroids
   (c) Chronic rejection
   (d) Coexisting rejection and ATN
9. Fever, tenderness of the grafted region, decreased urine volume, and increased creatinine are observed 1 week after kidney transplantation. Moreover, slow uptake, obvious parenchymal retention, and decreased excretion in a swelling kidney are observed in the ^{99m}-Tc-MAG3 renography. What is the most probable diagnosis?
   (a) Cell-mediated rejection
   (b) Renal vein thrombosis
   (c) Acute pyelonephritis
   (d) CMV infection

10. What is the Page kidney phenomenon in transplanted kidney?
    (a) Primary stages of ATN
    (b) Chronic rejection
    (c) Graft suppression with hematoma
    (d) Inflammatory reaction
11. ^{99m}-TC-sulfur colloid is used for differentiating ATN from acute rejection. What is the mechanism of sulfur colloid accumulation in acute rejection?
    (a) Phagocytosis by reticuloendothelial tissue
    (b) Trapping in thrombus fibrin
    (c) Interstitial leakage
    (d) Uptake by inflammatory tissue
12. This quantitative index for the evaluation of renal graft function is calculated by renal vascular transit time. Its normal value is less than 12.8 s.
    (a) Quantitation of parenchymal retention
    (b) Perfusion index
    (c) Cortical perfusion index
    (d) Deconvolution analysts of renal blood flow
13. ^{99m}Tc-MAG3 scan is performed on a transplanted kidney. The perfusion status is better than function, uptake is slow, and Tmax is reached at the end of the study. What is the most probable diagnosis?
    (a) ATN
    (b) Elongated obstructive uropathy
    (c) Chronic rejection
    (d) Pyelonephritis
14. ERPF and GFR are evaluated on a patient who underwent kidney transplantation. The reduction of ERPF is greater than that of GFR. What is the most probable diagnosis?
    (a) ATN
    (b) Renal artery stenosis
    (c) Rejection of the transplanted kidney
    (d) Glomerulonephritis
15. Decreased uptake and clearance are observed in the ^{99m}Tc-DTPA renography of a child 5 months after transplantation. An increased uptake is observed by the ^{99m}Tc-sulfur colloid. What is the most probable diagnosis?
    (a) Chronic rejection
    (b) Vasomotor nephropathy
    (c) Acute rejection
    (d) Cyclosporine-induced nephrotoxicity
16. Which of the following findings on a transplanted kidney is indicative of emergency surgery?
    (a) Hematoma
    (b) Abscess
    (c) Urinary leakage
    (d) Lymphocele

17. A ^{99m}Tc-EC renal scan is performed on a patient with transplanted kidney and now presenting with a gradual elevation of creatinine in the first 3 days after renal transplantation. On semiquantitative analysis, Tmax and *20 min/3 minute* count *ratio* are increased. In the follow-up scan performed 2 weeks later, a reduced Tmax and parenchymal transit time are observed. What is the most probable diagnosis?
    (a) Acute tubular necrosis
    (b) Acute cell-mediated rejection
    (c) Obstruction due to hematoma
    (d) Chronic nephropathy
18. Which of the following transplanted kidney complications usually appears in 2–4 months after surgery?
    (a) Abscess
    (b) Hematoma
    (c) Lymphocele
    (d) Urinary leakage
19. A 10-year-old child underwent kidney transplantation last week because of renal failure. The creatinine level increases the day after surgery. The quantitative perfusion factors on the kidney scintigraphy are as follows: vascular transit time, 8 s, and graft blood flow, 12% of the cardiac output. What is the most probable diagnosis?
    (a) Acute tubular necrosis
    (b) Acute rejection
    (c) Cyclosporine toxicity
    (d) Vascular hypertension due to hematoma
20. The perfusion of transplanted kidney in a child is less than 5% of the cardiac output. What is the most probable diagnosis?
    (a) ATN
    (b) Rejection
    (c) Renal artery thrombosis
    (d) Normal
21. The perfusion of a transplanted kidney is low, but function is relatively good. What is the most probable diagnosis?
    (a) ATN
    (b) Acute rejection
    (c) Chronic rejection
    (d) Page kidney
22. A significant decrease in perfusion with acceptable function is observed on the renal scan of a patient who underwent kidney transplantation less than 1 week ago. What is the most probable cause of this finding?
    (a) ATN
    (b) Rejection
    (c) Hematoma
    (d) Lymphocele

23. A 74-year-old man with a transplanted kidney is referred with increased creatinine. Normal perfusion and parenchymal retention are observed on the ^{99m}Tc-MAG3 dynamic scan. Furthermore, a mild increase in uptake in the transplanted kidney is found on the ^{99m}Tc-SC scan. What is the most probable diagnosis?
    (a) Acute tubular necrosis
    (b) Acute rejection
    (c) Chronic rejection
    (d) Renal infection
24. Which of the following factors best represents the function of a transplanted kidney on a renal scan?
    (a) Initial uptake
    (b) Renal excretion of the radiotracer
    (c) Excretory activity
    (d) Renal perfusion
25. ^{99m}Tc-DTPA scan is performed on an 18-year-old girl who underwent kidney transplantation 2 months ago. A mild decreased perfusion but severe decreased function is reported. The scan findings are suggestive of:
    (a) Acute tubular necrosis
    (b) Cyclosporine toxicity
    (c) Arterial stenosis
    (d) Rejection
26. What is the pattern of renography in the early stages of renal vein thrombosis?
    (a) Small kidney, decreased perfusion, normal function
    (b) Small kidney, decreased perfusion and function
    (c) Large kidney, decreased function, normal perfusion
    (d) Large kidney, decreased perfusion and function
27. Which of the complications of kidney transplantation usually occurs 5 days to 3 months after transplantation?
    (a) Acute tubular necrosis
    (b) Acute rejection
    (c) Chronic rejection
    (d) Hyperacute rejection
28. Which of the complications of kidney transplantation is most commonly observed in a cadaveric kidney?
    (a) Acute rejection
    (b) Acute tubular necrosis
    (c) Chronic rejection
    (d) Hyperacute rejection
29. Intravascular thrombosis is observed in … after kidney transplantation.
    (a) Acute tubular necrosis
    (b) Acute rejection
    (c) Chronic rejection
    (d) Hyperacute rejection

30. Arteriolar endothelial proliferation is reported in … after kidney transplantation.
    (a) Acute tubular necrosis
    (b) Acute rejection
    (c) Chronic rejection
    (d) Hyperacute rejection
31. An increased uptake in the transplanted kidney is observed on the ^{111}In-platelet scan. What is the most probable diagnosis?
    (a) Acute tubular necrosis
    (b) Acute rejection
    (c) Cyclosporine toxicity
    (d) Renal infarction
32. About the 20 min/peak ratio (in the third min) for a transplanted kidney:
    (a) Decreases in acute rejection.
    (b) This ratio is less than 0.8 in a healthy transplanted kidney.
    (c) It is higher than normal in chronic rejection.
    (d) It is normal in ATN.
33. The patient experiences severe pain and anuria 2 h after the completion of kidney transplantation. ^{99m}Tc-DTPA renal scintigraphy is immediately conducted, and it shows the absence of the transplanted kidney. Which of the following diseases is NOT possible?
    (a) Renal artery emboli
    (b) Renal vein thrombosis
    (c) ATN
    (d) Hyperacute rejection
34. In a transplanted kidney, the scan pattern of … is similar to that of severe nephrotoxicity due to cyclosporine A.
    (a) Acute rejection
    (b) ATN
    (c) RAS (renal artery stenosis)
    (d) Chronic rejection
35. Which of the following situations can be mistaken for hyperacute rejection of a kidney transplant?
    (a) Vascular obstruction
    (b) Acute tubular necrosis
    (c) Cyclosporine toxicity
    (d) Acute rejection
36. Which of the following diseases is characterized by hypoperfusion but with a relatively good function of the renal transplant?
    (a) ATN
    (b) External pressure to the kidney transplant
    (c) Drug toxicity
    (d) Chronic rejection

37. All of the following statements regarding scintigraphy of the transplanted kidney are correct *except*:
    (a) Problems on the renal scan appear a few days before the biochemical findings.
    (b) There is NO specific isotopic agent for each complication.
    (c) Serial scans are required for the evaluation of graft, although assessment on only vascular thrombosis and urinary leakage is possible with a single scan.
    (d) The average functioning time for a transplanted kidney (conserving of 50% of function) from a living donor is 7–8 years.
38. Which of the following radiotracers is NOT indicated for the study of flow phase in a transplanted kidney?
    (a) ^{123}I
    (b) ^{131}I
    (c) ^{99m}Tc
    (d) a and b
39. All of the following statements regarding perfusion index (PI) are true *except*:
    (a) PI can generally differentiate between arterial and parenchymal phases.
    (b) The normal value of PI is below 150.
    (c) All other criteria can differentiate between normal and rejected graft, but only PI can distinguish rejection from acute tubular necrosis (ATN).
    (d) The greater the time interval between normal iliac peak and graft peak is, the higher the probability of rejection.
40. All of the following statements regarding T1/2 on the scintigraphy of a renal graft are true *except*:
    (a) If T1/2 is longer than 10 s for aortic or iliac arteries, the radiotracer will NOT be injected properly. This finding is independent of the volume of injection.
    (b) T1/2 of the descending phase of perfusion curve is normally less than 18 s, which increases to 18–28 s in ATN and to longer than 28 s in rejection.
    (c) Vascular transit time is an appropriate criterion because of its similarity among subjects.
    (d) Distinguishing among ATN, rejection, and cyclosporine toxicity is an important issue on renal graft scintigraphy.
41. All of the following statements regarding renal transplant rejection are true *except*:
    (a) Lymphocyte infiltration is observed in the cellular type.
    (b) The vascular form is due to obstruction.
    (c) Cell-mediated rejection is similar to cyclosporine A toxicity.
    (d) The sensitivity and specificity of the perfusion index for the differentiation between cellular and vascular rejection are 86 and 94%, respectively.
42. What is the radiotracer of choice for renal graft scintigraphy?
    (a) ^{99m}Tc-Glucoheptonate
    (b) ^{99m}Tc-DTPA
    (c) ^{99m}Tc-MAG3
    (d) ^{99m}I-OIH

43. Which of the following diseases does NOT necessarily cause retention in the parenchymal system of a renal graft?
    (a) Cyclosporine A toxicity
    (b) Acute tubular necrosis (ATN)
    (c) Acute rejection
    (d) Dehydration
44. What is the most commonly used index in renal drainage?
    (a) Time of peak in a renogram
    (b) Time of elimination of half-activity
    (c) Blood clearance curve
    (d) Time of appearance of the bladder
45. Which of the following items about the application or definition of accumulation index (AI) and elimination index (EI) is NOT correct?
    (a) They are used in children.
    (b) AI represents perfusion.
    (c) EI represents retention.
    (d) EI can represent an effective renal plasma flow (ERPF).
46. After kidney transplantation … is NOT common in the first month.
    (a) Acute tubular necrosis (ATN)
    (b) Acute rejection
    (c) Urologic complications
    (d) Cyclosporine A toxicity
47. Which of the following statements regarding renal graft artery stenosis is NOT correct?
    (a) Short-segment stenosis is usually due to rejection.
    (b) Captopril renal scan is the best method for the diagnosis of renal graft artery stenosis.
    (c) The definite diagnosis of renovascular hypertension (RVH) is confirmed with improvement after revascularization.
    (d) Angiography is indicated only after an abnormal scan.
48. All of the following statements regarding the complications of kidney transplantation are correct *except*:
    (a) Hyperacute rejection is due to the previous formation of antibodies, and the scan pattern is photopenic.
    (b) Hypertension during surgery is one of the risk factors for acute tubular necrosis (ATN).
    (c) The severity of cyclosporine A toxicity is different among subjects, but it is inversely related to the age of the donor.
    (d) Acute rejection never occurs before 5 days.
49. Graft rupture rarely occurs in kidney transplantation, and it is associated with:
    (a) Graft vein thrombosis and acute rejection
    (b) Acute rejection and cyclosporine A toxicity
    (c) Graft vein thrombosis and arteriovenous fistula
    (d) Acute rejection and arteriovenous fistula

50. Which of the following complications of kidney transplantation exhibits a different scan pattern in comparison with the other items?
    (a) Cyclosporine A toxicity
    (b) New disease in renal graft
    (c) Chronic rejection
    (d) Graft vein thrombosis
51. The following situations are the differential diagnoses of renal graft infarction *except*:
    (a) Perirenal fluid
    (b) Hematoma
    (c) Lymphocele
    (d) Arteriovenous fistula
52. All of the following items regarding arteriovenous fistula are correct *except*:
    (a) It is formed because of biopsy.
    (b) It is presented with the clinical symptoms of high output cardiac failure.
    (c) Scan shows decreased activity in the perfusion phase with the early appearance of the inferior vena cava.
    (d) It is self-limited in most cases.
53. All of the following statements regarding renal graft rejection are correct *except*:
    (a) Radionuclide methods can differentiate between cellular and humoral rejections.
    (b) Graft function may be affected by the function of the original kidney (e.g., renin secretion from the original kidney).
    (c) A renal graft with poor function may NOT show a dilation response to obstruction and fail to respond to furosemide stimulation. Therefore, system dilatation is NOT necessarily required for the diagnosis of obstruction.
    (d) Graft rejection is one of the causes of ureteral stenosis.
54. A patient with renal graft complains about flank pain. Scan shows an abnormal increase in uptake outside the urinary tract with a poorly defined margin. What is the most probable diagnosis?
    (a) Rejection
    (b) Urinoma
    (c) Hematoma
    (d) Lymphocele
55. The incidence of false-positive findings is high in the evaluation of acute rejection of renal graft with typical radiotracers. Therefore, more specific radiotracers are preferred. All of the following radiotracers are specific *except*:
    (a) ^{125}I-fibrinogen
    (b) ^{99m}Tc-sulfur colloid
    (c) ^{67}Ga
    (d) ^{111}In-WBC

56. The labeling of which cells is the most appropriate for the diagnosis of acute rejection?
    (a) RBC
    (b) Lymphocytes
    (c) Platelets
    (d) Leukocytes
57. How long after kidney transplantation does accelerated rejection occur?
    (a) Minutes to hours postoperatively
    (b) After 5 days
    (c) 1–5 days
    (d) Second to fourth month postoperatively
58. Which type of renal graft rejection is irreversible?
    (a) Hyperacute
    (b) Accelerated
    (c) Chronic
    (d) a and c
59. Prolonged transit time is defined as the appearance of renal peak after the … min or the appearance of the pelvis after the … min on a renal scan.
    (a) 6th, 8th
    (b) 8th, 6th
    (c) 8th, 8th
    (d) 6th, 6th
60. What causes a Page kidney, and what is the scan pattern of this disease?
    (a) Compression effect of the lymphocele on the kidney, poor perfusion, relatively good function
    (b) Compression effect of hematoma on the kidney, good perfusion, relatively good function
    (c) Compression effect of the lymphocele on the kidney, relatively good perfusion, poor function
    (d) Compression effect of hematoma on the kidney, poor perfusion, poor function
61. Perfusion of the kidney is relatively better than its function. The uptake of the tracer is impaired, and clearance is diminished. What is the most appropriate diagnosis?
    (a) Acute rejection
    (b) ATN
    (c) Cyclosporine toxicity
    (d) Chronic rejection
62. All of the following statements regarding renal graft scan indices are correct *except*:
    (a) Vascular transit time (VTT) in ATN is 5.4 ± 3.1 min.
    (b) VTT in acute rejection is 20.6 ± 6.4 min.
    (c) Peak activity appears approximately in the 10th min.
    (d) Time of half-activity from peak is 5–6 min.

63. The graft is enlarged with impaired perfusion and uptake and has prolonged parenchymal transit and decreased excretion. What is the most probable diagnosis?
    (a) ATN
    (b) Acute rejection
    (c) Cyclosporine toxicity
    (d) Chronic rejection
64. The graft has a thin cortex with mild hydronephrosis and low tracer uptake but has normal parenchymal transit with absent or minimal cortical retention (normal Tmax with low GFR and ERPF). What is the best diagnosis?
    (a) ATN
    (b) Acute rejection
    (c) Cyclosporine toxicity
    (d) Chronic rejection
65. The scintigraphic patterns of mild and severe toxicity of cyclosporine A are similar to those of … and …, respectively.
    (a) Minor acute rejection (AR), chronic rejection
    (b) Chronic rejection, ATN
    (c) Chronic rejection, minor AR
    (d) Minor AR, hyperacute rejection
66. All of the following statements regarding renal graft scintigraphy are correct *except*:
    (a) Captopril renal scan is indicated for distinguishing renovascular hypertension (RVH) due to renal artery stenosis (RAS) from chronic rejection.
    (b) The pattern of RVH due to RAS is similar to that of acute rejection on the captopril renal scan.
    (c) Although cortical lesions are observed in the early images, they are nonspecific and require confirmation with other imaging methods and biopsy.
    (d) There is NO difference in the perfusion patterns between ^{99m}Tc-MAG3 and ^{99m}Tc-DTPA.
67. … scan is recommended for the differentiation of acute rejection from cyclosporine A toxicity in pediatrics. However, … scan provides high sensitivity but low specificity.
    (a) ^{99m}Tc-DTPA, ^{99m}Tc-SC
    (b) ^{99m}Tc-SC, ^{111}In-WBC
    (c) ^{111}In-RBC, ^{131}I-fibrinogen
    (d) ^{67}Ga, ^{111}In-Platelet
68. Which of the following tumors is the most probable in a patient with kidney transplantation?
    (a) Hemangioma
    (b) Angiosarcoma
    (c) Lymphangioleiomyomatosis
    (d) Kaposi's sarcoma

69. Which of the following scan indices is used for the evaluation of a pancreas graft?
   (a) T1/2
   (b) First-pass curve
   (c) Accumulation index
   (d) Elimination index

8.13.1 Answer

	A	B	C	D
1				*
2				*
3	*			
4			*	
5				*
6				*
7			*	
8			*	
9	*			
10			*	
11		*		
12				*
13	*			
14	*			
15			*	
16			*	
17		*		
18			*	
19	*			
20		*		
21				*
22			*	
23	*			
24	*			
25		*		
26				*
27		*		
28		*		
29				*
30			*	
31		*		
32		*		
33			*	
34		*		
35	*			
36		*		

37				*
38		*		
39	*			
40			*	
41			*	
42			*	
43				*
44		*		
45				*
46				*
47	*			
48		*		
49	*			
50				*
51				*
52			*	
53			*	
54		*		
55				*
56			*	
57			*	
58				*
59				*
60	*			
61		*		
62			*	
63		*		
64				*
65		*		
66				*
67	*			
68				*
69		*		

8.14 Genital Tract

1. The halo sign is seen in all of the following *except*:
   (a) Henoch–Schonlein purpura
   (b) Hematoma
   (c) Spermatocele
   (d) Non-infected hydrocele
2. An 18-year-old child is referred for a testicular scan. He developed sudden pain in the left testis 10 h ago, but the pain has slightly been attenuated in recent hours. Physical examination shows slight swelling and tenderness. Testicular scintigraphy reveals a normal angiography phase but a small hyperemia of the left testis in the static phase. What is the most probable diagnosis?
   (a) Spontaneous detorsion
   (b) Idiopathic scrotal edema
   (c) Acute hydrocele
   (d) Orchitis after the administration of an analgesic
3. The bull's eye sign on a scrotal scan is rare in:
   (a) Hematoma
   (b) Varicocele
   (c) Late missed torsion
   (d) Testicular abscess
4. What is the best test for the diagnosis of hydrocele?
   (a) Real-time sonography (RTUS)
   (b) Tc-99m-pertechnetate scintigraphy
   (c) CT Scan
   (d) Doppler
5. Which of the following modalities is commonly used for the evaluation of the scrotum?
   (a) Doppler sonography
   (b) Isotopic scan
   (c) Sonography
   (d) MRI
6. A 9-year-old boy with acute testicular pain is referred to the emergency room. Increased perfusion and radioactive accumulation in the left hemiscrotum with a margin of photon deficiency are observed on the testicular scan. What is the most probable diagnosis?
   (a) Acute torsion
   (b) Testicular appendage torsion
   (c) Epididymo-orchitis
   (d) Thrombotic varicocele
7. About the diagnosis of testicular torsion with ^{99m}Tc-pertechnetate:
   (a) Asymmetrical reduction of perfusion and decrease in parenchymal uptake
   (b) Asymmetrical increase in perfusion and increase in parenchymal uptake
   (c) Asymmetrical increase in blood circulation and central photopenia in the parenchymal phase
   (d) Symmetrical perfusion and parenchymal uptake in the scrotum

8. Scrotal scintigraphy of acute hemiscrotum is performed. What is indicated by a diffuse increase in perfusion and blood pool without photopenic regions?
   (a) Primary phase of testicular torsion
   (b) Delayed phase of testicular torsion or hydrocele
   (c) Torsion of appendix of the testis
   (d) Delayed phase of hematoma or missed torsion
9. Scrotal scintigraphy of acute hemiscrotum is performed. What is indicated by a diffuse decrease in perfusion and blood pool?
   (a) Primary phase of testicular torsion
   (b) Delayed phase of testicular torsion or hydrocele
   (c) Torsion of appendix of the testis
   (d) Delayed phase of hematoma or missed torsion
10. Scrotal scintigraphy of acute hemiscrotum is performed. What is indicated by a photopenic region with a marginal increase in activity (doughnut sign)?
    (a) Primary phase of testicular torsion
    (b) Delayed phase of testicular torsion or hydrocele
    (c) Torsion of appendix of the testis
    (d) Delayed phase of hematoma or missed torsion
11. Which of the following diseases is diagnosed with the nubbin sign on scrotal scintigraphy?
    (a) Epididymitis
    (b) Hydrocele
    (c) Torsion
    (d) Hematoma
12. An 18-year-old boy with a history of severe pain in the right testis since yesterday is referred. Hyperemia of the sclerotal zone in the flow phase and photopenia of the right testis with a marginal increased uptake in the static phase are obtained from the scan. What is the most probable diagnosis?
    (a) Acute torsion
    (b) Early missed torsion
    (c) Late missed torsion
    (d) Spontaneous torsion
13. An 8-year-old boy is referred with pain and edema of the right hemiscrotum after football. A diffuse decrease in the radiotracer uptake in the hemiscrotum is observed on the scan. What is the best answer if you are asked about whether surgery is necessary?
    (a) Surgery is not required with high probability
    (b) Surgery is required with high probability
    (c) Delayed images are required for further evaluation
    (d) The scan must be repeated

14. In which of the following conditions is scrotal scan preferred over sonography for the evaluation of acute scrotal dysfunction?
    (a) A 78-year-old man with sudden onset pain in the right hemiscrotum after trauma
    (b) A 22-year-old man with pain in the left hemiscrotum after urinary infection
    (c) A 42-year-old man with pain in the left hemiscrotum after urinary infection
    (d) A 60-year-old man with pain in the right hemiscrotum 12 h after urinary catheter
15. A patient with a history of epididymitis is referred to the emergency room because of sudden pain and scrotal edema. A diffusely increased activity in the perfusion phase and a rim activity in the right hemiscrotum in the static phase are found on the testicular scan. What is the most probable diagnosis?
    (a) Abscess
    (b) Acute torsion
    (c) Missed torsion
    (d) Hydrocele
16. Which of the following views in radionuclide hysterosalpingography (RNHSP) have been suggested to help separate anatomic structures?
    (a) Caudal angulation
    (b) Lateral oblique images
    (c) Tail on detector views
    (d) All of the above
17. A crescent sign of a reduced uptake in the lateral hemiscrotum is observed on scrotal scintigraphy. What is the most probable diagnosis?
    (a) Hydrocele
    (b) Scrotal torsion
    (c) Epididymitis
    (d) Abscess
18. A 5-year-old boy is subjected to a scrotal scan because of pain and edema of the hemiscrotum from 4 h ago. A region with a reduced uptake is observed on the scan. Which of the following diagnoses is the LEAST possible?
    (a) Testicular torsion
    (b) Hydrocele
    (c) Testicular appendages torsion
    (d) Hemangioma
19. Which of the following testicular problems presents a diffusely increased blood flow and blood pool without photopenic defect on scrotal scintigraphy?
    (a) Acute torsion
    (b) Abscess
    (c) Epididymitis
    (d) Testicular appendage torsion

20. Which of the following testicular problems presents a focal increase in blood flow and blood pool on scrotal scintigraphy?
    (a) Acute torsion
    (b) Abscess
    (c) Epididymitis
    (d) Testicular appendage torsion
21. Which of the following testicular problems presents a central photopenic defect with a marginal increase in activity on scrotal scintigraphy?
    (a) Acute torsion
    (b) Abscess
    (c) Epididymitis
    (d) Testicular appendage torsion
22. In which of the following conditions is the scrotal isotopic scan the method of choice for diagnosis?
    (a) Acute pain and edema of the testis after trauma
    (b) Ectopic testis
    (c) Acute pain and edema of the testis without trauma
    (d) Painless enlargement of the testis
23. What is the pattern of chronic torsion on a scrotal scan?
    (a) Increased uptake in the perfusion phase, decreased uptake in the static phase, small size of the testes
    (b) Normal uptake in the perfusion phase, normal uptake in the static phase, asymmetric size of the testes
    (c) Decreased uptake in the perfusion phase, increased uptake in the static phase, asymmetric size of the testes
    (d) Normal uptake in the perfusion phase, decreased uptake in the static phase, small size of the testes
24. Which statement about testicular appendage torsion is NOT correct?
    (a) It is a surgical case similar to testicular torsion.
    (b) The scan is normal in some cases.
    (c) Its clinical presentation is similar to that of acute scrotum.
    (d) Scan results in abnormal cases are similar to those of epididymitis.
25. The diagnosis of hydrocele is presumed for a patient with acute scrotal pain and edema. Which of the following scan methods is beneficial for a more accurate diagnosis?
    (a) Posterior caudal view
    (b) Anterior recumbent view with marker
    (c) Upright view
    (d) Anterior view with complete leg abduction
26. What happens to the sensitivity and specificity of a scan for the diagnosis of testicular torsion if the scan is performed more than 12 h after the onset of clinical presentation?
    (a) Decreased sensitivity, no change in specificity
    (b) No change in sensitivity, decreased specificity
    (c) Increased sensitivity, decreased specificity
    (d) Increased sensitivity, increased specificity

27. Which of the following torsions can be presented with symptoms similar to those of testicular torsion?
    (a) Torsion of testicular appendage
    (b) Torsion of paradidymis
    (c) Torsion of vas aberrans
    (d) All of the above
28. All of the following arteries are the main testicular arteries with different origins *except*:
    (a) Testicular artery from the aorta
    (b) Vassal artery from the internal iliac artery
    (c) Cremasteric artery from the inferior epigastric artery
    (d) Pudendal arteries from the renal artery
29. Which of the following statements about testicular torsion is NOT correct?
    (a) Torsion occurs commonly among adolescents with a history of strong physical activity or minor trauma and previous episodes of scrotal pain.
    (b) Extravaginal torsion occurs dominantly in children or in adults, whereas intravaginal torsion occurs dominantly in neonates.
    (c) Bell clapper deformity is the coverage of the whole testis by tunica vaginalis, which is usually bilateral.
    (d) A scan is NOT indicated for a perfusion study after detorsion or orchiopexy.
30. Which of the following symptoms is rare in testicular torsion?
    (a) Abdominal pain
    (b) Nausea and vomiting
    (c) Fever
    (d) Pyuria
31. Which of the following statements about testicular torsion is NOT correct?
    (a) Necrosis is induced in 100% of cases of extravaginal torsion.
    (b) Scrotal scintigraphy consists of two phases.
    (c) Converging and pinhole collimators are commonly used in adults and children, respectively.
    (d) The perfusion phase of the scan is the most important.
32. All of the following items describe the scan pattern in intravaginal torsion *except*:
    (a) Hypoperfusion of the whole testis in the primary phase (5–7 h) of the scan.
    (b) Rim activity in the medial phase (7–24 h) of scan.
    (c) Infarct (rim activity) is always observed in the late phase (>24 h) of the scan (missed torsion).
    (d) The nubbin sign is a common and specific sign of torsion.
33. The rim sign (halo or bull's eye sign) on testicular scintigraphy indicates:
    (a) Testicular necrosis, but the testis can be recovered if the pattern is NOT highly intense
    (b) Testicular necrosis, and the testis is NOT recoverable
    (c) Hypoactivity in the spermatic cord (matched with the obstruction site) because of a sudden vascular cutoff after branching from the internal iliac artery
    (d) Hyperactivity in the lateral region of the testis

34. Which of the following statements about epididymo-orchitis is NOT correct?
    (a) It is common in adults.
    (b) Gradually increasing of pain that peaks in 1–2 days.
    (c) Fever and pyuria are rarely observed.
    (d) It is related to sexual activity.
35. About epididymo-orchitis:
    (a) The scan pattern is an increase in flow and hypoactivity in the involved region.
    (b) ^{111}In-WBC scan is beneficial for the diagnosis.
    (c) ^{111}In-WBC scan can help in emergency cases.
    (d) The scan pattern of epididymitis is similar to the hyperactivity of the medial testis.
36. All of the following statements regarding testicular appendage torsion are correct *except*:
    (a) It is self-limiting.
    (b) The peak prevalence is at the age of 10–13 years.
    (c) Increased flow and hyperactivity of the involved region are the common findings of the scan.
    (d) The hot dot sign is a very specific finding (about 100%).
37. All of the following diseases present a cold lesion *except*:
    (a) Hydrocele
    (b) Spermatocele
    (c) Hernia
    (d) Henoch–Schonlein purpura
38. The rim sign is observed in all of the following diseases *except*:
    (a) Hematoma
    (b) Missed torsion
    (c) Abscess
    (d) Testicular cyst
39. Which of the following statements regarding the role of scan and sonography in testicular torsion is NOT correct?
    (a) Scintigraphy is a relatively sensitive and very specific test for testicular torsion.
    (b) The combination of sonography and scintigraphy increases the accuracy of the diagnosis of torsion.
    (c) Doppler sonography at the prepuberty ages is difficult and is NOT diagnostic.
    (d) A cold lesion indicates torsion in 63% of cases.
40. Surgery is required in:
    (a) Positive clinical symptoms, normal activity in both hemi-scrotums
    (b) Positive clinical symptoms, hyperactivity in the lateral scrotum
    (c) Positive clinical symptoms, unilateral increase in flow and blood pool
    (d) Positive clinical symptoms, small focal lesion

41. Which of the following statements about testicular scintigraphy is NOT correct?
    (a) Oral potassium or sodium perchlorate (8 mg/kg with a maximum dose of 500 mg, 15–30 min before scan) is indicated for some cases.
    (b) 10 mCi of ^{99m}Tc-pertechnetate is indicated for the scan.
    (c) The stomach receives the maximum radiation in this scan.
    (d) Converging low-energy collimator is recommended for adults.

8.14.1 Answer

	A	B	C	D
1	*			
2	*			
3		*		
4	*			
5	*			
6			*	
7	*			
8			*	
9	*			
10				*
11			*	
12		*		
13		*		
14	*			
15	*			
16				*
17	*			
18			*	
19			*	
20				*
21		*		
22			*	
23		*		
24	*			
25			*	
26		*		
27				*
28				*
29				*
30				*
31				*
32				*
33	*			
34			*	
35		*		

36			*	
37				*
38				*
39	*			
40	*			
41				*

Suggested Readings

1. Ahmadzadehfar H, Biersack HJ, Freeman LM, Zuckier L. Clinical nuclear medicine. 2nd ed. Berlin: Springer; 2018.
2. Ell PJ, Gambhir SS. Nuclear medicine in clinical diagnosis and treatment. 3rd ed. Edinburgh, NY: Churchill Livingstone; 2004.
3. Sandler MP, Coleman RE, Patton JA, Wackers FJT, Gottschalk A. Diagnostic nuclear medicine. 4th ed. Philadelphia: Lippincott & Williams Wilkins; 2003.
4. Henkin RE. Nuclear medicine. 2nd ed. Philadelphia: Mosby Elsevier; 2006.

9 Basic Sciences

9.1 Cell Biology Fundamentals

1. What is the ranking of the cell cycle?
   (a) S, G2, G1, M
   (b) S, G2, M, G1
   (c) S, M, G1, G2
   (d) S, G1, G2, M
2. The myc oncogene is associated with:
   (a) Breast cancer
   (b) Lung cancer
   (c) Acute myeloid leukemia
   (d) Pancreas
3. All of the following items regarding RNA interference (RNAi) are true *except*:
   (a) It is a single-stranded antisense RNA.
   (b) A high degree of specific gene silencing with less effort.
   (c) Highly potent and effective.
   (d) Target-dependent amplification of interfering molecules.
4. Which phase of the cell cycle is the most sensitive to ionizing radiation?
   (a) M
   (b) G1
   (c) S
   (d) G2

9.1.1 Answer

	A	B	C	D
1		*		
2			*	
3	*			
4	*			

M. Assadi et al., *Principles of Nuclear Medicine*,
https://doi.org/10.1007/978-3-319-91701-6_9

9.2 Radionuclide Production

1. This radionuclide is a reactor-produced agent:
   (a) ^{51}Cr
   (b) ^{201}Tl
   (c) ^{67}Ga
   (d) ^{111}In
2. Which of the following factors affects the transient equilibration time between parent and daughter nuclei?
   (a) Number of milking
   (b) Radionuclidic impurities of parent
   (c) Half-lives of parent and daughter
   (d) The difference in the half-lives between parent and daughter
3. Which substance is used in a molybdenum–technetium generator?
   (a) Manganese oxide
   (b) Aluminum oxide
   (c) Magnesium oxide
   (d) Calcium oxide
4. The activity of a generator is 1 Ci on Saturday at 8:00 am. If the generator is eluted once a day for 5 days, what is the total activity?
   (a) 2 Ci
   (b) 2.4 Ci
   (c) 4.2 Ci
   (d) 3.2 Ci
5. About the production of radionuclides in a cyclotron:
   (a) Electrons are accelerated and hit the target.
   (b) Negatively charged ions are accelerated and hit the target.
   (c) Positively charged ions are accelerated and hit the target.
   (d) Neutrons are accelerated and hit the target.
6. Which item is NOT a source of radionuclide production?
   (a) Nuclear reactors
   (b) Generators
   (c) Deuteron and proton accelerators
   (d) Neutron accelerators
7. Which statement about the presence of ^{99}Mo in a $^{99}Mo/^{99m}Tc$ generator is correct?
   (a) Generators containing ^{99}Mo from neutron bombarding require a smaller column than those containing ^{99}Mo from uranium fission.
   (b) Generators containing ^{99}Mo from neutron bombarding require a higher elution volume than those containing ^{99}Mo from uranium fission.
   (c) The unrequired radiation from ^{99}Mo radionuclide impurities in the neutron bombarding of ^{99}Mo is greater than that from uranium fission.
   (d) The specific activity of ^{99}Mo from neutron bombarding is higher than that from uranium fission.

8. ^{124}I causes undesirable effect on imaging because of the production of high-energy gamma photons. What is the recommended process to prevent ^{124}I impurities during ^{123}I production in a cyclotron?
   (a) ^{123}I production with proton bombarding of 124I
   (b) ^{123}I production with proton bombarding of 127I
   (c) ^{123}I production with proton bombarding of 130I
   (d) High-speed centrifugation
9. What is the reason for the higher specific activity of radioisotopes produced by fission than that of radioisotopes produced by neutron activation?
   (a) Carrier presence in fission products
   (b) Carrier presence in neutron activation products
   (c) Radionuclide impurity in fission products
   (d) Radionuclide impurity in neutron activation products
10. What is the advantage of radionuclides produced by the fission method over those produced by neutron capture?
    (a) Higher specific activity
    (b) Easier purification
    (c) User-friendly
    (d) Easier waste storage
11. About generators:
    (a) The difference in physical properties between parent and daughter radionuclide is used for their separation in generators.
    (b) The difference in chemical properties between parent and daughter radionuclide is used for their separation in generators.
    (c) The difference in physicochemical properties between parent and daughter radionuclide is used for their separation in generators.
    (d) The difference in radiochemical properties between parent and daughter radionuclide is used for their separation in generators.
12. Which of the following methods does NOT produce carrier-free radioisotopes?
    (a) Fission product
    (b) Neutron capture
    (c) Cyclotron
    (d) Radionuclide generator
13. If a Mo/Tc generator with activity of 200 mCi is at a steady state, how long does it take for technetium activity to reduce it to half? (T1/2 Mo, 66 h; T1/2 Tc, 6 h)
    (a) 8 h
    (b) 44 h
    (c) 66 h
    (d) 324 h
14. How long should a 99Mo/^{99m}Tc generator be stored before discarding it?
    (a) 8 days
    (b) 22 days
    (c) 46 days
    (d) 60 days

15. The production of which radioisotope in a cyclotron requires high proton energy?
    (a) ^{18}O (p, n) ^{18}F
    (b) ^{123}Te (p, n) ^{123}I
    (c) ^{68}Zn (p, 2n) ^{67}Ga
    (d) ^{111}Cd (p, n) ^{111}In
16. Which of the following radioisotopes is considered a reactor poison because of its extensive surface area during the 235 uranium fission?
    (a) ^{89}Sr
    (b) ^{103}Ru
    (c) ^{131}I
    (d) ^{135}Xe
17. When is the most appropriate time for the second elution of the Mo/^{99m}Tc generator if the goal is to obtain the maximum technetium activity?
    (a) 24 h after the first elution
    (b) 12 h after the first elution
    (c) 8 h after the first elution
    (d) 4 h after the first elution
18. If a target is bombarded for the time of T in the process of radioactive production, the obtained activity is related to:
    (a) Mass number
    (b) Inverse relative frequency of a bombarded isotope
    (c) Atomic number
    (d) Inverse density of a neutron flux
19. Regarding ^{99m}Tc generators:
    (a) They can be eluted every 24 h.
    (b) They are eluted with distilled water.
    (c) ^{99m}Tc is the parent radionuclide.
    (d) The effective life of these generators is about 67 h.
20. Which of the following equations describes the radioactive equilibrium in a $^{99}Mo/^{99m}Tc$ generator?
    (a) $dN1/dt = \lambda 2N2 - \lambda 1N1$
    (b) $dN1/dt = \lambda 1N1 - \lambda 2N2$
    (c) $dN2/dt = \lambda 1N1 - \lambda 2N2$
    (d) $dN1/dt = -\lambda 1N2$

9.2.1 Answer

	A	B	C	D
1	*			
2			*	
3		*		
4				*
5			*	
6				*
7		*		
8		*		
9		*		
10	*			
11		*		
12		*		
13			*	
14				*
15		*		
16				*
17	*			
18				*
19	*			
20			*	

9.3 Fundamentals of Radiochemistry

1. ^{99m}Tc-cold kits are usually supplied by manufactures with stability of typically 12 months, which is sometimes shorter as in the case of:
   (a) ECD
   (b) HMPAO
   (c) DTPA
   (d) MDP
2. Paper chromatography is used in:
   (a) Radionuclide purity
   (b) Chemical purity
   (c) Radiochemical purity
   (d) Biological purity
3. What is the maximum limit of chemical impurity in a ^{99m}Tc generator?
   (a) 1 μg/ml
   (b) 10 μg/ml
   (c) 5 μg/ml
   (d) 2 μg/ml
4. There is 20 mCi of ^{99m}Tc with a volume of 0.1 cm^3. If we increase the volume to 0.2 cm^3 with distilled water, what happens (fold change) to the specific radioactivity?
   (a) 0.35
   (b) 0.75
   (c) No change
   (d) 4
5. To minimize the Tc-99 competition with the Tc-99m in binding to the chelator:
   (a) The amount of 99-Mo in the generator should be increased.
   (b) Sn in kits should be used.
   (c) Oxygen content and moisture should be minimized.
   (d) Freshly eluted solutions should be used.
6. Which of the following kits does NOT contain $SnCl_2$ as a reducing agent?
   (a) MIBI
   (b) DTPA
   (c) MAA
   (d) Sulfur colloid
7. Which of the following items is NOT considered a radionuclidic impurity?
   (a) A small amount of ^{99m}Tc-sulfur colloid in a ^{99m}Tc-sulfur colloid solution
   (b) ^{127}I (nonradioactive iodine) in a ^{125}I (radioactive iodine) sample
   (c) ^{99}Mo in a generator-eluted solution of ^{99}Mo-^{99m}Tc
   (d) A small amount of ^{124}I in a sample of ^{123}I

8. What is the core component of complexing with ^{99m}Tc?
   (a) Reducing agent
   (b) Na-pertechnetate
   (c) Ligand
   (d) Preservative
9. Which method is used to determine radiopharmaceutical purity?
   (a) Spectroscopy
   (b) Chromatography
   (c) Gamma spectroscopy
   (d) Chemical reaction
10. What problems are observed when chemically radioactive impurities exist in the formulation?
    (a) Low quality of the image
    (b) Increased exposure
    (c) Misdiagnosis of the disease
    (d) All of the above
11. Apyrogenicity is required for:
    (a) Radiopharmaceuticals administered orally
    (b) Radiopharmaceuticals administered through IV
    (c) Radiopharmaceuticals administered intrathecally
    (d) Radiopharmaceuticals administered through IM
12. What are the main chemically radioactive impurities in ^{99m}Tc?
    (a) $^{99m}TcO2$ and $^{99m}Tco4$
    (b) Radiotracer and $^{99m}TcO2$
    (c) Radiotracer and $^{99m}TcO4$
    (d) Ligand-bound ^{99m}Tc
13. Which of the following quality control tests is retrospectively evaluated for radionuclides?
    (a) Radionuclide properties
    (b) Radiochemical properties
    (c) Sterility and bacterial endotoxin
    (d) Half-life
14. The existence of ^{201}Pb in a thallium radiotracer ($^{201}TlCl$) is considered a … impurity.
    (a) Radionuclide
    (b) Radiochemical
    (c) Chemical
    (d) Biologic

15. Na-^{99m}TcO4 is produced by washing the 99Mo/^{99m}Tc generator. What are the radionuclide, radiochemical, and chemical impurities of this generator, respectively?
    (a) ^{99}Mo, ^{99m}TcO2, Al
    (b) ^{201}Pb, ^{99m}TcO2, ^{99m}TcO4
    (c) ^{131}I, ^{99m}TcO2, Al
    (d) ^{99}Mo, ^{99m}TcO2, ^{99m}TcO4
16. Which method is preferred for the iodination of drugs containing proteins with aromatic amino acids (e.g., tyrosine)?
    (a) Indirect
    (b) Direct (electrophilic substitution)
    (c) Isotopic exchange
    (d) Addition of iodine to the double-bound method
17. A patient has received a sufficient amount of ^{99m}Tc-tetrofosmin. The scan shows no cardiac uptake but rather a homogenous uptake in other organs. What is the reason for such a finding?
    (a) The patient's heart is healthy with no problems.
    (b) An undefined complex is produced during the preparation of the radiopharmaceutical.
    (c) A suboptimal dose of the radiopharmaceutical.
    (d) The radiopharmaceutical is NOT prepared at a suitable temperature.
18. What is the permitted amount of ^{99}Mo impurities in an eluted solution from a ^{99}Mo-^{99m}Tc generator?
    (a) 0.15 μCi in each mCi of ^{99m}Tc
    (b) 11.5 μCi in each mCi of ^{99m}Tc
    (c) 25 μCi in each mCi of ^{99m}Tc
    (d) 225 μCi in each mCi of ^{99m}Tc
19. ^{101}Mo impurities are obtained from ^{98}Mo production with the neutron bombarding of $_{98}$Mo. Which method is used to eliminate such impurities?
    (a) Sublimation
    (b) Chemical
    (c) Centrifuge
    (d) Time for spontaneous decay
20. The culture medium of *Streptomyces griseus* is used for the biological synthesis of:
    (a) ^{14}C-urea
    (b) ^{57}Co-Vit B12
    (c) ^{75}Sc-selenomethionine
    (d) ^{131}I-iodomethyl-norcholesterol
21. In the radioiodine labeling of complexes, which method produces a low specific activity?
    (a) Chloramine-T
    (b) Iodogen
    (c) Peroxidase
    (d) Exchange reaction

22. What is the most commonly used agent for the quality control of radiopharmaceuticals with chromatography methods?
    (a) ITLC-SG
    (b) Aluminum oxide
    (c) Whatman No. I
    (d) (CH2)18
23. A vial contains 500 ml of 500 mCi pertechnetate. About … ml of this solution containing … mCi of ^{99}Mo is required for a patient.
    (a) 120 ml; 19 mCi
    (b) 76 ml; 12 mCi
    (c) 250 ml; 60 mCi
    (d) 400 ml; 56 mCi
24. What is the recommended intervention for reducing the autoradiolysis of ^{99m}Tc-DMSA?
    (a) Application of the minimum required activity for labeling.
    (b) Storage of the labeled kit in a refrigerator.
    (c) Its labeling is performed in a humid environment.
    (d) Labeling in a dark room.
25. What is the maximum allowed ^{99}Mo radionuclide impurity in a Mo/Tc generator with activity of 400 mCi in the first elution?
    (a) 0.04 mCi
    (b) 0.12 mCi
    (c) 0.08 mCi
    (d) 0.06 mCi
26. What is the main reason for the lyophilization of technetium-containing radiotracer kits?
    (a) Inhibition of bacterial growth.
    (b) Chelating radiotracers are sensitive to moisture and are degraded during time.
    (c) Stanochloride is very sensitive to moisture and oxygen.
    (d) Technetium undergoes hydrolysis in moisture and forms variable capacities.

9.3.1 Answer

	A	B	C	D
1		*		
2			*	
3		*		
4			*	
5				*
6				*
7		*		
8			*	
9		*		
10				*
11			*	
12	*			
13			*	
14	*			
15	*			
16		*		
17		*		
18	*			
19				*
20		*		
21				*
22	*			
23				*
24	*			
25				*
26			*	

9.4 Radiopharmacy

1. Most commercial radiopharmaceuticals have a recommended storage of:
   (a) −2 °C to +15 °C
   (b) 2 °C to 25 °C
   (c) −5 °C to +2 °C
   (d) 5 °C to 15 °C
2. Which radiopharmaceutical is stable at room temperature?
   (a) ^{99m}Tc-MAG3
   (b) ^{99m}Tc-MAA
   (c) ^{123}I-MIBG
   (d) ^{99m}Tc-MIBI
3. All of the following agents can reduce the bone uptake of ^{99m}Tc-MDP *except*:
   (a) Cortisone
   (b) Dextrose
   (c) Nifedipine
   (d) Erythromycin
4. Adverse drug reactions (ADRs) occur with radiopharmaceuticals, and they have an estimated prevalence of:
   (a) 1–6/1000
   (b) 1–6/10000
   (c) 1–6/100000
   (d) 1–6/1000000
5. About 5% of a radionuclide decays each hour. How long is its mean life?
   (a) 20 h
   (b) 45 h
   (c) 12 h
   (d) 120 h
6. Mortality is reported for:
   (a) Tc-99m-DMSA
   (b) Denatured serum albumin
   (c) Tc-99m-MDP
   (d) Ga-67-citrate
7. If the goal is to label RBC for children, which one is the most suitable?
   (a) In vivo technique
   (b) Semi in vitro
   (c) Sn-MDP kit
   (d) Ultratag kit
8. If equilibrium is achieved between parent and daughter elements in a technetium–molybdenum generator, how much technetium exists per each mCi of molybdenum? (The half-lives of Tc and Mb are 6 h and 66 h, respectively.)
   (a) 4.6 mCi
   (b) 2.5 mCi
   (c) 1.1 mCi
   (d) 14 mCi

9. What happens if a Tc-99m generator is eluted before equilibrium is achieved?
   (a) Increase in radionuclide impurities
   (b) Increase in chemical impurities
   (c) Decrease in eluted activity
   (d) Decrease in the life of the generator
10. How long should breastfeeding be paused after the administration of ^{99m}Tc?
   (a) 1 day
   (b) 3 days
   (c) 8 days
   (d) 14 days
11. Which statement is correct?
   (a) ^{177}Lu decays by positron emission.
   (b) ^{177}Lu has a higher tissue range in the immunotherapy of soft and small tumors than ^{90}Y.
   (c) ^{177}Lu-labeled peptide is used for imaging and treating tumors.
   (d) ^{90}Y-labeled peptide is used for imaging and treating tumors.
12. Air exposure is effective in the labeling of:
   (a) ^{99m}Tc-MAG3
   (b) ^{99m}Tc-HMPAO
   (c) ^{99m}Tc-ECD
   (d) ^{99m}Tc-DMSA
13. Pure beta emitter radioactive agents are suitable for treatment because of:
   (a) Short half-life
   (b) Do not harm healthy tissue
   (c) Simultaneous imaging
   (d) Less tissue range in soft tissue
14. What is the mechanism of radiopharmaceutical substitution on a pulmonary perfusion scan?
   (a) Phagocytosis
   (b) Active transport
   (c) Cellular elimination
   (d) Capillary obstruction
15. Which chemical is commonly used as a Tc-reducing agent in the preparation of ^{99m}Tc kits?
   (a) Ascorbic acid
   (b) Ferrous chloride ($FeCl_2$)
   (c) Sodium borohydride ($NaBH_4$)
   (d) Stannous chloride ($Sncl_2$)
16. A ^{99}Mo/^{99m}Tc generator is calibrated on Thursday at 7:00 am (^{99}Mo: 30 GBq; 8 am; Thursday). If the eluted generator on Saturday at 8:00 am provides 12 GBq of pertechnetate, what is the rate of efficiency of the generator?
   (a) 60%
   (b) 70%
   (c) 45%
   (d) 86%

17. The labeled analog of … is used for the evaluation of the adrenal cortex.
    (a) Norepinephrine
    (b) Guanethidine
    (c) Cholesterol
    (d) Adrenalin
18. These radiopharmaceuticals are prepared by ligand exchange:
    (a) ^{99m}Tc-tetrofosmin, ^{99m}Tc-ECD
    (b) ^{99m}Tc-DTPA, ^{99m}Tc-ECD
    (c) ^{99m}Tc-MAG3, ^{99m}Tc-HMPAO
    (d) ^{99m}Tc-MIBI, ^{99m}Tc-MDP
19. MIBG vials are frozen when delivered to nuclear medicine centers. What is the recommended condition for defreezing?
    (a) Incubation at 37 °C for 45 min
    (b) Incubation at 45 °C for 10 min
    (c) Incubation at 45 °C for 45 min
    (d) Incubation at 37 °C for 10 min
20. Technetium must be fresh (less than 2 h after elution), and the generator must be eluted at least once during the last 24 h for:
    (a) ^{99m}Tc-ECD
    (b) ^{99m}Tc-HMPAO
    (c) ^{99m}Tc-MAA
    (d) ^{99m}Tc-BRIDA
21. What is the storage condition for ^{153}Sm-EDTMP?
    (a) 18 °C
    (b) 0 °C
    (c) 4–10 °C
    (d) 25 °C
22. This radiopharmaceutical is used to determine the plasma volume:
    (a) ^{121}I-HAS
    (b) ^{51}Cr-RBC
    (c) ^{99m}Tc-RBC
    (d) ^{57}Co-Vit B12
23. What is the radiopharmaceutical of choice for the imaging of hypoxia?
    (a) ^{11}C-colchicine
    (b) ^{11}C-daunorubicin
    (c) ^{18}F-fluoromisonidazole
    (d) ^{99m}Tc-tetrofosmin
24. Dilution with normal saline after the addition of ^{99m}Tc results in instability of the radiopharmaceutical and the formation of free technetium in:
    (a) Sulfur colloid kit
    (b) MAA kit
    (c) Phytate kit
    (d) MDP kit

25. Which drug decreases the efficiency of ^{99m}Tc-RBC labeling by destroying tin (Sn) in the kit?
   (a) Propranolol
   (b) Heparin
   (c) Methyldopa
   (d) Omnipaque
26. Which of the following does NOT require a blood sample for WBC labeling?
   (a) ^{99m}Tc-HMPAO
   (b) ^{111}In-oxine
   (c) ^{18}F-FDG
   (d) ^{99m}Tc-NeutroSpec
27. Which characteristic is required for a technetium radiopharmaceutical for a brain scan?
   (a) Colloidal
   (b) Electric charge
   (c) High molecular weight
   (d) Lipophilicity and lack of electric charge
28. A WBC viability test is requested. What is the next step after WBC labeling with ^{111}In?
   (a) Colorimetric assay with alizarin indicator
   (b) Chromatography assays
   (c) LAL test
   (d) Tripan blue indicator
29. Which of the following activities is allowed in radioactivity storage and workplace?
   (a) Eating and drinking
   (b) Storage of edible materials
   (c) Smoking
   (d) Handwashing
30. Blue color is observed after the addition of ^{99m}Tc to the HMPAO ligand in the radiopharmaceutical preparation for a brain scan. What is the most appropriate action?
   (a) The radiopharmaceutical is not injectable and must be discarded.
   (b) The radiopharmaceutical is injectable.
   (c) More amount of ^{99m}Tc-pertechnetate must be added to HMPAO kit.
   (d) More amount of HMPAO ligand is required for labeling with ^{99m}Tc.
31. What happens if excessive heat is applied for the denaturation of RBC?
   (a) Increased pulmonary uptake
   (b) Decreased hepatic uptake
   (c) Increased stomach uptake
   (d) Decreased splenic uptake

32. A vial contains 240 mCi of ^{153}Sm-EDTMP in 6 cc on Saturday at 10:00 am. 2 cc of the radiopharmaceutical is wasted on Monday 8:00 am during the preparation of the radiopharmaceutical. How much is the remaining radiopharmaceutical?
    (a) 60 mCi
    (b) 80 mCi
    (c) 140 mCi
    (d) 240 mCi
33. A ^{99m}Tc-damaged RBC scan is requested for the evaluation of an alternative spleen in a woman with platelet fall due to ITP after splenectomy. A suspicious activity and a minor activity in the LUQ are noted. Moreover, despite the normal blood pool, a significant increase in liver activity is observed. Which of the following items can cause such a scan view?
    (a) Incubation of the blood sample at a temperature below the standard
    (b) Incubation of the blood sample at a temperature above the standard
    (c) Heating of a high volume of the sample
    (d) Low specific activity of the sample
34. Which one does NOT form a complex through chelation?
    (a) ^{67}Ga
    (b) ^{99m}Tc
    (c) ^{111}In
    (d) ^{14}C
35. Which of the following radiotracers has the smallest particle size?
    (a) ^{99m}Tc-Sb2S3
    (b) ^{99m}Tc-SnO colloid
    (c) ^{99m}Tc-sulfur colloid
    (d) ^{99m}Tc-Ca-phytate
36. Which of the following drugs does NOT decrease the efficiency of RBC labeling with technetium?
    (a) Heparin
    (b) Methyldopa
    (c) Hydralazine
    (d) Captopril
37. About ^{67}Ga:
    (a) It is produced by the bombarding of ^{68}Zn in a reactor.
    (b) It is readily dialyzable.
    (c) 75% of the radiotracer is excreted in urine in 24 h.
    (d) It has more affinity for binding to transferrin than to lactoferrin.
38. Which cell does NOT uptake gallium?
    (a) RBC
    (b) Neutrophil
    (c) Lymphocyte
    (d) Monocyte

39. What is the suitable condition for storage and transport of the Quadramet radiopharmaceutical?
    (a) −20 °C
    (b) 0 °C
    (c) 2–4 °C
    (d) 25 °C
40. Which of the following kits must be used in 30 min after preparation?
    (a) ^{99m}Tc-MIBI
    (b) ^{99m}TC-HMPAO
    (c) ^{99m}Tc-sulfur colloid
    (d) ^{99m}Tc-DTPA
41. Which statement about the synthesis and development of MAG3 for renal scintigraphy is NOT correct?
    (a) DADA (diamide disulfide) derivatives are the first complexes to show tubular secretion similar to hyporan.
    (b) MAG3 derivatives are synthesized with the addition of a carboxylic group in the non-chiral carbon of DADS.
    (c) The SH-thiol group in MAG3 is very reactive and protected by a benzyl group.
    (d) MAG3 is readily reabsorbed in renal tubules because of the acidic pKa caused by the carboxylic group.
42. Which of the following statements about labeling by exchange is NOT correct?
    (a) It includes a transient binding of technetium to a weak ligand and then exchange with the main ligand.
    (b) It is used for labeling when the main ligand is poorly water-soluble.
    (c) Binding of technetium to a weak ligand inhibits its re-reduction.
    (d) An increase in TcO2 production is considered a disadvantage of this method.
43. Which of the following statements about the ^{99m}Tc-MIBI kit for cardiac imaging is NOT correct?
    (a) The methoxy isobutyl group induces the highest myocardial uptake.
    (b) The methoxy isobutyl group of MIBI is very toxic, volatile, and malodorous.
    (c) An intermediate technetium citrate complex is formed as a ligand exchange.
    (d) The methoxy isobutyl isonitrile group of MIBI is stable as Zn(I) tetrafluoroborate.
44. What is the role of sodium hypochlorite in the in vitro labeling of RBC?
    (a) Plays a role in Sn2+ binding to RBC
    (b) Plays a role in TcO4 binding to RBC
    (c) Plays a role in the oxidation of RBC-bound Sn
    (d) Plays a role in the oxidation of free Sn

45. It is a Tc-tagged radiopharmaceutical:
    (a) ^{99m}Tc-ISA derivative
    (b) ^{99m} Tc-HYNIC TOC
    (c) ^{99m} Tc-MAA
    (d) ^{99m} Tc-MAG3
46. It is NOT normally accumulated in the lacrimal glands:
    (a) ^{99m}Tc-HMPAO
    (b) ^{67}Ga
    (c) ^{131}I-MIBG
    (d) ^{99m}Tc-MIBI
47. Which of the following insoluble particles has the highest affinity for free ligand?
    (a) Chalk
    (b) Charcoal
    (c) Resin
    (d) Polyethylene glycol
48. What is the most appropriate radiopharmaceutical for the evaluation of hypersplenism?
    (a) ^{111}In-WBC
    (b) ^{99m}Tc-SC
    (c) ^{52}Fe
    (d) ^{51}Cr-RBC
49. This radiopharmaceutical requires shaking before injection:
    (a) ^{99m}Tc-sulfur colloid
    (b) ^{99m}Tc-Sb_2S_3
    (c) ^{99m}Tc-MAA
    (d) ^{99m}Tc-Sno
50. The presence of Al^{+3} ion in a generator-eluted pertechnetate solution mainly interferes with the preparation of:
    (a) ^{99m}Tc-EC
    (b) ^{99m}Tc-ECD
    (c) ^{99m}Tc-HIDA
    (d) ^{99m}Tc-sulfur colloid
51. What is the most appropriate radiotracer for the evaluation of the mitochondrial metabolism of fatty acids?
    (a) ^{15}O-CO
    (b) ^{18}F-FDG
    (c) ^{11}C-octanoate
    (d) ^{13}N-ammonia
52. What is the best method to prevent radioiodine sublimation?
    (a) Solutions with acidic pH
    (b) Solutions with alkaline pH
    (c) Solutions with neutral pH
    (d) Oxidative agents

53. Fresh $^{99m}TcO4$ solution is required for the labeling of some kits. The addition of … to $^{99m}TcO4$ after elution removes this limitation.
  (a) Sodium iodide
  (b) Gentisic acid
  (c) Cobalt chloride
  (d) Ethanol

9.4.1 Answer

	A	B	C	D
1		*		
2				*
3				*
4			*	
5	*			
6		*		
7				*
8			*	
9			*	
10	*			
11			*	
12	*			
13				*
14				*
15				*
16		*		
17			*	
18	*			
19	*			
20		*		
21				*
22	*			
23			*	
24				*
25			*	
26				*
27				*
28				*
29				*
30		*		
31				*
32		*		
33		*		
34				*
35	*			
36				*

	A	B	C	D
37		*		
38	*			
39	*			
40		*		
41				*
42				*
43				*
44				*
45			*	
46				*
47		*		
48				*
49			*	
50				*
51			*	
52		*		
53		*		

9.5 Basic Physics and the Detection and Counting of Radiation in Nuclear Medicine

1. What is the parent of ^{81m}Kr?
   (a) ^{113}Sn
   (b) ^{81}Rb
   (c) ^{87}Y
   (d) ^{195m}Hg
2. Which of the following common scintillators is the most efficient?
   (a) Csl(Na)
   (b) CSF
   (c) BGO
   (d) LSO
3. In which of the following conditions does a decrease in the efficiency of PHA for the elimination of scattered photons occur?
   (a) Scattered photons in narrow angles
   (b) Increased energy of primary photons
   (c) Decreased PHA window
   (d) Decreased spatial resolution
4. How many should the "counting" be to achieve 2% of the risk ratio with 95% confidence?
   (a) 10,000
   (b) 60,000
   (c) 80,000
   (d) 100,000
5. What is the number of existing atoms in 1 mCi of ^{201}TI with a half-life of 3.04 days?
   (a) 6.2×10^{13}
   (b) 3.8×10^{14}
   (c) 1.4×10^{13}
   (d) 2.8×10^{12}
6. What type of equilibrium is formed between ^{81}Rb and its daughter ^{81m}Kr?
   (a) Transient.
   (b) Stable.
   (c) No equilibrium is achieved.
   (d) Stable after 20 min.
7. What is the relationship between the stopping power of the alpha particle and atomic number (Z) in a material medium?
   (a) Z
   (b) 1/Z
   (c) Z^2
   (d) $1/Z^2$

8. In the ^{67}Ga spectrum, the 156 keV peak corresponds to:
   (a) Backscatter
   (b) Coincidence
   (c) Iodine escape
   (d) Characteristic X-ray
9. On thyroid scintigraphy, if we increase the patient distance from the detector:
   (a) The intrinsic efficiency of the detector will increase.
   (b) The intrinsic efficiency of the detector will not change.
   (c) The geometric efficiency will increase.
   (d) The photopeak efficiency will decrease.
10. The decay constant of a radionuclide:
    (a) Depends on the number of nuclei
    (b) Decreases over time
    (c) Is constant for different isotopes
    (d) Is independent of physicochemical variables
11. In the decay equation of $^{236}{}_{92}U \rightarrow {}^{131}{}_{53}I + {}^{A}{}_{Z}X + 3n$, the X nucleus is:
    (a) $^{102}{}_{39}X$
    (b) $^{101}{}_{38}X$
    (c) $^{101}{}_{39}X$
    (d) $^{102}{}_{38}X$
12. An increased uptake of the tracer in an organ results in:
    (a) Enhanced sensitivity
    (b) Improved spatial resolution
    (c) Decreased noise
    (d) Decreased energy resolution
13. With the increase in patient distance to the collimator:
    (a) Sensitivity in the parallel collimators will improve.
    (b) Sensitivity in the pinhole collimators will decrease.
    (c) Spatial resolution in the parallel collimators will not change.
    (d) Spatial resolution in the pinhole collimators will not change.
14. If the atomic number increases, what will happen to the binding energy per nucleon?
    (a) Decrease
    (b) Increase
    (c) Increase and then decrease
    (d) No change
15. If a pinhole collimator is used instead of a parallel hole on thyroid scintigraphy:
    (a) Sensitivity increases.
    (b) A better resolution is achieved.
    (c) Noise decreases.
    (d) Scattered radiation increases.

16. If photon energy increases in a diagnostic range (100–510 KeV):
    (a) The scattered radiation increases.
    (b) The photoelectric event increases.
    (c) The intrinsic sensitivity of the detector increases.
    (d) The absorbed dose in the unit of activity increases.
17. If the maximum energy of beta particles of a radioactive agent is 1.8 MeV, how much is the average energy of the particles?
    (a) 1.8 MeV
    (b) 560 KeV
    (c) 345 KeV
    (d) 460 KeV
18. What is the advantage of alpha particles over beta particles in their application in therapeutic nuclear medicine?
    (a) Lower absorbed dose in healthy organs
    (b) Lower absorbed dose in blood
    (c) Higher OER
    (d) Higher absorbed dose in small tumors
19. Which of the following radioactive agents produces the highest X-ray energy?
    (a) ${}^{201}_{81}Tl$
    (b) ${}^{123}_{53}I$
    (c) ${}^{111}_{49}In$
    (d) ${}^{67}_{31}Ga$
20. Which of the following decay methods produces the Auger electron radiation?
    (a) Alpha
    (b) Positive beta
    (c) Negative beta
    (d) Internal conversion
21. Which of the following items best describes the arrow-marked peak?
    (a) Backscatter
    (b) Iodine escape
    (c) Compton edge
    (d) Single escape
22. In isomeric transition:
    (a) The atomic number increases.
    (b) The mass number increases.
    (c) The atomic and mass numbers remain constant.
    (d) The atomic and mass numbers decrease one unit.
23. What happens on scintigraphy when the produced photons per each MeV of gamma absorption increase?
    (a) Noise increases.
    (b) Spatial resolution decreases.
    (c) Intrinsic efficiency of the detector increases.
    (d) Sensitivity decreases.

24. About parallel-hole collimators:
    (a) They are suitable for the imaging of superficial structures.
    (b) Spatial resolution is not constant in the whole sample volume.
    (c) Magnification occurs.
    (d) Spatial resolution remains unaffected by the changes in patient distance from the collimator.
25. Which of the following changes in the nucleus should occur to form a new element?
    (a) Changes in energy level
    (b) Changes in the number of protons
    (c) Changes in the number neutrons
    (d) Changes in the number of electrons
26. How long is the physical half-life of a radionuclide if the mean effective half-life and the biological half-life are 2 h and 4 h, respectively?
    (a) 4 h
    (b) 6 h
    (c) 8 h
    (d) 2.5 h
27. What is the specific activity of 10 mCi of ^{99m}Tc?
    (a) 180 GBq/μg
    (b) 420 GBq/μg
    (c) 18 MBq/mol
    (d) 43 MBq/mol
28. How much is the energy of the backscatter peak if the photopeak energy of a radiation agent is 256 KeV?
    (a) 613 KeV
    (b) 104 KeV
    (c) 1020 KeV
    (d) 76 KeV
29. If the goal is to administer 10 mCi of a radiopharmaceutical with a specific activity of 80 mCi/ml, how much of the radiotracer is required after two half-lives?
    (a) 3 ml
    (b) 4 ml
    (c) 0.5 ml
    (d) 0.46 ml
30. If 10 mCi of a beta emitter with energy of 200 keV and mean effective life of 1 day is accumulated in a metastatic lesion weighing 10 g, how much is the absorbed dose?
    (a) 12.2 Gy
    (b) 147.6 Gy
    (c) 48.3 Gy
    (d) 92.34 Gy

31. If the M/P ratio of the liver to air is 1.8, how much is the liver absorption dose from 100 mR of gamma-radiating ^{99m}Tc?
    (a) 0.25 mGy
    (b) 1.56 mGy
    (c) 0.75 mGy
    (d) 15.55 mGy
32. Which of the following reactions is the most probable when neutrons hit the body?
    (a) Absorption and fission
    (b) Absorption and activation
    (c) Nonelastic
    (d) Elastic
33. Which free radical and ion are produced because of H_2O^+ decomposition in water radiolysis?
    (a) H^+, OH^o
    (b) OH^-, H^o
    (c) H_3O^+, OH^o
    (d) H_2O^-, H^o
34. The specific activity of 10 mCi of ^{99m}Tc is 180 MBq/ng. What happens to the specific activity if radioactivity decreases to half?
    (a) 6
    (b) 3
    (c) 0.75
    (d) No change
35. Which of the following events occurs because of strong nuclear power?
    (a) Alpha decay
    (b) β- decay
    (c) Gamma decay
    (d) β+ decay
36. About radiation and energy conversion in the nucleus:
    (a) Characteristic X-ray (Rontgen) interacts with the orbital electrons in internal conversion.
    (b) Auger electron radiation is the replacement of characteristic X-ray.
    (c) Metastable state and ground state are not different in terms of their energy.
    (d) Positron emission occurs when the energy difference between the parent and daughter nuclei is less than 1.02 MeV.
37. The activity of a radioactive agent decreases to 1/16 in 4 min. How long is the half-life of this radioisotope?
    (a) 1/2 min
    (b) 1/8 min
    (c) 1 min
    (d) 8 min

38. About the photoelectric effect:
    (a) The linear attenuation coefficient does NOT depend on energy for the photoelectric effect.
    (b) Photoelectric absorption is not a coherent process.
    (c) The possibility of a photoelectric effect directly depends on energy (E^3).
    (d) The photoelectric effect is indirectly related to the atomic number ($1/Z^3$).
39. Which of the following reactions is in the secular equilibrium state?
    (a) $^{99m}Mo \rightarrow {}^{99}Tc$
    (b) $^{226}Ra \rightarrow {}^{222}Ra$
    (c) $^{82}Sr \rightarrow {}^{82}Rb$
    (d) $^{89}Sr \rightarrow {}^{88}Sr$
40. About the external structure of an atom:
    (a) According to Bohr's law, each shell can contain only $2n^2$ electron.
    (b) According to Pauli's law, each shell can contain only $2n^2$ electron.
    (c) According to Bohr's law, each shell can contain only 2n electron.
    (d) According to Pauli's law, each shell can contain only $2n^2$ electron.
41. What type of equilibrium is achieved in $^{68}Ga \xrightarrow{280d} > {}^{68}Ga \xrightarrow{68m} > {}^{68}Zn$ decay?
    (a) Transient.
    (b) Secular.
    (c) Semi-secular.
    (d) No equilibrium is achieved.
42. In the interaction of gamma rays with the target:
    (a) No energy is transferred to the atom in the Rayleigh scatter.
    (b) A low proportion of photon energy is transferred to the atom in the photoelectric effect.
    (c) Auger electron is produced only in pair production.
    (d) The Compton scatter is the most useful phenomenon in nuclear medicine imaging.
43. About the sample count in a well counter:
    (a) The counting is NOT accurate when the activity of the particle is very high.
    (b) The ^{99m}Tc energy window for this system is 270–350 KeV.
    (c) The sample volume must be twice that of the standard.
    (d) Coincidence summing does NOT produce valuable information.
44. About the Anger camera:
    (a) Spatial nonlinearity is related to the errors in positioning of the scintillation event.
    (b) Event-to-event processing during data acquisition canNOT be used for distortion.
    (c) The sensitivity of a point source is constant from point to point during photopic change.
    (d) About 50–70% of counting events are associated with the photoelectric phenomenon in nuclear medicine.

45. Choose the correct item about alpha radiation.
 (a) ${}^{A}_{Z}X \rightarrow {}^{A-4}_{Z-4}X^{1} + (2P + 2n) + Q$
 (b) ${}^{A}_{Z}X \rightarrow {}^{A-4}_{Z-2}X^{1} + (2P + 2n) + Q$
 (c) ${}^{A}_{Z}X \rightarrow {}^{A-2}_{Z-2}X^{1} + 2^{4}\,\alpha + Q$
 (d) ${}^{A}Z\,X \rightarrow {}^{A-2}_{Z-4}X^{1} + 2^{4}\,\alpha + Q$
46. Which item about ^{131}I radioisotope decay is true? (υ: neutrino, ύ: antineutrino)
 (a) ${}^{131}_{53}I \rightarrow {}^{131}_{53}Xe + \beta^{+} + ύ$
 (b) ${}^{131}_{53}I \rightarrow {}^{131}_{54}Xe + \beta^{-} + υ$
 (c) ${}^{131}_{53}I \rightarrow {}^{131}_{54}Xe + \beta^{+} + υ$
 (d) ${}^{131}_{53}I \rightarrow {}^{131}_{54}Xe + \beta^{-} + ύ$
47. Electron capture occurs:
 (a) When the energy of the parent nucleus is higher than 2 $m_o c^2$
 (b) When the energy of the parent nucleus is exactly 3 $m_o c^2$ more than that of the daughter nucleus
 (c) When the energy of the parent nucleus is 4 $m_o c^2$ more than that of the daughter nucleus
 (d) When the energy of the parent nucleus is 2 $m_o c^2$ less than that of the daughter nucleus
48. Incubation at room temperature with pertechnetate solution is sufficient for the preparation of:
 (a) ^{99m}Tc-tetrofosmin
 (b) ^{99m}Tc-MIBI
 (c) ^{99m}Tc-MAG3
 (d) ^{99m}Tc-teboroxime
49. What proportion of pulmonary capillaries is filled with ^{99m}Tc-MAA particles during the pulmonary perfusion scan of an adult subject?
 (a) 1/10
 (b) 1/50
 (c) 1/100
 (d) 1/1000
50. If a vial containing 100 mCi of ^{64}Cu radioisotope (half-life: 693 min) breaks down at the center, how long does it take for the remaining activity to be 0.1 mCi?
 (a) $-1000 \times \text{Ln}\ 0.001$
 (b) $0.001 \times \text{Ln}\ 1000$
 (c) $1000 \times \text{Ln}\ 0.001$
 (d) $-0.001 \times \text{Ln}\ 1000$
51. Which radioisotope has the most appropriate photopic energy for imaging with a gamma camera?
 (a) ^{133}Xe
 (b) ^{123}I
 (c) ^{67}Ga
 (d) ^{201}Tl

52. What is the preferred decay procedure in nuclear medicine?
    (a) Alpha decay
    (b) Beta-minus decay
    (c) Fission
    (d) Isomeric transition
53. Which of the following forms of decay emits the characteristic X-ray?
    (a) β+
    (b) β-
    (c) Gamma
    (d) Electron capture
54. In which of the following interactions are photons slightly deviated without loss of energy?
    (a) Rayleigh
    (b) Compton
    (c) Photoelectric
    (d) Pair production
55. What happens to the spatial resolution in a gamma camera with the increase in crystal thickness?
    (a) Increase (poor resolution).
    (b) Decrease (better resolution).
    (c) No change.
    (d) It depends on the crystal type.
56. What is the relationship among Rs (system resolution), Ri (intrinsic resolution), and Rg (geometric resolution)?
    (a) Rs = Ri + Rg
    (b) $Ri^2 = Rs^2 + Rg^2$
    (c) Rg = Rs + Ri
    (d) $Rs^2 = Ri^2 + Rg^2$
57. Which decay occurs in specific conditions when the neutron-to-proton ratio is low?
    (a) Positive beta
    (b) Negative beta
    (c) Alpha
    (d) Gamma
58. What are the atomic and mass numbers of the Y nucleus in the following nuclear reaction, respectively? ${}^{A}_{Z}X \rightarrow {}^{?}_{?}Y + {}^{4}_{2}He$
    (a) A-6, Z-2
    (b) A-4, Z-2
    (c) A-2, Z-4
    (d) A-2, Z-2
59. The activity of ^{18}F-FDG is 110 mCi at 9:50 am. How much is the activity at 8:00 am on the same day?
    (a) $110e^{-0.693}$
    (b) $110e^{+0.693}$
    (c) $110e^{-0.693 \times 110}$
    (d) $110e^{+0.693 \times 110}$

60. What is the difference between X and gamma radiation?
    (a) Energy
    (b) Interaction with other materials
    (c) Origin of production
    (d) Distance range in materials
61. What is the phenomenon in which gamma emission from the nucleus encounters and expels the orbital electrons?
    (a) Beta emission
    (b) Positron emission
    (c) Internal conversion
    (d) Electron capture
62. What is the ratio of the detected photons to the received ones in a gamma camera?
    (a) Intrinsic efficiency
    (b) Geometrical efficiency
    (c) System efficiency
    (d) Collimator efficiency
63. Radioactivity administered for diagnostic nuclear medicine is in the range of … and for therapy is in the range of ….
    (a) 10^6 Bq and 10^9 Bq
    (b) 10^7 Bq and 10^{10} Bq
    (c) 10^8 Bq and 10^{10} Bq
    (d) 10^7 Bq and 10^9 Bq
64. If the radiopharmaceutical is administered orally, and excretions from urine, gastrointestinal, and respiration+ perspiration are 11.5%, 35%, and 3.5%, respectively, in 5 h, how long is the mean effective life? (physical half-life is 6 h)
    (a) 2.5 h
    (b) 3.5 h
    (c) 4.3 h
    (d) 8 h
65. If the pure parent radioactive nucleus (p) is converted to the daughter nucleus (d) after decay, when is the maximum activity of the daughter nucleus (Tmax) achieved?
    (a) $T_{max} = \lambda p \lambda d/(\lambda p - \lambda d)$
    (b) $T_{max} = (\lambda p - \lambda d)/\lambda p \lambda d$
    (c) $T_{max} = [1/(\lambda d - \lambda p)]\ln(\lambda d/\lambda p)$
    (d) $T_{max} = [1/(\lambda p - \lambda d)]\ln(\lambda p/\lambda d)$
66. If the physical half-life and mean effective life of a radiotracer are equal, the biological half-life is:
    (a) Shorter
    (b) Equal to them
    (c) Longer
    (d) Independent of these factors

67. The decay constant of a radioactive agent (λ) indicates:
    (a) Activity
    (b) Mean effective life
    (c) Biological half-life
    (d) Average life
68. What is the dominant form of interaction of gamma photons with the body in the energy range of nuclear medicine imaging (70–511 KeV)?
    (a) Coherent scatter
    (b) Photoelectric absorption
    (c) Compton scatter
    (d) Pair production
69. In transiently equilibrated systems at steady state:
    (a) The activities of the parent and daughter are equal.
    (b) The physical half-lives of the parent and daughter are equal.
    (c) The activity of the daughter is constant.
    (d) The activity of the parent is less than that of the daughter.
70. Delta rays:
    (a) Are secondary X-rays
    (b) Are secondary electrons
    (c) Are specific X-rays
    (d) Are primary electrons
71. Which energy range of gamma rays from ^{99m}Tc can be detected by a pulse height analyzer (PHA) with a window width of 20%?
    (a) Less than 140 KeV
    (b) More than 140 KeV
    (c) 126–154 KeV
    (d) 116–178 KeV
72. Which atomic parameter remains constant in beta-minus decay?
    (a) Atomic number
    (b) Number of neutrons
    (c) Number of orbital electrons
    (d) Number of nucleons
73. In a transient equilibrium at steady state:
    (a) The relative activity of the parent to the daughter is constant.
    (b) The relative activity of the parent to the daughter is one.
    (c) The activity of the daughter is constant.
    (d) The activity of the parent is minimal.
74. Carrier isotopes:
    (a) Occur along with fission parts
    (b) Decrease the specific activity
    (c) Can be separated by chemical procedures
    (d) Are side products of cyclotrons

75. Which of the following variables can affect the Compton scatter?
    (a) Atomic number
    (b) Mass number
    (c) Density
    (d) Angle of interaction
76. A photoelectric interaction occurs between a photon with energy of 80 keV and an electron with binding energy (Eb) of 60 KeV. How much is the energy of the photoelectron?
    (a) 20 KeV
    (b) 40 KeV
    (c) 120 KeV
    (d) 160 KeV
77. In which of the following regions is the possibility of a photoelectric event low during a scan?
    (a) Patient's body
    (b) Collimator
    (c) Detector
    (d) Protective layers
78. What is the unit of mass absorption coefficient?
    (a) Cm
    (b) Cm^{-1}
    (c) g/cm^2
    (d) Cm^2/g
79. Which statement about X-rays is NOT correct?
    (a) They are produced with the speed change of charged photons.
    (b) They are emitted from the nucleus of unstable atoms.
    (c) They can change the direction of charged photons.
    (d) They have wave–photon properties.
80. Which of the following variables is identical for two different radioisotopes with equal activity?
    (a) Decay constant
    (b) Physical half-life
    (c) Number of unstable nuclei
    (d) Decay frequency
81. Which characteristic of the parent and daughter atoms is equal in beta-minus emission?
    (a) Atomic mass
    (b) Atomic mass and energy
    (c) Atomic number
    (d) Number of neutrons
82. Which radioactive agent has a physical half-life of 5.2 days and gamma energy of 81 KeV and decays with beta emission?
    (a) ^{32}P
    (b) ^{125}I
    (c) ^{133}Xe
    (d) ^{68}Ga

83. In positron emission:
    (a) The atomic number increases.
    (b) It happens in nuclei with low neutrons.
    (c) The minimum level of nucleus energy is 1.2 MeV.
    (d) The amount of energy transferred to neutrino and antineutrino must be considered in the dosimetry.
84. Which of the following events does NOT occur in the photon interaction with an atom?
    (a) Photoelectric
    (b) Pair production
    (c) Bremsstrahlung
    (d) Compton electron
85. Which term is used to describe the $^{100}{}_{44}Ru$, $^{99}{}_{43}Tc$, and $^{98}{}_{42}Mo$ nuclides?
    (a) Isotone
    (b) Isobar
    (c) Isomer
    (d) Isotope
86. If N is the number of half-value layers (HVL), how much is the required N to decrease the initial photon density to 1%?
    (a) 2/log2
    (b) Log20/log2
    (c) 0.01log2/2
    (d) 100log2/log100
87. The physical half-life of ^{131}I is 8 days. How long is the mean life?
    (a) 4 days
    (b) 12 days
    (c) 16 days
    (d) 11.5 days
88. What is a photonuclear reaction?
    (a) Expelling of an electron from the orbital after interacting with a high-energy photon.
    (b) Nucleon emission after interacting with a high-energy photon.
    (c) Positron emission after interacting with a photon.
    (d) It is equivalent to the photoelectric phenomenon.
89. Which of the following statements describes the characteristic X-ray?
    (a) An electromagnetic radiation produced by replacing an emitted electron with another electron
    (b) The radiation produced following the interaction of an electron with a photon
    (c) The radiation produced following internal conversion
    (d) The radiation produced following the emission of an electron from the last orbital

90. Technetium and ^{99m} technetium are:
   (a) Isobars
   (b) Isomers
   (c) Isotones
   (d) Stable isotopes
91. What is the presumed condition of the nucleus in Bohr's atomic model?
   (a) Ovoid movement only
   (b) Substituted movement
   (c) Circular movement
   (d) Stationary
92. What type of power is a nuclear force?
   (a) Mechanical
   (b) Gravitational
   (c) Nuclear specific
   (d) Electromagnetic
93. How are electrons converted?
   (a) They are beta particles emitted from the nucleus.
   (b) They are produced by the bremsstrahlung interaction with electrons.
   (c) They are produced by the emission and interaction of gamma rays.
   (d) They are produced by beta particle interaction.
94. How much is the requisite difference in the energy between the parent and the daughter nuclei for positron emission?
   (a) 2 $m_o c^2$
   (b) Less than 2 $m_o c^2$
   (c) 1 $m_o c^2$
   (d) 3 $m_o c^2$
95. How much is the requisite energy of the parent nucleus for electron capture?
   (a) More than 2 $m_o c^2$
   (b) Less than 2 $m_o c^2$
   (c) More than 3 $m_o c^2$
   (d) Equal to 2 $m_o c^2$
96. Which wave or particle is usually accompanied with beta-minus (β^-) decay?
   (a) Negatron
   (b) Positron
   (c) Antineutrino
   (d) Neutrino
97. Which of the following items best describes the decay constant?
   (a) The proportion of atoms that decay in one half-life
   (b) The proportion of atoms that decay in a unit of time
   (c) Decay count in one half-life
   (d) Decay count in 1 s
98. Which of the following equations represents the mean effective life? (Te, mean effective life; Tb, biological half-life; Tp, physical half-life)
   (a) Te: $(Tb + Tp)/[(Tp + Tb)^2]$
   (b) Te: $(Tb + Tp)/(Tp \times Tb)$
   (c) Te: $(Tb \times Tp)/(Tp + Tb)$
   (d) Te: $(Tb \times Tp)/[(Tp - Tb)^2]$

99. How much is 1 mCi in MBq?
    (a) 30 MBq
    (b) 33 MBq
    (c) 35 MBq
    (d) 37 MBq
100. Which of the following radioisotopes has the highest exposure rate constant?
    (a) ^{131}I
    (b) ^{123}I
    (c) ^{137}Cs
    (d) ^{125}I
101. A high-count rate mediates which event in the ^{99m}Tc spectrum?
    (a) Tailing in high energy
    (b) Widening of peak
    (c) Tailing in high energy and widening of energy peak
    (d) No change
102. What happens to the proportion of scatter photons in tissue with increased energy higher than 100 KeV?
    (a) Increases
    (b) No change
    (c) Decreases
    (d) Intermittently increases and decreases
103. Which of the following equations describes the relationship between half-life and decay constant?
    (a) $\lambda = 0.693/T$
    (b) $\lambda = T/0.693$
    (c) $\lambda = 0.693T$
    (d) $\lambda = 1.44T$
104. Two isomers have:
    (a) Equal atomic numbers, different Z
    (b) Different atomic numbers, equal Z
    (c) Equal atomic numbers, equal Z
    (d) Different atomic numbers, different Z
105. Mass defect is the:
    (a) Difference in nucleus mass between the excited and non-excited states
    (b) Difference between the proton mass and the neutron mass in the nucleus
    (c) Difference between the nucleus mass and the summation of mass of components
    (d) Difference between the proton + neutrino mass and neutrons
106. Which of the following phenomena absorbs approximately all incident photons in the material?
    (a) Compton scattering
    (b) Pair production
    (c) Photoelectric effect
    (d) Rayleigh scattering

107. What is the initial intensity value of a batch of X-ray after crossing from three half-value layers (HVL)?
   (a) 12.5%
   (b) 45%
   (c) 85%
   (d) 35%
108. A process in which a neutral atom is converted into a charged one:
   (a) Photoelectric
   (b) Excitation
   (c) Internal conversion
   (d) Ionization
109. What is the unit of activity in SI?
   (a) Ci
   (b) Sv
   (c) Gy
   (d) Bq
110. What is the photon energy threshold in pair production?
   (a) 0.511 keV
   (b) 0.511 MeV
   (c) 1.022 MeV
   (d) 1.022 keV
111. The value of $e^{-\mu X}$ is independent of the … for a batch of gamma rays. (X, thickness of the material; μ, linear attenuation coefficient)
   (a) Density of the absorbent
   (b) Intensity of the radiation
   (c) Atomic number of the absorbent
   (d) Effective energy of radiation
112. If both parent and daughter nuclei are radioactive with a T1/T2 ratio of two, how long does it take for these nuclei to reach the same level of activity?
   (a) T2
   (b) T1
   (c) 4T2
   (d) 4T1
113. What is the difference between ^{131}I and ^{125}I radioisotopes?
   (a) Atomic number
   (b) Number of electrons
   (c) Number of protons
   (d) Number of neutrons
114. A gamma photon with energy of 140 keV interacts with an electron of the K orbital of iodine with a photoelectric event. How much is the energy of the released electron? (The binding energy of the K orbital in this atom is 32 keV.)
   (a) 88 keV
   (b) 108 keV
   (c) 150 keV
   (d) 184 keV

115. Electron capture decay produces:
    (a) Gamma
    (b) Beta minus
    (c) Characteristic X
    (d) Positron
116. The radiation intensity of a point radioactive source is 200 roentgens in a 10 cm distance. How much is the radiation intensity in a 50 cm distance from this source?
    (a) 8 roentgens
    (b) 30 roentgens
    (c) 25 roentgens
    (d) 4 roentgens
117. The initial activity of a radioactive source is 32 MBq. Twenty-four hours later, the activity is 4 MBq. How much is the activity of this source after another 8 h?
    (a) 16 MBq
    (b) 2 MBq
    (c) 14 MBq
    (d) 8 MBq
118. After how many half-lives is the activity of a radioactive sample less than 1% of the primary value?
    (a) 6
    (b) 8
    (c) 4
    (d) 7
119. The physical half-life of a radiotracer depends on:
    (a) Decay form
    (b) Dose
    (c) Type of radioactive atoms
    (d) Chemical formula of the radiotracer
120. A total of 360 ergs of gamma-ray energy is absorbed in 3 g of tissue. How much is the absorbed dose?
    (a) 120 cGy
    (b) 12 cGy
    (c) 0.12 cGy
    (d) 1.20 cGy
121. How much is the cumulative activity of a source organ with ^{99m}Tc activity of 3 mCi? (organ weight, 55 g; mean effective life of the radioisotope, 5 h)
    (a) 934 mCi/h
    (b) 4440 mCi/h
    (c) 31600 μCi/h
    (d) 8657 μCi/h

122. A total of 10 mCi of a ^{131}I radioisotope with a physical half-life of 8 h is injected into a patient. How much is the exposure of a subject with 2 m of distance from the patient? (exposure rate constant of the source is 2.2 R/(h. mCi) in a 1 cm distance from the source)
 (a) 1.24 R/h
 (b) 0.55 mR/h
 (c) 0.234 R/h
 (d) 0.077 mR/h
123. The wavelength of photon A in a medium is one-half of the wavelength of photon B in the same medium. What is the relation between the energy of A and that of B (Ea/Eb)?
 (a) 2
 (b) 1/16
 (c) 1/2
 (d) 8
124. What happens to the atomic and mass numbers after gamma emission, respectively?
 (a) Decrease, decrease
 (b) Increase, increase
 (c) Decrease, increase
 (d) Constant, constant
125. Which of the following absorption and scattering phenomena mostly occurs in energies lower than 0.05 MeV?
 (a) Triplet production and pair production
 (b) Pair production and Compton scattering
 (c) Rayleigh scattering and photoelectric
 (d) Compton scattering and triplet production
126. Regarding energy peaks in the ^{99m}Tc spectrum, which is performed with a thin NaI crystal:
 (a) The iodine scape peak is located in energies > 20 keV.
 (b) The iodine scape peak is located after the photopeak.
 (c) The iodine scape peak is located before the Pb X-ray and in energies of 40 keV.
 (d) The iodine scape peak is located in the energies of 100–120 keV.
127. Which of the following nuclear reactions regarding the production of ^{67}Ga is true?
 (a) ^{66}Zn (p, n) ^{67}Ga
 (b) ^{66}Zn (p, 2n) ^{67}Ga
 (c) ^{68}Zn (p, 2n) ^{67}Ga
 (d) ^{66}Zn (d, 2n) ^{67}Ga
128. Bremsstrahlung:
 (a) Radiation that is emitted from the nucleus
 (b) Does NOT depend on the atomic number (Z)
 (c) Has a direct relationship with the mass of the charged particle
 (d) Increases with the increase in energy of the charged particle

129. What is the formula for mass attenuation? (A, mass number; Z, atomic number; m, nuclear mass)
    (a) (m-A)c^2
    (b) (m-Z)c^2
    (c) (2Z-A)c^2
    (d) (2Z-A-m)c^2
130. Which item regarding nuclear medicine radioisotopes is correct?
    (a) ${}^{235}_{92}U + {}^{1}_{0}n \rightarrow {}^{236}_{92}U + {}^{131}_{53}I + {}^{102}_{39}Y + 3\ {}^{1}_{1}p$.
    (b) ${}^{68}{}_{30}Zn\ (p, n){}^{68}{}_{31}Ga$.
    (c) ${}^{130}Te\ (p, n)\ {}_{131}Te \rightarrow {}^{131}I$.
    (d) Transient equilibrium of technetium–molybdenum and maximum produced ${}^{99m}Tc$ is obtained after two half-lives of ${}^{99m}Tc$.
131. What is the purpose of applying multiple windows?
    (a) Increasing the sensitivity of the gamma camera on myocardial scintigraphy with ${}^{99m}Tc$
    (b) Simultaneous imaging of multiple radioisotopes that are injected concurrently
    (c) Separation of only one energy of a radioisotope such as ${}^{67}Ga$
    (d) Separation of the asymmetric peak in myocardial imaging
132. The N/Z ratio is a critical factor for the stability of the nucleus. Which of the following items about this ratio is correct?
    (a) N/Z = 1.2 for ${}^{12}_{6}C$, ${}^{14}_{7}N$, and ${}^{16}_{8}O$.
    (b) N/Z ratio increases with the increase in atomic number.
    (c) N/Z ratio decreases with the increase in atomic number in atoms with a low Z.
    (d) All atoms with a high N/Z ratio are on the line of stability.
133. How many counting is required for accuracy of 2% in data acquisition?
    (a) 2500
    (b) 7250
    (c) 3450
    (d) 5550
134. The neutron dissociation energy in a nucleus with a mass number of A and atomic number of Z is calculated by (B is the binding energy of the nucleus):
    (a) Sn = B(A,Z)/A-Z
    (b) Sn = B(A,Z)/A
    (c) Sn = B(A,Z)-B(A-1,Z)
    (d) Sn = [M(A-1,Z)-M(A,Z)]C^2
135. The uranium nucleus ${}^{238}_{92}u$ before stabilization needs repeated decay, and it emits eight alpha and six negative beta particles. What is the final stable nucleus?
    (a) ${}^{200}_{76}A$
    (b) ${}^{216}_{86}B$
    (c) ${}^{206}_{82}C$
    (d) ${}^{224}_{72}D$

136. In the radiologic voltage ranges, scattering is associated with the … event. Is it dependent on the atomic number (Z)?
   (a) Photoelectric, yes
   (b) Thomson, yes
   (c) Compton, no
   (d) Pair production (PP), no
137. All of the following processes cause ionization *except*:
   (a) Compton scattering
   (b) Photoelectric effect
   (c) Coherent scattering
   (d) Photodisintegration
138. A thyroid patient is given a ^{131}I-NaI capsule to measure the 24-h thyroid uptake. The 2-min counts are standard, 200,000; room background, 7000; thyroid, 70,000; and thigh, 8000. What is the percentage of the thyroid uptake?
   (a) 32%
   (b) 42%
   (c) 35%
   (d) 38%
139. If a radionuclide decays at a rate of 40%/h, how long is the half-life?
   (a) 1.73 h
   (b) 3.41 h
   (c) 2.44 h
   (d) 3.83 h
140. How many counts should be collected for a radioactive sample to have a 2% error at a 95% confidence level?
   (a) 1,000,000
   (b) 2,000,000
   (c) 10,000
   (d) 40,000
141. A radioactive sample and the background are counted for 5 min and are found to give 10,000 counts and 2000 counts, respectively. What is the net count rate?
   (a) 1700 cpm
   (b) 1600 cpm
   (c) 1660 cpm
   (d) 2800 cpm
142. A 2.5-Ci ^{99}Mo-^{99m}Tc generator calibrated for Thursday noon was received on Wednesday afternoon. Assuming a transient equilibrium between ^{99}Mo and ^{99m}Tc at the time of elution and an 85% elution, how much would the ^{99m}Tc activity, which would be eluted at 8:00 AM on Friday, yield?
   (a) 2865 mCi
   (b) 1646 mCi
   (c) 1665 mCi
   (d) 2784 mCi

143. If the HVL of lead for the 140 keV photons of ^{99m}Tc is 0.03 cm of lead, how thick is the tenth-value layer (TVL)?
  (a) 0.0877 cm
  (b) 0.0996 cm
  (c) 0.4400 cm
  (d) 0.0453 cm
144. Which of the following changes in photon energy and atomic number increase the probability of a photoelectric event?
  (a) Increase in the photon energy and atomic number of the matter
  (b) Increase in the photon energy and decrease in the atomic number of matter
  (c) Decrease in the photon energy and increase in the atomic number of matter
  (d) Decrease in the photon energy and atomic number of the matter
145. What was the previous unit of exposure?
  (a) Rem
  (b) Roentgen
  (c) Rad
  (d) Curie
146. Which of the following parameters is used for radiation protection?
  (a) Kerma
  (b) Equivalent dose
  (c) Effective equivalent dose
  (d) Absorbed dose
147. Which of the following rays has the longest wavelength?
  (a) X
  (b) Visible
  (c) Ultraviolet
  (d) Infrared
148. Which of the following factors is generally equivalent between the nucleus and the electrons of an atom?
  (a) Energy
  (b) Mass
  (c) Speed
  (d) Electric charge
149. In $^{131}_{53}$I, 131 represents the:
  (a) Atomic number
  (b) Mass number
  (c) Electron number
  (d) Neutron number
150. Which of the following tissues demonstrates the highest rate of photoelectric absorption?
  (a) Muscle
  (b) Fat
  (c) Lung
  (d) Bone

151. What happens following a photoelectric event?
   (a) Positron emission
   (b) Electron emission
   (c) X radiation
   (d) Gamma radiation
152. What happens to gamma rays after crossing the half-value layer (HVL)?
   (a) The type of ray changes.
   (b) Decrease in energy to half.
   (c) Decrease in wavelength to half.
   (d) Decrease in intensity to half.
153. What happens to the nucleus after gamma emission?
   (a) Decrease in atomic number.
   (b) Increase in atomic number.
   (c) Decrease in mass number.
   (d) The nucleus becomes more stable.
154. A photoelectric event is the emission of an electron from the atom that occurs because of the interaction of:
   (a) Positron and electron
   (b) Electron and material
   (c) Photon and material
   (d) Proton and material
155. Which of the following items best describes the specific activity?
   (a) Activity in unit of volume
   (b) Activity in unit of mass
   (c) Decay in unit of time
   (d) Decay in one half-life
156. If the physical half-life of a radioactive substance is longer than its biological half-life, the mean effective life is:
   (a) Close to the physical half-life
   (b) Close to the biological half-life
   (c) Equal to the physical half-life
   (d) Equal to the biological half-life
157. The production date of a ^{131}I sample is 40 days ago with activity of 400 mCi. How much is the activity at the present?
   (a) 12.5 mCi
   (b) 55 mCi
   (c) 70 mCi
   (d) 122 mCi
158. Which of the following items properly demonstrates the wavelength of different radiations?
   (a) X-ray < visible < infrared < radio waves
   (b) Infrared < visible < ultraviolet < X-ray
   (c) X-ray < visible < ultraviolet < radio waves
   (d) Radio waves < ultraviolet < visible < X-ray

159. Which of the following radiations produces more exposure assuming the equal energy of the rays?
    (a) X
    (b) Gamma
    (c) Beta
    (d) Neutron
160. The absorbed dose is:
    (a) The dose that passes through the unit of mass
    (b) The dose received by unit of mass
    (c) The dose that produces a defined level of energy in unit of mass
    (d) The dose that produces a defined level of flow in unit of mass
161. Which of the following events produces bremsstrahlung radiation?
    (a) Interaction of high-energy X-rays with an atom and expelling of orbital electrons
    (b) Transfer of high-energy electrons from the nuclear field of the atom
    (c) Transfer of high-energy electrons from the electron field of the atom
    (d) Interaction of high-energy electrons with an atom and change in orbital electrons
162. What is the unit of kerma?
    (a) C/kg
    (b) Gy
    (c) Sv
    (d) MeV/kg
163. According to the Medical Internal Radiation Dose (MIRD), absorption fraction (Φ) depends on:
    (a) Gamma radiation energy, biological half-life, distance between source and target organ
    (b) Gamma radiation energy, mean effective life, shape of the organ
    (c) Gamma radiation energy, shape of organ, distance between source and target organ
    (d) Gamma radiation energy, physical half-life, distance between source and target organ
164. Which of the following variables decreases the clinical application of a radionuclide with a short half-life?
    (a) Counting rate
    (b) Patient dose
    (c) Scattering
    (d) Biological clearance
165. Regarding X-ray interaction with a matter:
    (a) The mass energy transfer coefficient represents the absorbed dose of the substance.
    (b) The linear mass attenuation coefficient in a high-energy spectrum (pair production) is inversely related to Z.
    (c) The mass absorption coefficient is equal to the mass energy transfer coefficient in the absence of bremsstrahlung events.
    (d) The probability of bremsstrahlung event decreases with the increase in electron energy.

166. The interaction of X-ray or megavoltage gamma rays with the body is mostly:
    (a) Compton
    (b) Photoelectric
    (c) Coherent
    (d) a and b
167. Nuclear power depends on:
    (a) The type of electrical charge of particles
    (b) Mass of the charged particles
    (c) Distance between the charged particles
    (d) All of the above
168. Activity decreases to 1/8 of the initial value after … half-lives.
    (a) 3
    (b) 4
    (c) 9
    (d) 2
169. What is the main reason behind the widespread application of ^{99m}Tc in nuclear medicine?
    (a) Favorable half-life and energy
    (b) Gamma emission with different energies
    (c) Beta particles with favorable energy
    (d) Extensive diagnostic and therapeutic application
170. What happens to the range of a particle in a specific material if the electrical charge is doubled?
    (a) Increases by 8 times
    (b) Decreases to 1/4
    (c) Increases by 16 times
    (d) Decreases to 1/16
171. Ionic avalanche:
    (a) Occurs in the ionization chamber and shows the flow
    (b) Occurs in the proportions counter and shows the photon energy
    (c) Occurs in the Geiger–Muller counter and results in detection
    (d) Occurs in scintillates and results in photo production
172. Which of the following parameters determines the residual activity of ^{99}Mo/^{99m}Tc generator on a weekend?
    (a) Initial activity of molybdenum
    (b) The number of elutions
    (c) The half-life of ^{99m}Tc
    (d) The half-life of ^{99}Tc
173. The photon attenuation of three TVL (tenth-value layer) is … times that of HVL (half-value layer).
    (a) 6
    (b) 10
    (c) 18
    (d) 25

174. The half-life of 125I is 60 days. What happens to the decay constant after 120 days?
 (a) Decay constant decreases to half.
 (b) Decay constant does NOT change.
 (c) Decay constant increases by two times.
 (d) Decay constant increases by four times.
175. Which statement is correct?
 (a) Alpha particles show more deviation in each interaction than beta particles.
 (b) The tissue range of nuclear particles is directly related to their mass.
 (c) The tissue range of nuclear particles is directly related to their electrical charge.
 (d) The specific ionization of alpha particles is higher than that of beta particles.
176. The stability of the nucleus depends on:
 (a) The number and energy of neutrons
 (b) The number of electrons and energy of orbitals
 (c) The number and energy of protons
 (d) The ratio of neutrons to protons
177. If the attenuation constant of aluminum is 6.93 cm, how thick is the tenth-value layer (TVL) of aluminum?
 (a) 0.43 cm
 (b) 0.693 cm
 (c) 2.3 cm
 (d) 6.8 cm
178. What is the main reason for the instability of radioactive nuclei?
 (a) Elimination of electromagnetic power between protons
 (b) Elimination of nuclear power between protons
 (c) Elimination of nuclear power between protons and neutrons
 (d) Imbalance of nuclear and electromagnetic powers
179. Which statement is correct?
 (a) The number of electrons in each shell is 2l+1.
 (b) Each major shell contains $2n^2$ electrons.
 (c) According to Pauli's law, at least three quantum numbers are equal in every two electrons.
 (d) The shell nuclear model is similar to the surface tension in a drop of water.
180. How thick is the half-value layer (HVL) of a material with a linear attenuation coefficient (μ) of $0.22\ cm^{-1}$?
 (a) 3.15 cm
 (b) 6.16 cm
 (c) 5.8 cm
 (d) 2.15 cm

181. Which type of decay is used on a myocardial thallium scan?
(a) Isomeric radiation
(b) Internal conversion
(c) β decay
(d) Electron capture
182. Which of the following formulas describes the percentage of standard deviation in a Poisson model of photon distribution?
(a) $(n/\sqrt{n}) \times 100$
(b) $(\sqrt{n}/n) \times 100$
(c) $[n/\sqrt{(n-1)}] \times 100$
(d) $[\sqrt{(n/(n-1))}] \times 100$
183. If the maximum photon energy of β emission from $^{32}_{15}P$ is 1.71 keV, how much is the average energy of this photon?
(a) 0.52 MeV
(b) 0.44 MeV
(c) 0.57 MeV
(d) 0.14 MeV
184. How long does it take for the activity of a ^{131}I sample (half-life, 8.1 days) to decrease to less than 1% of the initial value?
(a) 97.7 days
(b) 56.7 days
(c) 43.3 days
(d) 33.3 days
185. Sievert is the unit of … and is … fold of the previous unit.
(a) Exposure, 10
(b) Equivalent dose, 100
(c) Absorbed dose, 20
(d) Radiation intensity, 2.78
186. 11.1×10^{10} Bq is … Ci.
(a) 3.0
(b) 8.7
(c) 16.6
(d) 47.0
187. What is the unit of radiation exposure in the International System of Units (SI)?
(a) Gray (Gy)
(b) Coulomb/kg (C/kg)
(c) Roentgen®
(d) Rem
188. What is the maximum electron capacity of the M shell in Bohr's model?
(a) 6 electrons
(b) 16 electrons
(c) 18 electrons
(d) 32 electrons

189. Which of the following phenomena is described by the change in electron arrangement with a constant number of electrons in the atom?
(a) Excitation
(b) Thermionic
(c) Photoelectric
(d) Ionization
190. What is the reason for the utilization of targets with a high atomic number (Z) in the production of bremsstrahlung X-ray?
(a) Higher yield of X-ray production
(b) Production of low scatter radiation
(c) Higher heat tolerance
(d) Production of more specific rays
191. If $^{A}_{Z}X$ nucleus decays with alpha radiation and the kinetic energies of the daughter nucleus and the alpha particle after disintegration are T and Tα, respectively, what is the relationship between T and Tα?
(a) T = 0
(b) T = Tα
(c) T = (4/A)Tα
(d) T = [4/(A-4)]Tα
192. Which between $^{56}_{26}Fe$ and $^{57}_{26}Fe$ nuclei has higher neutron separation energy, and what is the reason for this difference?
(a) $^{56}_{26}Fe$, because of fusion energy
(b) Equal, because these nuclei are isotopes
(c) $^{56}_{26}Fe$, because of its lower mass
(d) $^{57}_{26}Fe$ because of the even–odd ratio of the atomic and mass numbers
193. How much is the kinetic energy of the Auger electron produced in the transfer of electron from the L orbital to K in Au atom if the electron binding energies in the L and K orbitals are 13.335 keV and 80.713 keV, respectively?
(a) 12.654 KeV
(b) 32.231 KeV
(c) 54.043 KeV
(d) 65.765 KeV
194. How long does it take for 5 mCi of ^{131}I (half-life = 8.05 days) and 2 mCi of ^{32}P (half-life = 14.3 days) to reach an equal level of activity?
(a) 29.12 days
(b) 24.34 days
(c) 48.86 days
(d) 118.12 days
195. Regarding the even–even effect in the nucleus:
(a) The frequency of even nucleons (odd N and Z) in nature is greater than those of other forms.
(b) The relative frequency of nuclei with even nucleons (odd N and Z) is greater than those of other forms.
(c) The nuclei with even neutrons and protons are more stable.
(d) The nuclei with equal N and Z with magic numbers are more stable.

196. How long does the degradation of 7/8 of $^{24}_{11}Na$ radioisotope take? (half-life = 15 h)
 (a) 45 h
 (b) 34 h
 (c) 23 h
 (d) 86 h
197. Regarding the mass energy transfer coefficient:
 (a) $\mu_{tr}/p = \mu_{en}/p\ (1-g)$, where g is the ratio of energy transfer in *bremsstrahlung* radiation.
 (b) $\mu_{tr}/p = [(\mu_{en}/p)/(1-g)]$, where g is the ratio of energy transfer in *bremsstrahlung* radiation.
 (c) $\mu_{tr}/p = \mu_{en}/p\ (1-g)$ is the ratio of photon energy that exits as radiation.
 (d) $\mu_{tr}/p = [(\mu_{en}/p)/(1-g)]$ is the ratio of photon energy that exits as radiation.
198. If a radioactive nuclide is produced at a constant rate of n through neutron bombarding, what is the number of produced nuclei after t seconds?
 (a) $(n/\lambda) + (N_0\ n/\lambda)\ e^{-\lambda t}$
 (b) $[N_0 -(n/\lambda)]\ e^{-\lambda t}$
 (c) $N_0\ e^{-\lambda t}$
 (d) $(N_0\ n/\lambda)\ e^{-\lambda t}$
199. Which of the following experimental findings of β decay is the base of the neutrino hypothesis?
 (a) Electrons always accompany neutrinos.
 (b) Stability of magic nuclei.
 (c) Continuous energy spectrum of the produced nucleus.
 (d) Direct detection of the neutrino in lab.
200. Which of the following radiations has the highest range in water?
 (a) Gamma ray with energy of 1 MeV
 (b) Beta ray with energy of 1 MeV
 (c) Alpha
 (d) Proton
201. Where in the spectrum of ^{99m}Tc is the Compton edge located with a NaI scintillation detector?
 (a) After the main peak toward higher energies
 (b) Between the main peak and the backscatter peak
 (c) Between PbK-specific radiation and the backscatter peak
 (d) Between zero energy and the backscatter peak
202. If gamma photons encounter one TVL and one HVL, what percentage of them is attenuated?
 (a) 45%
 (b) 65%
 (c) 95%
 (d) 15.5%

9.5.1 Answer

	A	B	C	D		A	B	C	D		A	B	C	D
1		*			81	*				161		*		
2	*				82			*		162		*		
3	*				83		*			163			*	
4	*				84			*		164		*		
5			*		85	*				165			*	
6	*				86	*				166	*			
7	*				87				*	167			*	
8			*		88		*			168	*			
9		*			89	*				169	*			
10				*	90		*			170		*		
11	*				91				*	171			*	
12			*		92			*		172	*			
13		*			93			*		173		*		
14			*		94	*				174		*		
15		*			95		*			175				*
16	*				96			*		176				*
17		*			97		*			177			*	
18				*	98			*		178				*
19	*				99				*	179		*		
20				*	100			*		180	*			
21	*				101				*	181	*			
22			*		102			*		182		*		
23			*		103			*		183			*	
24		*			104			*		184		*		
25		*			105			*		185		*		
26	*				106			*		186	*			
27	*				107	*				187		*		
28			*		108				*	188			*	
29			*		109				*	189	*			
30		*			110			*		190	*			
31		*			111		*			191				*
32				*	112		*			192				*
33	*				113				*	193			*	
34				*	114		*			194		*		
35	*				115			*		195			*	
36		*			116	*				196	*			
37			*		117		*			197		*		
38		*			118				*	198	*			
39		*			119			*		199			*	
40				*	120				*	200	*			
41		*			121			*		201		*		
42	*				122			*		202			*	
43	*				123	*								
44	*				124				*					

45		*			**125**			*						
46				*	**126**				*					
47				*	**127**			*						
48	*				**128**				*					
49				*	**129**	*								
50	*				**130**		*							
51		*			**131**		*							
52				*	**132**		*							
53				*	**133**	*								
54	*				**134**			*						
55	*				**135**			*						
56				*	**136**			*						
57	*				**137**			*						
58		*			**138**	*								
59		*			**139**	*								
60			*		**140**			*						
61			*		**141**		*							
62	*				**142**		*							
63	*				**143**	*								
64			*		**144**			*						
65			*		**145**		*							
66			*		**146**			*						
67				*	**147**				*					
68			*		**148**				*					
69				*	**149**		*							
70		*			**150**				*					
71			*		**151**			*						
72				*	**152**				*					
73	*				**153**				*					
74		*			**154**			*						
75			*		**155**		*							
76	*				**156**		*							
77	*				**157**	*								
78				*	**158**	*								
79		*			**159**				*					
80				*	**160**			*						

9.6 Nuclear Medicine Imaging Instrumentation

1. For a general-purpose collimator, system resolution at 10 cm is approximately:
   (a) 4 mm
   (b) 9.5 mm
   (c) 15 mm
   (d) 20 mm
2. If the energy resolution of a NaI crystal for ^{99m}Tc is about 10%, how much is this value in 151 keV of energy?
   (a) 19%
   (b) 6%
   (c) 16%
   (d) 10%
3. On scintigraphy with ^{99m}-Tc, if the photopeak energy is mistakenly set to 160 keV, which one is the most probable with the same window?
   (a) Scattered photons increase.
   (b) The image is smoothened.
   (c) Sensitivity decreases.
   (d) Spatial resolution remains unaffected.
4. Which of the following group of factors affects the amplitude of the received pulses of PHA?
   (a) Type of radioactive agent, type of detector crystal, type of PMP lamp, enhancing efficiency
   (b) Type of radioactive agent, type of detector crystal, type of PMP lamp
   (c) Type of detector crystal, type of PMP lamp, enhancing efficiency, administered dose, enhancing efficiency
   (d) Administered dose, enhancing efficiency
5. What is the advantage of LSO over BGO?
   (a) Shorter scintillation time
   (b) Higher atomic number
   (c) Higher density
   (d) Higher energy resolution
6. On thyroid scintigraphy with a pinhole collimator with a small diameter:
   (a) Sensitivity does NOT change.
   (b) Smaller nodules are detectable.
   (c) Decrease in magnification to distance ratio.
   (d) A smoother image is obtained.

7. If paralyzable detectors are used instead of non-paralyzable ones:
   (a) Noise increases and smoothness improves.
   (b) Energy resolution improves.
   (c) The efficiency of the detector does NOT change.
   (d) Intrinsic sensitivity increases.
8. Which statement is correct about determining the sensitivity of a gamma camera if the distance of a vial containing 5 mCi of ^{99m}Tc from a gamma camera is 10 cm?
   (a) Determination of sensitivity is performed without error.
   (b) Sensitivity is overestimated.
   (c) Error depends on the counting time.
   (d) Error depends on the smoothness test.
9. In which of the following collimators can the spatial resolution of the system be lower than the intrinsic spatial resolution (without a collimator)?
   (a) Parallel hole
   (b) Convergent
   (c) Divergent
   (d) Pinhole
10. The specific curve of two filters in a frequency space is presented. The cutoff frequency ratio to the Nyquist frequency is 0.5. Which of the curves represents the Hamming filter?
   (a) A
   (b) B
   (c) C
   (d) D

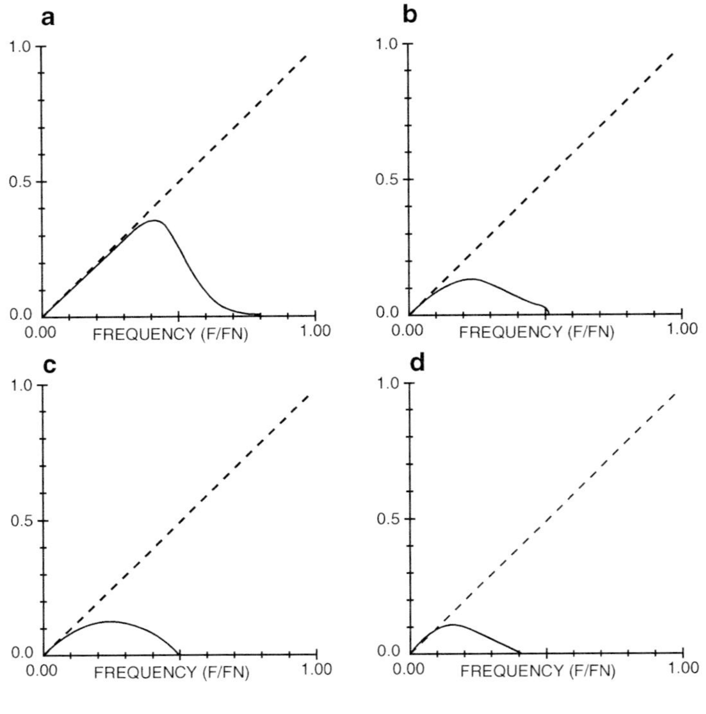

11. The changes in spatial resolution relative to the distance from the collimator is presented for different parallel-hole collimators. The arrow-marked curve corresponds to which item?
    (a) General purpose
    (b) High resolution
    (c) High sensitivity
    (d) Ultrahigh sensitivity

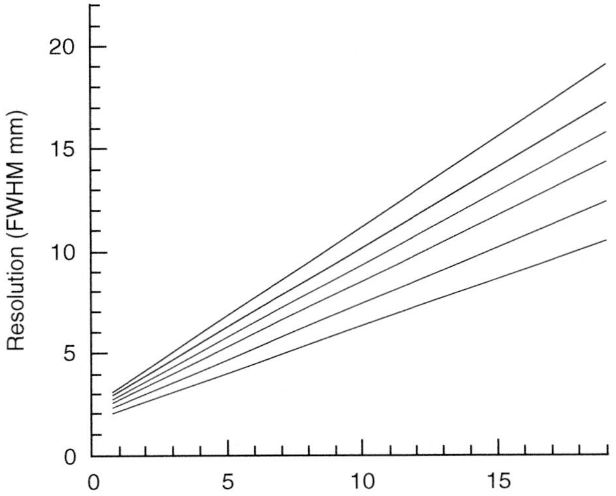

12. The following image describes the changes in some parallel-hole collimators with respect to the patient's distance from the collimator. Which item corresponds to the high-resolution collimator?
    (a) A
    (b) B
    (c) C
    (d) D

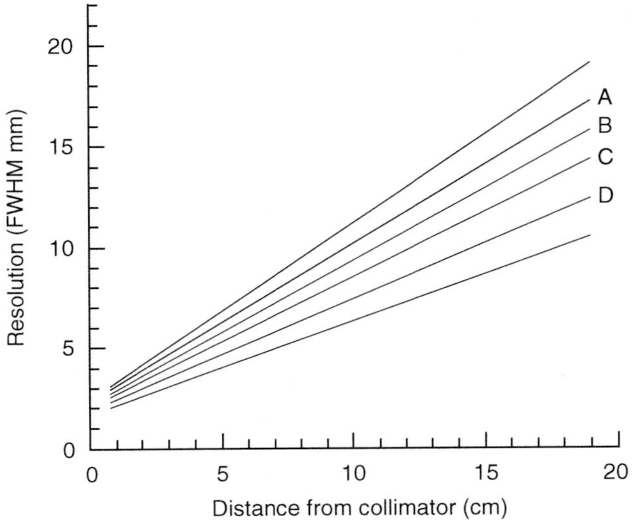

13. Which of the following items affects the energy resolution efficiency of the gamma camera?
    (a) Energy of the photons
    (b) Thickness of the detector
    (c) Type of collimator
    (d) Patient's distance from the collimator
14. Which of the following items affects the photopeak range?
    (a) Intrinsic efficiency of the detector
    (b) Geometrical efficiency of the detector
    (c) Photon interaction with the detector
    (d) Cutoff frequency of filters
15. What happens to sensitivity if the diameter of a parallel-hole collimator is doubled?
    (a) Sensitivity increases by twofold.
    (b) Sensitivity increases by fourfold.
    (c) Sensitivity decreases to one-half.
    (d) Sensitivity decreases to one-fourth.
16. Which of the following factors affects the height of pulses that reach PHA?
    (a) Time of imaging
    (b) Physical half-life of the radionuclide
    (c) Administered dose
    (d) Type of the radionuclide
17. The patient distance from the collimator is increased from 10 cm to 30 cm. Which of the following parallel-hole collimators shows the most change in spatial resolution?
    (a) Low energy, general purpose (LEGP)
    (b) High sensitivity, low energy (HSLE)
    (c) Medium sensitivity, general purpose (MSGP)
    (d) High resolution, general purpose (HRGP)
18. A vial containing 10 mCi of ^{99m}Tc is located in front of a gamma camera. Which part of the spectrum changes if the same dose is injected into a patient and imaging is repeated?
    (a) Counting of Compton edge
    (b) Photopeak height
    (c) Photopeak energy
    (d) Photopeak range
19. About image resolution in nuclear medicine:
    (a) If spatial resolution is rapidly degraded for surfaces near the focal plane, the collimator is high field.
    (b) Determining the spatial resolution of the collimator is NOT possible with a single-point image source.
    (c) The FWHM or LSF in the width of a linear source does NOT result in spatial resolution.
    (d) Geometric resolution is directly related to the thickness of the collimator.

20. In which of the following conditions does the PHA analyzing system have an output pulse? (E1, lower balance; E2, higher balance)
    (a) Input pulse lower than E1.
    (b) Input pulse between E1 and E2.
    (c) Input pulse higher than E2 (anticoincidence system).
    (d) Each pulse can be produced in any condition.
21. What is the main factor for a radioactive pileup?
    (a) Pulse height analyzer
    (b) 1–5 μs light decay in NaI crystal
    (c) Sample volume
    (d) Amplifier system and energy window
22. About collimator resolution:
    (a) The FWHM of a counting profile in the width of a linear radioactive source is used to determine the spatial resolution of a camera.
    (b) Geometrical resolution is the single determinant of spatial resolution.
    (c) Sensitivity increases linearly with the increase in spatial resolution.
    (d) Spatial resolution only depends on intrinsic resolution.
23. In a well-designed well-counter system with an approximately equal activity between the standard and the sample, what is the acceptable counting rate?
    (a) 5000 C/s
    (b) 20,000 C/s
    (c) 30,000 C/s
    (d) 100,000 C/s
24. Which method is used to eliminate the nonuniformity of resolution?
    (a) Taking the average of numerous photons
    (b) Application of a collimator that provides a uniform resolution at the object field
    (c) Application of fixed focused collimators
    (d) Imaging without a collimator
25. What is the ideal energy window of radioisotope photons for imaging?
    (a) 80–150 keV
    (b) 100–250 keV
    (c) 80–250 keV
    (d) 100–150 keV
26. What is the purpose of the PMT application in a scintillator detector?
    (a) Photon conversion to visible light
    (b) Amplification of visible light
    (c) Visible conversion to electrical signal
    (d) Amplification of electrical signal
27. If the crystal thickness increases in a gamma camera, what happens to the sensitivity and resolution of the system, respectively?
    (a) Increase, better
    (b) Decrease, worse
    (c) Increase, worse
    (d) Decrease, better

28. What happens to the energy resolution when the photon energy is reduced in a gamma camera?
    (a) Improves (decreases).
    (b) Deteriorates (increases).
    (c) It depends on the electronic system.
    (d) It has no relationship with energy.
29. Which source is preferred for the intrinsic uniformity test of a gamma camera?
    (a) Point source with a 10 cm distance
    (b) Point source with a distance of less than 1 FOV
    (c) A point source on the detector
    (d) A point source with a minimum distance of 1.5 FOV
30. What happens if the intrinsic resolution of the detector is better than the collimator resolution in a gamma camera system?
    (a) The image has very good quality.
    (b) The image of the collimator holes appears.
    (c) The resolution of the images decreases.
    (d) The sensitivity of the system increases.
31. The Metz filter is a … filter.
    (a) Low-pass
    (b) High-pass
    (c) Restoration
    (d) Inverse
32. The noise distribution in nuclear medicine complies with which type of statistical distribution?
    (a) Poisson
    (b) Gaussian
    (c) Normal
    (d) Bertoli
33. Which type of collimator results in the better quality of images in brain imaging?
    (a) Pinhole
    (b) LEHR
    (c) LEGP
    (d) Fan beam
34. What is the reason for applying Butterworth and Metz filters, respectively, in nuclear medicine?
    (a) Noise reduction, resolution restoration
    (b) Resolution restoration, noise reduction
    (c) Noise reduction, noise reduction
    (d) Noise increase, resolution restoration

35. What happens when the statistical oscillations are reduced in photon gathering and light production in scintillator detectors?
    (a) Energy resolution improves.
    (b) Efficiency increases.
    (c) Intrinsic efficiency improves.
    (d) Geometric efficiency improves.
36. What happens to the resolution and sensitivity when the source distance from the head increases with the parallel-hole collimator?
    (a) Decrease, no change
    (b) Decrease, increase
    (c) No change, decrease
    (d) Increase, no change
37. In which organ does attenuation correction with Chang's algorithm results in a good response?
    (a) Kidney
    (b) Brain
    (c) Heart
    (d) Pubis
38. The FWHM of a collimator with a 10 cm source distance from the head is 8 mm and that of the detector is 2 mm. What is the total FWHM of the system?
    (a) 4 mm
    (b) 12 mm
    (c) 8.2 mm
    (d) 10.4 mm
39. The aim is to decrease the FWHM to only half by changing the diameter of the collimator holes. Sensitivity is then reduced to:
    (a) 1/8
    (b) 1/32
    (c) 1/4
    (d) 1/16
40. The FWTM is seven times more than the FWHM in a collimator:
    (a) The geometric resolution of this collimator is low.
    (b) The sensitivity of the collimator is not acceptable.
    (c) Penetration into this collimator wall is high.
    (d) This is an ideal collimator.
41. The FWHM of tomographic imaging is 8 mm. The pixel size in a 128 × 128 matrix is 3.56. Which zooming factor is recommended for a 64 × 64 matrix according to the Nyquist theorem?
    (a) Zoom = 10
    (b) Zoom = 2.34
    (c) Zoom = 1.73
    (d) Zoom = 2

42. Which of the following collimators results in a two to three times increase in sensitivity in comparison with a parallel collimator with a similar resolution?
    (a) Fan beam
    (b) Pinhole
    (c) Converging
    (d) Cone beam
43. The final quality of a nuclear medicine image is determined by:
    (a) Resolution
    (b) Sensitivity
    (c) Uniformity of response across the detector
    (d) All of the above
44. About gamma camera collimators in nuclear medicine:
    (a) The geometric coefficient of multiple focused collimators is the subtraction of geometric coefficient in all focuses.
    (b) In multiple focused collimators, the geometric coefficient is constant for all points in the Z plate and field of view.
    (c) Divergent-hole collimators have a magnification effect.
    (d) The system resolution of parallel-hole collimators is calculated by $R_s = \sqrt{R_i \times R_g}$, where R_i is the intrinsic resolution and R_g is the geometric resolution.
45. About the resolution of collimators:
    (a) The FWHM of the counting profile in a linear radioactivity source is used to determine the spatial resolution.
    (b) Geometric resolution is the only determinant of spatial resolution.
    (c) Sensitivity is linearly increased with the increase in spatial resolution.
    (d) Spatial resolution depends only on intrinsic resolution.
46. Which item decreases the density of data in the image in linear scanners?
    (a) Decrease in distance between the lines
    (b) Increase in speed
    (c) Increase in the administered dose
    (d) Increase in the energy window width
47. The increase of which variable can enhance spatial resolution in a gamma camera?
    (a) Height of the collimator hole
    (b) Range of the PHA window
    (c) Crystal thickness
    (d) Patient's distance from the collimator
48. Which collimator produces the largest and inverse image in a gamma camera?
    (a) Parallel
    (b) Pinhole
    (c) Convergent
    (d) Divergent

49. Which item is caused by the pileup effect?
    (a) Decreased range of energy window
    (b) Improvement of energy resolution
    (c) Decreased spatial resolution
    (d) Increased sensitivity of the system
50. What happens to the counting rate when the source activity in a non-paralyzable counter is increased?
    (a) Primarily increases followed by a constant rate
    (b) Linearly increases
    (c) Primarily increases followed by a decrease
    (d) Primarily increases followed by a sudden drop to zero
51. Which item is induced by low-pass filters in the frequency range?
    (a) Increase in contrast
    (b) Decrease in noise
    (c) Better distinction of edges
    (d) Decrease in data density
52. In which working area of gas detectors is the response of a detector independent of the applied voltage?
    (a) Recombination
    (b) Saturation
    (c) Proportional
    (d) Limited proportion
53. The geometric efficiency of the detector depends on:
    (a) Type of source decay
    (b) Source decay constant
    (c) Distance of the source from the detector
    (d) Specific activity of the source
54. Photon fraction is the proportion of gamma photons that:
    (a) Interacts with the crystal
    (b) Produces a photoelectric interaction with the crystal
    (c) Is emitted with an angle of 180°
    (d) Passes through the crystal without any interaction
55. The energy resolution of a gamma camera system with energy of 140 keV is equal to the FWHM of 10%. What is the photopic range?
    (a) 126–154 keV
    (b) 133–147 keV
    (c) 140–154 keV
    (d) 130–150 keV
56. What happens in a gamma camera when crystal thickness increases?
    (a) Decrease in efficiency
    (b) Decrease in gamma photon scatter
    (c) Increase in light photon scatter
    (d) Increase in spatial resolution

57. Which of the following variables markedly affects the counting efficiency of a gamma camera?
    (a) Shape of the holes
    (b) Diameter of the holes
    (c) Length of the holes
    (d) Thickness of the holes
58. If the counting rate in a gamma camera is 10^6 count/min, what is the system error rate?
    (a) 0.1%
    (b) 11%
    (c) 1.5%
    (d) 2.5%
59. Which part of a gamma camera light photon is converted to electron during the production of an electric signal?
    (a) Photocathode
    (b) Crystal
    (c) Dynode
    (d) Amplifier
60. In the quality control of gamma camera uniformity, the extrinsic method has … compared with the intrinsic method.
    (a) Shorter procedure
    (b) More accuracy
    (c) Higher radiation exposure of the technician
    (d) Lower counting rate
61. Which parameter is critical in measuring a sample activity with a calibrator dose?
    (a) Calibration coefficient
    (b) Decay constant
    (c) Type of emission
    (d) Radiation energy
62. Septal penetration causes:
    (a) Decreased sensitivity
    (b) Increased spatial resolution
    (c) Increased patient dose
    (d) Decreased contrast
63. In comparing different imaging systems, which variable shows a better spatial resolution when increased?
    (a) FWHM
    (b) PSF
    (c) LSF
    (d) MTF
64. What is the most suitable filter to decrease blurring induced by scatter photons?
    (a) High-pass
    (b) Low-pass
    (c) Medium-pass
    (d) Restoration

65. Which of the following regions in a converging collimator provides the highest resolution?
    (a) The region with the highest sensitivity
    (b) The plate crossing from the presumed intersection of holes
    (c) The back of the collimator on a crystal
    (d) Collimator surface
66. What happens to the counting rate (sensitivity) and resolution if the length of the collimator hole in a parallel-hole collimator increases by three times?
    (a) The count rate decreases to 1/9, and the resolution increases.
    (b) The count rate increases nine times, and the resolution decreases.
    (c) The count rate does not change, and the resolution increases nine times.
    (d) The count rate does not change, and the resolution decreases to 1/9.
67. What is the most appropriate collimator for imaging an organ smaller than the scintillation detector surface?
    (a) Parallel-hole collimator
    (b) Slant-hole collimator
    (c) Converging collimator
    (d) Diverging collimator
68. The line spread function (LSF) is used for the estimation of:
    (a) Pulse height analyzer
    (b) Sensitivity
    (c) Uniformity
    (d) Resolution
69. Quartz fiber electrometers work the … zone of the ionization chamber.
    (a) Recombination
    (b) Proportional
    (c) Geiger
    (d) Saturation
70. In the energy range of 20–40 keV, … mediates the absorption of maximum energy in the gamma photon interaction.
    (a) Compton
    (b) Pair production
    (c) Rayleigh scatter
    (d) Photoelectric
71. If the goal is to distinguish pulses originating from alpha, beta, and gamma radiations, which functional part of a gas detector is the most suitable?
    (a) Ionization chamber
    (b) Proportional
    (c) Geiger
    (d) Recombination
72. Which of the following counting methods can be used to determine the maximum counting rate in a sample?
    (a) Differential mode
    (b) Average of the integral and differential modes
    (c) Integral mode
    (d) Subtraction of integral and differential modes

73. Which of the following adjustments increases the spatial resolution?
    (a) Decrease in crystal thickness and decrease in the number of PMTs
    (b) Decrease in crystal thickness and increase in the number of PMTs
    (c) Increase in crystal thickness and increase in the number of PMTs
    (d) Increase in crystal thickness and decrease in the number of PMTs
74. A point source is used for the quality control of a SPECT apparatus. How far is the minimum distance for this source assuming that the vertical positioning of the source to the visual center?
    (a) 5 CFOV
    (b) 5 UFOV
    (c) 2 UFOV
    (d) 2 CFOV
75. If the goal is to measure the intensity of emitted radiations in a gas detector, which of the following variables is recorded?
    (a) Released ions by radiation
    (b) All existing molecules in the sensitive material
    (c) Produced lights in the sensitive material
    (d) Produced heat by radiation
76. What happens when the object distance increases from a collimator in cameras with a converging-hole collimator?
    (a) Distortion of image
    (b) Decrease in visual field of the camera
    (c) Decrease in spatial resolution
    (d) Increase in absorbed dose
77. In a gamma camera, energy resolution depends on the:
    (a) Diameter of the detector
    (b) Distance from the collimator
    (c) Activity of the source
    (d) Photon energy
78. The increase in which variable decreases the sensitivity of a camera with a convergent collimator?
    (a) Efficiency of the photomultiplier lamp
    (b) Patient's distance from the camera
    (c) Thickness of the collimator
    (d) Thickness of the NaI (Tl) crystal
79. Energy resolution depends on the … in gamma camera.
    (a) Type of collimator
    (b) Intensity of radiation
    (c) Photon energy
    (d) Thickness of the crystal
80. What is the geometric efficiency rate if the distance of a gamma-radiating agent is 10 cm from a 4-cm^2-wide detector?
    (a) 2%
    (b) 0.75%
    (c) 8%
    (d) 4%

81. What is the function of a photomultiplier lamp in a scintillation detector?
    (a) Absorption of gamma rays, electron production, and amplification
    (b) Absorption of emitted light from the scintillator, electron production, and amplification
    (c) Absorption of gamma rays and production of light
    (d) Absorption and amplification of emitted light from the scintillator
82. The quenching mechanism is commonly used in:
    (a) Gas flow proportional counter
    (b) Geiger–Muller counter
    (c) Dose calibrator
    (d) Pocket dosimeter
83. Which of the following systems provides the highest resolution?
    (a) Geiger counter
    (b) Scintillation counter
    (c) Proportional counter
    (d) Semiconductor detector
84. What is the main function of a slant-hole collimator in nuclear medicine?
    (a) Increase the total resolution of the imaging system
    (b) Increase the total sensitivity of the imaging system
    (c) Better rotation and relocation of the patient
    (d) Inhibition of the rotation and relocation of the patient
85. Which of the following collimators has a large field of view (FOV) in a 10 cm distance?
    (a) Parallel hole
    (b) Converging hole
    (c) Pinhole
    (d) Diverging hole
86. Which statement is correct?
    (a) The number of PMT in a gamma camera has NO effect on the x–y coordination of pulses
    (b) Fan-beam collimators are convergent holes in one dimension and parallel holes in the other.
    (c) Attenuation correction and scatter correction are required on 180° SPECT but NOT on 360° SPECT.
    (d) The ramp filter does NOT amplify the image frequencies in regions dominated by noise.
87. Which statement is correct?
    (a) All data are used in each iteration in the ordered-subset expectation maximization (OSEM).
    (b) Axial resolution describes the blurring in axis alignment.
    (c) On a ^{99m}Tc brain SPECT, the emitted rays from the central regions of the brain show NO attenuation in comparison with those emitted from lateral regions.
    (d) NO difference can be found in photon attenuation between a coincidence system and a single-photon system.

88. This formula (all counts in the entire spectrum/number of radiations impinging on the detector) gives the:
    (a) Photopeak efficiency
    (b) Photofraction
    (c) Geometric efficiency
    (d) Intrinsic efficiency
89. The modulation transfer functions (MTFs) at a certain spatial frequency of the detector, the PM tubes, and the PHA of a gamma camera are 0.7, 0.5, and 0.5, respectively. What is the overall MTF?
    (a) 0.175
    (b) 0.342
    (c) 1.7
    (d) 0.017
90. Which of the following tools is utilized in a TLD reader?
    (a) Diode detector
    (b) Scintillation counter
    (c) Geiger counter
    (d) Photomultiplier tube
91. Which of the following parameters describes the capability of a gamma camera to detect photons?
    (a) Linearity of energy
    (b) Accuracy
    (c) Resolution
    (d) Sensitivity
92. Which of the following parameters is critical in the intrinsic nonuniformity of a camera?
    (a) Collimator damage
    (b) PMT malfunction
    (c) Nonuniformity of the radioactive source
    (d) Deterioration of the energy resolution
93. If the spatial resolution of the collimator and the intrinsic spatial resolution of the system are 10 mm and 4.6 mm, respectively, what is the total spatial resolution of the camera?
    (a) 9 mm
    (b) 10 mm
    (c) 11 mm
    (d) 12 mm
94. The spatial resolution and sensitivity of a gamma camera are 10 mm and 5000 cpm/mCi, respectively. How much is the sensitivity of the system if the collimator is replaced with another one that has spatial resolution of 5 mm?
    (a) 12,500 cpm/mci
    (b) 275,000 cpm/mci
    (c) 654,000 cpm/mci
    (d) 9250 cpm/mci

95. A decreased dead time in a gamma camera causes:
    (a) Increased energy resolution
    (b) Decreased spatial resolution
    (c) Decreased scattered photons
    (d) Increased system efficiency
96. The pulse height analyzer (PHA) in nuclear imaging increases:
    (a) Detecting efficiency
    (b) Scattered photons
    (c) Counting rate
    (d) Signal-to-noise ratio
97. What happens after dose calibration in a calibrator?
    (a) Accuracy of measurement increases.
    (b) Measurement error decreases.
    (c) Statistical error decreases.
    (d) Validity does NOT change.
98. Which item is NOT a scintillating detector?
    (a) Well counter
    (b) Gamma counter
    (c) Dose calibrator
    (d) PET scanner
99. Which of the following detectors has a high rate of photon detection?
    (a) Gas detector
    (b) Scintillation detector
    (c) Semiconductive detector
    (d) Proportional detector
100. Gas amplification occurs in the … region of gas detectors.
    (a) Recombination
    (b) Ionization
    (c) Proportional
    (d) Geiger–Muller
101. If a gas detector is used for imaging, the detector must operate in the:
    (a) Ionization chamber
    (b) Proportional
    (c) Rearrangement
    (d) Geiger–Muller

9.6.1 Answer

	A	B	C	D		A	B	C	D
1		*			53			*	
2		*			54		*		
3			*		55		*		
4		*			56			*	
5			*		57				*
6		*			58	*			

7				*	**59**	*			
8		*			**60**	*			
9				*	**61**	*			
10		*			**62**				*
11			*		**63**				*
12				*	**64**				*
13	*				**65**				*
14			*		**66**	*			
15		*			**67**			*	
16				*	**68**				*
17		*			**69**				*
18	*				**70**				*
19				*	**71**	*			
20		*			**72**			*	
21		*			**73**		*		
22			*		**74**		*		
23				*	**75**	*			
24		*			**76**			*	
25		*			**77**				*
26			*		**78**			*	
27			*		**79**			*	
28		*			**80**				*
29				*	**81**		*		
30		*			**82**		*		
31			*		**83**				*
32	*				**84**				*
33				*	**85**				*
34	*				**86**		*		
35	*				**87**		*		
36	*				**88**				*
37		*			**89**	*			
38			*		**90**				*
39				*	**91**				*
40			*		**92**		*		
41				*	**93**			*	
42				*	**94**	*			
43				*	**95**				*
44		*			**96**				*
45	*				**97**		*		
46		*			**98**			*	
47	*				**99**			*	
48		*			**100**			*	
49			*		**101**		*		
50	*								
51		*							
52		*							

9.7 Nuclear Medicine Computers: Basic Principle

1. A disk can store … times as many 64 × 64 images as 256 × 256.
   (a) 4
   (b) 8
   (c) 16
   (d) 32
2. To increase the difference in the mass attenuation coefficient between bone and tissue, we must:
   (a) Decrease the photon energy
   (b) Increase the photon count
   (c) Decrease the radiation dose
   (d) Decrease the geometric efficiency of the detector
3. Which quality control test of gamma cameras requires daily checks?
   (a) Uniformity
   (b) Spatial resolution
   (c) Linearity
   (d) a and c
4. What is the difference between the images obtained by 64 × 64 × 16 and those obtained by 64 × 64 × 8 matrices?
   (a) Higher resolution
   (b) Smoother image
   (c) Application of a filter with lower cutoff frequency
   (d) Lower noise
5. If the diameter of a crystal is 32 cm and the image matrix is 128 × 128, how much is the Nyquist frequency?
   (a) 3.9 cycle/mm
   (b) 0.2 cycle/mm
   (c) 0.76 cycle/mm
   (d) 0.85 cycle/mm
6. About the variables in imaging software:
   (a) A large matrix is required in static evaluation to inhibit the decrease in resolution.
   (b) Frame change after the initiation of data acquisition is possible with most software.
   (c) In gated studies, if the heart rate is 60, RR interval is 1000 ms, and 20 frames are obtained for each RR interval, the time for each frame will be 10 ms.
   (d) The list mode is used for reformatting and for applying numbers with special characteristics.

7. About nuclear imaging and radioisotopic data acquisition:
   (a) A small matrix size is used in static evaluation to inhibit the deterioration of resolution.
   (b) A physiologic signal is used only for the synchronization of data acquisition in gated studies.
   (c) The RR interval is instantly used to determine the frames in a gated study.
   (d) The required storage capacity for the list mode is lower than that for the frame mode.
8. Which of the following parameters affects pixel size?
   (a) The distance of collimator from source of radiation
   (b) Gantry angle
   (c) Distance of gantry from center of rotation
   (d) Zooming factor
9. Which scan requires more storage capacity?
   (a) Dynamic
   (b) List mode
   (c) SPECT
   (d) Gated SPECT
10. In nuclear medicine image display, the process of mapping the counts in the image to the available colors is called:
    (a) Scaling
    (b) Thresholding
    (c) Sampling theorem
    (d) Linear interpolation
11. If 400 counts are recorded per mm^2, what is the signal-to-noise ratio in each mm^2?
    (a) 600/1
    (b) 200/1
    (c) 60/1
    (d) 20/1
12. A 256 × 256 matrix is used for the imaging of a field of view of 25 cm in SPECT imaging. What is the pixel size in this test?
    (a) $0.5 \times 0.5\ mm^2$
    (b) $1 \times 1\ mm^2$
    (c) $4 \times 4\ mm^2$
    (d) $8 \times 84\ mm^2$
13. Useful field of view (UFOV) includes:
    (a) The pixels with activity content of about 95% of the central pixel
    (b) The pixels with activity content of about 1/3 of the central pixel
    (c) The pixels with activity content equal to or more than 50% of the central pixel
    (d) The pixels with activity content of less than 25% of the central pixel

14. In comparing paralyzable and non-paralyzable systems (r, observed count rate; R, true count rate),
    (a) r increments (increases stepwise) with the increase in R in paralyzable systems.
    (b) r decreases with the increase in R in non-paralyzable systems.
    (c) r increases with the increase in R until saturation in paralyzable systems.
    (d) r increases with the increase in R until saturation in non-paralyzable systems.
15. Which statement is correct?
    (a) On ^{99m}Tc SPECT, the proportion of scatter events to the total counting events is low.
    (b) Energy window manipulation is NOT indicated for scatter correction.
    (c) Spillover has NO relationship or similarity with the partial volume effect.
    (d) Recovery coefficient is the ratio of true count density to the reconstructed count density.
16. The image of a material in a linear imaging system is mathematically the result of:
    (a) Material convolution and point spread function (PSF)
    (b) Material deconvolution and PSF
    (c) Material convolution, PSF, and noise
    (d) Material deconvolution, PSF, and noise
17. What is the main advantage of reconstructing with OSEM rather than with MLEM?
    (a) More accurate reconstruction
    (b) Decreased noise
    (c) Faster reconstruction
    (d) Reconstruction of more slices

9.7.1 Answer

	A	B	C	D
1			*	
2	*			
3	*			
4	*			
5		*		
6	*			
7		*		
8				*
9		*		
10	*			
11				*
12		*		
13			*	
14				*
15				*
16			*	
17			*	

9.8 Nuclear Medicine Computers: Applications

1. It determines the rate at which the filter amplitude falls off:
   (a) Order
   (b) Power
   (c) Modulation transfer function (MTF)
   (d) Nyquist frequency
2. If the cutoff frequency increases, which of the followings occurs?
   (a) Better image resolution, lower noise.
   (b) Lower image resolution, higher noise.
   (c) Smoother image.
   (d) Both image resolution and noise will increase.
3. Which of the following filters provides the highest smoothness and the lowest noise?
   (a) RAMP
   (b) Butterworth
   (c) Hamming
   (d) Parzen
4. Which of the following items reduces noise in imaging?
   (a) Increase in cutoff frequency of the filter
   (b) Decrease in matrix size
   (c) Decrease in thickness of the crystal detector
   (d) Decrease in PHA window
5. If a significant level of radiation is found in the studied zone, which of the following filters gives the highest image resolution?
   (a) Butterworth filters at a Nyquist cutoff frequency of 3%
   (b) Butterworth filters at a Nyquist cutoff frequency of 4%
   (c) Parzen
   (d) Ramp
6. Which of the following items increases noise?
   (a) Decreased cutoff frequency
   (b) Decreased matrix size
   (c) Increased filter degree
   (d) Decreased PHA window
7. Which of the following items affects the amplitude of PHA-arriving pulses?
   (a) Time of imaging
   (b) Mean effective life
   (c) Dose of the radiotracer
   (d) Type of radiotracer
8. Which of the following affects spatial resolution efficiency, smoothness, and linearity of SPECT images?
   (a) Time of imaging
   (b) PMT efficiency
   (c) Administered dose of the radiotracer
   (d) Cutoff frequency of the filter

9. Which of the following filters is described as follows: "high resolution and maximum elimination of background counting and higher noise"?
   (a) Parzen
   (b) Butterworth
   (c) Ramp
   (d) Hamming
10. What happens in ^{99m}Tc imaging if the photopeak energy increases from 140 to 155, while the PHA window remains constant?
    (a) Scattered photons decrease.
    (b) Noise decreases.
    (c) Sensitivity decreases.
    (d) Spatial resolution increases.
11. The maximum and minimum counts are 2900 and 2100, respectively, in the uniformity test with a 512 × 512 matrix. What is the integral uniformity value?
    (a) 18
    (b) 16
    (c) 1.2
    (d) 2.8
12. Filtering can be applied to which of the following item(s)?
    (a) 2D image dataset
    (b) 3D image dataset
    (c) A curve
    (d) All of the above
13. The gamma camera image of which radiopharmaceutical has low quality because of inappropriate photon energy?
    (a) ^{123}I
    (b) ^{67}Ga
    (c) ^{111}In
    (d) ^{99m}Tc
14. Which of the following parameters can exclusively show the quality of SPECT imaging?
    (a) Linearity
    (b) Resolution
    (c) Uniformity
    (d) Center of rotation
15. What is the function of a pulse height analyzer (PHA) in a gamma camera?
    (a) Analyze and interpret the signals produced in the head of the camera
    (b) Increase the amplifying gain of the system
    (c) Correct the dead time counting
    (d) Analyze the count rate
16. What is the formula for image contrast (C) on scintigraphy? (A and B are the density of the recorded counts between two neighboring regions, respectively)
    (a) C = (A + B)/A
    (b) C = A − B
    (c) C = (A − B)/A
    (d) C = AB

9.8.1 Answer

	A	B	C	D
1	*			
2				*
3				*
4		*		
5				*
6				*
7				*
8		*		
9			*	
10			*	
11		*		
12				*
13		*		
14			*	
15	*			
16				*

9.9 Single-Photon Emission Computed Tomography

1. If the distance from the point source is r, then the final back-projected value is:
   (a) r^2
   (b) $1/r^2$
   (c) $1/r$
   (d) $2 r^2$
2. If the count density in a reconstruction is 400 counts/pixel with roughly 2000 resolution elements, the signal-to-noise ratio (SNR) for the reconstruction is:
   (a) 4
   (b) 3
   (c) 6
   (d) 8
3. Which method is used on SPECT to obtain smoother images?
   (a) Adjustment of the efficiency of PMT lamps
   (b) Averaging of many images
   (c) Adjustment of the photopeak energy
   (d) Adjustment of the energy window
4. About the partial volume phenomenon:
   (a) Changes in spatial resolution relative to the sample volume.
   (b) Changes in energy resolution relative to the sample volume.
   (c) Zones with low radioactivity are underestimated.
   (d) Zones with low radioactivity are overestimated when surrounded by high-activity zones.
5. On SPECT:
   (a) The energy window must always be confirmed in cameras with auto peaking.
   (b) The counting of a flood source for SFOV is higher than that for LFOV in a uniformity test.
   (c) Collimators must be evaluated annually.
   (d) COR in a SPECT camera is the evaluation of the alignment of two different views. An error of 3 mm in alignment does NOT significantly change the resolution.
6. About sampling and reconstruction of images in a SPECT system:
   (a) Reconstruction depends on the shape and size of the object.
   (b) Attenuation correction is NOT important in the reconstruction of SPECT.
   (c) Nonuniformity of resolution relative to depth is not available for parallel-hole collimators.
   (d) The minimum angle of sampling on SPECT is 10°.
7. Which test is used for detecting collimator dysfunction on SPECT?
   (a) Intrinsic uniformity
   (b) Collimator penetration
   (c) Linearity test
   (d) Extrinsic uniformity

8. What is the advantage of having a low-energy resolution on SPECT?
   (a) Increased sensitivity
   (b) Elimination of scatter photons
   (c) Increased time resolution
   (d) Decreased dead time
9. What happens to the intrinsic peak efficiency on SPECT when energy is increased?
   (a) Increases.
   (b) Decreases.
   (c) No change.
   (d) It depends on the thickness of the crystal.
10. What is the recommended collimator if SPECT is performed with high-energy radioisotopes and requires extremely high resolution?
    (a) HEGP
    (b) HEHS
    (c) HEUHR
    (d) HEHR
11. What is the recommended imaging method for the detection of ring artifacts in a SPECT system?
    (a) Planar with a point source and without a collimator
    (b) SPECT with a point source and with a collimator
    (c) SPECT phantom with a collimator
    (d) Planar with flood phantom and a collimator
12. Which gamma calibration is specific for SPECT?
    (a) Uniformity
    (b) Spectrometry
    (c) Linearity
    (d) COR
13. ... calibration is required if concentric rings are observed in the reconstructed image.
    (a) Uniformity
    (b) Spectrometry
    (c) Linearity
    (d) COR
14. Which of the following gamma cameras is the most suitable for the myocardial SPECT study with a 180° rotation?
    (a) Gamma camera with two 90° detectors
    (b) Gamma camera with two 120° detectors
    (c) Gamma camera with two 180° detectors
    (d) Gamma camera with one detector
15. The center of rotation (COR) correction for a SPECT gamma camera should be performed:
    (a) Every week
    (b) Every day
    (c) Every month
    (d) With uniformity correction

16. Which of the following methods is used for the fusion of PET or SPECT images?
    (a) MRI and CT
    (b) MRI and angiography
    (c) CT and angiography
    (d) Sonography and angiography
17. Regarding brain SPECT scan:
    (a) The shape of the head in a single-head SPECT does NOT affect the obtained images.
    (b) Increasing the number of heads does NOT change the sensitivity of the system.
    (c) The distance of the camera edge from the crystal edge is a critical factor in data acquisition.
    (d) The collimator type does NOT affect the obtained image in new cameras.
18. Which of the following measurements is appropriate for the uniformity test of a gamma camera (SPECT or planar)?
    (a) Integral uniformity in UFOV
    (b) Integral uniformity in CFOV
    (c) Differential uniformity in UFOV
    (d) Differential uniformity in CFOV
19. In SPECT systems:
    (a) Collimators with magnification are more sensitive.
    (b) An increased resolution does NOT enhance image contrast.
    (c) The artifacts of 180° and 360° imaging methods are similar.
    (d) Bladder fullness does NOT interfere with abdominal imaging.
20. In SPECT imaging:
    (a) Data acquisition from one section must be performed with different directions.
    (b) The spatial resolution of this method is usually higher than that of computed tomography.
    (c) The concurrent detection of gamma rays produced from pair annihilation is performed through this method.
    (d) Imaging usually takes less than 2 min.
21. Which of the following amendments increases the quality of brain SPECT images?
    (a) LEGP
    (b) High-pass window filtering
    (c) Fan-beam collimator
    (d) Single-head camera
22. Which types of matrices can be normally used in SPECT imaging?
    (a) 64 and 128
    (b) 128 and 256
    (c) 256 and 512
    (d) 512 and 1024

23. The application of … color distribution increases the resolution of high-count pixels.
    (a) Linear
    (b) Exponential
    (c) Logarithmic
    (d) Semilogarithmic
24. What happens in a gamma camera imaging when the matrix size is increased from 64 × 64 to 128 × 128? (all other variables are assumed constant)
    (a) System efficiency increases.
    (b) System efficiency decreases.
    (c) Noise decreases.
    (d) Noise increases.
25. What is the reason behind SPECT imaging having more details than a gamma camera?
    (a) Higher spatial resolution
    (b) Higher counting efficiency
    (c) Rapid imaging procedure
    (d) Separation of images of overlapping tissues
26. Which of the following errors on SPECT produces a loop image from a point source?
    (a) Nonuniformity
    (b) Nonlinearity
    (c) Energy window calibration error
    (d) Misalignment of the mechanical center of rotation and electrical center of the system

9.9.1 Answer

	A	B	C	D
1			*	
2		*		
3	*			
4				*
5	*			
6	*			
7				*
8		*		
9		*		
10			*	
11			*	
12				*
13	*			
14	*			
15				*
16	*			

17			*	
18	*			
19	*			
20	*			
21			*	
22	*			
23			*	
24				*
25				*
26				*

9.10 Positron Emission Tomography

1. The following are characteristics of 3D PET *except*:
   (a) Improves image quality in low-count studies
   (b) Reduces the administered radiation dose
   (c) Reduces scanning time in clinical studies
   (d) Reduces scattered coincidences
2. Which radionuclide used in PET provides the best spatial resolution?
   (a) ^{11}C
   (b) ^{18}F
   (c) ^{15}O
   (d) ^{82}Rb
3. Where in the spectrum is the backscatter peak for ^{18}F radioparticle located?
   (a) 90 keV
   (b) 170 keV
   (c) 285 keV
   (d) 340 keV
4. Which of the following radionuclides has the shortest positron range?
   (a) ^{18}F
   (b) ^{11}C
   (c) ^{13}N
   (d) ^{15}O
5. Which one is considered an advantage of PET/CT over PET?
   (a) Decreases the time of attenuation correction
   (b) Better spatial resolution of PET
   (c) Increased PET sensitivity
   (d) Decreases noise in PET
6. Which one is the key feature of PET?
   (a) Notable decrease in scattered photons.
   (b) Absence of collimators.
   (c) Attenuation correction is not required.
   (d) High spatial resolution.
7. What happens when the crystals against both BMT lamps in a PET system are divided into smaller crystals?
   (a) Sensitivity increases.
   (b) Random events decrease.
   (c) True events increase.
   (d) Localization of photons improves.
8. Which of the following parameters decreases with the increase in sensitivity of PET system imaging?
   (a) Magnification
   (b) Signal-to-noise ratio
   (c) Contrast
   (d) Energy resolution

9. Which of the following somatostatin analogues is used in the PET imaging of neuroendocrine tumors?
   (a) ^{99m}Tc-labeled somatostatin analogues
   (b) 111-In-labeled somatostatin analogues
   (c) ^{68}Ga-labeled somatostatin analogues
   (d) ^{177} Lu-labeled somatostatin analogues
10. Which of the following groups of radionuclides decays by positron emission and is identified as physiological tracers?
    (a) ^{13}N, ^{11}C, ^{15}O
    (b) ^{18}F, ^{111}In, ^{68}Ga
    (c) ^{15}O, ^{11}C, ^{14}N
    (d) ^{11}C, ^{13}N, ^{16}O
11. Which difference between normal and tumoral tissue is studied by PET in oncology?
    (a) Anatomic
    (b) Metabolic
    (c) Density
    (d) Hormonal
12. In PET and SPECT imaging:
    (a) Convulsion subtraction is used to compensate for scattering.
    (b) The statistical precision of SPECT does NOT depend on counting or volume.
    (c) Positron range does NOT affect the blurring of PET images, and this effect is acceptable up to FWHM of 3 mm.
    (d) High-sensitivity collimators increase the sensitivity of a camera by 30% in PET imaging.
13. What are the main physical limiting factors for spatial resolution in PET imaging?
    (a) Crystal thickness and positron range
    (b) Photon energy and deviation of 511 keV photons from a 180° alignment
    (c) Positron range and deviation of 511 keV photons from a 180° alignment
    (d) Crystal thickness and photon energy
14. What is the common scintillation crystal at the time of flight in the PET system?
    (a) BGO
    (b) BaF_2
    (c) NaI
    (d) CSF
15. Which item is considered a limitation of the PET system?
    (a) Increased energy of the emitted photons.
    (b) The positron travel path; the longer the positron pathway, the lesser the resolution.
    (c) The remnant kinetic energy of positron; the higher the level of this energy, the better the achieved resolution.
    (d) Lack of a parallel-hole collimator.

16. About the detector efficiency of the BGO scintillation system in PET:
    (a) BGO is commonly used in PET systems because of its stationary capability.
    (b) BGO with 1 cm thickness can counteract 90% of the gamma radiation.
    (c) BGO has a very short decay time.
    (d) BGO has a very high light output.
17. Which parameter is affected the most by the crystal size in the detector of a PET apparatus?
    (a) Contrast
    (b) Scatter ratio
    (c) Conformity of resolution
    (d) Spatial resolution
18. Which phenomenon in PET is described by the transmission of photon from one crystal and the absorption on the other without any interaction?
    (a) Intercrystal scatter
    (b) Penetration
    (c) Parallax
    (d) Interaction
19. Which coincidence phenomenon is recorded because of the annihilation of two positrons?
    (a) Random coincidence
    (b) True coincidence
    (c) Scatter coincidence
    (d) Triple coincidence
20. Resolution and count rate tests of a PET scanner should be performed:
    (a) Daily
    (b) Weekly
    (c) Monthly
    (d) Annually
21. Which item is NOT considered an advantage of CT images for the attenuation correction of PET images?
    (a) Low administered dose
    (b) Rapid transitional scan
    (c) Accurate tumor localization
    (d) Decrease in noise
22. The error of positron range increases with the increase of:
    (a) Diameter of the detector loop
    (b) Energy of the emitted positron
    (c) Crystal dimensions
    (d) Number of detectors
23. In a PET system, what is the effect of time of flight technique on image quality?
    (a) Increase in contrast
    (b) Increase in resolution
    (c) Decrease in contrast
    (d) Decrease in resolution

24. In PET imaging, what is the easiest and most common method of eliminating scatter photons?
    (a) Software
    (b) Adjustment of energy window
    (c) Deconvulsion
    (d) OSEM rearrangement
25. Which type of coincidence shows more increase with the increase in administered dose?
    (a) Correction coincidence
    (b) Scatter coincidence
    (c) Random coincidence
    (d) Scatter and random coincidences
26. In PET imaging, which parameter is mostly affected by the size of the detector crystal?
    (a) Contrast
    (b) Regional resolution
    (c) Scatter ratio
    (d) Uniformity of regional resolution
27. How is the sensitivity of 2D PET imaging compared with that of 3D PET?
    (a) Higher.
    (b) Lower.
    (c) Equal.
    (d) It depends on the target organ.
28. Which of the following coincidences is the most likely to be eliminated with the decrease in time window in the data acquisition of PET?
    (a) Scatter coincidences
    (b) True coincidences
    (c) Random coincidence
    (d) True and random coincidences
29. What is the advantage of the application of the time of flight (TOF) method on a PET/CT scan?
    (a) Increased spatial resolution
    (b) Increased contrast
    (c) Increased sensitivity
    (d) Increased energy resolution
30. If the goal is to improve the spatial resolution of PET, which variable should be increased?
    (a) Time window width
    (b) Energy window width
    (c) Positron range
    (d) Number of collinear photons
31. Which phenomenon is identified as the base of PET?
    (a) Pair production
    (b) Annihilation
    (c) Photoelectric absorption
    (d) Compton effect

32. What is the reason for applying the transmission scan in PET?
    (a) Shortening of the main imaging procedure
    (b) Background subtraction
    (c) Attenuation correction
    (d) Center of rotation (COR) correction
33. Which of the following events plays the main role in image formation in PET?
    (a) Random coincidence
    (b) Coincidence resolving time
    (c) Scattered coincidence
    (d) Positron range finding
34. In which of the following positron emitters is the proximity of the imaging center with cyclotron required?
    (a) ^{18}F
    (b) ^{82}Rb
    (c) ^{15}O
    (d) ^{62}Cu
35. If attenuation correction is NOT performed on a PET scan, the diagnosis of which tumors is the most problematic?
    (a) Head and neck
    (b) Thorax
    (c) Abdomen
    (d) Pelvis
36. Compared with CT scan and magnetic resonance images (MRIs), PET images appear:
    (a) More blurry.
    (b) Noisier.
    (c) Detector resolution is poorer.
    (d) All of the above.
37. The scintillators for PET photon detection have better efficacy with:
    (a) Low stopping power
    (b) High decay constant
    (c) High light production
    (d) Low intrinsic resolution
38. All statements are correct about PET imaging *except*:
    (a) Most of the lesions can be observed without attenuation correction.
    (b) Deep structures in the body center or near the regions with intense uptake of FDG are more likely to be overlooked if attenuation correction is NOT performed.
    (c) Filtered back-projection is more common than the iterative method for image processing.
    (d) 3D FDG-PET requires a higher dose of FDG than 2D FDG-PET.
39. Although 2D PET is more commonly used in most of cancers, 3D PET provides better images with a low FDG dose and less noise in … cancers.
    (a) Brain
    (b) Heart
    (c) Adrenal
    (d) Lung

40. Describe the resolution and sensitivity of PET imaging compared with those of coincidence imaging with a dual-head gamma camera.
    (a) Comparable resolution, higher sensitivity of coincidence imaging
    (b) Higher resolution and sensitivity of coincidence imaging
    (c) Similar resolution and sensitivity
    (d) Comparable resolution, lower sensitivity of coincidence imaging
41. What happens in PET when the positron energy decreases?
    (a) Energy resolution is enhanced.
    (b) Energy resolution is decreased.
    (c) Spatial resolution is enhanced.
    (d) Spatial resolution is decreased.
42. What happens in PET imaging when time resolution is enhanced?
    (a) Scattered coincidence is decreased.
    (b) Random coincidence is decreased.
    (c) Scattered coincidence is increased.
    (d) Random coincidence is increased.

9.10.1 Answer

	A	B	C	D
1				*
2		*		
3		*		
4	*			
5	*			
6		*		
7				*
8			*	
9			*	
10	*			
11		*		
12	*			
13			*	
14		*		
15		*		
16	*			
17				*
18			*	
19	*			
20				*
21	*			
22		*		
23		*		
24		*		
25			*	
26		*		
27				*

28			*	
29		*		
30				*
31		*		
32			*	
33		*		
34			*	
35	*			
36				*
37			*	
38				*
39	*			
40				*
41			*	
42		*		

9.11 Molecular Imaging Fundamentals

1. This type of molecular imaging has 2–3 mm spatial resolution, <1 cm depth, second-to-minute temporal resolution, and 10^{-9}–10^{-12} mol/l best estimate sensitivity.
   (a) PET
   (b) Optical bioluminescence imaging
   (c) Optical fluorescence imaging
   (d) MRI
2. Which items have the maximum and least absorption rate of X-ray, respectively?
   (a) Air, fat
   (b) Bone, soft tissue
   (c) Bone, air
   (d) Soft tissue, air
3. Which tissue density on CT scan (Hounsfield scale) is not correct?
   (a) Kidney: +40
   (b) Liver: +80
   (c) Muscle: +45
   (d) Fat: −80
4. What is the main purpose of the phase 1 of clinical studies for drug discovery?
   (a) Animal experiments for evaluating the possibility of human studies
   (b) Determination of dose range for phases 2 and 3
   (c) Identification of tumors for which the drug may be efficient
   (d) Comparison of a new drug with a standard in a small population for the possibility of designing the next phases
5. What is the main advantage of MRI over CT scan?
   (a) Contrast
   (b) Resolution
   (c) Imaging time
   (d) Depth of imaging
6. What is the main reason for applying contrast media in MRI?
   (a) To decrease T1 and imaging time
   (b) To increase T1 and signal-to-noise ratio (SNR)
   (c) To decrease T1 and signal-to-noise ratio (SNR)
   (d) To decrease T1 and increase imaging time
7. In a malignant lesion, T1 and T2 … because of …
   (a) Increase, water
   (b) Decrease, temperature
   (c) Increase, temperature
   (d) Decrease, water

8. Which of the following parameters is critical in the determination of the thickness of slice on CT scan?
   (a) Matrix size
   (b) Pixel size
   (c) Field of view (collimation) of detectors
   (d) Imaging time
9. Total imaging time in MRI is independent of:
   (a) The number of frequency encoding steps
   (b) The number of phase encoding steps
   (c) The repetition time (TR)
   (d) The number of data acquisitions
10. The absorption of ultrasound waves in tissue depends on:
   (a) Relaxation time and frequency
   (b) Viscosity and frequency
   (c) Relaxation time and viscosity
   (d) Viscosity and attenuation coefficient

9.11.1 Answer

	A	B	C	D
1			*	
2			*	
3			*	
4		*		
5	*			
6	*			
7	*			
8			*	
9	*			
10	*			

9.12 Radiation Protection and Dosimetry in Clinical Practice

1. What is the unit of exposure in the International System of Units (SI)?
   (a) Bq
   (b) Ci
   (c) Coulomb/kg
   (d) Gy
2. A 20 g mouse receives 2 Gray radiation. The absorbed energy is:
   (a) 0.04 J
   (b) 0.8 J
   (c) 1.9 J
   (d) 1.0 J
3. If the charge of a particle is doubled, what (fold change) will be the tissue range?
   (a) 0.25
   (b) 0.75
   (c) 6
   (d) 2
4. What is the main mechanism of the biological damage of ionizing rays?
   (a) Indirect effect from hydroxyl free radicals
   (b) Indirect effect from hydrogen free radicals
   (c) Direct effect on DNA molecules
   (d) Direct effect on protein molecules
5. A patient receives 5 rad of alpha, 10 rad of beta, and 20 rad of gamma radiation. What is the equivalent dose?
   (a) 1.3 Sievert
   (b) 4.6 Sievert
   (c) 3.2 Sievert
   (d) 8.2 Sievert
6. Which of the following adjustments decreases the shoulder of the survival curve?
   (a) Reduction of dose settings
   (b) Augmentation of LET
   (c) Reduction of tissue oxygen
   (d) Replacing beta with gamma ray
7. What is the unit of mass attenuation coefficient?
   (a) Cm^{-1}
   (b) Cm^2/gr
   (c) Cm^3/gr
   (d) gr/Cm^3
8. The radiation weighting factor is used for the calculation of:
   (a) Absorbed dose
   (b) Equivalent dose
   (c) Exposure
   (d) Effective dose

9. What is the unit of cumulative radiation in the Medical Internal Radiation Dose (MIRD) method?
   (a) mCi. hour
   (b) mCi/h
   (c) mCi
   (d) mSv/h
10. The dose–response curve of cataract induced by ionizing rays is:
   (a) Linear with threshold
   (b) Linear without threshold
   (c) Sigmoid with threshold
   (d) Sigmoid without threshold
11. A patient receives 200 mCi of radioactive iodine. If another individual stands beside him for 15 min with a distance of 10 cm, how much of the radiation dose will this person absorb?
   (a) 1.27
   (b) 0.8
   (c) 2.4
   (d) 8.2
12. Which of the following values can describe the society absorbed dose in diagnostic nuclear medicine?
   (a) Absorbed dose
   (b) Effective dose
   (c) Equivalent effective dose
   (d) Cumulative effective dose
13. Which item is the most efficient to reduce the exposure of personnel who apply ^{90}Sr on patients?
   (a) Maintain appropriate distance.
   (b) Use rubber gloves.
   (c) Use a syringe shield.
   (d) Use a lead apron.
14. ^{32}P emits:
   (a) Gamma ray
   (b) X- and gamma rays
   (c) X- and beta rays
   (d) Beta ray
15. Absorbed dose is:
   (a) Absorbed energy per unit of volume
   (b) Absorbed energy per unit of mass
   (c) Produced electric charge per unit of volume
   (d) Produced electric charge per unit of mass

16. If 1.2 Gray of neutron is required for erythema and the RBE for rapid neutron radiation is 1.8, what is the required dose for X-ray (250 kvp) to produce the same effect?
    (a) 216 rad
    (b) 16 rad
    (c) 12 rad
    (d) 220 rad
17. If equal amounts of the following radiopharmaceuticals are administered, which one produces the highest absorption dose?
    (a) ^{201}TlCl
    (b) ^{111}In-DTPA
    (c) ^{99m}Tc-SC
    (d) ^{67}Ga-citrate
18. What is the equivalent dose in an individual standing for 0.5 h with a 10 cm distance from a patient who has received 100 mCi of ^{131}I?
    (a) 11.3 mSev
    (b) 8.6 mSev
    (c) 6.2 mSev
    (d) 22.2 mSev
19. Which of the following cancers can be a consequence of radiation?
    (a) CML
    (b) Hodgkin's disease
    (c) Non-Hodgkin's lymphoma
    (d) CLL
20. LET is defined as:
    (a) Energy release in unit of length
    (b) Ratio of absorbed photons in unit of length
    (c) Thickness of materials that decreases the number of photons to 50%
    (d) Pattern of absorbed dose in unit of length
21. What is the unit of collective effective dose?
    (a) C/Kg.Sv
    (b) C/Kg.Gy
    (c) Man.Gy
    (d) Man.Sv
22. The equivalent dose of a radiology worker is 100 millisieverts. Assuming that the worker is exposed only to ^{131}I, how much is the absorbed dose?
    (a) 40 rad
    (b) 20 milligray
    (c) 0.1 Gray
    (d) 5 rem
23. About the stochastic effects of ionizing radiation:
    (a) Response is dose dependent.
    (b) The dose–response curve is always sigmoid.
    (c) The threshold dose is zero.
    (d) Response is linear with a threshold.

24. If the quality factors for X-ray, rapid neutrons, and alpha particles are 1, 20, and 20, respectively, how much is the equivalent dose of a subject exposed to 0.9 Gy X-ray, 0.03 Gy rapid neutron, and 0.06 Gy alpha radiation?
    (a) 0.027 Sv
    (b) 0.27 Sv
    (c) 2.7 Sv
    (d) 27 Sv
25. About radiobiological variables and detector systems:
    (a) The F factor depends on energy.
    (b) The daughter nuclei of radon (^{218}Polonium and ^{214}Polonium) do NOT play a role in carcinogenicity.
    (c) Film badge has a lower dose range for X and gamma radiations.
    (d) The Geiger–Müller counter is NOT a very sensitive detector of contamination.
26. Which of the following studies produces high exposure (mR/h with 1 m distance)?
    (a) ^{99m}Tc-RBC cardiac-gated imaging, 20 mCi
    (b) Tumor imaging by ^{67}Ga-citrate, 3 mCi
    (c) ^{201}Tl-chloride myocardial perfusion, 3 mCi
    (d) ^{99m}Tc-MDP bone scan, 25 mCi
27. A breastfeeding mother receives 5 μCi of ^{131}I for thyroid evaluation. How long must she pause breastfeeding?
    (a) Approximately 3 days
    (b) Approximately 1 week
    (c) Approximately 3 weeks
    (d) Approximately 10 weeks
28. A patient with thyroid cancer receives 100 mCi of ^{131}I. If all radioprotection parameters are noted, what is the required equivalent dose limit for his discharge?
    (a) Equal to or less than 50 μSv/h (5 mrem/h) in a 1 m distance
    (b) Equal to or less than 15 μSv/h in a 1 m distance
    (c) Equal to or less than 5 μSv/h in a 1 m distance
    (d) Equal to or less than 1 μSv/h in a 1 m distance
29. If the half-life of a radioactive particle is less than 65 days, how long is the required time for this particle to be characterized as ordinary garbage?
    (a) One half-life
    (b) 3 half-lives
    (c) 7 half-lives
    (d) 10 half-lives

30. About the assessment of internal dose:
    (a) Cumulated activity indicates the total counting for a specific radioactive particle in a source organ.
    (b) S factor indicates the total biologic harm of a cumulated activity of the source organ in CGy/μCi.h.
    (c) If the physical and biological half-lives are equal, the mean effective life is equal to the physical half-life.
    (d) The distribution of radioisotope in the organ is considered nonhomogenous when the goal is to calculate the internal dose by the MIRD method.
31. About the effects of ionizing radiation on human biological systems:
    (a) Stochastic effects have a specific threshold dose.
    (b) The threshold for deterministic effects in the primary embryonic life is 5–15 mGy.
    (c) Abortion must be considered if the fetus is exposed to more than 150 mGy radiation because of high statistical risk.
    (d) Stochastic effects are observed in much higher doses than those applied in diagnostic nuclear medicine.
32. How long is the required time of breastfeeding discontinuation after ^{67}Ga administration?
    (a) 4 h
    (b) 4 days
    (c) 4 weeks
    (d) 4 months
33. Which of the following equations is used for the calculation of mean life? (τ, mean life; Teff, mean effective life; Tbio, biological half-life; Tph, physical half-life)
    (a) $\tau = T_{eff} + T_{bio}$
    (b) $\tau = 0.693\ T_{eff}$
    (c) $\tau = 1.44\ T_{1/2\ eff}$
    (d) $\tau = 1.44\ T_{ph}$
34. … has a high-quality factor (QF) and therefore high biological harm in an equal condition.
    (a) X and gamma radiation
    (b) Positive beta radiation
    (c) Negative beta radiation
    (d) Neutron and positron
35. Which of the following radiopharmaceuticals induces the highest biological harm per 1 mCi of activity?
    (a) ^{99m}Tc-DTPA
    (b) ^{111}In-DTPA
    (c) ^{131}I-NaI (35% uptake)
    (d) ^{67}Ga-citrate

36. Which item about the discontinuation of breastfeeding after the administration of radionuclides is NOT correct?
    (a) 10 mCi of ^{99m}Tc-Na-pertechnetate, discontinuation for 24 h
    (b) 10 mCi of ^{67}Ga-citrate, discontinuation for 4 weeks
    (c) 3 mCi of ^{201}Tl-chloride, discontinuation for 3 weeks
    (d) 10 mCi of ^{131}I-Na citrate, discontinuation for 6 weeks
37. The exposure rate is 40 mR/h in a 1 m distance from a thyroid cancer patient who has received 200 mCi of ^{131}I, and it is 6 mR/h after hospitalization. How much is the remaining activity 2 days after hospitalization?
    (a) 125 mCi
    (b) 30 mCi
    (c) 45 mCi
    (d) 70 mCi
38. External radiation of a 17 Ci ^{99}Mo/^{99m}Tc generator is measured at the time of delivery. How much is the allowed surface dose rate?
    (a) <200 millirem/h
    (b) <400 millirem/h
    (c) <440 millirem/h
    (d) <550 millirem/h
39. If one lead gown decreases radiation transfer by 95%, what is the transfer rate from two lead gowns?
    (a) 0.25%
    (b) 0.5%
    (c) 1%
    (d) 1.25%
40. Which of the following formula is used to determine the effective dose of X-ray?
    (a) $H.W_R.D$
    (b) $W_T.W_R.S_E$
    (c) $D.W_R.W_T$
    (d) D.Q
41. If the radiation of a technologist's hands is 300 milligray during radiopharmaceutical injection, how much will the radiation be if he uses a syringe shield?
    (a) 40 milligray
    (b) 60 milligray
    (c) 250 milligray
    (d) 440 milligray
42. Compare the tissue range of different particles assuming equal energy among α, β, and γ rays.
    (a) $\gamma < \beta < \alpha$
    (b) $\gamma = \beta = \alpha$
    (c) $\alpha < \gamma < \beta$
    (d) $\alpha < \beta < \gamma$

43. In … phase of cell cycle, the cells are more susceptible to ionizing radiation.
    (a) G2, M
    (b) G1, S
    (c) S, M
    (d) G2, S
44. How much will the radiation exposure be if the distance from radiation source increases by four times?
    (a) 1/32
    (b) 1/8
    (c) 1/4
    (d) 1/16
45. The cell survival curve in low LET radiation is distinguished from that in high LET radiation based on:
    (a) Shoulder
    (b) Higher slope
    (c) Lower survival ratio with equal doses
    (d) Identical slope with equal doses
46. About random events of ionizing radiation:
    (a) The incidence of these events has a threshold.
    (b) The probability of these events is zero in lower energies.
    (c) It includes the genetic effects of radiation.
    (d) The incidence of these events is independent of dose.
47. How much is the cumulative effective dose (CED) limit for the whole body of a 37-year-old subject with previous occupational exposure?
    (a) 77 mSv
    (b) 370 mSv
    (c) 65 mSv
    (d) 850 mSv
48. What is the detector of choice for the evaluation of radioisotopic contamination?
    (a) Film badge
    (b) Thermoluminescence
    (c) Pen
    (d) Geiger
49. About relative biological effectiveness:
    (a) It is constant for each ray.
    (b) It is defined for a specific biological event.
    (c) Sievert is the unit in SI.
    (d) It has an inverse relationship with radiation LET.
50. A 36-year-old breastfeeding woman is subjected to a myocardial scan with ^{201}Tl. How long must she discontinue her breastfeeding?
    (a) 1 week
    (b) 2 weeks
    (c) 3 weeks
    (d) 4 weeks

51. A gamma beam with 10,000 photons passes through absorbent media. How many photons are absorbed if the attenuation coefficients for the photoelectric and Compton events are 0.02 and 0.05, respectively?
    (a) 200
    (b) 800
    (c) 600
    (d) 7300
52. A worker has been exposed to 10 mR/h of radiation with a 2 m of distance from the source. How long is the distance from the source if the equivalent absorbed dose is 2.5 mR/h?
    (a) 19 m
    (b) 14 m
    (c) 6 m
    (d) 4 m
53. Radiation-induced teratogenesis is defined as:
    (a) Congenital defects due to radiation of productive cells before fertilization
    (b) Congenital defects due to radiation of fetus
    (c) Cancer due to ionizing rays
    (d) Body damage due to low exposure
54. The lethal dose for humans is usually:
    (a) LD50/30
    (b) LD60/30
    (c) LD90/30
    (d) LD120/30
55. Most of radiation-induced mutations:
    (a) Are somatic
    (b) Appear in the first generation
    (c) Are radiation-specific spontaneous mutations
    (d) Are autosomal recessive mutations
56. Which of the following tools is NOT suitable for the individual monitoring of nuclear medicine technicians?
    (a) Film badge
    (b) Thermoluminescence dosimeter
    (c) Pocket dosimeter
    (d) Geiger–Müller counter
57. Which of the following items about the Geiger–Müller counter is NOT correct?
    (a) It is a suitable device for the detection of contamination.
    (b) Dead time is a problem of this device.
    (c) It can detect energy aside from radioactivity.
    (d) It is NOT suitable for the detection of a very high amount of radioactivity.

58. The dose rate near the ^{131}I storage vault is 160 mR/h. How thick should the required lead shield be if the goal is to decrease the dose rate to 10 mR/h? (lead HVL, 1.25 cm)
    (a) 5.5 cm
    (b) 6 cm
    (c) 5 cm
    (d) 8 cm
59. Gray (Gy) is the unit for:
    (a) Biological damage
    (b) Absorbed dose
    (c) Exposure
    (d) Exposure and biological damage
60. If the energy of gamma photons is 100 keV, the F factor is high for:
    (a) Muscle
    (b) Fat
    (c) Bone
    (d) Blood
61. Doubling dose is defined as:
    (a) The dose that causes a twofold increase in the incidence of natural mutations
    (b) The dose that causes a twofold increase in the incidence of cancer
    (c) The dose that causes a twofold increase in the incidence of congenital disorders
    (d) A twofold increase in the permitted dose
62. A total of 500 MBq of ^{131}I is used for the treatment of hyperthyroidism. If the thyroid uptake is 50%, how much is the approximate radiation of the ovary and testes, respectively?
    (a) 6 rad, 4 rad
    (b) 8 rad, 2 rad
    (c) 2 rad, 0.8 rad
    (d) 25 rad, 8 rad
63. The stochastic effects of ionizing rays include:
    (a) Erythema
    (b) Permanent sterility
    (c) Cataract
    (d) Leukemia
64. Which organ of radiology workers has a low annual dose limit?
    (a) Whole body
    (b) Eye
    (c) Skin
    (d) Thyroid
65. In radioisotope tests, organ dose is independent of:
    (a) Organ shape
    (b) Imaging time
    (c) Organ size
    (d) Amount of administered activity

66. What is the annual dose limit of the eye lens of radiology workers?
    (a) 50 mSv (5 rem)
    (b) 75 mSv (7.5 rem)
    (c) 100 mSv (10 rem)
    (d) 150 mSv (15 rem)
67. Abortion is recommended in the absorbed dose of:
    (a) 0.1 CGy
    (b) 1 CGy
    (c) 10 CGy
    (d) 100 CGy
68. How long is the required time for discontinuation of breastfeeding after the administration of 10 mCi of ^{99m}Tc-pertechnetate or 5 μCi of radioiodine, respectively?
    (a) 17 h for technetium, 10 h for radioiodine
    (b) 24 h for technetium, 2 months for radioiodine
    (c) 10 h for technetium, 2 weeks for radioiodine
    (d) 48 h for technetium, 3 days for radioiodine
69. About the transfer and concentration of ^{131}I in milk:
    (a) Its concentration in milk is about 33% of the plasma level.
    (b) Its concentration in milk is about 3.3-folds of the plasma level.
    (c) Its concentration in milk is about 13-folds of the plasma level.
    (d) Its concentration in milk is about 33-folds of the plasma level.
70. How much is the radiation of a vial containing 1.1 GBq (30 mCi) of ^{201}Tl at a 25 cm distance? ($\Gamma = 0.45$ Rcm^2/mCi.h at 1 cm)
    (a) 21.6 mR/h
    (b) 17.7 mR/h
    (c) 3.15 mR/h
    (d) 2.45 mR/h
71. If the physical half-life of a radiotracer is 6 h and the organ has NO biological elimination, how much is the cumulative activity after the bolus injection of 6 mCi of the radiotracer?
    (a) 24.5 mCi.h
    (b) 4.23 mCi.h
    (c) 51.84 mCi.h
    (d) 6.43 mCi.h
72. Which group of radiations has the highest weighing factor in the measurement of radiation dose and biological damage?
    (a) Gamma and X photons in all energies, and electrons in all energies
    (b) Neurons with energy of 2–20 MeV
    (c) Protons with energy of higher than 2 MeV
    (d) Alpha particles and fission fragments

73. What percentage of radiation exposure decreases with the application of a syringe shield during radiotracer preparation?
    (a) 20%
    (b) 40%
    (c) 60%
    (d) 80%
74. Which of the following indices in cell survival curves provides more information on radiosensitivity?
    (a) Dq
    (b) Do
    (c) Extrapolation number
    (d) Curve shoulder
75. In radiation protection, quality factor (QF) is associated with:
    (a) Relative biologic effectiveness (RBE)
    (b) Linear energy transfer (LET)
    (c) Restricted mass stopping power
    (d) Tissue weighting factor
76. Two materials of A and B with atomic numbers of 12 and 8, respectively, are exposed to a single energy of gamma ray. What is the ratio of mass attenuation coefficient with respect to their atomic numbers (A/B)?
    (a) $(8/12)^2$
    (b) $(8/12)^3$
    (c) $(12/8)^2$
    (d) $(12/8)^3$
77. … describes the radiosensitivity of a specific type of cells.
    (a) Cell survival curve
    (b) Hypoxic cell ratio
    (c) Water radiolysis
    (d) Dose–response curve
78. A nuclear medicine physician received a whole body absorbed dose of 0.2 rad. How much is the equivalent dose?
    (a) 0.6 mSV
    (b) 2 mSV
    (c) 4 mrem
    (d) 4.5 mrem
79. What happens when the linear energy transfer (LET) increases in terms of the radiosensitivity of tissues?
    (a) The oxygen enhancement ratio (REO) increases.
    (b) The relative biological effect (RBE) increases.
    (c) RBE decreases.
    (d) Both OER and RBE decrease.
80. Regarding the radiosensitivity of cells in different phases of the cell cycle:
    (a) Cells demonstrate the highest radiosensitivity in mitosis or near mitosis.
    (b) The radiosensitivity of cells is constant in the G1 phase.
    (c) The radiosensitivity of cells is equal between mitosis and G1 phases.
    (d) The radiosensitivity of cells is independent of the cell cycle.

81. The stochastic effects of radiation include:
    (a) Cataract
    (b) Shortened lifetime
    (c) Renal failure
    (d) Impotency
82. Regarding the deterministic effects of radiation:
    (a) A threshold dose exists.
    (b) The higher the radiation dose is, the higher the probability of incidence of deterministic effects.
    (c) The severity of these effects is dose independent.
    (d) They induce malignancy because of cellular transformations.
83. How much is the maximum permitted weekly exposure for radiology and nuclear medicine workers?
    (a) 1 mSv
    (b) 5 mSv
    (c) 10 mSv
    (d) 50 mSv
84. Most radiation-induced damages are due to the:
    (a) Compton effect on RNA
    (b) Direct effect on cells
    (c) Indirect effect on cells
    (d) Photoelectric effect on DNA
85. Regarding radiation-induced mutagenesis:
    (a) Low doses of ionizing rays do NOT induce mutation.
    (b) Radiation-induced mutagenesis is a non-stochastic effect.
    (c) Radiation-induced mutagenesis is non-specific and undesirable.
    (d) Radiation-induced mutagenesis is reported only in fruit flies.
86. The relative biological effect (RBE) depends on all of the following variables *except*:
    (a) Linear energy transfer (LET)
    (b) Radiation dose
    (c) Number of treatment sessions
    (d) Type of tissue
87. What is the principal mechanism of the biological effects of ionizing rays?
    (a) Accumulated electrical charge in the substance
    (b) Distortion of the chemical structure of molecules
    (c) Increase in temperature due to radiation exposure
    (d) Mechanical shock of the substance due to bombarding
88. Which of the following variables is critical for the intensity of radiation-induced biological damages?
    (a) Type of radiation
    (b) Type of cell
    (c) Duration of exposure
    (d) All of the above

89. What happens to the oxygen enhancement ratio (OER) when the linear energy transfer (LET) is increased?
    (a) Increases.
    (b) Decreases.
    (c) Does NOT change.
    (d) It is constant at first and then increases.
90. Amifostin is used for radioprotection, but it does NOT provide any protection in:
    (a) Brain cancers
    (b) Bone marrow cancers
    (c) Pulmonary cancers
    (d) Salivary gland cancers
91. Which of the following variables considers the sensitivity to radiation of different organs?
    (a) Linear energy transfer
    (b) Dose equivalent
    (c) Quality factor
    (d) Effective dose equivalent
92. The F factor is used for the conversion of the exposure rate to the absorbed dose of a tissue. This factor depends on:
    (a) Type of tissue and photon energy
    (b) Type of tissue and absorption coefficient of air
    (c) Relative density of bone to water
    (d) Relative density of tissue to air
93. Which of the following tools is suitable for identifying a lost radioactive source or a low amount of contamination?
    (a) Geiger–Müller dosimeter
    (b) Proportional counter
    (c) Ionization chamber
    (d) Thermoluminescence dosimeter
94. What are the monthly and total radiation dose limits for a fetus, respectively?
    (a) 1 and 12 mSv
    (b) 0.5 and 12 mSv
    (c) 0.5 and 5 mSv
    (d) 5 and 50 mSv
95. Regarding chromosomal disorders:
    (a) Duplication is the inverse fusion of the broken end to the same chromosome.
    (b) Dysenteric fragment is the fusion of broken ends from two different chromosomes.
    (c) Chromatid aberrations occur when the cells are subjected to ionizing rays in the G1 phase.
    (d) Chromosome aberrations occur when the cells are subjected to ionizing rays in the G1 phase.

96. Which of the following statements regarding radiation-induced mutation is NOT correct?
    (a) It is probably noncumulative and specific.
    (b) It is probably cumulative and often undesirable.
    (c) It is probably cumulative and specific.
    (d) It is probably noncumulative and often undesirable.
97. The lethal effect of …radiation is dependent on the presence of oxygen.
    (a) Beta
    (b) Gamma
    (c) Neutron
    (d) Alpha
98. Which phase of the cell cycle demonstrates the most resistance to ionizing rays?
    (a) G1
    (b) G2
    (c) S
    (d) M
99. Compare the radiosensitivity of different cell lines.
    (a) Spermatogonia > spermatocyte > fibroblast
    (b) Spermatocyte > spermatogonia > fibroblast
    (c) Fibroblast > spermatogonia > spermatocyte
    (d) Fibroblast > spermatocyte > spermatogonia
100. Which tissues demonstrate the most susceptibility to radiation-induced carcinogenicity?
    (a) Brain, bone marrow
    (b) Brain, thyroid
    (c) Bone marrow, thyroid
    (d) Brain, bone marrow, thyroid
101. What is the most effective radioprotective shield against ^{99m}Tc?
    (a) Lead, cadmium
    (b) Tungsten, boron
    (c) Lead, tungsten
    (d) Tungsten, cadmium
102. Protection against radiations with a … dose response is critical in radioprotection.
    (a) Nonlinear, non-threshold
    (b) Linear, non-threshold
    (c) Linear, threshold
    (d) Nonlinear, threshold
103. Which statement regarding the waste storage of samples with low-level activity is correct?
    (a) They must never be discarded.
    (b) They must be discarded and burned immediately.
    (c) They must be stored for four half-lives.
    (d) They must be stored for 10 half-lives.

104. Radiation-induced apoptosis occurs in the … of mitosis.
    (a) Prophase
    (b) Interphase
    (c) Metaphase
    (d) Telophase
105. Cells in the … show high radiosensitivity to ionizing rays.
    (a) Prophase
    (b) Metaphase
    (c) Anaphase
    (d) Telophase
106. The probability of gross malformation is high in:
    (a) Late fetal stage
    (b) Early organogenesis
    (c) Late organogenesis
    (d) Early fetal stage
107. The calculated values of the probability of causation (PC) analysis are dependent on:
    (a) The type of cancer
    (b) The sex and age of the person at the time of diagnosis
    (c) The time elapsed since the radiation exposure
    (d) All of the above
108. Cataract due to ionizing rays is a (an) … effect.
    (a) Early non-deterministic and without threshold
    (b) Early deterministic and with threshold
    (c) Delayed deterministic and with threshold
    (d) Late non-deterministic and without threshold
109. What is the relationship between LET (linear energy transfer) and RBE (relative biological effect)?
    (a) The highest RBE is induced by LET of 100 keV/μm.
    (b) RBE increases linearly with the increase in LET.
    (c) RBE decreases linearly with the increase in LET.
    (d) RBE does NOT change in LET over 100 KeV/μm.
110. In the new guidelines of the International Commission on Radiological Protection (ICRP), the maximum permitted dose (MPD) is replaced by:
    (a) Maximum limit
    (b) Effective dose equivalent limit
    (c) Maximum dose limit
    (d) Maximum dose
111. How long is the daily permitted work time for a nuclear medicine worker in the gamma radiation field with an exposure rate of 0.01 mSv/h? (the annual dose limit is 20 mSv; each year consists of 50 weeks with 5 work days in each)
    (a) 8 h
    (b) 6 h
    (c) 4 h
    (d) 2 h

112. Regarding the cell survival curve:
   (a) The slope of survival curve decreases with the increase in D0.
   (b) The slope of survival curve increases with the increase in D0.
   (c) The shoulder of survival curve decreases with the increase in quasi-threshold dose (Dq).
   (d) The shoulder of survival curve decreases with the increase in extrapolation number.
113. Regarding the 10-day rule:
   (a) For women, all radiologic studies are permitted only in the first 10 days after menstruation.
   (b) For women, all nonemergency radiologic studies are permitted only in the first 10 days after menstruation.
   (c) For women in reproductive age, all nonemergency radiologic studies are permitted only in the first 10 days after menstruation.
   (d) For women, all radiologic studies are permitted only 10 days after the menstrual period.
114. What is the most important advantage of a pocket dosimeter over a film badge for individual dosimetry?
   (a) Price
   (b) Continuous recording of radiation
   (c) Real-time dosimetry
   (d) User-friendliness
115. A dead cell in radiobiology is defined as a cell:
   (a) Incapable of DNA synthesis
   (b) Incapable of communicating with surrounding cells
   (c) Incapable of unlimited proliferation
   (d) That has shrunk because of cytoplasm condensation and loss of water
116. A patient has received 120 mCi of ^{131}I, and the dosimeter shows radiation of 80 mrem/h in a 1 m distance. The dose rate decreases to 40 mrem/h after 12 h. How much is the remaining activity in this patient's body?
   (a) 36.6 mCi
   (b) 76 mCi
   (c) 70 mCi
   (d) 60 mCi
117. Protection is NOT required if …particles are used for external radiation.
   (a) Neutron
   (b) Beta
   (c) Alpha
   (d) Proton

118. A radiology worker has received 14 mGy of homogenous external radiation of the whole body from gamma rays. This worker has also received 8 mGy of internal radiation from alpha particles in the lungs and 180 mGy of beta particles in the thyroid. How much is the effective dose? (W_R for alpha, beta, and gamma rays are 20, 1, and 1, and W_T for the lung, thyroid, and whole body are 0.12, 0.05, and 1, respectively)
    (a) 83 mSv
    (b) 42 mSv
    (c) 22 mSv
    (d) 15.3 mSv
119. Assuming the equal energy of rays, which of the following radiations demonstrate a low tissue range?
    (a) Neutron
    (b) Electron
    (c) Deuteron
    (d) Proton
120. Which of the following parameters is described by the amount of energy transfer of alpha particles in unit of length?
    (a) LET
    (b) Rad
    (c) Rem
    (d) RBE
121. The exposure rate is 10 mrem in a 1 m distance from the source. How far must the distance be to decrease the exposure rate to 2.5 mrem?
    (a) 45 cm
    (b) 2 m
    (c) 6 m
    (d) 10 m
122. How much is the annual dose limit for hands?
    (a) 7 rem
    (b) 15 rem
    (c) 75 rem
    (d) 75 rem
123. How much is the maximum permitted dose of radiology workers for whole-body exposure to X- and gamma rays according to the last ICRP guidelines?
    (a) 0.05 Sv annually
    (b) 0.12 Sv annually
    (c) 20 mSv annually
    (d) 70 mSv annually
124. The absorbed dose of a 26-year-old radiology worker is 25 Rem. How much will the annual dose limit for this worker for the subsequent year?
    (a) 72 rem
    (b) 50 rem
    (c) 20 rem
    (d) 2 rem

125. Potentially lethal is defined as:
   (a) An irreversible or untreatable damage that leads to cell death
   (b) A damage that is treatable unless another sublethal damage occurs
   (c) A damage capable of inducing cell death unless the medium condition changes
   (d) A damage that is treatable unless the medium condition changes
126. What is the relationship between effective dose and absorbed dose?
   (a) Effective dose is absorbed dose multiplied by radiation weighting factor.
   (b) Effective dose is absorbed dose multiplied by tissue weighting factor.
   (c) Effective dose is absorbed dose multiplied by radiation and tissue weighting factors.
   (d) Effective dose is equal to absorbed dose.
127. What is the main reason for the decrease in slope of the tumoral cell survival curve with an increased radiation rate (increased D0)?
   (a) Decreased ratio of hypoxic to oxygenated cells
   (b) Increased ratio of hypoxic to oxygenated cells
   (c) The balance between hypoxic and oxygenated cells
   (d) Sudden decrease in oxygenation of tumoral cells
128. Radiation exposure in which phase of the cell cycle induces chromosomal aberration?
   (a) Mitosis
   (b) Anaphase
   (c) Prophase
   (d) Interphase
129. What type of dose response does leukemia follow?
   (a) Linear, without threshold
   (b) Linear, with threshold
   (c) Nonlinear, without threshold
   (d) Nonlinear, with threshold
130. A region with a radiation exposure of 0.6 mSv/h is considered a:
   (a) Radiation zone
   (b) High-radiation zone
   (c) Very high-radiation zone
   (d) Dangerous-radiation zone
131. The presence of a shoulder in the cell survival curve in radiation indicates … assuming that the radiation energy of is constant.
   (a) Increased D37 and radiosensitivity
   (b) Increased D37 and decreased radiosensitivity
   (c) Decreased D37 and increased radiosensitivity
   (d) Decreased D37 and radiosensitivity

132. Radiation-induced biophysical changes include:
    (a) Delayed onset of DNA synthesis, short S phase, and general decrease in DNA synthesis
    (b) Rapid onset of DNA synthesis, prolonged S phase, and general decrease in DNA synthesis
    (c) Rapid onset of DNA synthesis, prolonged S phase, and general increase in DNA synthesis
    (d) Delayed onset of DNA synthesis, prolonged S phase, and general decrease in DNA synthesis
133. What is the most effective radioprotective shield against neutrons?
    (a) Lead
    (b) Graphite
    (c) Aluminum
    (d) Titanium
134. In high LET radiations such as alpha particles, the oxygen enhancement ratio (OER) is:
    (a) Maximum
    (b) Absent
    (c) Minimum
    (d) Moderate
135. Which of the following sources of rays has the least percentage in the annual effective dose received by an average member of the population?
    (a) Radon
    (b) Cosmic rays
    (c) Terrestrial radiation
    (d) Internal
136. If D0 for the decrease in hematopoietic cells is 100 rad, what percentage of the bone marrow cells survives after 400 rad of radiation?
    (a) 20%
    (b) 18%
    (c) 56%
    (d) 60%
137. Which of the following models demonstrates a survival curve with a wide shoulder?
    (a) Single-hit, single target
    (b) Multiple-hit, single target
    (c) Single-hit, multiple targets
    (d) Multiple-hit, multiple targets
138. What is the main cause of the indirect biological effects of ionizing rays?
    (a) Free radicals
    (b) Free ions
    (c) Oxygen
    (d) Hydrogen

139. What is the most basic method for radioprotection in external radiation?
   (a) Decreased exposure time, shielding, decreased distance from the source
   (b) Decreased intensity, shielding, decreased radiation intensity of the source
   (c) Decreased exposure time, shielding, increased distance from the source
   (d) Decreased intensity, shielding, increased distance from the source
140. Which type of individualized dosimeter can be applied for rapid determination of the exposure rate of a technician?
   (a) Film badge
   (b) Thermoluminescence
   (c) Pocket ion chamber
   (d) Ring dosimeter
141. What is the relationship between the dose and the frequency of radiation-induced chromosomal aberrations (dysenteric and loop)?
   (a) Two parametric nonlinear relationships with dose
   (b) Linear relationship with a square dose
   (c) Two parametric linear relationships with dose
   (d) Nonlinear relationship with a square dose
142. Which of the following parameters must be used for the total risk assessment for radiation of workers and the general population according to the guidelines of the International Commission on Radiological Protection (ICRP-60)?
   (a) Permitted dose limit
   (b) Upper dose limit
   (c) Effective dose limit
   (d) Minimum equivalent dose
143. Which of the following dosimeters is the best document for the legal demonstration of radiation exposure?
   (a) Film badge
   (b) Thermoluminescent dosimeter (TLD)
   (c) Pocket dosimeter
   (d) Semiconductive dosimeter
144. The stochastic effects of ionizing rays:
   (a) Include cancer.
   (b) Have a threshold.
   (c) The intensity and severity of effects are dose dependent.
   (d) Include cell death.
145. Which of the following parameters is used to determine the maximum radiation of a critical organ in radiotherapy?
   (a) Therapeutic dose
   (b) Tolerable dose
   (c) Deep dose
   (d) LD50

146. Regarding the radioprotection of a patient, what is the main advantage of high-energy photons?
    (a) High deep dose, low dermal dose
    (b) High deep dose, large half-shadow
    (c) Low dermal dose, large half-shadow
    (d) High deep-dose, low dermal dose, large half-shadow
147. What happens to the absorbed dose if the biological half-life of a radiopharmaceutical decreases to half?
    (a) It decreases by 50%.
    (b) It shows more than 50% reduction.
    (c) It shows less than 50% reduction.
    (d) It shows NO change.
148. The fetal LD50 is similar to that of adults in:
    (a) Preimplantation
    (b) Organogenesis
    (c) Fetal
    (d) At birth
149. The dose to the nursing staff from patients returning to the ward after a nuclear medicine procedure depends on:
    (a) The radiopharmaceutical administered
    (b) Its activity
    (c) The degree of care required by the patient
    (d) All of the above
150. The equivalent dose is greater than the absorbed dose for:
    (a) X- and gamma rays
    (b) Neutrons
    (c) Positrons
    (d) Electrons
151. In which phases of mitosis do chromosomal and chromatidal aberrations occur, respectively, when the cell is exposed to ionizing rays?
    (a) Late interphase, early interphase
    (b) Early interphase, late interphase
    (c) Early metaphase, late metaphase
    (d) Late metaphase, early metaphase
152. What is the most effective radioprotective shield against neutron and beta radiations, respectively?
    (a) Hydrogen-containing agents, lead
    (b) Hydrogen-containing agents, plastic
    (c) Copper, glass
    (d) Aluminum, glass
153. Radiation weighing factor (W_R):
    (a) Is used for converting Sievert to Gray
    (b) Increases with higher LET rays
    (c) Is independent of particle mass
    (d) Increases for sensitive organs

154. Survival curves with a high slope and curves with a wide shoulder indicate … and …, respectively.
   (a) High radiosensitivity, low radiotolerance
   (b) High radiotolerance, low radiosensitivity
   (c) High radiosensitivity, high radiotolerance
   (d) Low radiosensitivity, high radiotolerance
155. The OER of alpha particles is … than that of X- and gamma rays because the biological damage of these particles occurs through … effects.
   (a) Lower, direct
   (b) Lower, indirect
   (c) Higher, direct
   (d) Higher, indirect

9.12.1 Answer

	A	B	C	D		A	B	C	D
1			*		94			*	
2	*				95				*
3	*				96		*		
4	*				97		*		
5	*				98			*	
6		*			99	*			
7		*			100			*	
8		*			101			*	
9	*				102		*		
10			*		103				*
11			*		104		*		
12				*	105		*		
13		*			106		*		
14			*		107				*
15		*			108			*	
16	*				109	*			
17				*	110		*		
18	*				111	*			
19	*				112	*			
20	*				113			*	
21		*			114			*	
22			*		115			*	
23			*		116				*
24			*		117			*	
25	*				118	*			
26	*				119	*			
27				*	120	*			
28	*				121		*		
29				*	122				*

30	*				123			*	
31			*		124				*
32			*		125			*	
33			*		126			*	
34				*	127		*		
35			*		128				*
36				*	129	*			
37		*			130	*			
38	*				131		*		
39	*				132				*
40			*		133		*		
41		*			134		*		
42				*	135				*
43	*				136		*		
44				*	137				*
45	*				138	*			
46			*		139			*	
47		*			140			*	
48				*	141			*	
49		*			142			*	
50			*		143	*			
51	*				144	*			
52				*	145		*		
53		*			146	*			
54		*			147		*		
55			*		148			*	
56				*	149				*
57			*		150		*		
58			*		151		*		
59		*			152		*		
60				*	153		*		
61	*				154			*	
62			*		155	*			
63				*					
64	*								
65		*							
66				*					
67			*						
68		*							
69				*					
70	*								
71			*						
72				*					
73				*					
74		*							
75	*								
76				*					

77	*								
78		*							
79		*							
80	*								
81		*							
82	*								
83	*								
84			*						
85			*						
86				*					
87		*							
88				*					
89		*							
90	*								
91				*					
92	*								
93	*								

9.13 Clinical Decision-Making: An Introductory Quantitative Approach to Diagnostic Investigations

1. The kappa score is used in:
   (a) Reproducibility
   (b) Reliability
   (c) Agreement
   (d) Positive likelihood
2. What is the error level if 10,000 counting events are performed with 95% confidence?
   (a) 1%
   (b) 4%
   (c) 2%
   (d) 5%
3. What is the accuracy of the test if 10,000 counting events are performed in 1 min?
   (a) 0.1%
   (b) 12%
   (c) 41%
   (d) 1%
4. A clinical study is designed to determine the maximum tolerance dose of a new radionuclide agent. Patients with several types of refractory cancers undergoing standard therapy are included. The patients have a normal organ function.
   (a) This is a phase I clinical trial.
   (b) This is a phase II clinical trial.
   (c) This is a phase III clinical trial.
   (d) This is a descriptive study.
5. Which of the following studies compares the odds of past exposure between cases and controls and uses the exposure odds ratio to estimate the relative risk?
   (a) Cohort studies
   (b) Clinical trial studies
   (c) Case-control studies
   (d) Descriptive studies
6. The predictive value results from:
   (a) Sensitivity
   (b) Specificity
   (c) Prevalence
   (d) All of the above
7. Mean ± standard deviation includes … of the sample size.
   (a) 50%
   (b) 68.3%
   (c) 95.5%
   (d) 99%

8. The positive likelihood ratio [sensitivity/(1-specificity)] of myocardial perfusion imaging (MPI) for the diagnosis of coronary artery disease (CAD) is defined in the literature. What other information is required to estimate the possibility of CAD in a patient who comes to the clinic?
   (a) Positive predictive value of MPI
   (b) Prevalence of CAD
   (c) Pretest probability of CAD in the patient
   (d) Negative predictive value of MPI
9. In the diagnosis of coronary artery disease (CAD), all of the following statements regarding myocardial perfusion imaging (MPI) are true *except*:
   (a) In geographic regions with a high prevalence of CAD, the positive predictive value of MPI is high.
   (b) In geographic regions with a high prevalence of CAD, the accuracy of MPI is high.
   (c) In geographic regions with a low prevalence of CAD, the negative predictive value of MPI is high.
   (d) Clinicians use positive and negative predictive values more than accuracy to make decisions on the ordering of MPI.
10. In a study that evaluates the diagnostic value of myocardial perfusion imaging (MPI) in the diagnosis of coronary artery disease (CAD) on 1000 participants, both MPI and coronary angiography (CA) were carried out, and the following results were obtained. What is the prevalence of CAD based on coronary angiography?
   (a) 20%
   (b) 67%
   (c) 80%
   (d) 90%

	Angiography		
MPI	Positive CAD	Negative CAD	Total
Positive CAD	160	80	240
Negative CAD	40	720	760
Total	200	800	1000

11. What is the sensitivity of myocardial perfusion imaging (MPI) for the diagnosis of coronary artery disease (CAD)?
   (a) 20%
   (b) 67%
   (c) 80%
   (d) 90%
12. What is the specificity of myocardial perfusion imaging (MPI) for the diagnosis of coronary artery disease (CAD)?
   (a) 20%
   (b) 67%
   (c) 80%
   (d) 90%

13. What is the positive predictive value of myocardial perfusion imaging (MPI) for the diagnosis of coronary artery disease (CAD)?
    (a) 20%
    (b) 67%
    (c) 80%
    (d) 90%
14. What is the negative predictive value of myocardial perfusion imaging (MPI) for the diagnosis of coronary artery disease (CAD)?
    (a) 20%
    (b) 67%
    (c) 80%
    (d) 95%
15. Selective internal radiation therapy (SIRT) with ^{90}Y-SIR-Spheres microspheres for non-resectable colorectal metastases in the liver was performed in a study. The results of the study show that mortality decreases from 52% to 44%. What is the absolute risk reduction obtained by this procedure?
    (a) 1.18%
    (b) 8%
    (c) 10%
    (d) 40%
16. How many patients must be treated with selective internal radiation therapy (SIRT) to prevent one death?
    (a) 20
    (b) 12.5
    (c) 16
    (d) 44
17. The implementation of a repeat brain perfusion SPECT on the following day in a patient showed the same findings. According to this finding, which of the following screening test parameters is the most likely checked?
    (a) Acceptability
    (b) Repeatability
    (c) Validity
    (d) Specificity
18. Previous studies indicate that risk factor X requires 30 years for the induction of an uncommon cancer Y. What is the most appropriate study design to identify the etiologic relationship between factor X and cancer Y?
    (a) Cohort
    (b) Case-control
    (c) Cross-sectional
    (d) Descriptive
19. Which epidemiologic study is NOT analytical?
    (a) Descriptive
    (b) Ecologic
    (c) Cross-sectional
    (d) Case-control

20. Confidence interval (CI):
    (a) Evaluates the role of variables in a study.
    (b) Is independent of sample size.
    (c) The greater the CI is, the more reliable the study.
    (d) Is directly related to bias.
21. The sensitivity of a test is defined as:
    (a) The probability of positive findings when the disease is present
    (b) The probability of negative findings when the disease is absent
    (c) The ratio of findings with correct prediction
    (d) All of the above
22. What is the most appropriate definition of cumulative incidence?
    (a) The fraction of cases in a study that captures a disease in a specific time span
    (b) The fraction of cases in a study with a disease at a specific time
    (c) The fraction of cases in a study with a disease in a specific time span
    (d) The fraction of cases in a study that captures a disease at a specific time
23. If the Pearson's correlation between two quantitative variables $r = -0.20$, then:
    (a) A complete direct relationship exists between the two variables.
    (b) A complete inverse relationship exists between the two variables.
    (c) A partial inverse relationship exists between the two variables.
    (d) A partial direct relationship exists between the two variables.
24. Assuming a constant variance and sample size, what happens when the confidence level increases?
    (a) Confidence interval decreases.
    (b) Confidence interval increases.
    (c) Standard deviation decreases.
    (d) Standard deviation increase.
25. The prevalence of a disease is 20% in a random sample with 400 participants. What is the approximate standard deviation of the prevalence?
    (a) 0.08
    (b) 0.04
    (c) 0.32
    (d) 0.02

9.13.1 Answer

	A	B	C	D
1			*	
2		*		
3				*
4	*			
5	*			
6				*
7		*		

8			*	
9		*		
10	*			
11		*		
12				*
13		*		
14				*
15		*		
16		*		
17		*		
18		*		
19	*			
20	*			
21	*			
22			*	
23			*	
24		*		
25				*

9.14 Decision Analysis Fundamentals

1. It is used to denote the final outcomes of the branching pathways in decision analysis:
   (a) Decision node
   (b) Chance node
   (c) Terminal node
   (d) Decision tree
2. Captopril-enhanced renal scintigraphy is NOT a suitable method for the screening and diagnosis of hypertension secondary to renal artery stenosis in the normal population. Conversely, it is an appropriate method for the diagnosis of the same disease in high-risk patients (old patients with peripheral vascular disease). Which factor of the scan is different between the two groups of patients?
   (a) Sensitivity
   (b) Specificity
   (c) Positive predictive value
   (d) Negative predictive value
3. A 79-year-old man is referred with the diagnosis of differentiated thyroid carcinoma after surgery. His son asks you NOT to tell the truth to his father and to tell the father that he has undergone surgery because of a thyroid nodule. What is the best decision on this issue?
   (a) The patient must be aware of the truth regardless of his relatives' point of view.
   (b) Given the age and the condition of the patient, the patient can be kept away from the truth.
   (c) His son must be informed and convinced about the benefits and importance of telling the truth.
   (d) If hiding the truth is NOT ethical, then the patient can be referred to another physician.

9.14.1 Answer

	A	B	C	D
1			*	
2			*	
3			*	

Suggested Readings

1. Ahmadzadehfar H, Biersack HJ, Freeman LM, Zuckier L. Clinical nuclear medicine. 2nd ed. Berlin: Springer; 2018.
2. Saha GB. Physics and radiobiology of nuclear medicine. 4th ed. New York: Springer-Verlag; 2013.
3. Ell PJ, Gambhir SS. Nuclear medicine in clinical diagnosis and treatment. 3rd ed. Edinburgh, NY: Churchill Livingstone; 2004.
4. Sandler MP, Coleman RE, Patton JA, Wackers FJT, Gottschalk A. Diagnostic nuclear medicine. 4th ed. Philadelphia: Lippincott & Williams Wilkins; 2003.
5. Henkin RE. Nuclear medicine. 2nd ed. Philadelphia: Mosby Elsevier; 2006.

Index

M. Assadi et al., *Principles of Nuclear Medicine*,
https://doi.org/10.1007/978-3-319-91701-6

B

E

G

J